PN Adult Medical Surgical Nursing
Review Module Edition 8.0

Contributors

Audrey Knippa, MS, MPH, RN, CNE
Nursing Education Coordinator and
  Content Project Leader

Sheryl Sommer, PhD, MSN, RN, CNE
Director, Nursing Curriculum and
  Education Services

Brenda Ball, MEd, BSN, RN
Nursing Education Specialist

Lois Churchill, MN, RN
Nursing Education Specialist

Carrie B. Elkins, DHSc, MSN, PHCNS, BC
Nursing Education Specialist

Mary Jane Janowski, MA, BSN, RN
Nursing Resource Specialist

Sharon R. Redding, EdD, RN, CNE
Nursing Education Specialist

Karin Roberts, PhD, MSN, RN, CNE
Nursing Education Coordinator

Mendy G. Wright, DNP, MSN, RN
Nursing Education Specialist

Chris Crawford, BS Journalism
Product Developer and Editorial Project Leader

Derek Prater, MS Journalism
Lead Product Developer

Johanna Barnes, BA Journalism
Product Developer

Joey Berlin, BS Journalism
Product Developer

Hilary E. Groninger, BS Journalism
Product Developer

Megan E. Herre, BS Journalism
Product Developer

Amanda Lehman, BA English
Product Developer

Spring Lenox, BS Journalism
Product Developer

Robin Nelson, BA English
Product Developer

Joanna Shindler, BA Journalism
Product Developer

Morgan Smith, BS Journalism
Media Developer

Brant L. Stacy, BS Journalism, BA English
Product Developer

Mandy Tallmadge, BS Communication
Product Developer

Karen D. Wood, BS Journalism
Product Developer

Katherine Wood-Raclin, BA English, Mass
Communications
Product Developer

Consultants

Christi Blair, MSN, RN

Pam DeMoss, MSN, RN

Penny Fauber, RN, BSN, MS, PhD

Major Susan Lynn Hillhouse, RN, DNP, USAFR

Deb Johnson-Schuh, MSN, RN

Terri Lemon, MSN, RN

Beth Schultz, RN, MSN

Gale P. Sewell RN MSN CNE

INTELLECTUAL PROPERTY NOTICE

IMPORTANT NOTICE TO THE READER

USER'S GUIDE

Welcome to the Assessment Technologies Institute® PN Adult Medical Surgical Nursing Review Module Edition 8.0. The mission of ATI's Content Mastery Series® review modules is to provide user-friendly compendiums of nursing knowledge that will:

- Help you locate important information quickly.

- Assist in your remediation efforts.

- Provide exercises for applying your nursing knowledge.

- Facilitate your entry into the nursing profession as a newly licensed PN.

Organization

This review module is organized into units covering the foundations of nursing care (Unit 1), body systems and physiological processes (Units 2 to 13), and perioperative nursing care (Unit 14). Chapters within these units conform to one of three organizing principles for presenting the content:

- Basic concepts

- Procedures (diagnostic and therapeutic)

- Systems disorders

Basic concepts chapters begin with an overview describing the central concept and its relevance to nursing. Subordinate themes are in outline form to demonstrate relationships and present the information in a clear, succinct manner.

Procedures chapters include an overview describing the procedure(s) covered in the chapter. These chapters will provide you with nursing knowledge relevant to each procedure, including indications, interpretations of findings, client outcomes, nursing actions, and complications.

Systems disorders chapters include an overview describing the disorder(s) and/or disease process. These chapters may provide information on health promotion and disease prevention before addressing data collection, including risk factors, subjective data, and objective data. Next, you will focus on collaborative care, including nursing care, medications, interdisciplinary care, therapeutic procedures, surgical interventions, care after discharge, and client outcomes. Finally, you will find complications related to the disorder, along with nursing actions in response to those complications.

Application Exercises

At the end of each chapter there are questions you can use to practice applying your knowledge. The Application Exercises include both NCLEX-style questions, such as multiple-choice and multiple-select items, and questions that ask you to apply your knowledge in other formats, such as short-answer and matching items. After completing the Application Exercises, go to the Application Exercise Answer Key to check your answers and rationales for correct and incorrect answers.

NCLEX® Connections

To prepare for the NCLEX-PN, it is important for you to understand how the content in this review module is connected to the NCLEX-PN test plan. You can find information on the detailed test plan at the National Council of State Boards of Nursing's Web site: https://www.ncsbn.org/. When reviewing content in this review module, regularly ask yourself, "How does this content fit into the test plan, and what types of questions related to this content should I expect?"

To help you in this process, we've included NCLEX Connections at the beginning of each unit and with each question in the Application Exercises Answer Keys. The NCLEX Connections at the beginning of each unit will point out areas of the detailed test plan that relate to the content within that unit. The NCLEX Connections attached to the Application Exercises Answer Keys will demonstrate how each exercise fits within the detailed content outline.

These NCLEX Connections will help you understand how the detailed content outline is organized, starting with major client needs categories and subcategories and followed by related content areas and tasks. The major client needs categories are:

- Safe and Effective Care Environment
  - Management of Care
  - Safety and Infection Control
- Health Promotion and Maintenance
- Psychosocial Integrity
- Physiological Integrity
  - Basic Care and Comfort
  - Pharmacological and Parenteral Therapies
  - Reduction of Risk Potential
  - Physiological Adaptation

An NCLEX Connection might, for example, alert you that content within a unit is related to:

- Reduction of Risk Potential
  - Diagnostic Tests
    - Reinforce client teaching about diagnostic test.

Icons

Throughout the review module you will see icons that will draw your attention to particular areas. Keep an eye out for these icons:

 This icon indicates an Overview, or introduction, to a particular subject matter. Descriptions and categories will typically be found in an Overview.

 This icon indicates Application Exercises and Application Exercises Answer Keys.

 This icon indicates NCLEX connections.

 This icon indicates gerontological content. When you see this icon, take note of information that is specific to the aging process or the care of older adult clients.

 This icon indicates content related to safety. When you see this icon, take note of safety concerns or steps that nurses can take to ensure client safety and a safe environment.

 This icon indicates that a media supplement, such as a graphic, an animation, or a video, is available. If you have an electronic copy of the review module, this icon will appear alongside clickable links to media supplements. If you have a hardcopy version of the review module, visit www.atitesting.com for details on how to access these features.

Feedback

ATI welcomes feedback regarding this review module. Please provide comments to: comments@atitesting.com.

Table of Contents

Unit 8   Nursing Care of Clients with Renal System Disorders

Unit 9   Nursing Care of Clients with Reproductive Disorders

Unit 14   Nursing Care of the Perioperative Client

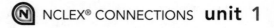

UNIT 1: FOUNDATIONS OF NURSING CARE FOR ADULT CLIENTS

- Health, Wellness, and Illness

- Emergency Nursing Principles and Management

NCLEX® CONNECTIONS
When reviewing the chapters in this section, keep in mind the relevant sections of the NCLEX® outline, in particular:

CLIENT NEEDS: HEALTH PROMOTION AND MAINTENANCE

Relevant topics/tasks include:
- Health Promotion/Disease Prevention
  ○ Gather data on client health history and risk for disease.
- High Risk Behaviors
  ○ Reinforce client teaching related to client high-risk behavior.

CLIENT NEEDS: PHYSIOLOGICAL ADAPTATION

Relevant topics/tasks include:
- Alterations in Body Systems
  ○ Provide care to correct client alteration in body system.
- Medical Emergencies
  ○ Respond to a client life-threatening situation.

Overview

- Wellness involves the ability to adapt emotionally and physically to a changing state of health and the environment.

- Illness is an altered level of functioning in response to a disease process. Disease is a condition that results in the physiological alteration in the composition of the body.

- Nurses must understand the variables affecting health/wellness/illness and how they relate to a client's health needs.

Health and Wellness

- Aspects of health and wellness

  - Physical – Able to perform activities of daily living

  - Emotional – Adapt to stress; express and identify emotions

  - Social – Interact successfully with others

- A client's state of health and wellness is constantly changing and adapting to a continually fluctuating external and internal environment.

  - The external environment

    - Social – Crime versus safety, poverty versus prosperity, and social unrest versus peace

    - Physical – Access to health care, sanitation, availability of clean water, and geographic isolation

  - The internal environment includes cumulative life experiences, cultural and spiritual beliefs, age, gender, and other support systems.

- The level of health and wellness is unique to each individual and relative to the individual's usual state of functioning.

  - For example – A person with rheumatoid arthritis who has a strong support system and positive outlook may consider himself healthy while functioning at an optimal level with minimal pain.

- Variables
  - Modifiable – May be changed such as smoking, nutrition, health education and awareness, and exercise
  - Nonmodifiable – Cannot be changed, such as gender, age, developmental level, and genetic traits
- Desired outcomes are to obtain and maintain optimal state of wellness and function.
  - Can be achieved through health education and positive action (smoking cessation, weight loss, seeking health care)
- The health/wellness/illness continuum is an assessment tool that is used to measure the level of wellness.
  - It is used as a model to compare the present state of health of a client to that of his previous state of health. It may be useful as an assessment guide and also as a tool to set goals and find ways to improve the client's state of health. The health care professional can assist the client to see at what point he is at on the continuum and seek ways to move toward optimal wellness.
  - The degree of wellness is relative to the usual state of wellness for a client.
  - The range of health to illness runs from optimal wellness to severe illness.
  - At the center of the continuum is the client's normal state of health.
  - Level of health/illness is assessed in comparison to the norm for a client.

Illness

- Response to disease may be influenced by:
  - Degree of physical changes as a result of the disease process.
  - Perceptions by self and others of the disease, which may be influenced by various reliable and unreliable sources of information, such as friends, magazines, TV, and the Internet.
  - Cultural values and beliefs.
  - Denial or fear of illness.
  - Social demands and time constraints.

Nursing Care

- Evaluate the health needs of a client and create strategies to meet those needs.
- Health/wellness data collection
  - Physical assessment
  - Evaluating health perceptions
  - Identifying risks to health/wellness
  - Identifying access to health care

- Identifying obstacles to adherence

  o Perceptions of illness – Awareness of the severity of the illness

  o Confidence in the provider

  o Belief in the prescribed therapy

    ▪ For example – A person who has had a negative experience with the health care system, may not trust the health care provider and may not follow the advice and comply with the treatment prescribed.

  o Availability of support systems

  o Family role and function (One member of the family may be the family caregiver and may neglect caring for him/herself.)

  o Financial restrictions that may lead to prioritized health care (A parent may seek medical care for children, but not for him/herself.)

- Health promotion and disease prevention – Use health education and awareness to reduce risk factors and promote health care.

- Interventions

  o Provide resources to strengthen coping abilities.

  o Encourage use of support systems during times of illness and stress.

  o Identify obstacles to health and wellness and create strategies to reduce these obstacles.

  o Identify ways to reduce health risks and improve compliance.

  o Develop health education methods to improve health awareness and reduce health risks.

Ⓐ APPLICATION EXERCISES

1. A nurse in a provider's office is collecting data from an older adult client who has a long history of rheumatoid arthritis and reports she that has morning stiffness and pain upon movement. Which of the following data collected from the client is a modifiable variable? The client

   A. is overweight.

   B. is female.

   C. experienced onset of the disorder at age 46.

   D. has a family history of the disorder.

2. A nurse in a community clinic has been asked to take clients' vital signs and mark their level of wellness on a health-wellness-illness continuum tool prior to being seen by the provider. Which of the following clients should be placed at the center of the continuum?

   A. A young adult client with influenza-like symptoms

   B. A woman who is pregnant and has a urinary tract infection

   C. An older adult who is newly diagnosed with diabetes mellitus

   D. An older adult with a long history of well-controlled rheumatoid arthritis

3. The nurse is caring for a middle-aged woman diagnosed with terminal breast cancer. While the client's family frequently visits the client, the oldest daughter sleeps at the hospital and provides much of the client's personal care. The nurse should take which of the following actions with the daughter?

   A. Request the daughter allow the staff to provide the client's personal care.

   B. Ensure the daughter gets enough rest, fluids, and nutrition.

   C. Tell the daughter that visitors are not allowed to stay at night.

   D. Ask the daughter if she would like to hire a sitter for her mother.

APPLICATION EXERCISES ANSWER KEY

1. A nurse in a provider's office is collecting data from an older adult client who has a long history of rheumatoid arthritis and reports she that has morning stiffness and pain upon movement. Which of the following data collected from the client is a modifiable variable? The client

   A. is overweight.

   B. is female.

   C. experienced onset of the disorder at age 46.

   D. has a family history of the disorder.

   A modifiable variable is one that can be changed. The client can lose weight; therefore this is a modifiable variable. Rheumatoid arthritis is more common in females and there is a genetic predisposition to the disorder. These are nonmodifiable variables. The onset of the disorder is often during middle adulthood and this is also a nonmodifiable variable.

   NCLEX® Connection: Reduction of Risk Potential, Illness Management

2. A nurse in a community clinic has been asked to take clients' vital signs and mark their level of wellness on a health-wellness-illness continuum tool prior to being seen by the provider. Which of the following clients should be placed at the center of the continuum?

   A. A young adult client with influenza-like symptoms

   B. A woman who is pregnant and has a urinary tract infection

   C. An older adult who is newly diagnosed with diabetes mellitus

   D. An older adult with a long history of well-controlled rheumatoid arthritis

   The center of the health, wellness, and illness continuum is the client's normal state of health, which is assessed in comparison to the norm for that client. While the older adult client who has rheumatoid arthritis has a chronic illness, this is considered the client's "new normal" since it is well controlled, and the client's level of wellness can be placed at the center of the continuum.

   NCLEX® Connection: Reduction of Risk Potential, Illness Management

PN ADULT MEDICAL SURGICAL NURSING

3. The nurse is caring for a middle-aged woman diagnosed with terminal breast cancer. While the client's family frequently visits the client, the oldest daughter sleeps at the hospital and provides much of the client's personal care. The nurse should take which of the following actions with the daughter?

    A. Request the daughter allow the staff to provide the client's personal care.

    B. Ensure the daughter gets enough rest, fluids, and nutrition.

    C. Tell the daughter that visitors are not allowed to stay at night.

    D. Ask the daughter if she would like to hire a sitter for her mother.

The nurse should recognize that the client's daughter has assumed the role of caregiver for the family. The daughter should be supported in her efforts to provide comfort care for her mother. The nurse should ensure the daughter gets adequate rest by providing a comfortable place to sleep as well as access to food and fluids so the daughter can remain healthy during this difficult time.

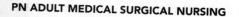 NCLEX® Connection: Reduction of Risk Potential, Potential for Complications from Surgical Procedures, and Health Alterations

UNIT 1	FOUNDATIONS OF NURSING CARE FOR ADULT CLIENTS
Chapter 2	Emergency Nursing Principles and Management

Overview

- Emergency nursing principles are the guidelines that nurses follow to assess and manage emergency situations for both a client and multiple clients.

- Nurses must have the ability to identify emergent situations and rapidly assess and intervene when life-threatening conditions exist. Emergent conditions are common to all nursing environments.

- Emergency nursing principles

  o Primary survey

  o Airway/cervical spine, breathing, circulation, disability, and exposure (ABCDE) principle

  o Triage guidelines

  o Basic First-Aid

  o Cardiac arrest and CPR

Primary Survey

- A primary survey is a rapid assessment of life-threatening conditions. It should take no longer than 60 seconds to perform.

- The primary survey should be completed systematically so conditions are not missed.

- Standard precautions attire – gloves, gowns, eye protection, face masks, and shoe covers must be worn to prevent contamination with bodily fluids.

- The ABCDE principle guides the primary survey.

ABCDE Principle

- Emergency care is guided by the principle of ABCDE.

- Airway/Cervical Spine

  o This is the most important step in performing the primary survey. If a patent airway is not established, subsequent steps of the primary survey are futile.

  o If clients are awake and responsive, the airway is open.

- ○ If the client's ability to maintain an airway is lost, it is important to inspect for blood, broken teeth, vomitus, or other foreign materials in the airway that may cause an obstruction.

- ○ If clients are unresponsive without suspicion of trauma, the airway should be opened with a head-tilt-chin-lift maneuver.

  - ▪ This is the most effective manual technique for opening a client's airway.

  - ▪ Do NOT perform this technique on clients who have a potential cervical spine injury.

  - ▪ The nurse should assume a position at the head of the client, place one hand on his forehead, and the other on his chin. His head should be tilted while his chin is lifted superiorly. This lifts the tongue out of the laryngopharynx and provides for a patent airway.

- ○ If the client is unresponsive with suspicion of trauma, the airway should be opened with a modified jaw thrust maneuver.

  - ▪ The nurse should assume a position at the head of the client, and place both hands on either side of the client's head. Locate the connection between the maxilla and the mandible. Lift the jaw superiorly while maintaining alignment of the cervical spine.

- ○ Once the airway is opened, it should be inspected for blood, broken teeth, vomitus, and secretions. If present, obstructions should be cleared with suction or a finger-sweep method.

- ○ The open airway can be maintained with airway adjuncts, such as an oropharyngeal or nasopharyngeal airway.

- ○ A bag-valve-mask with a 100% oxygen source is indicated for clients who need additional support during resuscitation.

- • Breathing

  - ○ Once a patent airway is achieved, the presence and effectiveness of breathing should be checked.

  - ○ Breathing assessment

    - ▪ Auscultation of breath sounds

    - ▪ Observation of chest expansion and respiratory effort

    - ▪ Notation of rate and depth of respirations

    - ▪ Identification of chest trauma

  - ○ If clients are not breathing or are breathing inadequately, manual ventilation should be performed by a bag-valve-mask with supplemental oxygen or mouth-to-mask ventilation until a bag-valve-mask can be obtained.

- • Circulation

  - ○ Once adequate ventilation is accomplished, circulation is checked.

  - ○ Nurses should check heart rate, blood pressure, and perfusion.

- o Interventions geared toward restoring effective circulation
    - CPR
    - Hemorrhage control (direct pressure should be applied to visible, significant external bleeding)
    - Monitoring infusion of fluids and/or blood. IV access is usually through a large-bore catheter into the antecubital fossa (bend of the elbow). Lactated Ringer's and 0.9% normal saline are typical resuscitation fluids.
- o Shock may develop if circulation is compromised. Shock is the body's response to inadequate tissue perfusion and oxygenation. It manifests with an increased heart rate and hypotension and may result in tissue ischemia and necrosis.
- o Interventions to alleviate shock include:
    - Administering oxygen.
    - Applying pressure to bleeding that is obvious.
    - Elevating the client's feet to shunt blood to vital organs.
    - Monitoring IV fluids and blood products as ordered.
    - Monitoring vital signs.
    - Remaining with clients and provide reassurance and support for anxiety.

- Disability

- o Disability is a quick assessment to determine the client's level of consciousness.
- o The AVPU mnemonic is useful.
    - A – Alert
    - V – Responsive to voice
    - P – Responsive to pain
    - U – Unresponsive
- o The Glasgow Coma Scale is another widely used method.
    - Components include eye opening, verbal response, and motor response.
- o Neurologic assessment must be repeated at frequent intervals to assure immediate response to any change.

- Exposure

- o Nurses should remove all of the client's clothing for a complete physical assessment.
- o Cut away clothing during a resuscitation situation.
- o Preserve evidence such as bullets, drugs, or weapons.
- o Hypothermia is a primary concern for clients. Hypothermia leads to vasoconstriction and impaired oxygenation.

- To prevent hypothermia
  - Remove wet clothing from the client.
  - Cover the client with blankets.
  - Increase the temperature of the room.
  - Monitor infusion of warmed fluids as prescribed.

Triage Guidelines

- Triage Under Usual Conditions
  - Triage guidelines ensure that clients with the highest acuity needs receive the quickest treatment.
  - Clients are categorized based upon their acuity. One example of a triage framework is the Emergent, Urgent, Nonurgent model.
    - Emergent triage indicates a life- or limb-threatening situation.
    - Urgent triage indicates that the client should be treated soon, but that the risk posed is not life-threatening.
    - Nonurgent cases can generally wait for an extended length of time without serious deterioration.
- Triage Under Mass Casualty Conditions
  - This is a military form of triage that is implemented with a focus of achieving the greatest good for the greatest number of people.
  - Classifications
    - Emergent or Class I – identified with a red tag indicating an immediate threat to life
    - Urgent or Class II – identified with a yellow tag indicating major injuries that require immediate treatment
    - Nonurgent or Class III – identified with a green tag indicating minor injuries that do not require immediate treatment
    - Expectant or Class IV – identified with a black tag indicating one who is expected and allowed to die

Basic First-Aid

- Complete the primary survey before performing First-Aid.
- Bleeding
  - Identify any sources of external bleeding and apply direct pressure to the wound site.
  - DO NOT remove impaled objects.
  - Internal bleeding may require intravascular volume replacement with fluids and/or blood products or surgical intervention.

- Fractures and Splinting
    - Check the site for swelling, deformity, and skin integrity.
    - Check temperature, distal pulses, and mobility.
    - Apply a splint to immobilize the fracture. Cover any open areas with a sterile cloth if available.
    - Recheck neurovascular status after splinting.

- Sprains
    - Refrain from weight-bearing.
    - Apply ice to decrease inflammation.
    - Apply a compression dressing to minimize swelling.
    - Elevate the affected limb.

- Heat Stroke
    - Identify heat stroke quickly and treat aggressively.
        - Signs and symptoms of a heat stroke include hypotension, tachypnea, tachycardia, anxiety, confusion, unusual behavior, seizures, and coma.
    - Provide for rapid cooling
        - Remove the client's clothing.
        - Place ice packs over the major arteries (axillae, chest, groin, neck).
        - Immerse clients in a cold-water bath.
        - Wet the client's body, then fan with rapid movement of air.

- Frostnip and Frostbite
    - Frostnip is a type of a superficial cold injury resulting in numbness and pain of the skin.
    - Frostnip can be easily treated by warming the affected area.
    - Frostnip does not cause tissue damage.
    - Common areas affected by frostnip are the nose, face, fingers, and toes.
    - Frostnip untreated can lead to frostbite.
    - Frostbite is the degree of tissue freezing resulting in tissue damage.
    - Frostbite can be superficial-, partial-, or full-thickness of the skin.
    - Frostbite presents as white, waxy areas on exposed skin, and tissue injury occurs.
    - Warm the affected area in a water bath 38° to 41° C (100.4° to 105.8° F).
    - Provide pain medication.
    - Administer a tetanus immunization.

PN ADULT MEDICAL SURGICAL NURSING

- Burns
  - Burns may result from an electrical current, chemicals, radiation, and/or flames.
    - Remove the agent (electrical current, radiation source, chemical).
    - Smother any flames that are present.
    - Perform a primary survey.
    - Cover the client and maintain NPO status.
    - Elevate the client's extremities, if not contraindicated (presence of a fracture).
    - Perform a head-to-toe assessment and estimate the surface area and thickness of burns.
    - Monitor IV fluids and a tetanus toxoid.
- Altitude-Related Illnesses
  - Clients may become hypoxic in high altitudes.
  - Signs and symptoms
    - Throbbing headache
    - Nausea
    - Vomiting
    - Dyspnea
    - Anorexia
  - Nursing interventions
    - Administer oxygen.
    - Descend to a lower altitude.
    - Provide pharmacological therapy, such as steroids and diuretics, if indicated.
  - Altitude sickness can progress to cerebral and pulmonary edema and should be treated immediately.

Cardiac Arrest and CPR

- Cardiac Arrest
  - Cardiac arrest, the sudden cessation of cardiac function, is characterized by the absence of a carotid pulse in the adult and child 1 year to adolescent. In infant's up to 1 year, cardiac arrest is the absence of a brachial pulse. If no brachial pulse, check the infant's carotid pulse. The brachial pulse is checked first because the carotid pulse may be difficult to palpate due to the fatty tissue of the infant's neck.

Data Collection

- The client's skin has an ashy appearance.
- The client has no respirations.
- The client's pupils are dilated.

○ Findings

- Ventricular fibrillation (VF) is the cause of sudden, nontraumatic cardiac arrest in 80 to 90% of victims.
- Cardiac arrest may also occur following respiratory arrest. Sometimes, electrical activity is present, but is not sufficient enough to stimulate effective cardiac contractions. This condition is called pulse-less electrical activity.
- In children and infants, cardiac arrest is often secondary to hypoxemia or shock.
- Without sufficient cardiac output, the brain will suffer cell anoxia (cell death) within 4 to 6 min, with death following shortly thereafter.
- An interdisciplinary team will provide care during in-facility cardiac arrests. This team should include nurses, physicians, respiratory therapists, laboratory personnel, and chaplain services.
- Management of cardiac arrest depends on prompt recognition of signs and symptoms and the introduction of therapeutic interventions directed at artificially sustaining circulation and ventilation.

○ Goals for management of cardiac arrest

- Rapid identification of the signs and symptoms of cardiac arrest
- Quick initiation of both circulatory and respiratory support
- Activation of the emergency medical system
- Use of emergency equipment and cardiac monitoring
- Stabilization of the client following the arrest
- Diagnosis and treatment of the cause of the cardiac arrest

○ CPR is the process of externally supporting the circulation and respirations of a client who has experienced a cardiac arrest. Defibrillation is used in the presence of ventricular fibrillation and ventricular tachycardia. Neither of these rhythms provide sufficient cardiac output to support life. CPR and defibrillation significantly increases the client's chances of survival when initiated immediately.

○ Prefacility care greatly improves the chance of survival for clients who have experienced cardiac arrest.

- CPR

  - CPR is a combination of basic interventions designed to sustain oxygen and circulation to vital organs until more advanced interventions can be initiated to correct the cause of the cardiac arrest.

  - Basic interventions can be delivered by trained citizens, but advanced interventions require more sophisticated training and certification and the use of emergency equipment.

  - CPR is a series of emergency procedures directed at artificially providing a client with circulation (chest compressions) and oxygenation (ventilations) in the absence of cardiac output.

  - CPR is a component of basic life support (BLS) and advanced cardiac life support (ACLS).

  - The goal of BLS is to provide oxygen to the vital organs until appropriate advanced resuscitation measures can be initiated or until resuscitative efforts are ordered to be stopped. BLS involves Airway, Breathing, and Circulation (ABCs) — the basis of CPR.

    - Airway

      - Confirm the absence of spontaneous respirations.

      - Establish a patent airway.

      - Perform the Heimlich maneuver if the client's airway is obstructed with a foreign object.

      - Use abdominal thrusts for clients who are unconscious.

    - Breathing

      - Provide artificial respirations (ventilations) to deliver oxygen into the blood in an attempt to prevent cell anoxia.

    - Circulation

      - Confirm the absence or presence of a pulse.

      - Provide external support of circulation (chest compressions) to transport oxygenated blood to the brain.

  - The goal of ACLS is the return of spontaneous breathing and circulation. In addition to the ABCs of BLS, ACLS involves the diagnosis and treatment of underlying cardiac dysrhythmias; insertion of an oropharyngeal or endotracheal airway with bag ventilation and supplemental oxygen; administration of IV fluids; and administration of IV antidysrhythmic medications.

  - The chain of survival is a series of interventions directed at the resuscitation of the cardiac arrest victim. It involves:

    - Early activation of emergency medical services.

    - Early CPR/early defibrillation.

    - Early ACLS care.

- Nursing Responsibilities During a Cardiac Arrest

  o The nurse assisting during a cardiac arrest must:

    ▪ Be knowledgeable about the facility's procedure for alerting members of the code team to the presence of an emergency.

    ▪ Use the current BLS guidelines from the American Heart Association (AHA).

    ▪ Be knowledgeable about facility policies/procedures and the location and operation of emergency equipment (crash cart).

    ▪ Have current certification for basic life support skills.

  o Nursing responsibilities

    ▪ Know the client's status regarding resuscitation (The nurse must know whether or not the client has a current Do-Not-Resuscitate order.).

    ▪ Maintain airway patency.

    ▪ Determine the depth and rate of respirations.

    ▪ Provide chest compressions at the proper rate and depth for age.

    ▪ Check vital signs for effectiveness of chest compressions and ventilations.

- The AHA guidelines for basic life support and advanced life support are updated on a regular basis. Go to http://www.americanheart.org/ for current guidelines.

- These updates are based on research and aggregate client outcomes.

- Since most cases of adult cardiac arrest are caused by ventricular fibrillation or ventricular tachycardia, early defibrillation is essential. When a defibrillator is immediately available (and ventricular fibrillation or ventricular tachycardia is confirmed) the client is defibrillated prior to the initiation of CPR. A standard defibrillator or an automated external defibrillator (AED) may be used. Although the occurrence of cardiac arrest is rare in the pediatric population, the nurse must also be prepared to use a defibrillator when indicated.

Emergency Medications

PHARMACOLOGICAL ACTION	THERAPEUTIC USE
epinephrine (Adrenaline)	
• Vasoconstriction	• Slows absorption of local anesthetics • Manages superficial bleeding • Reduces congestion of nasal mucosa • Increases blood pressure
• Increases heart rate • Strengthens myocardial contractility • Increases rate of conduction through the AV node	• Treatment of AV block and cardiac arrest
• Bronchodilation	• Asthma
dopamine (Intropin)	

• Increased
  ○ Heart rate
  ○ Myocardial contractility
  ○ Rate of conduction through the AV node
  ○ Blood pressure
	• Shock
	• Heart failure

Nursing Interventions and Client Education

- Monitor clients receiving medications by continuous IV infusion.

- Monitor clients for chest pain. Notify the provider if clients experience chest pain.

- Provide continuous ECG monitoring. Notify the provider if the client experiences tachycardia or dysrhythmias.

Client Outcomes

- The client will have improved tissue perfusion.

- The client will maintain adequate gas exchange.

- The client will have a patent airway.

- The client will have an improved mental status.

- The client will have an improved, adequate cardiac function.

APPLICATION EXERCISES

1. A nurse in a long-term care facility is called to the dining room to assist a client who fell from her chair to the floor while eating lunch. Which of the following should the nurse check first?

   A. The presence of injuries

   B. The client's airway

   C. The client's pulse

   D. The client's neurological status

2. A nurse in an urgent care clinic is providing care for a client with heat stroke. Which of the flowing interventions should the nurse take? (Select all that apply.)

   _____ Immerse the victim in cold water.

   _____ Encourage the client to take a slow walk with assistance.

   _____ Apply ice packs to the groin and axillae.

   _____ Keep clothing on to avoid sun exposure.

   _____ Administer a tetanus vaccination.

APPLICATION EXERCISES ANSWER KEY

1. A nurse in a long-term care facility is called to the dining room to assist a client who fell from her chair to the floor while eating lunch. Which of the following should the nurse check first?

   A. The presence of injuries
   B. The client's airway
   C. The client's pulse
   D. The client's neurological status

   Using the ABCDE priority-setting framework, checking the client's airway is the first action the nurse should take. Checking the client's pulse, neurological status, and presence of injuries are all important actions, but not the priority actions.

   NCLEX® Connection: Physiological Adaptation, Medical Emergencies

2. A nurse in an urgent care clinic is providing care for a client with heat stroke. Which of the flowing interventions should the nurse take? (Select all that apply.)

X	**Immerse the victim in cold water.**
	Encourage the client to take a slow walk with assistance.
X	**Apply ice packs to the groin and axillae.**
	Keep clothing on to avoid sun exposure.
	Administer a tetanus vaccination.

   Immersing the client in cold water and applying ice packs to the groin and axillae are appropriate interventions for heat stroke. The client should stop all activity to conserve energy. All clothing should be removed prior to immersing the client in cold water. A tetanus vaccination is not indicated for heatstroke, but is indicated for frostnip and frostbite.

   NCLEX® Connection: Physiological Adaptation, Medical Emergencies

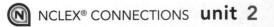

UNIT 2: NURSING CARE OF CLIENTS WITH NEUROSENSORY DISORDERS

- Diagnostic and Therapeutic Procedures
- Central and Peripheral Nervous System Disorders
- Sensory Disorders

NCLEX® CONNECTIONS

When reviewing the chapters in this section, keep in mind the relevant sections of the NCLEX® outline, in particular:

CLIENT NEEDS: BASIC CARE AND COMFORT

Relevant topics/tasks include:
- Mobility/Immobility
  - Maintain client correct body alignment.
- Nonpharmacological Comfort Interventions
  - Assist in planning comfort interventions for client with impaired comfort.
- Nutrition and Oral Hydration
  - Identify client potential for aspiration.

CLIENT NEEDS: PHARMACOLOGICAL THERAPIES

Relevant topics/tasks include:
- Adverse Effects/ Contraindications/Side Effects/Interactions
  - Identify a contraindication to the administration of prescribed over-the-counter medication to the client.
- Expected Actions/ Outcomes
  - Reinforce education to client regarding medications.
- Pharmacological Pain Management
  - Identify client need for pain medication.

CLIENT NEEDS: PHYSIOLOGICAL ADAPTATION

Relevant topics/tasks include:
- Alterations in Body Systems
  - Provide care for client experiencing increased intracranial pressure.
- Basic Pathophysiology
  - Identify signs and symptoms related to acute or chronic illness.
- Medical Emergencies
  - Notify primary health care provider about client unexpected response/emergency situation.

UNIT 2	NURSING CARE OF CLIENTS WITH NEUROSENSORY DISORDERS
Section	Diagnostic and Therapeutic Procedures
Chapter 3	Neurological Diagnostic Procedures

Overview

- Neurologic assessment and diagnostic procedures are used to evaluate neurologic function by testing indicators such as mental status, motor functioning, electrical activity, and intracranial pressure.

- Neurologic assessment and diagnostic procedures that nurses should be knowledgeable about

  ○ Cerebral angiogram

  ○ Cerebral computed tomography (CT) scan

  ○ Electroencephalography (EEG)

  ○ Glasgow Coma Scale (GCS)

  ○ Lumbar puncture (spinal tap)

  ○ Magnetic resonance imaging (MRI) scan

  ○ Positron emission tomography (PET) and single-photon emission computed tomography (SPECT) scans

  ○ Radiography (x-ray)

Cerebral Angiogram

- A cerebral angiogram provides visualization of the cerebral blood vessels.

  ○ Digital subtraction angiography "subtracts" the bones and tissues from the images, providing x-rays with only the vessels apparent.

  ○ The procedure is performed within the radiology department, because x-ray images provide documentation of blood vessel integrity.

- Indications

  ○ A cerebral angiogram is used to assess the blood flow to and within the brain, identify aneurysms, and define the vascularity of tumors (useful for surgical planning). It may also be used therapeutically to inject medications that treat blood clots or to administer chemotherapy.

- Interpretation of Findings
    - Blockages in the arteries or veins in the head and neck may indicate impaired blood flow.
    - Surgical procedure may be indicated to open blockage.
- Preprocedure
    - If clients are pregnant, a determination of the risks to the fetus versus the benefits of the information obtained by this procedure should be made.
    - Nursing Actions
        - Instruct clients to refrain from consuming food or fluids for 4 to 8 hr prior to the procedure.
        - Check for allergy to shellfish or iodine, which would require the use of a different contrast media. Any history of bleeding requires additional monitoring to assure clotting after the procedure.
        - Ensure that clients are not wearing any jewelry.
        - A mild sedative is usually administered prior to the procedure and vital signs are continuously monitored during the procedure.
    - Client Education
        - Instruct clients about the importance of not moving during the procedure and about the need to keep the head immobilized.
- Intraprocedure
    - The client is placed on a radiography table, where the client's head is secured.
    - A catheter is placed into an artery (usually in the groin or the neck), dye is injected, and x-ray pictures are taken.
    - The catheter is removed once all pictures are taken.
    - Additional sedation may be provided during the procedure, if required.
- Postprocedure
    - Nursing Actions
        - Closely monitor the site to assure that clotting occurs.
        - Restrict movements for 8 to 12 hr to prevent rebleeding at the catheter site.
- Complications
    - Bleeding
        - There is a risk for bleeding at the entry site.
        - Nursing Actions
            - Check the insertion site frequently.
            - If bleeding does occur, reinforce dressings without removing, apply pressure and notify the provider.

CT Scan

- A CT scan provides cross-sectional images of the cranial cavity. A contrast media may be used to enhance the images.

- Indications

  - A CT scan can be used to identify tumors and infarctions, detect abnormalities, monitor response to treatment, and guide needles used for biopsies.

- Interpretation of Findings

  - A surgical procedure may be indicated if a tumor or vascular abnormality is identified.

- Preprocedure

  - If clients are pregnant, a determination of the risks to the fetus versus the benefits of the information obtained by this procedure should be made.

  - Nursing Actions

    - If contrast media and/or sedation is expected:
      - Instruct clients to refrain from consuming food or fluids for 4 to 8 hr prior to the procedure.
      - Check for allergy to shellfish or iodine, which would require the use of a different contrast media.
      - Check renal function (BUN), because contrast media is excreted by the kidneys.

    - Because this procedure is performed with clients in a supine position, placing pillows in the small of the client's back may assist in preventing back pain. The head must be secured to prevent unnecessary movement during the procedure.

    - Ensure that the client's jewelry is removed prior to this procedure. In general, clients wear a hospital gown to prevent any metals from interfering with the x-rays.

- Intraprocedure

  - Clients must lie supine with the head stabilized during the procedure.

  - Although CT scanning is painless, sedation may be provided.

- Postprocedure

  - Nursing Actions

    - There is no follow-up care associated with a CT scan.

    - If contrast media is injected, monitor the site to assure clotting has occurred.

    - If sedation is administered, monitor clients until stable.

EEG

- This noninvasive procedure assesses the electrical activity of the brain and is used to determine if there are abnormalities in brain wave patterns.

- Indications

  o EEGs are most commonly performed to identify and determine seizure activity, but they are also useful for detecting sleep disorders and behavioral changes.

- Interpretation of Findings

  o Location of abnormal wave patterns may indicate site of brain that is stimulating seizure activity.

- Preprocedure

  o Nursing Actions

    ▪ Review medications with the provider to determine if they should be continued prior to this procedure.

  o Client Education

    ▪ Instruct clients to refrain from drinking fluids containing caffeine on the day of the test.

    ▪ Instruct clients to wash hair before (no oils or sprays) and after (to remove electrode glue) the procedure.

    ▪ If indicated, instruct clients to induce "sleep deprivation" the night before the procedure by awakening at 2 a.m. to 3 a.m. and staying awake for the rest of the night.

    ▪ Instruct clients to withhold medications that are stimulants or CNS depressants and antiepileptic medications, if instructed by provider.

    ▪ Inform clients that they may be asked to take deep breaths and/or will be exposed to flashes of light during the procedure.

    ▪ Inform clients the test will not be painful.

- Intraprocedure

  o The procedure generally takes 1 hr.

  o There are no risks associated with this procedure.

  o With clients resting in a chair or lying in bed, small electrodes are placed on the scalp and connected to a brain wave machine or computer.

  o Clients may be given sedation by IV infusion to induce sleep.

  o Electrical signals produced by the brain are recorded by the machine or computer in the form of wavy lines. This documents brain activity.

  o Notations are made when stimuli are presented or when sleep occurs. (Flashes of light or pictures may be used during the procedure to assess the client's response to stimuli.)

  o An EEG provides information about the ability of the brain to function and highlights areas of abnormality.

- Postprocedure

  - Client Education

    - Instruct clients that normal activities may be resumed.

GCS

- This assessment concentrates on neurologic function and is useful to determine the level of consciousness and monitor response to treatment. The GCS is reported as a number, which allows providers to immediately determine if neurologic changes have occurred.

- Indications

  - GCS scores are helpful in determining changes in the level of consciousness for clients with head injuries, space occupying lesions or cerebral infarctions, and encephalitis. This is important because complications related to neurologic injuries may occur rapidly and require immediate treatment.

- Interpretation of Findings

  - The best possible GCS score is 15. In general, total scores of the GCS correlate with the degree or level of coma.

  - Less than 8 – Associated with severe head injury and coma

  - 9 to 12 – Indicate a moderate head injury

  - Greater than 13 – Reflect minor head trauma

- Procedure

  - The GCS is calculated by using appropriate stimuli (a painful stimulus may be necessary) and then assessing the client's response in three areas.

    - Eye opening (E) – The best eye response, with responses ranging from 4 to 1

      - 4 = Eye opening occurs spontaneously

      - 3 = Eye opening occurs secondary to voice

      - 2 = Eye opening occurs secondary to pain

      - 1 = Eye opening does not occur

    - Verbal (V) – The best verbal response, with responses ranging from 5 to 1

      - 5 = Conversation is coherent and oriented

      - 4 = Conversation is incoherent and disoriented

      - 3 = Words are spoken, but inappropriately

      - 2 = Sounds are made, but no words

      - 1 = Vocalization does not occur

- Motor (M) – The best motor response, with responses ranging from 6 to 1
  - 6 = Commands are followed
  - 5 = Local reaction to pain occurs
  - 4 = There is a general withdrawal to pain
  - 3 = Decorticate posture (adduction of arms, flexion of elbows and wrists) is present
  - 2 = Decerebrate posture (abduction of arms, extension of elbows and wrists) is present
  - 1 = Motor response does not occur
- Responses within each subscale are added, with the total score quantitatively describing the client's level of consciousness. E + V + M = Total GCS
  - In critical situations, where head injury is present and close monitoring is required, subscale results may also be documented. Thus, a GCS may be reported as either a single number, indicating the sum of the subscales (3 to 15), or as 3 numbers, one from each subscale result, and the total (E3 V3 M4 = GCS 13). This allows providers to determine specific neurologic function.
  - Intubation limits the ability to use GCS summed scores. If intubation is present, the GCS may be reported as two scores, with modification noted. This is generally reported as "GCS 5t" (with the t representing the intubation tube).

Lumbar Puncture (Spinal Tap)

- A lumbar puncture is a procedure in which a small amount of cerebrospinal fluid (CSF) is withdrawn from the spinal canal and then analyzed to determine its constituents.

- Indications
  - This procedure is used to detect the presence of certain diseases (multiple sclerosis, syphilis), infection, and malignancies. A lumbar puncture may also be used to administer medication or chemotherapy directly to spinal fluid.

- Interpretation of Findings
  - Presence of red or white blood cells in CSF indicates an intracranial bleed or other vascular pathological process in the brain.
  - Elevated CSF readings can also indicate increased intracranial pressure.

- Preprocedure
  - The risks versus the benefits of a lumbar puncture should be discussed with clients prior to undertaking this procedure.
    - A lumbar puncture is associated with severe complications, especially when performed in the presence of increased ICP (brain herniation).
    - Lumbar punctures for clients with bleeding disorders or those taking anticoagulants may result in bleeding that compresses the spinal cord.

- Nursing Actions
  - Ensure that the client's jewelry has been removed and that clients are wearing only a hospital gown.
  - Instruct clients to void prior to the procedure.
  - Position clients to stretch the spinal canal. This may be done by having clients assume a "cannonball" position while on one side or by having clients stretch over an overbed table if sitting is preferred.

> **View Media Supplement:** Lumbar Puncture Positioning (Image)

- Intraprocedure
  - The area of the needle insertion is cleansed, and a local anesthesia is injected.
  - This is not a painful procedure; there should be little need for pain or relaxing medication other than the local anesthesia.
  - The needle is inserted and the CSF is withdrawn, after which the needle is removed.
  - A manometer may be used to determine the opening pressure of the spinal cord, which is useful if increased pressure is a consideration.
- Postprocedure
  - CSF is sent to the pathology department for analysis.
  - Nursing Actions
    - Monitor the puncture site. Have clients lie for several hours to ensure that the site clots.
  - Client Education
    - Once stable, advise clients that normal activities may be resumed.
- Complications
  - CSF leakage
    - If clotting does not occur, CSF may leak, resulting in a headache and increasing the potential for infection.

MRI Scan

- An MRI scan provides cross-sectional images of the cranial cavity. A contrast media may be used to enhance the images.
  - Unlike CT scans, MRI images are obtained using magnets, thus the consequences associated with radiation are avoided. This makes this procedure safer for women who are pregnant.

○ The use of magnets precludes the ability to scan a client who has an artificial device, (pacemakers, surgical clips, IV access port). If these are present, shielding may be done to prevent injury.

○ MRI-approved equipment must be used to monitor vital signs and provide ventilator/oxygen assistance to clients undergoing MRI scans.

- Indications

  ○ MRI scans may be used to detect abnormalities, monitor response to treatment, and guide needles used for biopsies.

  ○ MRIs are capable of discriminating soft tissue from tumor or bone. This makes the MRI scan more effective at determining tumor size and blood vessel location.

- Interpretation of Findings

  ○ Detailed three-dimensional pictures provide location and size of cranial pathology, such as tumors, arteriovenous malformations, and other vascular disorders.

- Preprocedure

  ○ Nursing Actions

    ■ Ensure that the client's jewelry is removed prior to this procedure. Have clients wear a hospital gown to prevent any metals from interfering with the magnet.

    ■ If sedation is expected, clients should refrain from food or fluids for 4 to 8 hr prior to the procedure.

    ■ Determine if clients have a history of claustrophobia and explain the tight space and noise.

    ■ Providers (and family members) who are in the scanning area while the magnet is on must remove all jewelry, pagers, and phones to prevent damage to themselves or the magnet.

    ■ Because this procedure is performed with clients in a supine position, placing pillows in the small of the client's back may assist in preventing back pain. The head must be secured to prevent unnecessary movement during the procedure.

- Intraprocedure

  ○ Clients must lie supine with his head stabilized.

  ○ MRI scanning is noisy, and earplugs or sedation may be provided.

- Postprocedure

  ○ Nursing Actions

    ■ No follow-up care is required after an MRI scan.

    ■ If contrast media is injected, monitor the site to assure clotting has occurred.

    ■ If sedation is administered, monitor clients until stable.

PET and SPECT Scans

- PET and SPECT scans are nuclear medicine procedures that produce three-dimensional images of the head. These images can be static (depicting vessels) or functional (depicting brain activity).

  - A glucose-based tracer is injected into the blood stream prior to the PET/SPECT scan. This initiates regional metabolic activity, which is then documented by the PET/SPECT scanner.

  - A CT scan may be performed after a PET/SPECT scan, as this provides information regarding brain activity and pathological location.

- Indications

  - A PET/SPECT scan captures regional metabolic activity and is most useful in determining tumor activity and/or response to treatment. PET/SPECT scans are also able to determine the presence of dementia, indicated by the inability of the brain to respond to the tracer.

- Interpretation of Findings

  - PET/SPECT scans are able to determine the areas of the brain that are and are not functioning.

  - This tool can help provide diagnostic evidence of dementia.

- Preprocedure

  - PET/SPECT scans use radiation, thus the risk/benefit consequences to any client who may be pregnant must be discussed.

  - Nursing Actions

    - Check for a history of diabetes mellitus. While this condition does not preclude a PET/SPECT scan, alterations in the client's medications may be necessary to avoid hyperglycemia or hypoglycemia before and after this procedure.

- Intraprocedure

  - While the pictures are being obtained, clients must lie flat with the head restrained.

  - This procedure is not painful and sedation is rarely necessary.

- Postprocedure

  - Nursing Actions

    - There is no follow-up care after a PET/SPECT scans.

    - Because the tracer is glucose based and short acting (less than 2 hr), it is broken down within the body as a sugar, not excreted.

Radiography (X-Ray)

- An x-ray uses electromagnetic radiation to capture images of the internal structures of an individual.

  o A structure's image is light or dark relative to the amount of radiation the tissue absorbs. The image is recorded on a radiograph, which is a black and white image that is held up to light for visualization. Some are recorded digitally and are available immediately.

  o X-rays must be interpreted by a radiologist, who documents the findings.

- Indications

  o X-ray examinations are done to diagnose possible skull or spinal fractures. They also determine the cause of paralysis or paresthesia and increasing neurological deficits.

- Interpretation of Findings

  o X-ray examinations of the skull and spine can reveal fractures, curvatures, bone erosion and dislocation, and possible soft-tissue calcification, all of which can damage the nervous system.

- Preprocedure

  o Nursing Actions

    ■ There is no special preprocedure protocol for x-rays that do not use contrast. X-rays are often the first diagnostic tool used after an injury (rule out cervical fracture in head trauma), and they can be done without any preparation.

    ■ Determine if female clients are pregnant.

    ■ Ensure that the client's jewelry is removed and that no clothes cover the area.

  o Client Education

    ■ Explain that the amount of radiation used in contemporary x-ray machines is very small.

- Intraprocedure

  o Client Education

    ■ Instruct clients to remain still during the procedure.

- Postprocedure

  o Nursing Actions

    ■ No postprocedure care is required.

  o Client Education

    ■ Inform clients when results will be available.

(A) APPLICATION EXERCISES

1. A nurse is caring for a client scheduled for a cerebral angiogram with contrast dye. Which of the following client responses should the nurse communicate to the provider? (Select all that apply.)

   _____ "I may be pregnant."

   _____ "I take Coumadin."

   _____ "I am on an antihypertensive."

   _____ "I am allergic to shellfish."

   _____ "I am allergic to latex."

2. A nurse is providing education to a client who is to undergo an electroencephalogram (EEG) the next day. Which of the following should the nurse include?

   A. Do not wash your hair the morning of the procedure.

   B. You will be given an analgesic prior to the test.

   C. The procedure will take approximately 15 min.

   D. You will need to lie flat for 4 hr after the procedure.

3. A nurse is collecting data from a client who was admitted to the medical-surgical unit 12 hr ago after falling off a ladder and hitting his head. The client is drowsy, but responds to verbal commands, and opens his eyes when the nurse calls his name. He is oriented to time, place, and person. The nurse should document that the client's Glasgow Coma Scale Score is which of the following?

   A. 15

   B. 14

   C. 13

   D. 12

(A) APPLICATION EXERCISES ANSWER KEY

1. A nurse is caring for a client scheduled for a cerebral angiogram with contrast dye. Which of the following client responses should the nurse communicate to the provider? (Select all that apply.)

    | X | "I may be pregnant." |
    | X | "I take Coumadin." |
    | ___ | "I am on an antihypertensive." |
    | X | "I am allergic to shellfish." |
    | ___ | "I am allergic to latex." |

    The provider should be notified of clients who are or could be pregnant due to the risks to the fetus secondary to exposure of radiation. Allergies to shellfish or iodine are also contraindications to contrast dye. A client taking warfarin (Coumadin) should also be reported to the provider due to the potential for bleeding postprocedure. There are no contraindications to contrast dye in clients who are on antihypertensives or are allergic to latex.

    (N) NCLEX® Connection: Reduction of Risk Potential, Potential for Complications of Diagnostic Tests/Treatments/Procedures

2. A nurse is providing education to a client who is to undergo an electroencephalogram (EEG) the next day. Which of the following should the nurse include?

    A. Do not wash your hair the morning of the procedure.

    B. You will be given an analgesic prior to the test.

    C. The procedure will take approximately 15 min.

    D. You will need to lie flat for 4 hr after the procedure.

    This test is noninvasive and does not cause any pain. There is no indication for pain medication prior to the test. The client may be given sedation by IV infusion to induce sleep. The client should be instructed to wash her hair prior to the procedure. An EEG usually takes approximately 1 hr and there are no activity restrictions postprocedure.

    (N) NCLEX® Connection: Reduction of Risk Potential, Potential for Complications of Diagnostic Tests/Treatments/Procedures

3. A nurse is collecting data from a client who was admitted to the medical-surgical unit 12 hr ago after falling off a ladder and hitting his head. The client is drowsy, but responds to verbal commands, and opens his eyes when the nurse calls his name. He is oriented to time, place, and person. The nurse should document that the client's Glasgow Coma Scale Score is which of the following?

    A. 15

    B. 14

    C. 13

    D. 12

The client's Glasgow Coma Scale Score is 14. Eye-opening response is 3 (secondary to voice). Verbal response is 5 (coherent and oriented to conversation). Motor response is 6 (follows commands.) 3+5+6=14

(N) NCLEX® Connection: Reduction of Risk Potential, Potential for Complications of Diagnostic Tests/Treatments/Procedures

UNIT 2	NURSING CARE OF CLIENTS WITH NEUROSENSORY DISORDERS
Section	Diagnostic and Therapeutic Procedures
Chapter 4	Pain Management

Overview

- Effective pain management includes the use of pharmacological and nonpharmacological pain management therapies. Invasive therapies such as nerve ablation may be appropriate for intractable cancer-related pain.

- Clients have a right to appropriate pain management. Nurses are accountable for the assessment of pain. A nurse's role is that of an advocate and educator for effective pain management.

- Nurses have a priority responsibility to continually collect data regarding a client's pain level and to provide individualized interventions. They should determine the effectiveness of the interventions 30 to 60 min after implementation.

Physiology of Pain

- Transduction is the conversion of painful stimuli to an electrical impulse through peripheral nerve fibers (nociceptors).

- Transmission occurs as the electrical impulse travels along the nerve fibers and is regulated by neurotransmitters.

- The point at which one feels pain is known as the pain threshold.

- The amount of pain one is willing to bear is known as pain tolerance.

SUBSTANCES THAT INCREASE PAIN TRANSMISSION AND CAUSE AN INFLAMMATORY RESPONSE	SUBSTANCES THAT DECREASE PAIN TRANSMISSION AND PRODUCE ANALGESIA
• Substance P • Prostaglandins • Bradykinin • Histamine	• Serotonin • Endorphins

- Perception or awareness of pain occurs in the brain and is influenced by thought and emotional processes.

- Modulation occurs in the spinal cord, causing muscles to contract reflexively, moving the body away from painful stimuli.

Pain Categories

ACUTE PAIN	CHRONIC PAIN
• Acute pain is protective, temporary, usually self-limiting, and resolves with tissue healing. • Physiological responses (sympathetic nervous system) are fight-or-flight responses (tachycardia, hypertension, anxiety, diaphoresis, muscle tension). • Behavioral responses include grimacing, moaning, flinching, and guarding. • Interventions include treatment of the underlying problem.	• Chronic pain is not protective; it is ongoing or recurs frequently, lasting longer than 6 months and persisting beyond tissue healing. • Physiological responses do not usually alter vital signs, but the client may experience depression, fatigue, and a decreased level of functioning. • Psychosocial implications may lead to disability. • Chronic pain may not have a known cause, and it may not respond to interventions. • Management of pain is aimed at symptomatic relief. • Chronic pain can be malignant or nonmalignant.
NOCICEPTIVE PAIN	NEUROPATHIC PAIN

• Nociceptive pain arises from damage to or inflammation of tissue other than that of the peripheral and central nervous systems.
• It is usually throbbing, aching, and localized.
• This pain typically responds to opioids and nonopioid medications.
• Types of nociceptive pain
  ○ Somatic – in bones, joints, muscles, skin, or connective tissues
  ○ Visceral – in internal organs such as the stomach or intestines. It can cause referred pain in other body locations not associated with the stimulus
  ○ Cutaneous – in the skin or subcutaneous tissue
	• Neuropathic pain arises from abnormal or damaged pain nerves.
	• It includes phantom limb pain, pain below the level of a spinal cord injury, and diabetic neuropathy.
	• Neuropathic pain is usually intense, shooting, burning, or described as "pins and needles."
	• This pain typically responds to adjuvant medications (antidepressants, antispasmodic agents, skeletal muscle relaxants).

- Causes of Acute and Chronic Pain

    ○ Trauma

    ○ Surgery

    ○ Cancer (tumor invasion, nerve compression, bone metastases, associated infections, immobility)

    ○ Arthritis

    ○ Fibromyalgia

- o   Neuropathy
- o   Diagnostic or treatment procedures (injection, intubation, radiation)
- The Pain Experience is Affected by:
  - o   Age.

    - ■   Older adult clients may have multiple pathologies that cause pain and limit function.
  - o   Fatigue, which can increase sensitivity to pain.
  - o   Genetic sensitivity, which can increase or decrease the amount of pain an individual can tolerate.
  - o   Cognitive function.
    - ■   Clients who are cognitively impaired may not be able to report pain or report it accurately.
  - o   Prior experiences, which can increase or decrease sensitivity depending on whether or not adequate relief was obtained.
  - o   Anxiety and fear, which can increase sensitivity to pain.
  - o   Support systems that are present and can decrease sensitivity to pain.
  - o   Culture, which may influence how clients express pain or the meaning given to it.

Data Collection

- According to noted pain experts Margo McCaffery and Chris Pasero, pain is whatever the person experiencing it says it is, and it exists whenever the person says it does. The client's report of pain is the most reliable diagnostic measure of pain.
- Pain should be assessed and recorded frequently, and may be considered the fifth vital sign.
- Subjective data can be obtained using a symptom analysis.

PARAMETERS	QUESTIONS TO ASK
The location is described using anatomical terminology and landmarks.	"Where is your pain? Does it radiate anywhere else?" "Can you point to where it hurts?"
Quality refers to how the pain feels. Feelings of pain include: Sharp, dull, aching, burning, stabbing, pounding, throbbing, shooting, gnawing, tender, heavy, tight, tiring, exhausting, sickening, terrifying, torturing, nagging, annoying, intense, and/or unbearable.	"What does the pain feel like?" Is the pain throbbing, burning, or stabbing?"

PARAMETERS	QUESTIONS TO ASK
Intensity, strength, and severity are "measures" of the pain. Visual analog scales (description scale, number rating scale) can be used to: • Measure pain. • Monitor pain. • Evaluate the effectiveness of interventions to relieve pain.	"How much pain do you have now?" • "What is the worst/best the pain has been?" • "How would you rate your pain on a scale of 0 to 10?"
Timing – onset, duration, frequency	"When did it start?" • "How long does it last?" • "How often does it occur?" • "Is it constant or intermittent?"
Setting – how the pain affects daily life or how ADLs affect the pain	"Where are you when the symptoms occur?" • "What are you doing when the symptoms occur?" • "How does the pain affect your sleep?" • "How does the pain affect your ability to work and do your job?"
Associated symptoms that should be noted include fatigue, depression, nausea, and anxiety.	"What other symptoms do you experience when you are feeling pain?"
Aggravating/relieving factors	• "What makes the pain better?" • "What makes the pain worse?" • "Are you currently taking any prescription, herbal, or over-the-counter medications?"

- Objective Data

  - Behaviors complement self-report and assist in pain assessment of clients who are nonverbal.

    - Facial expressions (grimacing, wrinkled forehead) and body movements (restlessness, pacing, guarding)

    - Moaning, crying

    - Decreased attention span

- Acute pain temporarily increases blood pressure, pulse, and respiratory rate. Eventually, increases in vital signs will stabilize despite the persistence of pain. Therefore, physiologic indicators may not be an accurate measure of pain over time.

Nonpharmacological Pain Management

- Cutaneous (skin) stimulation – transcutaneous electrical nerve stimulation (TENS), heat, cold, therapeutic touch, and massage

 View Media Supplement: TENS Unit (Video)

  - Interruption of pain pathways
  - Cold for inflammation
  - Heat to increase blood flow and to reduce stiffness
- Distraction
  - Includes ambulation, deep breathing, visitors, TV, and/or music
- Relaxation
  - Includes meditation, yoga, and/or progressive muscle relaxation
- Imagery
  - Focuses on a pleasant thought to divert focus
  - Requires an ability to concentrate
- Acupuncture – Tiny needles are inserted into the skin and subcutaneous tissues at specific points along energy meridians. If heat is applied to or near the needles, this is called moxibustion.
- Reduction of pain stimuli in the environment
- Elevation of extremities that are edematous help to promote venous return and decrease swelling

Pharmacological Interventions

- Analgesics are the mainstay for relieving pain. The three classes of analgesics are nonopioids, opioids, and adjuvants.
- Nonopioid analgesics, such as acetaminophen, ibuprofen, and aspirin, are appropriate for treating mild to moderate pain.
  - Acetaminophen has analgesic and antipyretic effects. NSAIDs have analgesic, anti-inflammatory, antiplatelet, and antipyretic effects.
  - Be aware of the hepatotoxic effects of acetaminophen. A client who has a healthy liver should take no more than 4 g/day. Be aware of opioids that contain acetaminophen, such as hydrocodone bitartrate 5 mg and acetaminophen 500 mg (Vicodin).
  - Monitor clients taking aspirin for salicylism (tinnitus, vertigo, decreased hearing acuity).

- ○ Prevent gastric upset in clients by administering the medication with food or antacids.

- ○ Monitor clients for bleeding with long-term NSAID use.

- Opioid analgesics (morphine sulfate, fentanyl [Sublimaze], codeine) are appropriate for treating moderate to severe pain (postoperative pain, MI pain, cancer pain).

  - ○ Manage a client's acute severe pain with short-term, (24 to 48 hr) around-the-clock opioids. Maintain consistency in timing and dosing to provide consistent pain control.

  - ○ Monitor clients receiving parenteral opioids for immediate, short-term relief of acute pain.

  - ○ Use the oral route for chronic, nonfluctuating pain.

  - ○ Monitor and intervene for adverse effects of opioid use.

    - ▪ Respiratory depression – Monitor the client's respiratory rate prior to and following administration of opioids (especially in clients who are opioid-naïve). Initial treatment of respiratory depression and sedation is generally a reduction in opioid dose. Notify the charge nurse of respiratory depression for administration of naloxone (Narcan).

    - ▪ Constipation – Use a preventative approach (monitoring of bowel movements, fluids, fiber intake, exercise, stool softeners); use stimulant laxatives, enemas when necessary.

    - ▪ Orthostatic hypotension – Advise clients to sit or lie down if symptoms of lightheadedness or dizziness occur. Instruct clients to avoid sudden changes in position by slowly moving from a lying to a sitting or standing position. Provide assistance with ambulation as needed.

    - ▪ Urinary retention – Monitor the client's I&O, check for distention, administer bethanechol (Urecholine), and catheterize as prescribed.

    - ▪ Nausea/vomiting – Administer antiemetics, advise clients to lie still and/or move slowly, and eliminate odors.

    - ▪ Sedation – Monitor the client's level of consciousness and take safety precautions. Sedation usually precedes respiratory depression.

- Adjuvant analgesics enhance the effects of nonopioids, help alleviate other symptoms that aggravate pain (depression, seizures, inflammation), and are useful for treatment of neuropathic pain.

  - ○ Adjuvant medications

    - ▪ Anticonvulsants – carbamazepine (Tegretol)

    - ▪ Antianxiety agents – diazepam (Valium)

    - ▪ Tricyclic antidepressants – amitriptyline (Elavil)

    - ▪ Antihistamine – hydroxyzine (Vistaril)

    - ▪ Glucocorticoids – dexamethasone (Decadron)

    - ▪ Antiemetics – ondansetron hydrochloride (Zofran)

- Patient-controlled analgesia (PCA) is a medication delivery system that allows clients to self-administer safe doses of opioid analgesics.

    o Constant plasma levels are maintained by small, frequent doses.

    o The client experiences less lag time between identified need and delivery of medication, which increases the client's sense of control and may decrease the amount of medication needed.

    o Commonly used opioids are morphine sulfate and hydromorphone (Dilaudid).

    o Monitor clients for sedation and respiratory depression.

    o The client is the only person who should push the PCA button to prevent inadvertent overdosing.

- Other strategies for effective pain management

    o Take a proactive approach by giving clients analgesics before pain becomes too severe. It takes less medication to prevent pain than to treat pain.

    o Instruct clients to report developing or recurrent pain and to not wait until pain is severe (for PRN orders of pain medication).

    o Reinforce with clients misconceptions about pain.

    o Assist clients to reduce fear and anxiety.

    o Contribute nonpharmacological and pharmacological pain relief measures to the plan of care.

Complications and Nursing Implications

- Undertreatment of pain is a serious complication and may lead to increased anxiety with acute pain and depression with chronic pain. Monitor clients for pain frequently, and intervene as appropriate.

- Sedation, respiratory depression, and coma can occur as a result of overdosing. Sedation always precedes respiratory depression.

- Identify clients who are high-risk (older adult clients, clients who are opioid-naïve).

- Carefully titrate doses while closely monitoring respiratory status.

- Notify the charge nurse to administer naloxone (Narcan) if the client's respirations are less than 8/min and shallow, or if the client is difficult to arouse.

APPLICATION EXERCISES

1. When caring for clients experiencing pain, the nurse should recognize that which of the following substances decrease pain transmission? (Select all that apply.)

    _____ Substance P

    _____ Serotonin

    _____ Bradykinin

    _____ Endorphins

    _____ Histamine

2. A nurse is performing a pain assessment on a client. Which of the following subjective data describes the quality of the client's pain?

    A. "My pain is so bad I cannot sleep at night."

    B. "My pain feels like a tight feeling in my chest."

    C. "My pain started last week after I went for a hike."

    D. "My pain feels better if I rest in an upright position."

3. A nurse is caring for a postoperative client who is receiving morphine for pain. For which of the following findings should the nurse monitor and report to the charge nurse? (Select all that apply.)

    _____ BP sitting 120/80 mm Hg, and when standing 100/70 mm Hg

    _____ Urinary output of 30 mL/hr

    _____ Reports of nausea

    _____ Frequent loose stools

    _____ Respiratory rate 10/min

4. A nurse is providing pain relief for a client who was diagnosed with peripheral neuropathy. Which of the following pain descriptions by the client is consistent with neuropathic pain?

    A. Aching

    B. Throbbing

    C. Burning

    D. Cramping

APPLICATION EXERCISES ANSWER KEY

1. When caring for clients experiencing pain, the nurse should recognize that which of the following substances decrease pain transmission? (Select all that apply.)

    _____   Substance P

    __X__   **Serotonin**

    _____   Bradykinin

    __X__   **Endorphins**

    _____   Histamine

    Serotonin and endorphins are natural substances within the body that decrease pain transmission. Substance P, bradykinin, and histamine all increase pain transmission.

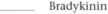 NCLEX® Connection: Physiological Adaptation, Pathophysiology

2. A nurse is performing a pain assessment on a client. Which of the following subjective data describes the quality of the client's pain?

    A. "My pain is so bad I cannot sleep at night."

    B. "My pain feels like a tight feeling in my chest."

    C. "My pain started last week after I went for a hike."

    D. "My pain feels better if I rest in an upright position."

    Option B describes the quality of the pain, referring to how the pain feels to the client. This is typically a description such as throbbing, sharp, dull, or tight. Option A describes associated symptoms such as difficulty sleeping, nausea, and anxiety. Option C describes the timing of the pain. Option D describes a relieving factor.

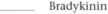 NCLEX® Connection: Reduction of Risk Potential, System-Specific Assessment

3. A nurse is caring for a postoperative client who is receiving morphine for pain. For which of the following findings should the nurse monitor and report to the charge nurse? (Select all that apply.)

   __X__   **BP sitting 120/80 mm Hg, and when standing 100/70 mm Hg**

   _____   Urinary output of 30 mL/hr

   __X__   **Reports of nausea**

   _____   Frequent loose stools

   __X__   **Respiratory rate 10/min**

Adverse effects of opioid analgesics include orthostatic hypotension, reports of nausea, and respiratory depression. Urinary output less than 30 mL/hr may indicate urinary retention, an adverse effect of opioids. Constipation rather than diarrhea is an adverse effect of opioids.

 NCLEX® Connection: Pharmacological Therapies, Adverse Effects/Contraindications/Side Effects/Interactions

4. A nurse is providing pain relief for a client who was diagnosed with peripheral neuropathy. Which of the following pain descriptions by the client is consistent with neuropathic pain?

A. Aching

B. Throbbing

C. Burning

D. Cramping

Neuropathic pain is usually described as burning, shooting, or a pins and needles feeling. Aching and throbbing pain is usually associated with nociceptive pain, and cramping pain with visceral pain.

 NCLEX® Connection: Reduction of Risk Potential, Potential for Alterations in Body Systems

UNIT 2	NURSING CARE OF CLIENTS WITH NEUROSENSORY DISORDERS
Section:	Central and Peripheral Nervous System Disorders
Chapter 5	Increased Intracranial Pressure Disorders

Overview

- Brain tumors occur in any part of the brain and are classified according to the cell or tissue of origin. Types of brain tumors include: malignant gliomas (neuroglial cells), benign meningiomas (meninges), pituitary tumors, and acoustic neuromas (acoustic cranial nerve).

- Brain tumors apply pressure to surrounding brain tissue, resulting in decreased outflow of cerebrospinal fluid, increased intracranial pressure, cerebral edema, and neurological deficits. Tumors that involve the pituitary gland may cause endocrine dysfunction.

- Head injuries can be classified as open (skull integrity is compromised – penetrating trauma) or closed (skull integrity is maintained – blunt trauma). Head injuries are also classified as mild, moderate, or severe, depending upon Glasgow Coma Scale (GCS) ratings and the length of time the client was unconscious.

- Head injuries may or may not be associated with hemorrhage (epidural, subdural, and intracerebral). Cerebrospinal fluid leakage is also possible. Any collection of fluid or foreign objects that occupies the space within the confines of the skull consequently poses a risk for cerebral edema, increased intracranial pressure, cerebral hypoxia, and brain herniation.

BRAIN TUMORS

Overview

- Primary malignant brain tumors originate from neuroglia tissue and rarely metastasize outside of the brain. Secondary malignant brain tumors are lesions that are metastases from a primary cancer located elsewhere in the body. Cranial metastatic lesions are most common from breast, kidney, and gastrointestinal tract cancers.

- Benign brain tumors develop from the meninges or cranial nerves and do not metastasize. These tumors have distinct boundaries and cause damage either by the pressure they exert within the cranial cavity and/or by impairing the function of the cranial nerve.

- Brain tumors that occur in the cerebral hemispheres above the tentorium cerebelli are classified as supratentorial tumors. Those below the tentorium cerebelli, such as tumors of the brainstem and cerebellum, are classified as infratentorial tumors.

Data Collection

- Risk Factors
  - The cause is unknown, but several risk factors have been identified including:
    - Genetics
    - Environmental agents
    - Exposure to ionizing radiation
    - Exposure to electromagnetic fields
    - Previous head injury
- Subjective and Objective Data
  - Physical Assessment Findings
    - Dysarthria
    - Dysphagia
    - Positive Romberg sign
    - Positive Babinski's sign
    - Vertigo
    - Hemiparesis
    - Cranial nerve dysfunction (inability to discriminate sounds, loss of gag reflex, loss of blink response)

SUPRATENTORIAL BRAIN TUMORS	INFRATENTORIAL BRAIN TUMORS
• Severe headache – worse upon awakening, but gets better over time • Visual symptoms (blurring, visual field deficit) • Seizures • Loss of voluntary movement or the inability to control movement • Change in cognitive function (memory loss, language impairment) • Change in personality, inability to control emotions • Nausea with or without vomiting	• Hearing loss or ringing in the ear • Facial drooping • Difficulty swallowing • Nystagmus, crossed eyes, or decreased vision • Autonomic nervous system (ANS) dysfunction • Ataxia or clumsy movements • Hemiparesis • Cranial nerve dysfunction (inability to discriminate sounds, loss of gag reflex, loss of blink response)

  - Laboratory Tests
    - CBC and differential to rule out anemia or malnutrition
    - Alcohol and illicit drug screen to rule out these as causes of abnormal physical examination
    - TB and HIV screening if social conditions warrant

○ Diagnostic Procedures

■ X-ray; computed tomography (CT) imaging, magnetic resonance imaging (MRI), brain, and position emission tomography (PET) scans; and cerebral angiography are all used to determine the size, location, and extent of the tumor.

■ Cerebral biopsy – performed to identify cellular pathology

□ Client Education

▸ Include specific instruction regarding medications.

▷ Instruct clients to continue antiepileptic medications to prevent seizure activity.

▷ Instruct clients to discontinue aspirin products at least 72 hr prior to the procedure to minimize the risk of intracerebral bleeding.

▷ Inform clients that preprocedure activities may be resumed after recovering from the general anesthetic.

▷ Instruct clients to keep the incision clean and dry. If sutures are in place, they need to be removed 1 to 7 days later.

▷ Encourage clients to avoid driving or other dangerous activities until follow-up appointment occurs and diagnosis is known.

Collaborative Care

● Nursing Care

○ Maintain airway (monitor oxygen levels, administer oxygen as needed, monitor lung sounds).

○ Monitor neurological status, in particular, observing for changes in level of consciousness, neurological deficits, and occurrence of seizures.

○ Maintain client safety (assist with transfers and ambulation, provide assistive devices as needed).

○ Implement seizure precautions.

○ Administer medications as prescribed.

● Medications

○ Nonopioid analgesics are used to treat headaches.

■ Opioid medications are avoided, as they tend to decrease the client's level of consciousness.

○ Corticosteroids are used to reduce cerebral edema.

■ Corticosteroid medications quickly reduce cerebral edema and may be rapidly administered to maximize their effectiveness.

■ Chronic administration is used to control cerebral edema associated with the presence or treatment of benign or malignant brain tumors.

- ○ Anticonvulsant medications are used to control or prevent seizure activity.

  - ■ Anticonvulsant medications suppress the neuronal activity within the brain, which prevents seizure activity.

- ○ H_2-receptor antagonists are used to decrease the acid content of the stomach, reducing the risk of stress ulcers.

  - ■ H_2-receptor antagonist medications are administered during acute or stressful periods, such as after surgery, at the initiation of chemotherapy, or during the first several radiation therapy treatments.

- ○ Antiemetics are used if nausea with or without vomiting is present.

  - ■ Nausea and vomiting may be present as a result of the increased intracranial pressure, the site of the tumor, or the treatment required.

  - ■ These medications are administered as prescribed, and may be provided as a preventative intervention, especially when the treatment is associated with nausea and/or vomiting.

- ● Interdisciplinary Care

  - ○ Request appropriate referrals (social services, support groups, medical equipment, and physical, speech, and occupational therapy).

  - ○ Treatments include steroids, surgery, chemotherapy, conventional radiation therapy, stereotactic radiosurgery, and clinical trials. Chemotherapy and/or conventional radiation therapy may be administered prior to surgery to reduce the bulk of the tumor.

  - ○ In cases where the tumor is a metastatic lesion from a primary lesion elsewhere in the body, treatments are palliative in nature. These treatments may consist of surgery, radiation, and chemotherapy, in any combination, and are aimed at controlling intracerebral lesions.

- ● Surgical Interventions

  - ○ Craniotomy – complete or partial resection of brain tumor through surgical opening in the skull

    - ■ Nursing Actions

      - □ Preoperatively

        - ▸ Explain the procedure to clients, answering all appropriate questions and providing emotional support.

        - ▸ Instruct clients to discontinue aspirin products at least 72 hr prior to the procedure.

□ Postoperatively

▸ Provide routine postoperative care to prevent complications

▸ Keep the client's head elevated 30° and placed in a neutral position.

▸ Assist clients to avoid straining activities (moving up in bed and attempting to have a bowel movement) to prevent increased intracranial pressure. Postoperative bleeding and seizure activity are the greatest risks.

- Client Outcomes

  ○ The client will be free from injury.

  ○ The client will be free from infection.

Complications

- Syndrome of inappropriate antidiuretic hormone (SIADH)

  ○ This is a condition where fluid is retained as a result of an overproduction of vasopressin or antidiuretic hormone (ADH) from the posterior pituitary gland.

  ○ The condition occurs when the hypothalamus has been damaged and can no longer regulate the release of ADH.

  ○ Treatment of SIADH consists of fluid restriction, desmopressin acetate tablets (DDAVP), and treatment of hyponatremia.

  ○ If SIADH is present, the client may be disoriented, report a headache, and/or vomit.

  ○ If severe or untreated, this condition may cause seizures and/or a coma.

- Diabetes insipidus (DI)

  ○ This is a condition where large amounts of urine are excreted as a result of a deficiency of ADH from the posterior pituitary gland.

  ○ The condition occurs when the hypothalamus has been damaged and can no longer regulate the release of ADH.

  ○ Treatment of DI consists of massive fluid replacement, careful attention to laboratory values, and replacement of essential nutrients as indicated.

HEAD INJURY

Overview

- Skull fractures are often accompanied by brain injury. Damage to the brain tissue may be the result of decreased oxygen supply, or the direct impact from the skull fracture, which caused the trauma. The glucose levels in the brain are negatively affected, resulting in an alteration in neurological synaptic ability.

- Open-head injuries pose a high risk for infection.

- A cervical spine injury should always be suspected when a head injury occurs. A cervical spine injury must be ruled out prior to removing any devices used to stabilize the cervical spine.

Data Collection

- Risk Factors

  - Males under 25 years of age

  - Motor vehicle or motorcycle crashes

  - Drug and alcohol use

  - Sports injuries

  - Assault

  - Gunshot wounds

  - Falls

- Subjective and Objective Data

  - Presence of alcohol or illicit drugs at time of injury

  - Amnesia (loss of memory) before or after the injury

  - Loss of consciousness – Length of time the client is unconscious is significant

  - Glasgow Coma Scale

    - Scores of:

      - Less than 8 – Associated with severe head injury and coma

      - 9 to 12 – Indicate a moderate head injury

      - Greater than 13 – Reflect minor head trauma

  - Signs of increased intracranial pressure

    - Severe headache

    - Deteriorating level of consciousness, restlessness, irritability

    - Dilated or pinpoint pupils that are slow to react or nonreactive

    - Alteration in breathing pattern (Cheyne-Stokes respirations, central neurogenic hyperventilation, apnea)

    - Deterioration in motor function, abnormal posturing (decerebrate, decorticate, or flaccidity)

    - Cushing reflex is a late sign characterized by severe hypertension with a widening pulse pressure (systolic – diastolic = pulse pressure) and bradycardia.

    - Cerebrospinal fluid leakage from the nose and ears ("halo" sign – yellow stain surrounded by blood on a paper towel; fluid tests positive for glucose)

    - Seizures

  - Laboratory Tests

    - ABGs

    - Alcohol level and drug screen

- CBC with differential and BUN
  - BUN is used to determine the client's renal status. This information is needed prior to administration of radiology contrast media.

  o Diagnostic Procedures
  - Cervical spine films are used to diagnose a cervical spine injury.
  - Computerized tomography (CT) and/or a magnetic resonance imaging (MRI) of the head and/or neck (with and without contrast if indicated).

Collaborative Care

- Nursing Care

  o There is a 1 hr "golden window" for treatment of head injuries. Emergency treatment provided during this time frame, especially for epidural hematomas, decreases the morbidity and mortality rates associated with these conditions.

  o Instruct the client's family on effective ways to communicate with the client (touch, talk, and assist with care as appropriate).

  o Monitor at regularly scheduled intervals
  - Respiratory status is the priority assessment.
    - The brain is dependent upon oxygen to maintain function and has little reserve available if oxygen is deprived. Brain function begins to diminish after 3 min of oxygen deprivation.
  - Cranial nerve function (eye-blink response, gag reflex, tongue and shoulder movement)
  - Pupillary changes (PERRLA, pinpoint, fixed/nonresponsive, dilated)
  - Signs of infection (nuchal rigidity occurs with meningitis)
  - Sensory and/or motor responses if spinal injury is present
  - Changes in level of consciousness, using the GCS, provides the earliest indication of neurological deterioration.
  - Intracranial pressure (ICP)
    - Expected reference range for ICP level is 10 to 15 mm Hg.
    - Implement actions that will decrease ICP:
      - Elevate head to reduce ICP and to promote venous drainage.
      - Avoid extreme flexion, extension or rotation of the head, and maintain the body in a midline neutral position, with the head of the bed elevated 30°.
      - Maintain a patent airway.
      - Administer oxygen as indicated to maintain an oxygen saturation level of greater than 95%.
      - Discourage coughing and blowing nose forcefully.

- ▸ Minimize endotracheal or oral tracheal suctioning. Do not routinely perform suctioning.

- ▸ Maintain cervical spine stability until cleared by an x-ray.

- ▸ Report presence of cerebrospinal fluid (CSF) from nose or ears to the provider.

- ▸ Provide a calm, restful environment (limit visitors, minimize noise).

- ▸ Implement measures to prevent complications of immobility (turn the client every 2 hr, footboard, and splints). Specialty beds can be used.

- ▸ Monitor fluid and electrolyte values and osmolarity to detect changes in sodium regulation, the onset of diabetes insipidus, or severe hypovolemia.

- ▸ Provide adequate fluids to maintain cerebral perfusion. When a large amount of IV fluids are prescribed, monitor the client carefully for excess fluid volume, which could increase ICP.

- ▸ Maintain client safety and seizure precautions (side rails up, padded side rails, call light within the client's reach).

- ▸ Even if the level of consciousness is decreased, explain to the client the actions being taken and why. Hearing is the last sense affected by a head injury.

- Medications

  - ○ Corticosteroids – Dexamethasone (Decadron) and methylprednisolone (Solu-Medrol)

    - ▪ Used to reduce cerebral edema

    - ▪ Nursing Considerations

      - □ Use with caution in the presence of diabetes mellitus, hypertension, glaucoma, or renal impairment. If these conditions exist, additional monitoring is required as corticosteroids disrupt the stability of those conditions and can require alterations in care.

  - ○ Mannitol (Osmitrol)

    - ▪ Osmotic diuretic used to treat acute cerebral edema

    - ▪ Nursing Considerations

      - □ Monitor clients receiving mannitol IV.

      - □ Insert indwelling urinary catheter to monitor fluid and renal status.

  - ○ Pentobarbital (Nembutal)

    - ▪ Pentobarbital is used to induce a barbiturate coma to decrease cerebral metabolic demands.

    - ▪ This treatment is performed when the ICP is refractory to treatment, has exceeded 25 mm Hg for 30 min, 30 mm Hg for 15 min, or 40 mm Hg for 1 min.

- A barbiturate coma is a treatment of last resort and aims to decrease elevated ICP by inducing vasoconstriction and decreasing cerebral metabolic demands.
- Nursing Considerations
  □ Monitor clients receiving pentobarbital.
  - Phenytoin (Dilantin)
    - Used prophylactically to prevent or treat seizures that can occur
      □ Nursing Considerations
        ▸ Check for medication interactions.
  - Morphine sulfate or fentanyl (Sublimaze)
    - Analgesics used to control pain and restlessness
    - Nursing Considerations
      □ Use opioids if client is receiving mechanical ventilation.
      □ Avoid the use of opioids due to the CNS depressant effect that will make a neurological assessment difficult.
- Interdisciplinary Care
  - Care for a client with a head injury should include professionals from other disciplines as indicated. This may include a physical, occupational, recreational and/or speech therapist due to neurological deficits that may occur secondary to the area of the brain damaged. Rehabilitation facilities are frequently used to compress the time required to recover from a head injury and support re-emergence into society.
  - Request referral for social services to provide links to social service agencies and schools.
- Surgical Interventions
  - Craniotomy
    - A craniotomy is the removal of nonviable brain tissue that allows for expansion and/or removal of epidural or subdural hematomas. It involves drilling a burr hole or creating a bone flap to permit access to the affected area. Treatment of intracranial hemorrhages require surgical evacuation.
    - Nursing Actions
      □ Provide routine postoperative care to prevent complications.

UNIT 2	NURSING CARE OF CLIENTS WITH NEUROSENSORY DISORDERS
Section:	Central and Peripheral Nervous System Disorders
Chapter 6	Meningitis

Overview

- Meningitis is an inflammation of the meninges, which are the membranes that protect the brain and spinal cord.

- Viral, or aseptic meningitis, is the most common form and commonly resolves without treatment.

- Bacterial, or septic meningitis, is a contagious infection with a high mortality rate. The prognosis depends on how quickly care is initiated.

Data Collection

- Risk Factors

  - Viral meningitis

    - Viral illnesses such as the mumps, measles, herpes, and arboviruses such as the mosquito-borne West Nile virus.

  - Bacterial meningitis

    - Bacterial-based infections, such as otitis media, pneumonia, or sinusitis, in which the infectious micro-organism is *Neisseria meningitidis*, *Streptococcus pneumoniae*, or *Haemophilus influenzae*

    - Immunosuppression

    - Invasive procedures, skull fracture, or penetrating head wound (direct access to CSF)

    - Overcrowded or communal living conditions

- Subjective Data

  - Excruciating, constant headache

  - Nuchal rigidity (stiff neck)

  - Photophobia (sensitivity to light)

- Objective Data

  - Physical Assessment Findings

    - Fever and chills

    - Nausea and vomiting

- Altered level of consciousness
- Disorientation to person, place, and time.
- Abnormal eye movements
- Alterations in motor function (hemiparesis, hemiplegia)
- Positive Kernig's sign (resistance and pain with extension of the client's leg from a flexed position)
- Positive Brudzinski's sign (flexion of extremities occurring with deliberate flexion of the client's neck)
- Hyperactive deep-tendon reflexes
- Tachycardia
- Seizures
- Red macular rash (meningococcal meningitis)
- Restlessness, irritability

o Laboratory Tests

- Urine, throat, nose, blood, and culture and sensitivity

  □ Perform culture and sensitivity of various body fluids to identify possible infectious bacteria and an appropriate broad-spectrum antibiotic. Not definitive for meningitis, but can guide initial selection of antimicrobial therapy.

- CBC

  □ Elevated WBC count

o Diagnostic Procedures

- Cerebrospinal fluid (CSF) analysis

  □ CSF analysis is the most definitive diagnostic procedure. CSF is collected during a lumbar puncture performed by the provider.

  □ Results indicative of meningitis

    ▸ Appearance of CSF – Cloudy (bacterial) or clear (viral)

    ▸ Elevated WBC

    ▸ Elevated protein

    ▸ Decreased glucose (bacterial)

    ▸ Elevated CSF pressure

  □ New enteroviral diagnostic test can be done on CSF to determine if infectious agent is viral or bacterial in 2.5 hr.

- CT scan and MRI

  □ A CT scan or an MRI may be performed to identify increased intracranial pressure (ICP) and/or an abscess.

Collaborative Care

- Nursing Care
  - Isolate clients as soon as meningitis is suspected.
  - Maintain isolation precautions (droplet precautions) per facility policy. This requires a private room or a room with cohorts, wearing of a surgical mask when within 3 ft of clients, appropriate hand hygiene, and use of designated equipment, such as a blood pressure cuff and thermometer. Continue until antibiotics have been administered for 24 hr.
  - Implement fever-reduction measures, such as a cooling blanket, if necessary.
  - Report meningococcal infections to the public health department.
  - Decrease environmental stimuli.
    - Provide a quiet environment.
    - Minimize exposure to bright light (natural and electric).
  - Maintain bed rest with the head of the bed elevated to 30°.
  - Maintain client safety, such as seizure precautions.
  - Monitor clients receiving IV fluids and electrolytes to maintain hydration.
  - Monitor older adult clients for secondary complications, such as pneumonia.
- Medications
  - Ceftriaxone (Rocephin) or cefotaxime (Claforan)
    - Give antibiotics until culture and sensitivity results are available, which are effective for bacterial infections.
  - Phenytoin (Dilantin)
    - Anticonvulsants are given if ICP increases or the client experiences a seizure.
  - Acetaminophen (Tylenol), ibuprofen (Motrin)
    - Analgesics are given for headache and/or fever – nonopioid to avoid masking changes in the level of consciousness
  - Ciprofloxacin (Cipro), rifampin (Rifadin)
    - Prophylactic antibiotics are given to individuals in close contact with clients.
- Care After Discharge
  - Client Education
    - Encourage adults who are immunocompromised, who have a chronic disease, who smoke cigarettes, or who live in a long-term care facility to receive the pneumococcal polysaccharide vaccine (PPSV).
    - Encourage residential college students, older adults, and those who have chronic illness to receive the meningococcal vaccine (MCV4) for *Neisseria meningitidis*.
    - Instruct clients to use an insect repellent when risk of being bitten by a mosquito exists.

- Client Outcomes

  o The client's ICP and neurological status will return to their premeningitis parameters.

  o The client's headache, photophobia, and nuchal rigidity will resolve.

Complications

- Increased ICP (possibly to the point of brain herniation)

  o Meningitis can cause ICP to increase.

  o Nursing Actions

    - Monitor for signs of increasing ICP (decreased level of consciousness, pupillary changes, and widening pulse pressure).

    - Provide interventions to reduce ICP (positioning and avoidance of coughing and straining).

- Syndrome of inappropriate antidiuretic hormone (SIADH)

  o SIADH can be a complication of meningitis.

  o Nursing Actions

    - Monitor for signs and symptoms (dilute blood, concentrated urine).

    - Provide interventions, such as the administration of demeclocycline (Declomycin) and restriction of fluid.

- Septic emboli (leading to disseminated intravascular coagulation or vascular compromise)

  o Septic emboli can form during meningitis and travel to other parts of the body, particularly the hands.

  o Development of gangrene will necessitate an amputation.

     View Media Supplement: Gangrenous Toe (Image)

  o Nursing Actions

    - Monitor circulatory status of extremities and coagulation studies.

    - Report any alterations immediately to the provider.

- Subjective and Objective Data
  - Generalized seizures – Loss of consciousness occurs with involvement of both cerebral hemispheres
    - Tonic-clonic seizure
      - It may begin with an aura (alteration in vision, smell, or emotional feeling).
      - Tonic phase – A 15- to 20-second episode of stiffening of muscles, loss of consciousness, cessation of breathing, dilated pupils and development of cyanosis.
      - Clonic phase – A 1- to 2-min episode of rhythmic jerking of the extremities, irregular respirations, biting of the cheek or tongue and bladder and bowel incontinence may occur.
      - Postictal phase – May last for several hours. Unconsciousness may last for 30 min at which time the client awakens slowly and is usually confused and disoriented. Reports of headache, fatigue, and muscle aches are not uncommon. Clients may have no memory of what happened just before the seizure.
    - Absence seizure
      - Absence seizures are most common in children.
      - The seizure consists of a loss of consciousness lasting a few seconds, accompanied by blank staring (appears to be daydreaming) and associated automatisms (behaviors that clients are unaware of, such as lip-smacking or picking at clothes).
      - Baseline neurological function is resumed after seizures, with no apparent sequela.
      - Clients are often unaware seizure is occurring.
  - Partial or focal/local seizure – Seizure activity begins in one cerebral hemisphere.
    - Complex partial seizure
      - Complex partial seizures have associated automatisms (behaviors that clients are unaware of, such as lip-smacking or picking at clothes).
      - The seizure can cause a loss of consciousness for several minutes.
      - Amnesia may occur immediately prior to and after the seizure.
    - Simple partial seizures
      - Consciousness is maintained throughout simple partial seizures.
      - Seizure activity may consist of unusual sensations, a sense of déjà vu, autonomic abnormalities, such as changes in heart rate and abnormal flushing, unilateral abnormal extremity movements, pain, or offensive smell.
  - Unclassified or idiopathic seizures do not fit into other categories. These types of seizures account for half of all seizures activities and occur for no known reason.

- o   Laboratory Tests
    - ■   Alcohol and illicit drug levels, HIV testing, and, if suspected, screen for the presence of toxins.
- o   Diagnostic Procedures
    - ■   Electroencephalogram (EEG)
        - □   An EEG records electrical activity and may identify the origin of seizure activity.
    - ■   Magnetic resonance imaging (MRI); computed tomography imaging (CT)/ computed axial tomography (CAT), and positron emission tomography (PET) scans; cerebrospinal fluid (CSF) analysis; and a skull x-ray can all be used to identify or rule out potential causes of seizures.

Collaborative Care

- ●   Nursing Care

    (M) **View Media Supplement:** Seizure Precautions (Video)

- o   During a seizure:
    - ■   Protect clients from injury.
        - □   Move furniture away.
        - □   Hold the client's head in lap if she is on the floor.
        - □   Position clients to provide a patent airway.
        - □   Turn clients to the side to decrease the risk of aspiration.
        - □   Be prepared to suction oral secretions.
        - □   Loosen restrictive clothing.
        - □   Do not attempt to restrain clients.
        - □   Do not attempt to open jaw or insert airway during seizure activity (may damage teeth, lips, and tongue). Do not use padded tongue blades.
    - ■   Document onset and duration of seizure and client findings/observations prior to, during, and following the seizure (level of consciousness, apnea, cyanosis, motor activity, incontinence).
- o   Post seizure:
    - ■   Maintain clients in a side-lying position to prevent aspiration and to facilitate drainage of oral secretions.
    - ■   Check vital signs.
    - ■   Check for injuries.
    - ■   Perform neurological checks.

- Allow clients to rest if necessary.

- Reorient and calm clients (may be agitated or confused).

- Institute seizure precautions including placing the bed in the lowest position and padding the side rails to prevent future injury.

- Determine if the client experienced an aura, which can possibly indicate the origin of seizure in the brain.

- Try to determine possible trigger.

- Medications

  - Antiepileptic drugs (AEDs) – diazepam (Valium), phenytoin (Dilantin), carbamazepine (Tegretol), valproic acid (Depakene), gabapentin (Neurontin), and fosphenytoin sodium (Cerebyx)

    - Nursing Considerations

      - Monitor therapeutic plasma levels. Be aware of therapeutic levels for medications prescribed. Notify the provider of results.

    - Client Education

      - Advise clients that treatment provides for control of seizures, not cure of the disorder.

      - Encourage clients to keep a seizure frequency diary to monitor the effectiveness of therapy.

      - Advise clients to take medications as prescribed, usually the same time every day. If a dose is forgotten, tell them to take the next scheduled dose. Extra doses should not be taken.

      - Advise clients to not stop taking medications without consulting the provider. Sudden cessation of medication may result in seizures.

      - Advise clients to avoid hazardous activities (driving, operating heavy machinery) until seizures are fully controlled.

      - Instruct clients not to take any unprescribed medications and to be aware of drug-drug and drug-food interactions (decreased effectiveness of oral contraceptives).

      - Advise clients of childbearing age to avoid pregnancy, as medications may cause birth defects and congenital abnormalities.

- Interdisciplinary Care

  - Request referrals for social service agencies to assist with school support as well as financial and employment issues.

- Surgical Interventions

  - Surgical interventions include placement of a vagal nerve stimulator and excision of the portion of the brain causing the seizures for intractable seizures.

- o Vagal nerve stimulator

  - This procedure is indicated for clients with simple or complex partial seizures. It is contraindicated for clients with generalized seizures.

  - This procedure is performed under general anesthesia.

  - The device is implanted into the left chest wall and connected to an electrode placed at the left vagus nerve. The device is then programmed to administer intermittent vagal nerve stimulation at a rate specific to the client's needs.

  - In addition to routine stimulation, clients may initiate vagal nerve stimulation by holding a magnet over the implantable device at the onset of seizure activity. This either aborts the seizure or lessens its severity.

- Care after Discharge

  - o Educate clients about the importance of periodic laboratory testing to monitor AED levels.

  - o Encourage medication adherence.

  - o Encourage clients to wear a medical alert bracelet or necklace at all times.

  - o Refer clients to the state's Department of Motor Vehicles to determine laws regarding driving for clients with seizure disorders.

- Client Outcomes

  - o The client will experience a decreased incidence of seizures.

  - o The client will be compliant with the medication regimen.

Complications

- Status epilepticus

  - o This is prolonged seizure activity occurring over a 30-min time frame. The complications associated with this condition are related to decreased oxygen levels, inability of the brain to return to normal functioning, and continued assault on neuronal tissue. This acute condition requires immediate treatment to prevent loss of brain function, which may become permanent.

  - o Nursing Actions

    - Call for assistance.

    - Maintain an airway, provide oxygen, and monitor pulse oximetry.

    - Assist with emergency care as appropriate.

  - o Client Education

    - Provide support for the family.

3. A nurse is reinforcing teaching to a client who has questions about taking phenytoin (Dilantin) for seizures. The client asks what he should do if he forgets to take a dose. Which of the following is the appropriate information to provide?

    A. "Take the missed dose as soon as possible and skip the next scheduled dose."

    B. "Take a double dose of the medication at the next scheduled time."

    C. "Wait until the next scheduled time and take the regular dose."

    D. "Take the skipped dose as soon as possible and another dose at the next scheduled time."

The client should not take an extra dose or miss any remaining doses for the day. It is important that anticonvulsant medication be taken on a regular basis to maintain a consistent blood level. Taking a double dose increases the risk of toxicity. The client should wait and take the next regularly scheduled dose if it is within 4 hr of the next dose.

NCLEX® Connection: Pharmacological Therapies, Expected Actions/Outcomes

4. A nurse is reinforcing client education regarding an EEG, which is scheduled for the next day. Which of the following instructions is appropriate to provide?

    A. Get a good night's sleep prior to the test.

    B. Do not drink caffeinated coffee the morning of the procedure.

    C. Do not wash hair prior to the procedure.

    D. Do not consume food the morning of the procedure.

Products containing caffeine should be avoided 6 to 9 hr prior to the EEG, but decaffeinated products and food may be consumed. Hair should be washed prior to the procedure and the client should not sleep the night prior if possible.

NCLEX® Connection: Reduction of Risk Potential, System-Specific Assessment

UNIT 2	NURSING CARE OF CLIENTS WITH NEUROSENSORY DISORDERS
Section:	Central and Peripheral Nervous System Disorders
Chapter 8	Parkinson's Disease

Overview

- Parkinson's disease (PD) is a progressively debilitating disease that grossly affects motor function. It is characterized by four primary symptoms – tremor, muscle rigidity, bradykinesia (slow movement), and postural instability. These symptoms occur due to overstimulation of the basal ganglia by acetylcholine.

- The secretion of dopamine and acetylcholine in the body produce inhibitory and excitatory effects on the muscles respectively.

- Overstimulation of the basal ganglia by acetylcholine occurs because degeneration of the substantia nigra results in decreased dopamine production. This allows acetylcholine to dominate, making smooth, controlled movements difficult.

- Treatment of PD focuses on increasing the amount of dopamine or decreasing the amount of acetylcholine in a client's brain.

- As PD is a progressive disease, there are 5 stages of involvement.

  o Stage 1 – Unilateral shaking or tremor of one limb.

  o Stage 2 – Bilateral limb involvement makes walking and balance difficult.

  o Stage 3 – Physical movements slow down significantly, affecting walking more.

  o Stage 4 – Tremors may decrease but akinesia and rigidity make day-to-day tasks difficult.

  o Stage 5 – Client is unable to stand or walk, is dependent for all care, and may exhibit dementia.

Data Collection

- Risk Factors

  o Onset of symptoms between age 40 to 70

  o More common in men

  o Genetic predisposition

  o Exposure to environmental toxins

- Subjective Data

  o Report of fatigue

  o Report of decreased manual dexterity over time

- Objective Data

 View Media Supplement: Clinical Manifestations of Parkinson's Disease (Video)

  o Physical Assessment Findings

  - Stooped posture

  - Slow, shuffling, and propulsive gait

  - Slow, monotonous speech

  - Tremors/pill-rolling tremor of the fingers

  - Muscle rigidity

  - Bradykinesia/akinesia

  - Mask-like expression

  - Autonomic symptoms (orthostatic hypotension, flushing, diaphoresis)

  - Difficulty chewing and swallowing

  - Drooling

  - Dysarthria

  - Progressive difficulty with ADLs

  - Mood swings

  - Cognitive impairment (dementia)

  o Laboratory Tests

  - There are no definitive diagnostic procedures.

  - Diagnosis is made based on symptoms, their progression, and by ruling out other diseases.

Collaborative Care

- Nursing Care

  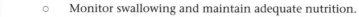

  o Administer the client's medications at prescribed times.

  o Monitor swallowing and maintain adequate nutrition.

  - Request a referral for a speech-language pathologist to assess swallowing if clients demonstrate a risk for choking.

- Consult the client's dietician for appropriate diet.
- Document the client's weight at least weekly.
- Keep a diet intake log.
- Encourage fluids and document intake.
- Provide smaller, more frequent meals.
- Add commercial thickener to thicken food.
- Provide supplements as prescribed.
  - Maintain client mobility for as long as possible.
    - Encourage exercise, such as yoga (may improve mental status as well).
    - Encourage the use of assistive devices as the disease progresses.
    - Encourage range-of-motion (ROM) exercises.
    - Reinforce to clients to stop occasionally when walking to slow down speed and reduce the risk for injury.
    - Pace activities by providing rest periods.
    - Assist clients with ADLs as needed (hygiene, dressing).
  - Promote client communication for as long as possible.
    - Instruct clients to use facial muscle strengthening exercises.
    - Encourage clients to speak slowly and to pause frequently.
    - Use alternate forms of communication as appropriate.
    - Request a referral for a speech-language pathologist.
  - Monitor a client's mental and cognitive status.
    - Observe for signs of depression and dementia.
    - Provide a safe environment (no throw rugs, encourage the use of an electric razor).
    - Determine personal and family coping with the client's chronic, degenerative disease.
    - Provide a list of community resources (support groups) to the client and the client's family.
    - Request a referral for a social worker or case manager as the condition advances (financial issues, long-term home care, and respite care).
- Medications
  - May take several weeks of use before improvement of symptoms is seen.
  - While the client is taking a combination of medications, maintenance of therapeutic medication levels is necessary for adequate control.

- o Dopaminergics
  - When given orally, medications, such as levodopa (Dopar), are converted to dopamine in the brain, increasing dopamine levels in the basal ganglia.
  - Dopaminergics may be combined with carbidopa (Sinemet) to decrease peripheral metabolism of levodopa, requiring a smaller dose to make the same amount available to the brain. Side effects are subsequently less.
  - Due to medication tolerance and metabolism, the client's dosage and administration times must be adjusted to avoid periods of poor mobility.
  - Nursing Considerations
    - □ Monitor for the "wearing-off" phenomenon and dyskinesias (problems with movement), which can indicate the need to adjust the dosage or time of administration or the need for a medication holiday.

- o Dopamine agonists
  - Dopamine agonists, such as bromocriptine (Parlodel) and pramipexole (Mirapex), activate the release of dopamine. May be used in conjunction with a dopaminergic for better results.
  - Nursing Considerations
    - □ Monitor for orthostatic hypotension, dyskinesias, and hallucinations.

- o Anticholinergics
  - Anticholinergics, such as benztropine (Cogentin) and trihexyphenidyl (Artane), help control tremors and rigidity.
  - Nursing Considerations
    - □ Monitor for anticholinergic effects (dry mouth, constipation, urinary retention).

- o Catechol O-methyltransferase (COMT) inhibitors
  - COMT inhibitors, such as entacapone (Comtan), decrease the breakdown of levodopa, making it more available to the brain as dopamine. It can be used in conjunction with a dopaminergic and dopamine agonist for better results.
  - Nursing Considerations
    - □ Monitor for dyskinesia/hyperkinesia when used with levodopa.
    - □ Check for diarrhea.
    - □ Reassure clients that dark urine is an expected finding.

- o Antivirals
  - Antivirals, such as amantadine (Symmetrel), stimulate the release of dopamine and prevent its reuptake.

- Nursing Considerations
  - Monitor for swollen ankles and discoloration of the skin.
- Interdisciplinary Care
  - During the later stages of the disorder, clients will need referrals to and support from such disciplines as speech, occupational, and physical therapists; social services; and finally, placement in a long-term care facility.
- Surgical Interventions
  - Stereotactic pallidotomy
    - Stereotactic pallidotomy is the destruction of a small portion of the brain within the globus pallidus through the use of brain imaging and electrical stimulation.
    - The target area is identified with a CT scan or an MRI.
    - Mild electrical stimulation is provided through a burr hole to a target area.
    - Client is assessed for a decrease in tremors and muscle rigidity.
    - When a decrease is elicited, a temporary lesion is formed and the client is reassessed.
    - If symptomatic relief is demonstrated, a permanent lesion is made.
  - Deep brain stimulation
    - An electrode is implanted in the thalamus.
    - A current is delivered through an implanted pacemaker generator.
    - The goal of the current is to interfere with electrical conduction in "tremor cells" decreasing tremors.
- Client Outcomes
  - The client will ambulate safely through the use of assistive devices.
  - The client will maintain adequate hydration and nutrition via appropriate diet and thickened liquids.

Complications

- Aspiration pneumonia
  - As PD advances in severity, alterations in chewing and swallowing will worsen, increasing the risk for aspiration.
  - Nursing Actions
    - Use swallowing precautions to decrease the risk for aspiration.
    - Follow the individual dietary plan based on the speech-language pathologist's recommendations.

- Have a nurse in attendance when the client is eating.

- Encourage clients to eat slowly and chew thoroughly before swallowing.

- Feed clients in an upright position and have suction equipment on standby.

- Altered cognition (dementia, memory deficits)

  - Clients in advanced stages of PD may exhibit altered cognition in the form of dementia and memory loss.

  - Nursing Actions

    - Acknowledge the client's feelings.

    - Provide for a safe environment.

(A) APPLICATION EXERCISES

Scenario: An older adult client was diagnosed with Parkinson's disease (PD) 1 year ago. He is currently living independently with his wife of 50 years and takes levodopa with carbidopa (Sinemet) to control his disease. Due to a recent episode of aspiration pneumonia, the client has been admitted to the hospital for IV antibiotic and respiratory therapies.

1. Which of the following findings should the nurse expect to find when collecting data? (Select all that apply.)

   _____ Decreased vision

   _____ Pill-rolling tremor of the fingers

   _____ Shuffling gait

   _____ High pitched, squeaky voice

   _____ Lack of facial expressions

   _____ Frequent periods of sleep

2. Which of the following questions should the nurse ask to determine if the medication is being given in appropriate dosages and at the appropriate times?

   A. "Is your weight staying the same?"

   B. "Can you see the television from a comfortable distance?"

   C. "Are you having periods when walking is more difficult?"

   D. "Are you experiencing any night sweats?"

3. The client has been prescribed bromocriptine (Parlodel) to obtain better management of the muscular rigidity. Which of the following instructions should the nurse give the client to manage a common side effect of bromocriptine?

   A. Rise slowly when standing up.

   B. Increase dietary fiber and fluid intake.

   C. Chew sugarless gum for dry mouth.

   D. Wear sunscreen when outdoors.

4. Which of the following is the priority intervention the nurse should recommend for inclusion on the client's plan of care?

   A. Assist the client to the restroom.

   B. Have assistive personnel assist the client with dressing.

   C. Have suction equipment at the bedside.

   D. Observe IV catheter insertion site for inflammation every 12 hr.

UNIT 2	NURSING CARE OF CLIENTS WITH NEUROSENSORY DISORDERS
Section:	Central and Peripheral Nervous System Disorders
Chapter 9	Alzheimer's Disease

Overview

- Alzheimer's disease (AD) is a nonreversible type of dementia (multiple cognitive deficits that impair memory and can affect language, motor skills, and/or abstract thinking) that progressively develops through seven stages over many years. A framework made up of seven stages has been designed to categorize the disease and its signs and symptoms. The framework is based on three general stages – Early stage, mid stage, and late stage.

- Some people die 4 to 6 years after diagnosis, but others can live with the disease for up to 20 years.

- Severe physical decline occurs along with deteriorating cognitive functions.

Data Collection

- Risk Factors

  - Advanced age

  - Genetic predisposition

  - Environmental agents (herpes virus, metal, or toxic waste)

  - Previous head injury

  - Apolipoprotein E.

- Subjective and Objective Data

STAGE	SIGNS AND SYMPTOMS
Stage 1: No impairment (Normal function)	• No memory problems
Stage 2: Very mild cognitive decline (May be normal age-related changes or very early signs of AD)	• Forgetfulness, especially of everyday objects (eyeglasses or wallet) • No memory problems evident to provider, friends, or coworkers

STAGE	SIGNS AND SYMPTOMS
Stage 3: Mild cognitive decline (Problems with memory or concentration may be measurable in clinical testing or during a detailed medical interview)	• Mild cognitive deficits, including losing or misplacing important objects • Decreased ability to plan • Short-term memory loss noticeable to close relatives • Decreased attention span • Difficulty remembering words or names • Difficulty in social or work situations
Stage 4: Moderate cognitive decline (Mild or early-stage AD; medical interview will detect clear-cut deficiencies)	• Personality changes – Appearing withdrawn or subdued, especially in social or mentally challenging situations • Obvious memory loss • Limited knowledge and memory of recent occasions, current events, or personal history • Difficulty performing tasks that require planning and organizing (paying bills or managing money) • Difficulty with complex mental arithmetic
Stage 5: Moderately severe cognitive decline (Moderate or mid-stage AD)	• Increasing cognitive deficits emerge • Inability to recall important details such as address, telephone number, or schools attended, but memory of information about self and family remains intact • Disorientation and confusion as to time and place
Stage 6: Severe cognitive decline (Moderately severe or mid-stage AD)	• Memory difficulties continue to worsen • Loss of awareness of recent events and surroundings • May recall own name, but unable to recall personal history • Significant personality changes are evident (delusions, hallucinations, and compulsive behaviors) • Wandering behavior • Requires assistance with usual daily activities such as dressing, toileting, and other grooming • Normal sleep/wake cycle is disrupted • Increased episodes of urinary and fecal incontinence
Stage 7: Very severe cognitive decline (Severe or late-stage AD)	• Ability to respond to environment, speak, and control movement is lost • Unrecognizable speech • General urinary incontinence • Inability to eat without assistance and impaired swallowing • Gradual loss of all ability to move extremities (ataxia)

- ○ Laboratory Tests
  - ■ Genetic testing for the presence of apolipoprotein E. can determine if late onset dementia is due to AD.
- ○ Diagnostic Procedures
  - ■ There is no definitive diagnostic procedure, except brain tissue examination upon death.
  - ■ Magnetic resonance imaging (MRI); computed tomography (CT) imaging/computed axial tomography (CAT), positron emission tomography (PET) scans; and electroencephalogram (EEG) may be performed to rule out other possible causes of symptoms.

Collaborative Care

- • Nursing Care
  - ○ Check cognitive status, memory, judgment, and personality changes.
  - ○ Initiate bowel and bladder program with clients based on a set schedule.
  - ○ Encourage clients and their families to participate in an AD support group.
  - ○ Provide a safe environment.
  - ○ Keep clients on a sleeping schedule and monitor for irregular sleeping patterns.
  - ○ Provide verbal and nonverbal ways to communicate with clients.
  - ○ Offer snacks or finger foods if clients are unable to sit for long periods of time.
  - ○ Check the client's skin weekly for breakdown.
  - ○ Provide cognitive stimulation.
    - ■ Offer varied environmental stimulations such as walks, music, or craft activities.
    - ■ Keep a structured environment and introduce change gradually (client's daily routine or a room change).
    - ■ Use a calendar to assist with orientation.
    - ■ Use short directions when explaining an activity or care clients need, such as a bath.
    - ■ Be consistent and repetitive.
    - ■ Use therapeutic touch.
  - ○ Provide memory training.
    - ■ Reminisce with clients about the past.
    - ■ Use memory techniques such as making lists and rehearsing.
    - ■ Stimulate the client's memory by repeating the client's last statement.
  - ○ Avoid overstimulation (keep noise and clutter to a minimum and avoid crowds).

- o Promote consistency by placing commonly used objects in the same location and using a routine schedule.
    - Reality orientation (early stages)
    - Easily viewed clock and single-day calendar
    - Pictures of family and pets
    - Frequent reorientation to time, place, and person
- o Validation therapy (later stages)
    - Acknowledge the client's feelings.
    - Don't argue with clients; this will lead to clients becoming upset.
    - Reinforce and use repetitive actions or ideas cautiously.
- o Promote self-care as long as possible. Assist clients with activities of daily living as appropriate.
- o Speak directly to clients in short, concise sentences.
- o Reduce agitation (use calm, redirecting statements; provide a diversion).
- o Provide a routine toileting schedule.

- Medications
    - o Most medications for clients who have dementia attempt to target behavioral and emotional problems, such as anxiety, agitation, combativeness, and depression and include antipsychotics, anxiolytics and antidepressants. Clients receiving these medications should be closely monitored for adverse effects.
    - o AD medications temporarily slow the course of the disease and do not work for all clients.
    - o Benefits for those clients who do respond to medication include improvements in cognition, behavior, and function.
    - o Donepezil (Aricept)
        - Prevents the breakdown of acetylcholine (ACh), which increases the amount of ACh available. This results in increased nerve impulses at the nerve sites.
        - Cholinesterase inhibitors help slow this process down.
        - Nursing Considerations
            - □ Observe clients for frequent stools and or upset stomach.
            - □ Monitor clients for dizziness and or headache. Clients may feel lightheaded or have an unsteady gait.
            - □ Use caution when administering this medication to clients who have asthma or COPD.

- Interdisciplinary Care

  - Request a referral for social services and case managers for possible adult day care or long-term care facilities.

  - Request a referral for clients to the Alzheimer's Association and community outreach programs. This can include in-home or respite care.

- Therapeutic Procedures

  - Alternative therapy

    - Ginkgo biloba, an herbal product taken to increase memory and blood circulation, can cause a variety of side effects and medication interactions. If a client is using ginkgo biloba or other nutritional supplements, that information should be shared with providers.

- Care after Discharge

  - Client Education

    - Reinforce to families/caregivers about illness, methods of care, and adaptation of the home environment.

    - Instruct families in home safety measures:
      - Remove scatter rugs.
      - Install door locks that cannot be easily opened, and place alarms on doors.
      - Keep a lock on the water heater and thermostat; keeping the water temperature turned down to a safe level.
      - Provide good lighting, especially on stairs.
      - Install handrails on stairs and marking step edges with colored tape.
      - Place the mattress on the floor.
      - Remove clutter and clearing hallways for walking.
      - Secure electrical cords to baseboards.
      - Keep cleaning supplies in locked cupboards.
      - Install handrails in the bathroom, at bedside, and in the tub; placing a shower chair in the tub.
      - Have clients wear a medical identification bracelet if living at home with caregiver.
      - Monitor for improvement in memory and the client's quality of life.

    - Support for caregivers
      - Review the resources available to the family as the client's health declines. Include long-term care options. A wide variety of home care and community resources, such as respite care, may be available to the family in many areas of the country, and these resources may allow clients to remain at home rather than in an institution.

- Client Outcomes

  S

  o   The client will remain free from injury.

  o   The client will sleep 5 to 6 hr every night.

  o   The client will be able to perform self-care independently with verbal assistance.

UNIT 2	NURSING CARE OF CLIENTS WITH NEUROSENSORY DISORDERS
Section:	Central and Peripheral Nervous System Disorders
Chapter 10	Cerebrovascular Accident

Overview

- Cerebrovascular accidents (CVAs) or strokes involve a disruption in the cerebral blood flow secondary to ischemia, hemorrhage, or embolism.

- There are three types of CVAs:

  - Hemorrhagic – These occur secondary to a ruptured artery or aneurysm.

  - Thrombotic – These occur secondary to the development of a blood clot on an atherosclerotic plaque in a cerebral artery that gradually shuts off the artery and causes ischemia distal to the occlusion. Symptoms of a thrombotic CVA evolve over a period of several hours to days.

  - Embolic – These occur secondary to an embolus traveling from another part of the body to a cerebral artery. Blood to the brain distal to the occlusion is immediately shut off causing neurologic deficits or a loss of consciousness to instantly occur.

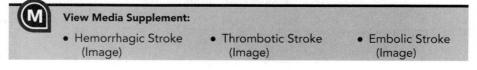

View Media Supplement:
- Hemorrhagic Stroke (Image)
- Thrombotic Stroke (Image)
- Embolic Stroke (Image)

Data Collection

- Risk Factors

  - Cerebral aneurysm

  - Arteriovenous malformation (AV)

  - Diabetes mellitus

  - Obesity

  - Hypertension

  - Atherosclerosis

  - Hyperlipidemia

  - Hypercoagulability

  - Atrial fibrillation

- o Use of oral contraceptives

- o Smoking

- o Cocaine use

- Subjective Data

  - o Some clients report transient symptoms such as dizziness, slurred speech, and a weak extremity.

  - o These symptoms may indicate a transient ischemic attack (TIA), which can be a warning of an impending CVA.

- Objective Data

  - o Physical Assessment Findings

    - ■ Symptoms will vary based on the area of the brain that is deprived of oxygenated blood.

      - □ The left cerebral hemisphere is responsible for language, mathematic skills, and analytic thinking.

      - □ Symptoms consistent with a left-hemispheric CVA

        - ‣ Expressive and receptive aphasia (ability to speak and understand language respectively)

        - ‣ Agnosia (unable to recognize familiar objects)

        - ‣ Alexia (reading difficulty)

        - ‣ Agraphia (writing difficulty)

        - ‣ Right extremity hemiplegia (paralysis) or hemiparesis (weakness)

        - ‣ Slow, cautious behavior

        - ‣ Depression, anger, and quick to become frustrated

        - ‣ Visual changes, such as hemianopsia (loss of visual field in one or both eyes)

        - ‣ One-sided neglect syndrome (ignore right side of the body – cannot see, feel or move affected side; so, client is unaware of its existence)

 View Media Supplement: Hemianopsia (Image)

      - □ The right cerebral hemisphere is responsible for visual and spatial awareness and proprioception.

        - ‣ Altered perception of deficits (overestimation of abilities)

        - ‣ One-sided neglect syndrome (ignore left side of the body – cannot see, feel, or move affected side; so, client is unaware of its existence) – more common with right-hemispheric CVAs

        - ‣ Loss of depth perception

- ▸ Poor impulse control and impaired judgment
- ▸ Short attention span
- ▸ Left hemiplegia or hemiparesis
- ▸ Visual changes, such as hemianopsia

- ○ Diagnostic Procedures

  - ■ A magnetic resonance imaging (MRI), computed tomography (CT) imaging, and/or a computed axial tomography (CAT) scan may be used to identify edema, ischemia, and necrosis.

  - ■ A magnetic resonance angiography (MRA) or a cerebral angiography are used to identify the presence of a cerebral hemorrhage, abnormal vessel structures (AV malformation, aneurysms), vessel ruptures, and regional perfusion of blood flow in the carotid arteries and brain.

  - ■ A lumbar puncture is used to assess for the presence of blood in the cerebrospinal fluid (CSF). A positive finding is consistent with a cerebral hemorrhage or ruptured aneurysm.

  - ■ The Glasgow Coma Scale score is used when clients have a decreased level of consciousness or orientation.

Collaborative Care

- Nursing Care

  - ○ Monitor for changes in the client's level of consciousness (increased ICP sign).

  - ○ Elevate the client's head of the bed approximately 30° to reduce ICP and to promote venous drainage. Avoid extreme flexion or extension of the neck, and maintain the client's head in the midline neutral position.

  - ○ Initiate seizure precautions.

  - ○ Assist with the client's communication skills if his speech is impaired.

    - ■ Identify the ability to understand speech by asking clients to follow simple commands.

    - ■ Observe for consistently affirmative answers when the client actually does not comprehend what is being said.

    - ■ Determine accuracy of yes/no responses in relation to closed-ended questions.

    - ■ Supply clients with a picture board of commonly requested items/needs.

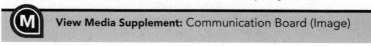

View Media Supplement: Communication Board (Image)

Ⓢ   ○   Assist with safe feeding.

- Check swallowing and gag reflexes before feeding. Follow recommendations of speech pathologist.

- Thicken clear liquids with a commercial thickener to avoid aspiration if a swallowing deficit is identified.

- Have clients eat in an upright position and swallow with the head and neck flexed slightly forward.

- Place food in the back of the mouth on the unaffected side.

- Have suction on standby.

- Maintain a distraction-free environment during meals.

○   Maintain skin integrity.

- Reposition clients frequently and use padding.

- Monitor bony prominences, paying particular attention to the affected extremities.

- If clients have one-sided neglect, teach them to protect and care for the affected extremity to avoid injuring it in the wheel of the wheelchair or hitting/smashing it against a doorway.

○   Encourage passive range of motion every 2 hr to the affected extremities and active range of motion every 2 hr to the unaffected extremities. Show clients how to use the unaffected side to exercise the affected side of the body.

○   Elevate the affected extremities to promote venous return and to reduce swelling. An elastic glove can be placed on the affected hand if swelling is severe. Show clients how to massage the affected hand by stroking it in a distal to proximal manner encouraging fluid in the hand to move back into the wrist and arm.

Ⓢ   ○   Maintain a safe environment to reduce the risk of falls. Use assistive devices during transfers such as transfer belts, sliding boards, and sit-to-stand lifts.

○   If clients have homonymous hemianopsia (loss of the same half of the visual field in both eyes) instruct them to use a scanning technique (turning head from the direction of the unaffected side to the affected side) when eating and ambulating.

○   Apply sequential compression stockings, implement frequent position changes, and encourage mobilization to prevent deep vein thrombosis and complications from immobility.

○   Provide assistance with ADLs as needed. Instruct clients to dress the affected side first and sit in a supportive chair that aids in balance. Have occupational therapy assess clients for adaptive aids, such as a plate guard, utensils with built-up handles, a reaching tool to pick things up, and shirts and shoes that have hook and loop fasteners/tape instead of buttons and ties.

○   Provide for frequent rest periods from sitting in the wheelchair by returning clients to bed after therapies and meals.

- o Support the affected arm while in bed, the wheelchair, or during ambulation with an arm sling or strategically placed pillows.

- o Support clients during periods of emotional lability and depression.

- Medications

  - o Anticoagulants (aspirin, heparin sodium, enoxaparin [Lovenox], warfarin [Coumadin])

    - These medications are usually given to clients who have experienced an embolic CVA to prevent development of additional emboli.

  - o Antiplatelets (ticlopidine [Ticlid], clopidogrel [Plavix])

    - These medications are usually given to clients who have experienced a thrombotic CVA to prevent extension of the CVA.

  - o Thrombolytic medications alteplase (Activase, tPA)

    - Can be given within 3 to 6 hr of onset of symptoms to dissolve embolism.

  - o Antiepileptic medications (phenytoin [Dilantin], gabapentin [Neurontin])

    - These medications are not commonly given following a CVA unless clients develop seizures.

    - Gabapentin can be given for paresthetic pain in an affected extremity.

- Interdisciplinary Care

  - o Recognize the need for speech and language therapists for language and swallowing evaluations.

  - o Request a referral for physical therapy for assistance with re-establishment of ambulation with or without assistive devices (single or quad cane, walker) or wheelchair support.

  - o Request a referral for occupational therapy for assistance with re-establishment of partial or full function of the affected hand and arm. If function does not return to the extremity, measures such as massage and elastic gloves will be prescribed by occupational therapy to prevent swelling of the extremity.

  - o Request a referral for social services to make arrangements for rehabilitation services and temporary placement on a skilled rehabilitation unit or extended-care facility during provision of these services. Prior to discharge, the social worker may make a home visit with selected therapists and nurses to evaluate the need for environmental alterations in the home and adaptive equipment needed for ADLs.

- Therapeutic Procedures

  - o Systemic or catheter-directed thrombolytic therapy restores cerebral blood flow. It must be administered within 3 hr of the onset of symptoms. It is contraindicated for treatment of a hemorrhagic CVA and for clients with an increased risk of bleeding due to anticoagulant therapy or another bleeding anomaly. Possibility of a hemorrhagic CVA is ruled out with an MRI prior to the initiation of thrombolytic therapy.

- Surgical Interventions

  - Carotid endarterectomy is performed to open the artery by removing atherosclerotic plaque. This procedure is performed when the carotid artery is blocked or when clients are experiencing TIAs.

- Care After Discharge

  - Client Education

    - Encourage clients to receive early treatment of hypertension and to adhere to the prescribed regimen.

    - Encourage clients who have diabetes mellitus to maintain blood glucose within expected range.

    - Recommend smoking cessation.

    - Recommend that clients maintain a healthy weight and participate in regular exercise.

- Client Outcomes

  - The client's transient neurological deficits will cease and he will not experience a CVA.

  - The client will use adaptive devices to compensate for neurological deficits.

Complications

- Dysphagia and aspiration

  - Dysphagia can result from neurological involvement of the cranial nerves that innervate the face, tongue, soft palate, and throat. As a result, the client's risk of aspiration is great.

  - Nursing Actions

    - Start clients on a prescribed diet and observe closely for choking. Have the suction equipment available. Initial feedings should be done by an RN.

    - Thicken oral liquids as prescribed. Use the appropriate amount of thickener to obtain the prescribed consistency.

  - Client Education

    - Reinforce to the client's family how to thicken liquids to the proper consistency.

    - Instruct clients to flex their head forward when swallowing to decrease the risk of choking.

- Unilateral neglect

  - Unilateral neglect is the loss of awareness of the side affected by the CVA. Clients cannot see, feel, or move the affected side of the body; therefore, they forget that it exists.

  - This lack of awareness poses a great risk for injury to the neglected extremities and creates a self-care deficit.

UNIT 2	NURSING CARE OF CLIENTS WITH NEUROSENSORY DISORDERS
Section:	Central and Peripheral Nervous System Disorders
Chapter 11	Spinal Cord Injuries

 Overview

- Spinal cord injuries (SCIs) involve the loss of motor function, sensory function, reflexes, and control of elimination. Injuries in the cervical region result in quadriplegia – paralysis/paresis of all four extremities and trunk. Injuries below T1 result in paraplegia – paralysis/paresis of the lower extremities. Truncal instability also results if the lesion is in the upper thoracic region.

 View Media Supplement: Spinal Cord (Image)

- Not all fractures of the vertebrae cause SCIs. Direct injury to the spinal cord secondary to the trauma or bone fragments in the spinal canal must occur for the spinal cord itself to become damaged.

- SCIs range from contusions or incomplete lesions of the spinal cord to complete lesions caused by a lesion that extends across the entire diameter of the cord, or an actual transection of the cord. Complete lesions result in the loss of all voluntary movement and sensation below the level of the injury. Incomplete lesions result in varying losses of voluntary movement, and sensation below the level of injury.

Health Promotion and Disease Prevention

- Client Education

  ○ Promote safe driving practices.

  ○ Promote swimming and diving safety.

Data Collection

- Risk Factors

  ○ Males age 16 to 30

  ○ High-risk activities (extreme sports or high-speed driving)

  ○ Active in impact sports (football or diving)

  ○ Acts of violence (gunshot and knife wounds)

○ Alcohol and/or drug abuse

○ Disease (metastatic cancer or arthritis of the spine)

○ Falls, especially in older adults

- Subjective Data

  ○ Report of lack of sensation of dermatomes below the level of the lesion

  ○ Report of neck or back pain

- Objective Data

  ○ Physical Assessment Findings

    - Inability to feel light touch when touched by a cotton ball, inability to discriminate between sharp and dull when touched with a safety pin or other sharp objects, and an inability to discriminate between hot and cold when touched with containers of hot and cold water.

    - Absent deep-tendon reflexes

    - Involuntary respirations can be affected due to a lesion at or above the phrenic nerve, or swelling from a lesion immediately below C4.

    - Impaired voluntary movement of muscles used in respiration (increase in depth or rate) may occur due to lesions in the cervical or upper thoracic area.

    - Spinal shock, which accompanies spinal trauma, causes a total loss of all reflexive and autonomic function below the level of the injury for a period of several days to weeks. Hypotension (that is more severe when clients are sitting in an upright position), dependent edema, and loss of temperature regulation (hyperthermia or hypothermia) are common findings.

    - Clients who have upper motor neuron injuries (above L1 and L2) will convert to a spastic muscle tone after spinal shock.

    - Paraplegics who have lower motor neuron injuries (below L1 and L2) will convert to a flaccid type of paralysis.

    - Varying degrees of loss of sensation and motor function will be experienced depending on whether the lesion is complete or incomplete.

    - Bowel and bladder

      □ Clients who have upper motor neuron injuries will develop a spastic bladder after the spinal shock resolves.

      □ Clients who have lower motor neuron injuries will develop a flaccid bladder.

    - Quadriplegics and other clients who have upper motor neuron lesions are usually capable of reflexogenic erections (erections secondary to manual manipulation). Ejaculation coordinated with emission may or may not occur. Clients who have lower motor neuron injuries are less able to have reflexogenic erections, but clients who have incomplete injuries may be able to have a combination of reflexogenic and psychogenic erections (erections stimulated by sexual thoughts and images).

- ○ Laboratory Tests
  - ■ Urinalysis, hemoglobin, ABGs
    - □ Used to monitor for undiagnosed internal bleeding (clients may not feel pain from internal injuries) and impaired respiratory exchange (due to phrenic nerve involvement and/or inability to voluntarily increase depth and rate of respirations).
- ○ Diagnostic Procedures
  - ■ X-rays, magnetic resonance imaging (MRI), and computed tomography (CT) imaging/computed axial tomography (CAT) scan can be used to assess the extent of the damage and the location of blood and bone fragments.

Collaborative Care

- • Nursing Care
  - ○ Maintain respiratory function
    - ■ Monitor the client's respiratory status.
    - ■ Provide the client with humidified oxygen and suction as needed.
    - ■ Assist with intubation and mechanical ventilation if necessary.
    - ■ Assist the client to cough by applying abdominal thrusts when the client is attempting to cough.
  - ○ Maintain tissue perfusion
    - ■ Transfer the client to a wheelchair in stages.
    - ■ Raise the client's head of the bed and be ready to lower the angle if the client reports dizziness.
    - ■ Transfer the client into a reclining wheelchair with the back of the wheelchair reclined.
    - ■ Be ready to lock and lean the wheelchair back to a fully reclined position if the client reports dizziness after the transfer. Do not attempt to return the client to bed.
    - ■ Monitor the client for signs of thrombophlebitis (swelling of extremity, absent/decreased pulses, and areas of warmth and/or tenderness). The client may be on anticoagulants to prevent development of lower extremity thrombi.
  - ○ Maintain NPO status several days if prescribed.
  - ○ Assist with the care of clients receiving IV fluids.
  - ○ Monitor clients for changes in neurological function.
  - ○ Monitor clients for changes in muscle strength in the affected extremities.
    - ■ Encourage active range of motion (ROM) exercises when possible, and assist with passive ROM if clients lack all motor function.

- Use measures to prevent skin breakdown. Use foam and air mattresses for beds and wheelchairs.
- Bladder and bowel function
  - Spastic neurogenic bladder – Bladder management options for male clients include condom catheters and stimulation of the micturition reflex by tugging on the pubic hair. Female clients will need to use an indwelling urinary catheter due to the unpredictability of the release of urine.
  - Flaccid neurogenic bladder – Bladder management options for males and females include intermittent catheterization and Credé's method (downward pressure placed on the bladder to manually express the urine).
  - Monitor for bowel sounds.
  - Neurogenic bowel functioning does not differ a lot between upper and lower motor neuron injuries. Daily use of stool softeners or bulk forming laxatives is recommended to keep the stool soft. A bowel movement can be stimulated daily or every other day by administration of a bisacodyl (Dulcolax) suppository or digital stimulation (stimulation of the rectal sphincter with a gloved and lubricated finger).
  - Development of a schedule as part of bladder and bowel training is critical for the establishment of a routine.
- Change the client's position every 2 hr while in bed and every 1 hr when in a wheelchair. Use pressure-relief devices in both the bed and wheelchair.
- Reinforce to clients the alterations in sexual function and possible adaptive strategies.
- Administer medications as prescribed.
- Medications
  - Glucocorticoids
    - Adrenocortical steroids such as dexamethasone (Decadron) aid in decreasing swelling of the spinal cord, which can increase pressure on the spinal cord, and subsequently, areas of ischemia.
  - Vasopressors
    - Norepinephrine and dopamine are given to treat postural hypotension, particularly during spinal shock.
    - Nursing Considerations
      - Ensure medication has been given 30 min prior to sitting clients up in a wheelchair.
  - Plasma expanders
    - Iron (Dextran) – Used to treat hypotension secondary to spinal shock.
    - Nursing Considerations
      - Observe clients for symptoms of fluid overload.

- ○ Muscle relaxants

  - Baclofen (Lioresal) and dantrolene sodium (Dantrium) – Given to clients who have severe muscle spasticity. Spasticity can be so severe that sitting in a wheelchair can be physically difficult.

- ○ Cholinergics

  - Bethanechol (Urecholine) – Decreases spasticity of the bladder allowing for easier bladder training and fewer accidents.

  - Nursing Considerations

    - □ Observe clients for urinary retention. Measure residual periodically.

- ○ Analgesics

  - Opioids, non-opioids, and NSAIDs are given for pain. Clients may or may not be able to feel pain from spinal cord injury. Clients who do have muscle spasticity may report feeling discomfort from the muscle spasms.

- ○ Anticoagulants

  - Heparin or low-molecular-weight heparins are used for deep vein thrombosis prophylaxis

  - Nursing Considerations

    - □ Monitor INR, PT, and aPTT for therapeutic levels of anticoagulation.

    - □ Observe for signs of gastrointestinal bleeding or bleeding secondary to unrecognized injury.

- ○ Stool softeners and bulk-forming laxatives

  - Docusate sodium (Colace) or polycarbophil (Fibercon) to prevent constipation and keep the stool soft

- ○ Vasodilators

  - Hydralazine (Apresoline) and nitroglycerin (Nitrostat) – Used PRN to treat episodes of hypertension during automatic dysreflexia

- Interdisciplinary Care

  - ○ Recognize the need for intensive occupational and physical therapy to learn how to perform ADLs and re-establish mobility using either a manual or electric wheelchair, or braces and crutches. Clients will also be fitted for splints to prevent contractures and/or provide wrist support for eating and manipulating a joy stick on an electric wheelchair.

  - ○ Request a referral for social services to determine the client's financial resources, home care needs, and adaptations needed in the home prior to discharge.

  - ○ Request a referral to an SCI support group to aid in emotionally adapting to changes in body image and role.

- Therapeutic Procedures
  - Application of immobilization devices and traction
    - Clients who have cervical fractures may be placed in a halo fixation device or cervical tongs. The purpose is to provide traction and/or immobilize the spinal column.

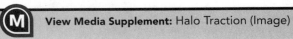
View Media Supplement: Halo Traction (Image)

    - Nursing Actions
      - Maintain body alignment and ensure that cervical tong weights hang freely.
      - Monitor skin integrity by providing pin care and assessing the skin under the halo fixation vest as appropriate.
    - Client Education
      - Provide instruction on pin and vest care if clients go home with a halo fixation device on.
      - Reinforce to clients signs of infection and skin breakdown.
- Surgical Interventions
  - Spinal Surgery
    - Spinal fusion is commonly done when a spinal fracture creates an area of instability of the spine.
    - Spinal fusions done in the cervical area are usually done using an anterior approach through the front of the neck.
    - Spinal fusions done in the thoracic or lumbar areas are done using a posterior approach and can be combined with a decompressive laminectomy.
    - A decompressive laminectomy is done by removing a section of lamina, accessing the spinal canal, and removing bone fragments, foreign bodies, or hematomas that may be placing pressure on the spinal cord.

View Media Supplement: Laminectomy (Image)

    - Donor bone is often obtained from the iliac crest and used to fuse together the vertebrae that are unstable.
    - Application of paravertebral rods can be used to mechanically immobilize several vertebral levels.
    - Client Education
      - Inform clients that an area of decreased range of motion will always exist in the area of fusion or paravertebral rods.
      - Inform clients that rods are usually not removed unless they cause pain. Removal can be done after the spine restabilizes.

- Care after Discharge
  - Client Education
    - Assist family members to learn about the aspects of the client's personal needs.
    - Provide emotional support to clients and their families.
- Client Outcomes
  - The client will integrate physiological changes in his body into a new, positive body image.
  - The client will be free of urinary complications.
  - The client will develop a regular routine for bowel movements.
  - The client will not experience autonomic dysreflexia.

Complications

- Orthostatic hypotension
  - Occurs when clients change position due to the interruption in functioning of the automatic nervous system and pooling of blood in lower extremities when clients are in an upright position.
  - Nursing Actions
    - Change client's positioning slowly and place clients in a wheelchair that reclines.
    - Use thigh-high elastic hose or elastic wraps to increase venous return. Elastic wraps may need to extend all the way up the client's legs and include the client's abdomen.
- Neurogenic shock
  - Neurogenic shock is a common response of the spinal cord following an injury.
  - Symptoms of bradycardia, hypotension, flaccid paralysis, loss of reflex activity below level of injury, and paralytic ileus accompany spinal shock due to the loss of autonomic function.
  - Nursing Actions
    - Monitor vital signs for hypotension and bradycardia.

- Autonomic dysreflexia

  ○ Occurs secondary to the stimulation of the sympathetic nervous system and inadequate compensatory response by the parasympathetic nervous system. Clients who have lesions below T6 do not experience dysreflexia because the parasympathetic nervous system is able to neutralize the sympathetic response.

  ○ Nursing Actions

    ▪ Determine and treat the cause.

      □ Sit clients up (to decrease blood pressure secondary to postural hypotension).

      □ Notify the provider.

      □ Determine the cause.

        ‣ Distended bladder is the most common cause (kinked or blocked urinary catheter, urinary retention, or urinary calculi)

        ‣ Fecal impaction

        ‣ Cold stress or drafts on lower part of the body

        ‣ Tight clothing

        ‣ Undiagnosed injury or illness (kidney infection or stone, lower extremity fracture)

      □ Treat the cause.

        ‣ Relieve the kink in the catheter or irrigate to remove blockage.

        ‣ Catheterize clients.

        ‣ Remove the impaction.

        ‣ Adjust the room temperature and block drafts.

        ‣ Remove tight clothing.

        ‣ Check for injury, such as lower extremity fracture or kidney/bladder infection.

    ▪ Monitor vital signs for severe hypertension and bradycardia.

  ○ Client Education

    ▪ Provide client education regarding potential causes of dysreflexia.

    ▪ Instruct clients to space out fluid intake and increase frequency of intermittent catheterizations if fluid intake is temporarily increased.

    ▪ Provide a list of possible actions to pursue if an episode of dysreflexia does occur.

Data Collection

- Risk Factors

  - The onset of MS is typically between 20 and 40 years of age and occurs twice as often in women. The etiology of MS is unknown. There is a family history (first-degree relative) of MS in many cases.

  - Since MS is an autoimmune disease, there are factors that trigger relapses.

    - Viruses and infectious agents

    - Living in a cold climate

    - Physical injury

    - Emotional stress

    - Pregnancy

    - Fatigue

    - Overexertion

    - Temperature extremes

    - Hot shower/bath

- Subjective and Objective Data

  - Fatigue – Especially of the lower extremities

  - Pain or paresthesia

  - Diplopia, changes in peripheral vision, decreased visual acuity

  - Uhthoff's sign (a temporary worsening of vision and other neurological functions commonly seen in clients with MS, or clients predisposed to MS, just after exertion or in situations where they are exposed to heat)

  - Tinnitus, vertigo, decreased hearing acuity

  - Dysphagia – Swallowing difficulties

  - Dysarthria (speech difficulties – Slurred and nasal speech)

  - Muscle spasticity

  - Ataxia and/or muscle weakness

  - Nystagmus

  - Bowel dysfunction (constipation, fecal incontinence)

  - Bladder dysfunction (areflexia, urgency, nocturia)

  - Cognitive changes (memory loss, impaired judgment)

  - Sexual dysfunction

- o Laboratory Tests
  - Cerebrospinal fluid analysis – Elevated protein level and a slight increase in WBCs
- o Diagnostic Procedures
  - Magnetic resonance imaging (MRI)
    - □ An MRI of the brain and spine is used to reveal plaques, which is mostly diagnostic.

Collaborative Care

- Nursing Care
  - o Nurses caring for clients who have MS should monitor:
    - Visual acuity
    - Speech patterns – Fatigue with talking
    - Swallowing
    - Activity tolerance
    - Skin integrity
  - o Encourage fluid intake and other measures to decrease the risk of developing a urinary tract infection. Assist clients with bladder elimination (intermittent self-catheterization, bladder pacemaker, Credé [placing manual pressure on abdomen over the bladder to expel urine]).
  - o Monitor cognitive changes and take interventions to maintain function (reorient clients, place objects used daily in routine places).
  - o Facilitate effective communication (dysarthria) through the use of a communication board.
  - o Apply alternating eye patches to treat diplopia. Show clients scanning techniques.
  - o Encourage clients to exercise and stretch involved muscles (avoid fatigue and overheating).
  - o Encourage clients to utilize energy conservation measures.
  - o Maintain a safe hospital environment to reduce the risk of injury (walk with wide base of support, assistive devices, skin precautions).
- Medications
  - o Azathioprine (Imuran) and cyclosporine (Sandimmune)
    - Use immunosuppressive agents to reduce the frequency of relapses.
    - Nursing Considerations
      - □ Monitor for long-term effects.
      - □ Be alert for signs and symptoms of infection.
      - □ Monitor for hypertension and kidney dysfunction.

- ○ Prednisone (Deltasone)
  - ▪ Use corticosteroids to reduce inflammation in acute exacerbations.
  - ▪ Nursing Considerations
    - □ Monitor for increased risk of infection, hypervolemia, hypernatremia, hypokalemia, hyperglycemia, gastrointestinal bleeding, and personality changes.
- ○ Dantrolene (Dantrium), tizanidine (Zanaflex), baclofen (Lioresal), and diazepam (Valium)
  - ▪ Use antispasmodics to treat muscle spasticity.
  - ▪ Intrathecal baclofen can be used for severe cases of MS.
  - ▪ Nursing Considerations
    - □ Observe for increased weakness.
    - □ Monitor for liver damage if taking tizanidine or dantrolene.
  - ▪ Client Education
    - □ Instruct clients to report increased weakness and/or jaundice to the provider.
    - □ Encourage clients to avoid stopping baclofen abruptly.
- ○ Interferon beta (Betaseron)
  - ▪ Use immunomodulators to prevent or treat relapses.
- ○ Carbamazepine (Tegretol)
  - ▪ Use anticonvulsants for paresthesia.
- ○ Docusate sodium (Colace)
  - ▪ Use stool softeners for constipation.
- ○ Propantheline (Pro-Banthine)
  - ▪ Use anticholinergics for bladder dysfunction.
- ○ Primidone (Mysoline) and clonazepam (Klonopin)
  - ▪ Use beta-blockers for tremors.
- • Interdisciplinary Care
  - ○ Request a referral for community resources and respite services for clients and their families.
  - ○ Request a referral for occupational and physical therapy for home environment assessment to determine safety and ease of mobility. Use adaptive devices to assist with ADLs.
  - ○ Request a referral for a speech language therapist for dysarthria and dysphagia.

- Care After Discharge

  - Client Education

    - Encourage family members to maintain a safe home environment to reduce the risk of injury (eliminate scatter rugs, keep electrical cords along baseboards, adequate lighting)

    - Encourage clients to use assistive devices for ambulation.

    - Encourage clients to adhere to the medication regimen.

- Client Outcomes

  - The client will be able to ambulate without assistance and independently perform ADLs.

  - The client will avoid triggers and exhibit fewer relapses.

AMYOTROPHIC LATERAL SCLEROSIS

Overview

- Amyotrophic lateral sclerosis (ALS) is a degenerative neurological disorder of the upper and lower motor neurons that result in deterioration and death of the motor neurons. This results in a progressive paralysis and muscle wasting that eventually causes respiratory paralysis and death. Cognitive function is not usually affected.

- Death usually occurs within 3 to 5 years of the initial symptoms due to respiratory failure. The cause of ALS is unknown and there is no cure.

Data Collection

- Risk Factors

  - ALS affects more men than women, often developing between the ages of 40 to 70.

- Subjective Data

  - Fatigue

  - Twitching and cramping of muscles

- Objective Data

  - Physical Assessment Findings

    - Muscle weakness – Usually begins in one part of the body

    - Muscle atrophy

    - Dysphagia

    - Dysarthria

- ○ Laboratory Tests
    - Creatine kinase (CK-BB) level – Increased
- ○ Diagnostic Procedures
    - Electromyogram (EMG)
        - □ Reduction in number of functioning motor units of peripheral nerves
    - Muscle biopsy
        - □ Reduction in number of motor units of peripheral nerves and atrophic muscle fibers

Collaborative Care

- Nursing Care
    - ○ Maintain a patent airway and suction as needed.
    - ○ Keep the head of the bed at 45°; turn, cough, and deep breathe every 2 hr; conduct incentive spirometry/chest physiotherapy.
    - ○ Facilitate effective communication (dysarthria) with the use of a communication board or a speech language therapist referral.
    - ○ Ensure safety with oral intake. Thicken fluids as needed.
    - ○ When no longer able to swallow, provide enteral nutrition as prescribed.
    - ○ Utilize energy conservation measures.
    - ○ Address the client's interest in the establishment of advance directives/living wills.
- Medications
    - ○ Riluzole (Rilutek)
        - Glutamate antagonist that can slow the deterioration of motor neurons by decreasing the release of glutamic acid. Must be taken early in disease process. Will add approximately 2 to 3 months of life to the client's overall lifespan.
        - Nursing Considerations
            - □ Monitor liver function tests – Hepatotoxic risk.
            - □ Observe for dizziness, vertigo, and somnolence.
        - Client Education
            - □ Suggest clients avoid drinking alcohol.
            - □ Instruct clients to take medication at evenly spaced regular intervals (every 12 hr).
            - □ Instruct clients to store medication away from bright light.
    - ○ Baclofen (Lioresal), dantrolene sodium (Dantrium), diazepam (Valium)
        - Use antispasmodics to decrease spasticity.

- Interdisciplinary Care

  o Request appropriate referrals (dietician, speech pathologist, social service, physical therapy, occupational therapy, clinical psychologist) for extended care in the home or a long-term care facility as client's condition deteriorates.

  o Consider hospice referral to provide support to the client and family coping with the terminal phase of the illness.

- Care After Discharge

  o Client Education

    ▪ Recommend genetic counseling for family members of clients who have ALS.

- Client Outcomes

  o The client will remain independent in ADLs until severe weakness and paralysis develops. The client will be able to remain in the home with support services available to meet needs.

  o The client will be free of infections (respiratory, urinary, integument).

Complications

- Pneumonia

  o Pneumonia can be caused by respiratory muscle weakness and paralysis contributing to ineffective airway exchange.

  o Nursing Actions

    ▪ Monitor respiratory status and provide antimicrobial therapy as indicated.

UNIT 2	NURSING CARE OF CLIENTS WITH NEUROSENSORY DISORDERS
Section:	Central and Peripheral Nervous System Disorders
Chapter 13	Guillain-Barré Syndrome and Myasthenia Gravis

Overview

- Guillain-Barré syndrome (GBS) develops in relation to acute destruction of the myelin sheath of peripheral nerves due to an autoimmune disorder that results in varying degrees of muscle weakness and paralysis.

 View Media Supplement: Nerve with Myelin Sheath (Image)

- After the acute phase, remyelination occurs and re-establishes nerve functions. However, aggregates of lymphocytes can cause secondary damage, which can delay recovery or result in permanent deficits.

- Chronic inflammatory demyelinating polyneuropathy (CIDP) is a different type of GBS that progresses over a very long period, and recovery is rare.

- Three stages characterize the course of GBS:

  o Initial period – 1 to 4 weeks; onset of symptoms until neurological deterioration stops

  o Plateau period – Several days to 2 weeks; no deterioration, and no improvement occurs

  o Recovery period – 4 to 6 months and up to 2 years; remyelination and return of muscle strength

- Etiology is unknown. Evidence indicates a cell-mediated immunologic reaction. A history of a recent viral event is reported by many clients.

Data Collection

- Risk Factors

  o Recent (within 1 to 3 weeks) history of:

    ▪ Acute illness (upper respiratory infection, gastrointestinal illness)

    ▪ Viruses such as Epstein-Barr virus (EBV) or cytomegalovirus (CMV)

    ▪ Vaccination (swine flu vaccination)

    ▪ Surgery

- Subjective Data

  o Clients report increasing weakness with no recollection of injury.

  o Clients report a virus within the previous 1 to 3 weeks.

- Objective Data

  o Acute progressive muscle weakness and paralysis

    ▪ Ascending (initially, bilateral lower extremity muscles are affected, then progresses upward through arms and thorax)

    ▪ Recovery is in descending order (initially, facial muscles recover, then improvement progresses downward)

  o Muscle flaccidity without muscle atrophy

  o Paresthesias – Creeping/crawling sensations across skin

  o Cranial nerve symptoms (diplopia, facial weakness, dysarthria, dysphagia)

  o Decreased/absent deep-tendon reflexes

  o Signs of respiratory compromise when muscle weakness reaches thorax

  o Autonomic dysfunction (fluctuating blood pressure, dysrhythmias)

  o Diagnostic Procedures

    ▪ Electromyography (EMG) and nerve conduction velocity (NCV)

      □ Shows evidence of denervation after 4+ weeks.

    ▪ WBC count

      □ Leukocytosis can develop.

    ▪ Lumbar puncture (LP)

      □ Shows an increase in protein within the cerebrospinal fluid without an increase in cell count, which is the distinguishing characteristic of GBS.

Collaborative Care

- Nursing Care

  o Monitor respiratory status (rate and depth of respirations, pulse oximetry, ABGs). Have oxygen, suction equipment, and intubation tray readily available.

  o Keep the head of the bed at 45°; have clients turn and cough, deep breathe, and use an incentive spirometer every 2 hr; institute chest physiotherapy if indicated.

  o Monitor heart rhythms for irregularities and bradycardia.

  o Monitor blood pressure and report fluctuations to the provider.

  o Provide alternatives for communication such as an alphabet board if clients can still use hands.

○ Check swallowing and gag reflexes before feeding. Follow recommendations of speech pathologist.

○ Take measures to prevent skin breakdown. Clients may not be able to change position or feel pain when skin breakdown is occurring.

○ Provide comfort measures (frequent repositioning, ice, heat, massage, distraction).

○ Identify support systems and coping abilities. Communicate appropriately because cognitive functions are not affected.

○ Administer medications as prescribed.

- Medications

  ○ Morphine

    ▪ An analgesic given for pain and paresthesias

    ▪ Nursing Considerations

      □ Monitor for respiratory depression and constipation.

  ○ IV Immunoglobulin (IVIg)

    ▪ Given to suppress attack on immune system

    ▪ Nursing Considerations

      □ Monitor for side effects such as chills, fever, myalgia, and for possible complications including anaphylaxis or renal failure.

  ○ Neurontin (Gabapentin)

    ▪ Given for neuropathic pain

    ▪ Nursing Considerations

      □ Monitor for confusion, depression, drowsiness, and ataxia.

- Interdisciplinary Care

  ○ Request appropriate referrals (social services, physical therapy, occupational therapy).

- Therapeutic Procedures

  ○ Plasmapheresis – A treatment where blood is removed from the body, run through a separator, and the circulating antibodies are removed from the plasma. This procedure decreases the attack against the myelin sheath. This may be done several times over a period of several weeks.

    ▪ Nursing Actions

      □ Preprocedure

        ‣ Check vital signs, laboratory values, and weight.

- □ Postprocedure
  - ▸ Apply pressure dressing to access site.
  - ▸ Monitor for infection at access site.
  - ▸ Monitor laboratory values.
    - ▹ Monitor for the possible complications of hypovolemia, hypokalemia, and hypocalcemia.
- ■ Client Education
  - □ Instruct clients that the procedure will typically last 2 to 5 hr.
- Care after Discharge
  - ○ Client Education
    - ■ Instruct clients to adhere to the medication regimen.
- Client Outcomes
  - ○ The client will be free from complications of immobility.
  - ○ The client will be able to resume ADLs.
  - ○ The client's muscle strength and functioning will return to baseline.

Complications

- Respiratory compromise
  - ○ Recognize progressing paralysis and be prepared to intervene promptly.
  - ○ Nursing Actions
    - ■ Monitor respiratory status (rate and depth of respirations, pulse oximetry, ABGs).
    - ■ Have oxygen, suction equipment, and intubation tray readily available.
    - ■ Provide assistance in mobilization and removal of secretions.

MYASTHENIA GRAVIS

Overview

- Myasthenia gravis (MG) is a progressive autoimmune disease that produces severe muscular weakness. It is characterized by periods of exacerbation and remission. Muscle weakness improves with rest.
- It is caused by antibodies that interfere with the transmission of acetylcholine at the neuromuscular junction.

Data Collection

- Risk Factors

    - Associated with rheumatoid arthritis, scleroderma, and systemic lupus erythematosus

    - Causes

        - Co-existing autoimmune disorder

        - Frequently associated with hyperplasia of the thymus gland

    - Factors that trigger exacerbations

        - Infection

        - Stress, emotional upset, and fatigue

        - Pregnancy

        - Increases in body temperature (fever, sunbathing, hot tubs)

- Subjective Data

    - Progressive muscle weakness

    - Diplopia (double vision)

    - Fatigue after exertion

- Objective Data

    - Physical Assessment Findings

        - Impaired respiratory status (difficulty managing secretions, poor respiratory effort)

        - Decreased swallowing ability

        - Poor muscle strength, especially of the face, eyes, and proximal portion of major muscle groups

        - Incontinence

        - Drooping eyelids – Unilateral or bilateral

        - Poor posture

    - Diagnostic Procedures

        - Tensilon testing

            - Baseline assessment of the cranial muscle strength is done.

            - Edrophonium chloride (Tensilon) is administered.

                - Medication inhibits the breakdown of acetylcholine, making it available for use at the neuromuscular junction. A positive test results in marked improvement in muscle strength that lasts approximately 5 min.

- ☐ Nursing Actions
    - ▸ Assist provider in administering the test.
    - ▸ Observe for complications such as fasciculations around the eyes and face, as well as cardiac arrhythmias.
    - ▸ Have atropine available, which is the antidote for edrophonium chloride (bradycardia, sweating, and abdominal cramps).
- ☐ Client Education
    - ▸ Explain purpose of the test to clients.
    - ▸ Encourage clients to follow the provider's directions in moving previously affected muscles.
    - ▸ Discourage clients from demonstrating improvement by increasing effort, which could skew the test results.
- ■ Electromyography
    - ☐ Shows the neuromuscular transmission characteristics of MG.
    - ☐ Decrease in amplitude of the muscle is demonstrated over a series of consecutive muscle contractions.

Collaborative Care

- • Nursing Care
    - o Monitor respiratory status (rate and depth of respirations, pulse oximetry, ABGs). Have oxygen, suction equipment, and intubation tray readily available.
    - o Check swallowing and gag reflexes before feeding. Follow recommendations of speech pathologist.
    - o Use energy conservation measures. Allow for periods of rest.
    - o Provide small, frequent high-calorie meals and schedule at times when medication is peaking.
    - o Have clients sit upright when eating and use thickener in liquids as necessary.
    - o Apply a lubricating eyedrop during the day and ointment at night if clients are unable to completely close their eyes. Clients may also need to patch or tape eye shut at night to prevent damage to the cornea.
    - o Encourage clients to wear a medical identification wristband or necklace at all times.
    - o Administer medications as prescribed and at specified times.
- • Medications
    - o Anticholinesterase agents
        - ■ Cholinesterase inhibitor medications are the first line in therapy.

- Nursing Considerations
  - Ensure that the medication is given at the specified time – usually 4 times a day.
  - If periods of weakness are observed, discuss change in administration times with the provider.
  - Use cautiously in clients who have a history of asthma or cardiac dysrhythmias.
- Client Education
  - Instruct clients to take with small amount of food to minimize gastrointestinal side effects.
  - Instruct clients to eat meals within 45 min of taking the medication to strengthen chewing and reduce the risk for aspiration.
  - Stress the importance of maintaining therapeutic levels and taking the medication at the same time each day.

- Pyridostigmine (Mestinon) and neostigmine (Prostigmin)
  - Used to increase muscle strength in the symptomatic treatment of MG. These medications inhibit the breakdown of acetylcholine and prolong its effects.
  - Nursing Considerations
    - Use cautiously in clients who have a history of asthma and cardiovascular disease.

- Immunosuppressants such as azathioprine (Imuran) and prednisone (Deltasone)
  - Use immunosuppressants during exacerbations when pyridostigmine is not adequately effective.
  - Since MG is an autoimmune disease, immunosuppressants decrease the production of antibodies.
  - A corticosteroid, such as prednisone, is the first medication of choice. Cytotoxic medications, such as azathioprine (Imuran), are given if corticosteroids are ineffective.
  - Nursing Considerations
    - Monitor for infection.
  - Client Education
    - Explain to clients the importance of slowly tapering off of a corticosteroid.
    - Tell clients to observe for signs of infection and take precautions against exposure to viruses and contaminants.

- IV immunoglobulins (IVIg) – Acute management
  - IVIg, an immunoglobulin, may be prescribed for MG that does not respond to the above treatments.

- Interdisciplinary Care

  o Request a referral for physical therapy for durable medical equipment needs.

  o Request a referral for occupational therapy for assistive devices to facilitate ADLs.

  o Request a referral to a speech and language therapist if weakening of facial muscles impacts communication or swallowing.

- Therapeutic Procedures

  o Plasmapheresis – Removes circulating antibodies from the plasma. This is usually done several times over a period of days and may continue on a regular basis for some clients.

- Surgical Interventions

  o Thymectomy – Removal of the thymus gland is done to attain better control or complete remission.

    ■ This may take months to years to see results due to the life of the circulating T cells.

- Client Outcomes

  o The client will not experience periods of fatigue that interfere with the ability to perform ADLs.

  o The client will verbalize the importance of taking medication regularly and at the prescribed time.

Complications

- Myasthenic crisis and cholinergic crisis

  o Myasthenic crisis occurs when clients are experiencing a stressor that causes an exacerbation of MG, such as infection, or are taking inadequate amounts of cholinesterase inhibitor.

  o Cholinergic crisis occurs when clients have taken too much cholinesterase inhibitor.

  o The symptoms of both can be very similar (muscle weakness, respiratory failure).

  o The client's highest risk for injury is due to respiratory compromise and failure.

- o Diabetic retinopathy – Microaneurysms

- o Macular degeneration – Loss of central vision

- o Eye infection, inflammation, or injury

- o Brain tumor

- Subjective Data

  - o Frequent headaches

  - o Frequent eye strain

  - o Blurred vision

  - o Poor judgment of depth

  - o Diplopia – Double vision

- Objective Data

  - o Tendency to close or favor one eye

  - o Poor hand-eye coordination

  - o Diagnostic Procedures

    - ■ Ophthalmoscopy

      - □ An ophthalmoscope is used to examine the back part of the eyeball (fundus), including the retina, optic disc, macula, and blood vessels.

    - ■ Visual acuity tests

      - □ Visual acuity tests include the Snellen chart and Rosenbaum Pocket Vision chart.

    - ■ Tonometry

      - □ Tonometry is used to measure intraocular pressure (IOP). IOP (normal is 10 to 21 mm Hg) is elevated with glaucoma, especially angle-closure glaucoma.

    - ■ Gonioscopy

      - □ Gonioscopy is used to examine the iridocorneal angle or anterior chamber of the eyes.

    - ■ Slit lamp

      - □ The slit lamp is used to examine the anterior portion of the eye, such as the cornea, anterior chamber, and the lens.

Collaborative Care

- Nursing Care
    - Use the Snellen chart or the Rosenbaum Pocket Vision Screener to check distance vision.
        - Have clients stand 20 ft from the Snellen chart.
        - Have clients hold the Rosenbaum chart 14 inches away from their eyes.
    - Identify how clients are adapting to their environment to maintain safety.
- Medications
    - Anticholinergics, such as atropine (Isopto Atropine ophthalmic solution)
        - Anticholinergics are used for intraocular exams/surgery. They provide mydriasis (dilation of the pupil) and cycloplegia (ciliary paralysis).
        - Client Education
            - Inform clients of adverse effects including reduced accommodation, blurred vision, and photophobia. With systemic absorption, there could be anticholinergic effects (tachycardia, decreased secretions).
- Interdisciplinary Care
    - Request referrals as appropriate to social services, support groups, and reduced-vision resources.
- Care after Discharge
    - Client Education
        - Recommend clients wear sunglasses to protect eyes.
        - Recommend clients wear eye protection to prevent injury to the eye.
        - Provide suggestions for home safety:
            - Increase the amount of light in a room.
            - Arrange the home to remove hazards, such as eliminating throw rugs.
            - Use phones with large numbers and/or auto dial.
        - Suggest clients use adaptive devices that accommodate for reduced vision.
            - Magnifying lens and large-print books/newspapers
            - Talking devices, such as clocks and watches
        - Recommend clients maintain blood pressure and cholesterol within appropriate reference range.
        - Recommend clients who have diabetes mellitus to maintain blood glucose levels within appropriate reference range.

■ Eat foods rich in antioxidants, such as green, leafy vegetables.

■ Encourage adults 40 or older to have an annual examination including a measurement of IOP.

- Client Outcomes

  o The client will be free of injury to the eye.

  o The client will maintain level of vision and report any changes.

  o The client will be free of pain and infection, and report any changes to his provider.

Complications

- Risk for Injury

  o Reduced vision places clients at a higher risk for injury. In particular, disturbed visual sensory perception is a well-known risk factor for injury and mortality in older adults.

  o Nursing Actions

  ■ Monitor for safety risks, such as the ability to drive safely, and intervene to reduce risks.

  o Client Education

  ■ Encourage annual eye examinations.

RETINAL DETACHMENT

Overview

- Retinal detachment is a painless separation of the retina from the epithelium, resulting in the loss of vision in fields corresponding to the separation.

- Retinal detachment is a medical emergency, and the assistance of a provider should be sought immediately.

Data Collection

- Risk Factors

  o Nearsightedness

  o Family history

  o Previous cataract surgery

  o Eye injury

  o Retinal tear – Trauma

  o Fibrous vitreous tissue – Pulls retina

  o Exudate – Forms under retina

- Subjective and Objective Data

    o The onset of retinal detachment is abrupt.

    o Bright flashes of light can occur.

    o Floating dark spots, commonly referred to as floaters, can be seen.

    o "Curtain drawing over visual field" sensation can occur.

    o An examination reveals a sudden loss of vision without pain.

    o Diagnostic Procedures

        ▪ A detached retina can be determined with an ophthalmoscope examination. Depending on the type of retinal tear, laser and/or surgery can be used as an intervention.

Collaborative Care

- Nursing Care

    o Restrict activity to prevent additional detachment.

    o Cover the affected eye with an eye patch.

- Medications

    o Terramycin with dexamethasone (TobraDex-ophthalmic solution)

        ▪ Antibiotic-steroid combination

        ▪ Prevents infection and decreases inflammation of the eye

        ▪ Client Education

            □ Remind clients to instill the drops as prescribed to prevent infection and inflammation.

- Interdisciplinary Care

    o Recognize the need for a retinal specialist for surgery.

    o Request referrals for services, such as community outreach programs, meals on wheels, and services for the blind as needed.

- Surgical Interventions

    o Scleral buckling

        ▪ Scleral buckling involves local or general anesthesia for the application of a silicone sponge held in place with stitches or an encircling band to promote attachment. An infiltration of a gas bubble can be done at the same time to push the retina back against the wall of the eye.

- ○ Retinal rebinding
  - ▪ The application of diathermy (high-frequency current), cryotherapy (freezing probes), or photocoagulation (laser beams) are used to create an inflammatory response for the purpose of rebinding the retina.
  - ▪ Nursing Actions
    - ☐ Provide information about the procedure for clients.
    - ☐ Rest the eye prior to the procedure.
    - ☐ An eye patch and shield are applied, and clients will lie with the affected eye up, or as prescribed, if a gas bubble is injected during the procedure.
    - ☐ Administer analgesics, antiemetics, antibiotics, and anti-inflammatory medications as prescribed.
  - ▪ Client Education
    - ☐ Avoid activities that cause rapid eye movement (reading, writing) for a specified period of time.
    - ☐ Wear sunglasses while outside or in brightly lit areas.
    - ☐ Rest the eye.
    - ☐ Contact the surgeon immediately if there is acute pain of the affected eye.
    - ☐ Contact the surgeon immediately if the eye has discharge or bleeds.
- Care after Discharge
  - ○ Client Education
    - ▪ Instruct clients to take precautions when engaging in sports that can cause a blow to the head or the eye.
    - ▪ Instruct clients to avoid activities that increase IOP
      - ☐ Bending over at the waist
      - ☐ Sneezing
      - ☐ Coughing
      - ☐ Straining
      - ☐ Vomiting
      - ☐ Head hyperflexion
      - ☐ Restrictive clothing, such as tight shirt collars
    - ▪ Clients should report if any changes occur, such as lid-swelling, decreased vision, bleeding or discharge, a sharp, sudden pain in the eye, and/or flashes of light or floating shapes.
- Client Outcomes
  - ○ The client will remain free from injury to the affected eye.
  - ○ The client will remain free from infection.

     o   The client will be pain free.

     o   The client will have improved vision as result of retinal surgery.

Complications

- Loss of vision

  o   The final visual result is not always known for several months postoperatively. More than one attempt at repair of the eye may be required.

  o   Client Education

  ▪   Instruct clients to seek professional help immediately if signs of detachment occur.

CATARACTS

 Overview

- A cataract is opacity in the lens of an eye that impairs vision.

- There are three types of cataracts:

  o   A subcapsular cataract begins at the back of the lens.

  o   A nuclear cataract forms in the center (nucleus) of the lens.

  o   A cortical cataract forms in the lens cortex and extends from the outside of the lens to the center.

(M) **View Media Supplement:** Cataracts (Image)

Data Collection

- Risk Factors

  o   Advanced age

  o   Diabetes mellitus

  o   Heredity

  o   Smoking

  o   Trauma

  o   Excessive exposure to the sun

  o   Chronic corticosteroid use

- Subjective Data

  - Decreased visual acuity (prescription changes, reduced night vision, loss of color perception)

  - Blurred vision

  - Diplopia – Double vision

  - Glare and light sensitivity – Photo sensitivity

  - History of visual problems

- Objective Data

  - Physical Assessment Findings

    - Progressive and painless loss of vision

    - Visible opacity

    - Absent red reflex

  - Diagnostic Procedures

    - Cataracts can be determined upon examination of the lens with an ophthalmoscope.

Collaborative Care

- Nursing Care

  - Check the client's visual acuity using the Snellen and Rosenbaum charts.

  - Examine the external and internal eye structures using an ophthalmoscope.

- Medications

  - Cholinesterase inhibitor (Atropine 1% ophthalmic solution)

    - This medication prevents pupil constriction for prolonged periods of time and relaxes muscles in the eye. It is used to dilate the eye preoperatively and for visualization of the eye's internal structures.

    - Nursing Considerations

      - The medication has a long duration, but a slow onset.

    - Client Education

      - Remind clients that the medication takes more than 24 hr to begin working.

  - Acetazolamide (Diamox – Oral medication)

    - Use acetazolamide preoperatively to reduce IOP, to dilate pupils, and to create eye paralysis to prevent lens movement.

    - Nursing Considerations

      - Always ask clients if they have an allergy to sulfa. Acetazolamide is a sulfa-based medication.

- Interdisciplinary Care

  o An ophthalmologist should be consulted for cataract surgery.

- Surgical Interventions

  o Surgical removal of the lens

    ▪ A small incision is made and the lens is either removed in one piece, or in several pieces after being broken up using sound waves. The posterior capsule is retained. A replacement or intraocular lens is inserted. Replacement lenses can correct refractive errors resulting in improved distant vision.

    ▪ Nursing Actions

      □ Postoperative care should focus on:

        ▸ Preventing infection.

        ▸ Administering ophthalmic medications.

        ▸ Providing pain relief.

        ▸ Teaching clients about self-care at home.

    ▪ Client Education

      □ Wear sunglasses while outside or in brightly lit areas.

      □ Report signs of infection, such as yellow or green drainage.

      □ Avoid activities that increase IOP.

      □ Limit activities.

        ▸ Avoid tilting the head back to wash hair.

        ▸ Limit cooking and housekeeping.

        ▸ Avoid rapid, jerky movements, such as vacuuming.

        ▸ Avoid driving and operating machinery.

        ▸ Avoid sports.

      □ Report pain with nausea/vomiting – indications of increased IOP or hemorrhage.

      □ Best vision is not expected until 4 to 6 weeks following the surgery.

      □ Clients should report if any changes occur, such as lid-swelling, decreased vision, bleeding or discharge, a sharp, sudden pain in the eye, and/or flashes of light or floating shapes.

- Care After Discharge

  o Client Education

    ▪ Recommend clients wear sunglasses to protect eyes.

    ▪ Recommend clients wear eye protection to prevent injury to the eye.

- ▪ Tonometry

  - ☐ Tonometry is used to measure IOP. IOP is elevated with glaucoma, especially angle-closure.

- ▪ Gonioscopy

  - ☐ Gonioscopy is used to determine the drainage angle of the anterior chamber of the eyes.

Collaborative Care

- Nursing Care

  - ○ Monitor clients for increased IOP.

  - ○ Monitor clients for decreased vision and light sensitivity.

  - ○ Check clients for aching or discomfort around the eye.

  - ○ Explain the disease process to clients and allow time for expression of feelings.

  - ○ Treat severe pain and nausea that accompanies angle-closure glaucoma with analgesics and antiemetics.

- Medications

  - ○ Timolol (Timoptic) – Topical nonselective beta blocker

  - ○ Betaxolol (Betoptic) – Topical cardiac selective beta blocker

    - ▪ Decreases IOP by reducing aqueous humor production.

  - ○ Brimonidine (Alphagan) – Topical

    - ▪ Alpha$_2$ adrenergic agonist that decreases production and may also decrease outflow of aqueous humor to lower IOP.

  - ○ Latanoprost (Xalatan) – Topical

    - ▪ Prostaglandin analog that increases aqueous humor outflow through relaxation of ciliary muscle.

  - ○ Acetazolamide (Diamox) oral

    - ▪ Anhydrase inhibitor that reduces production of aqueous humor by causing diuresis through renal effects

  - ○ Mannitol (Osmitrol) – IV mannitol is an osmotic diuretic used in the emergency treatment for angle-closure glaucoma to quickly decrease IOP.

- Interdisciplinary Care

  - ○ Recognize the need for a referral to an ophthalmologist if surgery is necessary.

  - ○ Request a referral for community outreach programs, meals on wheels, and services for the blind.

- Surgical Interventions
  - Glaucoma surgery
    - Laser trabeculectomy, iridotomy, or the placement of a shunt are procedures used to improve the flow of the aqueous humor by opening a channel out of the anterior chamber of the eye.
    - Nursing Actions
      - IOP is checked 1 to 2 hr postoperatively by the surgeon.
      - Instruct clients about the disease and the importance of adhering to the medication schedule to treat IOP.
    - Client Education
      - Instruct clients to:
        - Wear sunglasses while outside or in brightly lit areas.
        - Report signs of infection, such as yellow or green drainage.
        - Avoid activities that increase IOP.
        - Not lie on the operative side and to report severe pain or nausea (possible hemorrhage).
        - Report if any changes occur, such as lid-swelling, decreased vision, bleeding or discharge, a sharp, sudden pain in the eye and/or flashes of light or floating shapes.
        - Limit activities.
        - Report pain with nausea/vomiting – indications of increased IOP or hemorrhage.
        - Inform clients that best vision is not expected until 4 to 6 weeks postoperative.
- Care after Discharge
  - Client Education
    - Emphasize the importance of adhering to a medication schedule to treat IOP.
- Client Outcomes
  - The client will be free from injury, infection, and pain.
  - The client will have decreased IOP due to the eye surgery.

UNIT 2	NURSING CARE OF CLIENTS WITH NEUROSENSORY DISORDERS
Section:	Sensory Disorders
Chapter 15	Hearing Loss and Middle and Inner Ear Disorders

 Overview

- Disorders related to hearing and balance can be caused by injury, disease, and/or the aging process.

- Auditory problems that nurses should be knowledgeable about include:

  ○ Hearing loss

  ○ Middle and inner ear disorders

HEARING LOSS

 Overview

- Hearing loss is difficulty in hearing or accurately interpreting sounds due to a problem in the middle or inner ear.

- There are two types of hearing loss:

  ○ Conductive hearing loss occurs when there is an alteration in the middle ear and sound waves are blocked before reaching the inner ear.

  > **View Media Supplement:** External, Middle, and Internal Ear (Image)

  ○ Sensorineural hearing loss occurs when there is an alteration in the inner ear that involves cranial nerve VIII and/or cochlear damage.

Data Collection

- Risk Factors

  ○ Risk for and degree of hearing loss progressively advances with aging.

  ○ Conductive hearing loss

    ▪ History of middle ear infections

    ▪ Older age (otosclerosis)

○ Sensorineural hearing loss

- Prolonged exposure to loud noises

- Ototoxic medications to include antibiotics (gentamicin [Garamycin], amikacin [Amikin], or metronidazole [Flagyl]), diuretics (furosemide [Lasix]), NSAIDs (aspirin or ibuprofen [Advil]), and chemotherapeutic agents (cisplatin [Abiplatin])

- Infectious processes

- Age-related (presbycusis – Decreased ability to hear high-pitched sounds)

- Subjective and Objective Data

○ Conductive hearing loss

- Subjective

□ Reports hearing better in a noisy environment

- Objective

□ Clients speak softly

□ Obstruction in external canal visualized (packed cerumen is very common)

□ Abnormal tympanic membrane findings (holes, scarring)

□ Rinne test that demonstrates time of air conduction of sound is greater than or equal to time of bone conduction of sound

□ Weber test lateralizes to the affected ear

○ Sensorineural hearing loss

- Subjective

□ Tinnitus (ringing, roaring, or humming in ears)

□ Dizziness

□ Hears poorly in a noisy environment

- Objective

□ Clients speak loudly

□ Otoscopic exam shows no abnormalities

□ Rinne test that demonstrates time of air conduction of sound is less than time of bone conduction of sound.

□ Weber test lateralizes to the unaffected ear.

□ Diagnosis of acoustic neuroma (benign tumor cranial nerve VIII)

○ Diagnostic Procedures

- Weber test

□ Place a vibrating tuning fork stem on the center of the client's head

□ Ask the client to tell where the sound is heard the loudest.

- □ Expected finding – The sound is heard equally in both ears

- □ Unexpected finding – Lateralization to one ear

- ■ Rinne Test

    - □ Place a vibrating tuning fork stem on the client's mastoid process (bone conduction). When the client says he no longer hears the sound, move the tuning fork in front of the client's ear, and have the client say when he no longer hears the sound.

    - □ Expected finding – Air conduction is longer than or equal to bone conduction.

    - □ Unexpected finding – Bone conduction is longer than air conduction.

- ■ Audiometry

    - □ An audiogram identifies if hearing loss is sensorineural and/or conductive.

    - □ Nursing Actions

        - ▸ Minimize environmental sounds during testing.

        - ▸ Follow protocol to test a client's ability to hear various frequencies (high versus low pitch) at various decibels (soft versus loud tones).

        - ▸ Have clients wear audiometer headphones and face away from person performing test.

        - ▸ Plot responses on a graph for each ear and compare to expected findings based on age.

    - □ Client Education

        - ▸ Instruct clients to indicate when a tone is heard and in which ear by raising the hand on the corresponding side.

- ■ Tympanogram

    - □ A tympanogram measures the mobility of the tympanic membrane and middle ear structures relative to sound.

    - □ This test is effective in diagnosing disease of the middle ear.

- ■ Otoscopy

    - □ An otoscope is used to examine the external auditory canal, the tympanic membrane (TM), and malleus bone visible through the TM.

    - □ Nursing Actions

        - ▸ Use the appropriate size speculum and introduce into the external ear.

        - ▸ Pull up and back on the auricle to straighten out the canal and enhance visualization.

        - ▸ The tympanic membrane should be a waxy gray color and intact. It should provide complete structural separation of the outer and middle ear structures.

- ► The light reflex should be visible from the center of the TM anteriorly (5 o'clock right ear; 7 o'clock left ear).

- ► In the presence of fluid or infection in the middle ear, the TM will become inflamed and may bulge from the pressure of the exudate. This will also displace the light reflex, a significant diagnostic finding.

- ► Avoid touching the lining of the ear canal, which causes pain due to sensitivity.

- □ Client Education

- ► Warn clients that to see the TM clearly, the auricle may need to be pulled firmly.

Collaborative Care

- • Nursing Care

  - ○ Monitor the client's functional ability.

  - ○ Communication

    - ▪ Get the client's attention before speaking.

    - ▪ Stand/sit facing clients in a well-lit, quiet room without distractions.

    - ▪ Speak clearly and slowly to clients without shouting and without hands or other objects covering the mouth.

    - ▪ Arrange for communication assistance (sign-language interpreter, closed-captions, phone amplifiers, teletypewriter [TTY] capabilities) as needed.

  - ○ Check the hearing of clients receiving ototoxic medications for more than 5 days.

- • Interdisciplinary Care

  - ○ If abnormality is identified during audiometry, clients should be referred to an audiologist for more sensitive testing.

- • Therapeutic Procedures

  - ○ Hearing aid – Conductive hearing loss

    - ▪ Hearing aids are effective in treating conductive hearing loss.

    - ▪ Hearing aids amplify sounds, but do not help clients interpret what they are hearing.

    - ▪ Amplification of sound in a loud environment can be distracting and disturbing.

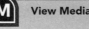 **View Media Supplement:** Hearing Aid (Image)

  - ○ Nursing Actions

    - ▪ Provide emotional support to clients using hearing aids for the first time.

- ○ Client Education
  - Instruct clients to use the lowest setting that allows hearing without feedback noise.
  - Tell clients to follow manufacturer's direction for cleaning and storing. To clean the ear mold, use mild soap and water while keeping hearing aid dry.
  - Remind clients to turn off hearing aids when not in use to conserve the life of the batteries. Replacement batteries should always be kept on hand.

- Surgical Interventions
  - ○ Tympanoplasty/myringoplasty – Conductive hearing loss
    - Tympanoplasty is a surgical reconstruction of the middle ear structures and myringoplasty is an eardrum repair.
    - Nursing Actions
      - □ Maintain sterile packing in the client's ear postoperatively.
      - □ Position clients flat with the operative ear facing up for 12 hr.
    - Client Education
      - □ Instruct clients to avoid forceful straining, coughing, sneezing with the mouth closed, and air travel.
      - □ Only wash hair if the ear is covered with a dressing. No water should enter the ear.
      - □ Remind clients that hearing will be impaired until packing is removed from the ear.

- Care After Discharge
  - ○ Client Education
    - Encourage clients not to place any objects in the ears, including cotton-tipped swabs.
    - Encourage clients to seek medical care if a foreign object is present in the ear or if ear is impacted with cerumen. Clients may use a commercial ceruminolytic (ear drops that soften cerumen) that can be instilled, followed by irrigation with warm water.
    - Encourage clients to wear ear protection for exposure to high-intensity noise and/or risk for ear trauma.
    - Encourage clients to keep volume as low as possible when wearing headphones.

- Client Outcomes
  - ○ The client will be able to accurately interpret speech and environmental sounds.
  - ○ The client will demonstrate proper care of the ears and adaptive devices.

MIDDLE AND INNER EAR DISORDERS

 Overview

- The middle ear consists of the tympanic membrane (eardrum), three bones (malleus, incus, and stapes), and connects to the oropharynx via the Eustachian tube.

- Middle ear infections are called otitis media.

- The inner ear consists of the oval window, cochlea (hearing organ), and the vestibular system (organ responsible for balance, which includes the semicircular canals).

- Middle and inner ear disorders cause many of the same symptoms due to their close proximity and adjoining structures.

- Inner ear problems are characterized by tinnitus (continuous ringing in ear), vertigo (whirling sensation), and dizziness.

- Labyrinthitis and Ménière's disease are inner ear problems.

    o Labyrinthitis is an infection of the labyrinth, usually secondary to otitis media.

    o Ménière's disease is a vestibular disease characterized by a triad of symptoms – tinnitus, unilateral sensorineural hearing loss, and vertigo.

        ▪ Benign paroxysmal vertigo (BPV) is a disorder that occurs in response to a change in position. It is thought to be due to a disturbance of crystals in the semicircular canals initiating vertigo that lasts from days to months.

- Visual, vestibular, and proprioceptive systems provide the brain with input regarding balance. Problems within any of these systems pose a risk for loss of balance.

Data Collection

- Risk Factors

    o Middle ear disorders

        ▪ Recurrent colds and otitis media

        ▪ Enlarged adenoids

        ▪ Trauma

        ▪ Changes in air pressure (scuba diving, flying)

    o Inner ear disorders

        ▪ Viral or bacterial infection

        ▪ Ototoxic medications

- Subjective Data
  - Middle ear disorders
    - Hearing loss
    - Feeling of fullness and/or pain in the ear
  - Inner ear disorders
    - Hearing loss
    - Tinnitus
    - Dizziness or vertigo
- Objective Data
  - Middle ear disorders
    - Red, inflamed ear canal and TM
    - Bulging TM
    - Fluid and/or bubbles behind TM
  - Inner ear disorders
    - Vomiting
    - Nystagmus
    - Poor balance
  - Diagnostic Procedures
    - Hearing acuity tests (Refer to tests performed for middle ear disorders.)
    - Electronystagmography (ENG)
      - ENG is done to determine the type of nystagmus elicited by the stimulation of the acoustic nerve.
      - Electrodes are placed around the eyes, and movements of the eyes are recorded when the ear canal is stimulated with cold water instillation or injection of air. Recording of eye movements can be interpreted by a specialist as either normal or abnormal.
      - Nursing Actions
        - Clients should be maintained on bed rest and NPO postprocedure until vertigo subsides.
      - Client Education
        - Instruct clients to fast immediately before the procedure and to restrict caffeine, alcohol, sedatives, and antihistamines 24 hr prior to the test.

- Caloric testing
    - Water (warmer or cooler than body temperature) is instilled into the ear in an effort to induce nystagmus.
    - The eyes' response to the instillation of cold and warm water is diagnostic of vestibular disorders.
    - This test can be done concurrently with ENG.
    - Nursing Actions
        - Clients should follow the same restrictions as those for an ENG.
    - Client Education
        - Inform clients of the above restrictions.

Collaborative Care

- Nursing Care
    - Monitor the client's functional ability and balance. Take fall-risk precautions as necessary.
    - Check the hearing of clients receiving ototoxic medications for more than 5 days.
    - Assist with ENG and/or caloric testing as needed.
    - Administer antivertigo and antiemetic medications as needed.
- Medications
    - Meclizine (Antivert)
        - Meclizine has antihistamine and anticholinergic effects and is used to treat the vertigo that accompanies inner ear problems.
        - Nursing Considerations
            - Contraindicated for clients who have closed-angle glaucoma.
            - Observe clients for sedation and take appropriate precautions to ensure safe ambulation.
        - Client Education
            - Warn clients about the sedative effects of meclizine (avoid driving, operating heavy machinery).
    - Antiemetics
        - Droperidol (Inapsine) is one of several antiemetics used to treat nausea and vomiting associated with vertigo.
        - Nursing Considerations
            - Observe clients for postural hypotension and tachycardia.
            - Tell clients to avoid abrupt changes in position.

- Client Education
  - Warn clients about the hypotensive effects of droperidol.
- Diphenhydramine (Benadryl) and dimenhydrinate (Dramamine)
  - Antihistamines are effective in the treatment of vertigo and nausea that accompany inner ear problems.
  - Nursing Considerations
    - Observe clients for urinary retention.
    - Observe clients for sedation and take appropriate precautions to ensure safe ambulation.
  - Client Education
    - Warn clients about the sedative effects (avoid driving, operating heavy machinery).
    - Inform clients that dry mouth is to be expected.
- Scopolamine (Transderm Scop)
  - Anticholinergics, such as scopolamine, are effective in the treatment of nausea that accompanies inner ear problems.
  - Nursing Considerations
    - Observe clients for urinary retention.
    - Observe clients for sedation and take appropriate precautions to ensure safe ambulation.
  - Client Education
    - Warn clients about the sedative effects of antihistamines (avoid driving, operating heavy machinery).
    - Inform the client that dry mouth is to be expected.
- Diazepam (Valium)
  - Diazepam is a benzodiazepine that has antivertigo effects.
  - Nursing Considerations
    - Observe for sedation and take appropriate precautions to ensure safe ambulation.
  - Client Education
    - Warn clients about the sedative effects of diazepam (avoid driving, operating heavy machinery).
    - Inform clients of diazepam's addictive properties and appropriate use of the medication.

- Interdisciplinary Care

    o Vestibular rehabilitation is an option for clients who experience frequent episodes of vertigo and/or are incapacitated due to the vertigo. A team of health care providers is used to treat the cause and teach clients exercises that can help clients adapt to and minimize the effects of vertigo. A combination of biofeedback, physical therapy, and stress management may be used. Postural education can teach clients positions to avoid, as well as positional exercises that can terminate an attack of vertigo.

- Therapeutic Procedures

    o Vertigo-reducing activities

        ■ Client Education

            □ Reinforce to clients to prevent stimulation/exacerbation of vertigo.

            □ Tell clients to space intake of fluids evenly throughout the day.

            □ Teach clients to decrease intake of salt and sodium-containing foods (processed meats, MSG).

            □ Have clients avoid caffeine and alcohol.

            □ Instruct clients to take a diuretic, if prescribed, to decrease the amount of fluid in semicircular canals.

            □ Tell clients to take these precautions when vertigo is present.

                ▸ Encourage clients to rest in a quiet, darkened environment when the symptoms are severe.

                ▸ Have clients use assistive devices as needed (cane, walker) for safe ambulation to assist with balance.

                ▸ Encourage clients to maintain a safe environment that is free of clutter.

- Surgical Interventions

    o Stapedectomy – Conductive hearing loss

        ■ A stapedectomy is a surgical procedure of the middle ear in which the stapes is removed and replaced with a prothesis.

        ■ The procedure is done when otosclerosis has developed and the bones of the middle ear fuse together.

        ■ Otosclerosis is one of the causes of conductive hearing loss in older adults.

        ■ Nursing Actions

            □ The procedure is done through the external ear canal and TM.

            □ The stapes is completely or partially removed and replaced with a prosthesis.

            □ The TM is repaired and sterile ear packing is placed in the ear postoperatively.

            □ Monitor clients for facial nerve damage.

            □ Intervene for vertigo, nausea, and vomiting (common findings following the procedure).

- Client Education

  □ Inform clients that hearing is initially worse but will improve as healing occurs.

  □ Instruct clients to avoid straining, coughing, sneezing with mouth closed, air travel, and rapid head movements.

  □ Instruct clients to cover ear when washing hair. Ensure that no water enters the ear.

- Cochlear implant – Sensorineural hearing loss

  - Cochlear implants consist of a microphone that picks up sound, a speech processor, a transmitter and receiver that converts sounds into electric impulses, and electrodes that are attached to the auditory nerve.

     View Media Supplement: Cochlear Implant (Image)

  - The implant's transmitter is located outside the head behind the ear and connects via a magnet to the receiver located immediately below it, under the skin.

  - Young children and adults who lost their hearing after speech development adapt to cochlear implants more quickly than those who were totally deaf at birth. Intensive and prolonged language training is necessary for individuals who did not develop speech.

  - Nursing Actions

    □ Placement of an implant can be done on an outpatient basis.

  - Client Education

    □ Inform clients that immediately after surgery the unit is not turned on.

    □ Tell clients that 2 to 6 weeks after surgery, the external unit is applied and the speech processor is programmed.

    □ Instruct clients on precautions to prevent infection.

    □ Instruct clients that MRIs must be avoided.

- Labyrinthectomy

  - A labyrinthectomy is a surgical treatment for vertigo that involves removal of the labyrinthine portion of the inner ear.

  - Nursing Actions

    □ The client will have severe nausea and vertigo postoperatively. Take appropriate safety precautions and give antiemetics as needed.

  - Client Education

    □ Inform clients that hearing loss is to be expected in the affected ear.

- Client Outcomes

  - The client will have decreased episodes of vertigo.

  - The client will be free from injury.

(A) APPLICATION EXERCISES

1. Identify unexpected findings for the Weber and Rinne tests.

2. A nurse is caring for a client in an extended care facility who has been diagnosed with sensorineural hearing loss. Which of the following findings in the client history are possible causative factors for the hearing loss? (Select all that apply.)

   _____ Age 81

   _____ History of vancomycin antibiotic therapy

   _____ Worked with heavy artillery in the Army 60 years ago

   _____ Presbyopia

   _____ Daily use of warfarin (Coumadin)

   _____ Presbycusis

   _____ History of IV furosemide (Lasix) therapy for heart failure

3. A client is newly fitted with a hearing aid. Which of the following client statements indicates a need for intervention by the nurse?

   A. "I have difficulty hearing in a loud environment."

   B. "I wash the earpiece of my hearing aid with alcohol."

   C. "I keep my hearing aid turned down low."

   D. "I turn my hearing aid off at night."

4. A client has been experiencing mild to moderate vertigo due to benign paroxysmal vertigo for several weeks. Which of the following actions should the nurse recommend to help control the vertigo? (Select all that apply.)

   _____ Take prescribed meclizine hydrochloride (Antivert).

   _____ Move head slowly when changing positions.

   _____ Avoid fruits high in potassium.

   _____ Use stress-management techniques.

   _____ Avoid beverages that contain caffeine.

5. A nurse has been assigned to care for a client diagnosed with Ménière's disease. Which of the following precautions should the nurse inform the assistive personnel (AP) about prior to the AP providing morning care?

   A. Remove scopolamine patch during bath care.

   B. Encourage high intake of fluids.

   C. Ensure adequate lighting by keeping curtains open.

   D. Observe the client for dizziness when ambulating.

(A) APPLICATION EXERCISES ANSWER KEY

1. Identify unexpected findings for the Weber and Rinne tests.

    Weber test: Unexpected finding – Lateralization indicating the sound is heard loudest in one ear.

    Rinne test: Unexpected finding – Bone conduction is longer than air conduction.

    (N) NCLEX® Connection: Reduction of Risk Potential, Diagnostic Tests

2. A nurse is caring for a client in an extended care facility who has been diagnosed with sensorineural hearing loss. Which of the following findings in the client history are possible causative factors for the hearing loss? (Select all that apply.)

X	**Age 81**
X	**History of vancomycin antibiotic therapy**
X	**Worked with heavy artillery in the Army 60 years ago**
_____	Presbyopia
_____	Daily use of warfarin (Coumadin)
X	**Presbycusis**
X	**History of IV furosemide (Lasix) therapy for heart failure**

    All of the above factors can contribute to hearing loss except daily use of warfarin, an anticoagulant, and presbyopia, which is loss of near vision between the ages of 40 and 50.

    (N) NCLEX® Connection: Physiological Adaptation, Alterations in Body Systems

3. A client is newly fitted with a hearing aid. Which of the following client statements indicates a need for intervention by the nurse?

    A. "I have difficulty hearing in a loud environment."

    B. "I wash the earpiece of my hearing aid with alcohol."

    C. "I keep my hearing aid turned down low."

    D. "I turn my hearing aid off at night."

    The earpiece of a hearing aid should be cleaned with mild soap and water, not alcohol. The other statements do not indicate a need for intervention.

    (N) NCLEX® Connection: Basic Care and Comfort, Assistive Devices

4. A client has been experiencing mild to moderate vertigo due to benign paroxysmal vertigo for several weeks. Which of the following actions should the nurse recommend to help control the vertigo? (Select all that apply.)

    __X__ **Take prescribed meclizine hydrochloride (Antivert).**

    __X__ **Move head slowly when changing positions.**

    _____ Avoid fruits high in potassium.

    __X__ **Use stress-management techniques.**

    __X__ **Avoid beverages that contain caffeine.**

    Meclizine is an effective pharmacologic treatment for vertigo. Moving the head slowly when changing positions and stress management techniques can all lessen the incidence of vertigo. Instruct clients to avoid beverages that contain caffeine. Foods high in potassium have no effect on vertigo.

    (N) NCLEX® Connection: Physiological Adaptation, Alterations in Body Systems

5. A nurse has been assigned to care for a client diagnosed with Ménière's disease. Which of the following precautions should the nurse inform the assistive personnel (AP) about prior to the AP providing morning care?

    A. Remove scopolamine patch during bath care.

    B. Encourage high intake of fluids.

    C. Ensure adequate lighting by keeping curtains open.

    D. Observe the client for dizziness when ambulating.

    Clients who have Ménière's disease experience the triad of symptoms – tinnitus, unilateral hearing loss, and vertigo. Instruct the AP to observe the client for dizziness when ambulating the client. Do not remove the scopolamine patch, which is used to treat dizziness, during bath care. A high intake of fluids and bright lights may exacerbate the symptoms.

    (N) NCLEX® Connection: Physiological Adaptations, Alterations in Body Systems

UNIT 3: NURSING CARE OF CLIENTS WITH RESPIRATORY DISORDERS

- Diagnostic and Therapeutic Procedures
- Respiratory Systems Disorders

NCLEX® CONNECTIONS

When reviewing the chapters in this section, keep in mind the relevant sections of the NCLEX® outline, in particular:

CLIENT NEEDS: PHARMACOLOGICAL THERAPIES

Relevant topics/tasks include:
- Adverse Effects/ Contraindications/Side Effects/Interactions
  - Reinforce client teaching on possible effects of medications.
- Expected Actions/ Outcomes
  - Identify client expected response to medication.
- Medication Administration
  - Identify client need for PRN medications.

CLIENT NEEDS: REDUCTION OF RISK POTENTIAL

Relevant topics/tasks include:
- Laboratory Values
  - Identify laboratory values for ABGs, BUN, cholesterol , glucose, hematocrit, hemoglobin, glycosylated hemoglobin, platelets, potassium, sodium, WBC, creatinine, PT, PTT, and APTT.
- Potential for Alterations in Body Systems
  - Reinforce client teaching on methods to prevent complications associated with activity level/ diagnosed illness/disease.
- Therapeutic Procedures
  - Assist with the performance of a diagnostic or invasive procedure.

CLIENT NEEDS: PHYSIOLOGICAL ADAPTATION

Relevant topics/tasks include:
- Alterations in Body Systems
  - Provide care to a client on a ventilator.
- Medical Emergencies
  - Notify primary health care provider about client unexpected response/emergency situation.
- Unexpected Response to Therapies
  - Recognize complications of acute or chronic illness and intervene.

UNIT 3	NURSING CARE OF CLIENTS WITH RESPIRATORY DISORDERS
Section:	Diagnostic and Therapeutic Procedures
Chapter 16	**Respiratory Diagnostic and Therapeutic Procedures**

Overview

- Respiratory diagnostic procedures are used to evaluate a client's respiratory status by checking indicators such as the oxygenation of the blood, lung functioning, and the integrity of the airway.

- Respiratory diagnostic procedures that nurses should be knowledgeable about include:

    o   Pulse oximetry

    o   ABGs

    o   Bronchoscopy

    o   Thoracentesis

- Chest tubes are a type of therapeutic procedure inserted into the pleural space to drain fluid, blood, or air; reestablish a negative pressure; facilitate lung expansion; and restore normal intrapleural pressure.

- Chest tubes can be inserted in the emergency department, at the client's bedside, or in the operating room through a thoracotomy incision.

- Chest tubes are removed when the lungs have reexpanded and/or there is no more fluid drainage.

Pulse Oximetry

- Pulse oximetry is a noninvasive measurement of the oxygen saturation of the blood, but it is not a replacement for ABG measurement.

    o   A pulse oximeter is a battery- or electric-operated device with a sensor probe that is attached securely onto the client's fingertip, toe, bridge of nose, earlobe, or forehead with a clip or band.

    o   Pulse oximetry measures arterial oxygen saturation (SaO_2) via a wave of infrared light that measures light absorption by oxygenated and deoxygenated Hgb in arterial blood. SaO_2 and SpO_2 are used interchangeably.

- Indications

  - Pulse oximetry is indicated for conditions or situations in which a client's respiratory status should be monitored, such as during a continuous opioid epidural infusion.

  - Client presentation

    - The following signs and symptoms indicate that oxygen saturation should be monitored in a client

      - Increased work of breathing

      - Wheezing

      - Coughing

      - Cyanosis

- Interpretation of Findings

  - The expected reference range for SaO_2 is 95% to 100%. Acceptable levels may range from 91% to 100%. Some illness states may even allow for an SaO_2 of 85% to 89%.

  - Values may be slightly lower in the older adult client and those with dark skin.

  - Additional reasons for low readings include hypothermia, poor peripheral blood flow, too much light (sun or infrared lamps), low Hgb levels, client movement, edema, and nail polish.

  - An SaO_2 below 91% requires interventions to help the client regain acceptable SaO_2 levels. An SaO_2 below 86% is an emergency. An SaO_2 below 80% is life-threatening. The lower the SaO_2 level, the less accurate the value.

  - Values obtained by pulse oximetry are unreliable in cardiac arrest, shock, and other states of low perfusion.

- Preprocedure

  - Nursing actions

    - Perform hand hygiene and provide privacy.

    - Find an appropriate probe site. It must be dry and have adequate circulation.

    - Be sure the client is in a comfortable position, supporting the arm if a finger is used as a probe site.

- Intraprocedure

  - Nursing actions

    - Apply the sensor probe to the site.

    - Press the power switch on the oximeter.

    - Note the pulse reading and compare it with the client's radial pulse. Any discrepancy warrants further data collection.

    - Allow time for the readout to stabilize, and then record this value as the oxygen saturation.

- ■ Remove the probe, turn off the oximeter, and store it appropriately.
- ■ If continuous monitoring is required, make sure the alarms are set for a low and a high limit, they are functioning, and that the sound is audible. Check the condition of the skin under the probe every 4 hr and move the sensor every 24 hr if indicated.

- Postprocedure
  - o Nursing actions
    - ■ Document the findings and report abnormal findings to the provider.
    - ■ If a client's SaO_2 is less than 90% (indicating hypoxemia):
      - □ Confirm that the sensor probe is properly placed.
      - □ Confirm that the oxygen delivery system is functioning and that the client is receiving prescribed oxygen levels.
      - □ Place the client in a semi-Fowler's or Fowler's position to maximize ventilation.
      - □ Encourage the client to deep-breathe.
      - □ Report significant findings to the provider.
      - □ Remain with the client and provide emotional support to decrease anxiety.

ABGs (Arterial Blood Gases)

- An ABG sample reports the status of oxygenation and acid-base balance of the blood.
  - o An ABG measures:
    - ■ pH – The amount of free hydrogen ions in the arterial blood (H^+).
    - ■ PaO_2 – The partial pressure of oxygen.
    - ■ $PaCO_2$ – The partial pressure of carbon dioxide.
    - ■ HCO_3 – The concentration of bicarbonate in arterial blood.
    - ■ SaO_2 – Percentage of oxygen bound to Hgb as compared to the total amount that can be possibly carried.
  - o ABGs can be obtained by an arterial puncture or through an arterial line.
- Indications
  - o Potential diagnoses
    - ■ Blood pH levels may be affected by any number of disease processes (respiratory, endocrine, or neurologic).
    - ■ These assessments are helpful in monitoring the effectiveness of various treatments (such as acidosis interventions), in guiding oxygen therapy, and in evaluating client responses to weaning from mechanical ventilation.

- Interpretation of Findings

ABG MEASURE	NORMAL RANGE
pH	7.35 to 7.45
PaO_2	80 to 100 mm Hg
$PaCO_2$	35 to 45 mm Hg
HCO_3^-	22 to 26 mEq/L
SaO_2	95 to 100%*

*Older adult values may be slightly lower.

  - Blood pH levels below 7.35 reflect acidosis, while levels above 7.45 reflect alkalosis.

- Complications

  - Hematoma, arterial occlusion

    - A hematoma occurs when blood accumulates under the skin at the IV site.

    - Nursing Actions

      - Observe the client for changes in temperature, swelling, color, loss of pulse, or pain.

      - Notify the provider immediately if symptoms persist.

      - Apply pressure to the hematoma site.

  - Air embolism

    - Air enters the arterial system during catheter insertion.

    - Nursing Actions

      - Monitor the client for a sudden onset of shortness of breath, decreases in SaO_2 levels, chest pain, anxiety, and air hunger.

      - Notify the provider immediately if symptoms occur, administer oxygen therapy, and obtain ABGs. Continue to assess the client's respiratory status for any deterioration.

Bronchoscopy

- Bronchoscopy permits visualization of the larynx, trachea, and bronchi through either a flexible fiberoptic or a rigid bronchoscope.

  - Bronchoscopy can be performed as an outpatient procedure, in a surgical suite under general anesthesia, or at the bedside under local anesthesia and moderate sedation.

  - Bronchoscopy can also be performed on clients who are receiving mechanical ventilation by inserting the scope through the client's endotracheal tube.

- Indications

  - Potential diagnoses

    - Visualization of abnormalities such as tumors, inflammation, and strictures

    - Biopsy of suspicious tissue (lung cancer)

      - Clients undergoing a bronchoscopy with biopsy have additional risks for bleeding and/or perforation.

    - Aspiration of deep sputum or lung abscesses for culture and sensitivity and/or cytology (pneumonia)

  - Note – Bronchoscopy is also performed for therapeutic reasons, such as removal of foreign bodies and secretions from the tracheobronchial tree, treating postoperative atelectasis, and to destroy and excise lesions.

- Interpretation of Findings

  - A bronchoscopy can identify airway problems, cancer and lung disease.

- Preprocedure

  - Nursing actions

    - Check clients for allergies to anesthetic agents or routine use of anticoagulants.

    - Verify that a consent form is signed by clients prior to the procedure.

    - Remove the client's dentures, if applicable, prior to the procedure.

    - Maintain the client on NPO status prior to the procedure as ordered, usually 8 to 12 hr, to reduce the risk of aspiration when the cough reflex is blocked by anesthesia.

    - Obtain baseline vital signs and place pulse oximeter for continuous monitoring during the procedure.

    - Administer preprocedure medications as prescribed, such as viscous lidocaine or local anesthetic throat sprays.

- Postprocedure

  - Nursing actions

    - Monitor clients returning from the PACU. Ensure gag reflex is present before resuming oral intake.

    - Monitor vital signs and pulse oximeter reading every 15 min until stable.

    - Monitor clients for development of significant fever (mild fever for less than 24 hr is not uncommon), productive cough, significant hemoptysis indicative of hemorrhage (a small amount of blood-tinged sputum is expected), and hypoxemia.

    - Provide oral hygiene to clients.

Ⓖ

- For older adult clients, encourage coughing and deep breathing every 2 hr. There is an increased risk of respiratory infection and pneumonia in older adult clients due to delay in return of the cough reflex, decreased cough effectiveness and decreased secretion clearance. Respiratory infections may be more severe and last longer in older adult clients.

  ○ Client education

    - Instruct clients that gargling with salt water or use of throat lozenges may provide comfort for soreness of the throat.

    - Discourage smoking, talking, and coughing for several hours.

- Complications

  ○ Laryngospasm

    - Laryngospasm is uncontrolled muscle contractions of the laryngeal cords (vocal cords) that impede the client's ability to inhale.

    - Nursing Actions

      □ Continuously monitor clients for signs of respiratory distress.

      □ Call for assistance if indicated.

      □ Maintain a patent airway by repositioning clients or inserting an oral or nasopharyngeal airway as appropriate.

      □ Administer oxygen therapy to clients as prescribed. Humidification can decrease the likelihood of laryngeal edema.

  ○ Aspiration

    - Aspiration can occur if clients choke on oral secretions.

    - Nursing Actions

      □ Prevent aspiration in clients by withholding oral fluids or food until the gag reflex returns (usually 2 hr).

      □ Perform suctioning as needed.

Thoracentesis

- Thoracentesis is the surgical perforation of the chest wall and pleural space with a large-bore needle. It is performed to obtain specimens for diagnostic evaluation, instill medication into the pleural space, and remove fluid (effusion) or air from the pleural space for therapeutic relief of pleural pressure.

  ○ Thoracentesis is performed under local anesthesia by a provider at the client's bedside, in a procedure room, or in a provider's office.

  ○ Use of an ultrasound for guidance decreases the risk of complications.

- Indications
  - Potential diagnoses
    - Transudates (heart failure, cirrhosis, nephrotic syndrome)
    - Exudates (inflammatory, infectious, neoplastic conditions)
    - Empyema
    - Pneumonia
    - Blunt, crushing, or penetrating chest injuries/trauma or invasive thoracic procedures, such as lung and/or cardiac surgery
  - Client presentation
    - Large amounts of fluid in the pleural space compress lung tissue and can cause pain, shortness of breath, cough, and other symptoms of pleural pressure.
    - Assessment of the effusion area may reveal decreased breath sounds, dull percussion sounds, and decreased chest wall expansion. Pain may occur due to the inflammatory process.

- Interpretation of Findings
  - Aspirated fluid is analyzed for general appearance, cell counts, protein and glucose content, the presence of enzymes such as lactate dehydrogenase (LDH) and amylase, abnormal cells, and culture.

- Preprocedure
  - Percussion, auscultation, radiography, or sonography is used to locate the effusion and needle insertion site.
  - Changes in fat deposition in many older adult clients may make it difficult for the provider to identify the landmarks for insertion of the thoracentesis needle.
  - Nursing actions
    - Verify that clients have signed the informed consent form.
    - Gather all needed supplies.
    - Obtain preprocedure x-ray as prescribed to locate pleural effusion and to determine needle insertion site.
    - Position clients sitting upright with his arms and shoulders raised and supported on pillows and/or on an overbed table, and with his feet and legs well-supported.
  - Client education
    - Instruct clients to remain absolutely still (risk of accidental needle damage) during the procedure and to not to cough or talk unless instructed by the primary care provider.

- Intraprocedure
  - Nursing actions
    - Assist the provider with the procedure (strict surgical aseptic technique).
    - Prepare clients for a feeling of pressure with needle insertion and fluid removal.
    - Monitor the client's vital signs, skin color, and oxygen saturation throughout the procedure.
    - Measure and record the amount of fluid removed from the client's chest.
    - Label specimens at the bedside and promptly send them to the laboratory.
  - Note – The amount of fluid removed is limited to 1 L at a time to prevent cardiovascular collapse.
- Postprocedure
  - Nursing actions
    - Apply a dressing over the puncture site and position clients on the unaffected side for 1 hr.
    - Monitor the client's vital signs and respiratory status (respiratory rate and rhythm, breath sounds, oxygenation status) hourly for the first several hours after the thoracentesis.
    - Encourage clients to deep breathe to assist with lung expansion.
    - Allow clients to resume normal activity after 1 hr if no signs of complications are present.
    - Obtain a postprocedure chest x-ray (check resolution of effusions, rule out pneumothorax).
    - Document the procedure to include the client's response; volume and character of fluid removed; and vital signs.
- Complications
  - Pneumothorax
    - Pneumothorax is a collapsed lung. It can occur due to injury to the lung during the procedure.
    - Nursing Actions
      - Monitor clients for signs and symptoms of pneumothorax, such as diminished breath sounds.
      - Monitor postprocedure chest x-ray results.
  - Bleeding
    - Bleeding can occur if clients are moved during the procedure or are at an increased risk for bleeding.

- Nursing Actions
  - Monitor clients for coughing and/or hemoptysis.
  - Monitor the client's vital signs and laboratory results for evidence of bleeding (hypotension, reduced Hgb level).
- Infection
  - Infection can occur due to the introduction of bacteria with the needle puncture.
  - Nursing Actions
    - Insure that sterile technique is maintained.
    - Monitor the client's temperature following the procedure.

Chest Tube Systems

- Types of chest drainage systems:
  - Single-chamber systems have a water seal and a drainage collection in the same chamber.
  - Two chamber systems have a water seal and a drainage collection in separate chambers, which allows for the collection of larger amounts of drainage.
  - Three chamber systems have a water seal, a drainage collection, and suction control in separate chambers.
  - Disposable chest tube drainage systems are now commonly used.

 View Media Supplement: Chest Tube Drainage System (Image)

- Water seals are created by adding sterile fluid to a chamber up to the 2 cm line. The water seal allows air to exit from the pleural space on exhalation and stops air from entering with inhalation.
  - To maintain the water seal, the chamber must be kept upright and below the chest tube insertion site at all times. The nurse should routinely monitor the water level due to the possibility of evaporation. The nurse should add fluid as needed to maintain the 2 cm water seal level.
  - The height of the water in the suction control chamber determines the amount of suction transmitted to the pleural space. A suction pressure of –20 cm H_2O is common. The application of suction results in continuous bubbling in the suction chamber. The nurse should monitor the fluid level and add fluid as needed to maintain the prescribed level of suctioning.
  - Tidaling (movement of the water level with respiration) is expected in the water seal chamber. With spontaneous respirations, the water level will rise with inspiration (increase in negative pressure in lung) and will fall with expiration. With positive-pressure mechanical ventilation, the water level will rise with expiration and fall with inspiration.
  - Cessation of tidaling in the water seal chamber signals lung reexpansion or an obstruction within the system.

Chest Tube Insertion

- Indications
  - Diagnoses
    - Pneumothorax (collapsed lung)
    - Hemothorax (blood in lung)
    - Postoperative chest drainage (thoracotomy or open-heart surgery)
    - Pleural effusion (fluid in lung)
    - Lung abscess (necrotic lung tissue)
  - Client presentation
    - Dyspnea
    - Distended neck veins
    - Poor circulation
    - Cough
- Client Outcomes
  - The client will maintain adequate gas exchange.
  - The client will be free from pain.
  - The client will remain free from infection.
- Preprocedure
  - Nursing actions
    - Verify that the consent form is signed.
    - Reinforce client teaching. Breathing will improve when the chest tube is in place.
    - Check for allergies to local anesthetics.
    - Assist clients into the desired position (supine or semi-Fowler's).
    - Prepare the chest drainage system prior to the insertion per the facilities protocol (fill the water seal chamber).
    - Administer pain and sedation medications as prescribed.
    - Prep the insertion site with povidone iodine (Check for iodine allergy.). Drape the insertion site.

- Intraprocedure

  o Nursing actions

    ▪ Assist the charge nurse and provider with insertion of the chest tube, application of a dressing to the insertion site, and setup of the drainage system.

      □ The chest tube tip is positioned up toward the shoulder (pneumothorax) or down toward the posterior (hemothorax or pleural effusion).

      □ The chest tube is then sutured to the chest wall and an airtight dressing is placed over the puncture wound.

      □ The chest tube is then attached to drainage tubing that leads to a collection device.

      □ Place the chest tube drainage system below the client's chest level with the tubing coiled on the bed. Ensure that the tubing from the bed to the drainage system is straight to promote drainage via gravity.

    ▪ Monitor the client's vital signs and response to the procedure.

 View Media Supplement: Chest Tube (Image)

- Postprocedure

  o Nursing actions

    ▪ Check the client's vital signs, breath sounds, SaO_2, color, and respiratory effort as indicated by the status of the client and at least every 4 hr.

    ▪ Encourage coughing and deep-breathing every 2 hr.

    ▪ Keep the drainage system below the client's chest level, including during ambulation.

    ▪ Monitor the chest tube's placement and function.

      □ Check the water seal level every 2 hr and add water as needed. The water level should fluctuate with respiratory effort.

      □ Document the amount and color of drainage hourly for the first 24 hr and then at least every 8 hr. Mark the date, hour, and drainage level on the container at the end of each shift. Report excessive drainage (greater than 70 mL/hr) or drainage that is cloudy or red to the provider. Drainage will often increase with position changes or coughing.

      □ Monitor the fluid in the suction control chamber and maintain the fluid level prescribed by the provider.

      □ Check for expected findings of tidaling in the water seal chamber and continuous bubbling only in the suction chamber.

    ▪ Routinely monitor tubing for kinks, occlusions, or loose connections.

    ▪ Monitor the chest tube insertion site for redness, pain, infection, and crepitus (air leakage in subcutaneous tissue).

- Position clients in the semi-Fowler's to high-Fowler's position to promote optimal lung expansion and drainage of the fluid from the lungs.

- Administer pain medications as prescribed.

- Obtain a chest x-ray to verify the chest tube's placement.

- Keep two enclosed hemostats, a bottle of sterile water, and an occlusive dressing located at the bedside at all times.

- Due to the risk of causing a tension pneumothorax, chest tubes are only clamped when ordered by the provider in specific circumstances, such as an air leak, during drainage system change, accidental disconnection of tubing, or damage to the collection device.

- Do not strip or milk tubing routinely; only perform this action when prescribed by the provider. Stripping creates a high negative pressure and can damage the client's lung tissue.

- Complications

  - Air leaks

    - Air leaks can result if a connection is not taped securely.

    - Nursing Actions

      - Monitor the water seal chamber for continuous bubbling (air leak finding). If observed, locate the source of the air leak and intervene accordingly (tighten the connection, replace drainage system).

        ‣ Check all of the connections.

        ‣ Call for assistance.

        ‣ Cross clamp close to client's chest. If bubbling stops, the leak is at the insertion site or within the thorax. If bubbling doesn't stop, methodically move clamps down the drainage tubing toward the collection device, moving one clamp at a time. When the bubbling stops, the leak is within the section of tubing or at that connection distal to the clamp.

  - Accidental disconnection, system breakage, or removal

    - Complications can occur at any time.

    - Nursing Actions

      - If a chest tube is accidentally dislodged from the client's chest, the nurse should immediately cover the insertion site with dry sterile gauze and notify the provider. This allows air to escape and reduces the risk for development of a tension pneumothorax.

      - If a chest tube disconnects from the drainage system, the nurse should immediately place the end of the tube in sterile water to restore the water seal. It is also important to keep the drainage system below the level of the client's chest.

- o Tension pneumothorax
  - Sucking chest wounds, prolonged clamping of the tubing, kinks in the tubing, or obstruction may cause a tension pneumothorax.

Chest Tube Removal

- Provide pain medication 30 min before removing chest tubes.

- Assist the provider with sutures and chest tube removal.

- The provider will instruct clients to take a deep breath, exhale, and bear down (Valsalva maneuver) or to take a deep breath and hold it (increases intrathoracic pressure and reduces the risk of air emboli) during chest tube removal.

- Apply airtight sterile petroleum jelly gauze dressing. Secure in place with a heavyweight stretch tape.

- Obtain chest x-rays as prescribed. This is performed to verify continued resolution of the pneumothorax, hemothorax, or pleural effusion.

- Monitor clients for excessive wound drainage, signs of infection, or recurrent pneumothorax.

- Disadvantages
  - The FiO$_2$ varies with the flow rate and the client's rate and depth of breathing.
  - Extended use can lead to skin breakdown and dry the mucous membranes.
  - The tubing is easily dislodged.
- Nursing Interventions
  - Check the patency of the nares.
  - Ensure that the prongs fit in the nares properly.
  - Use water-soluble gel to prevent dry nares.
  - Provide humidification for flow rates of 4 L/min and above.

○ Simple face mask (covers the client's nose and mouth)

- FiO$_2$ – 40% to 60% at flow rates of 5 to 8 L/min (the minimum flow rate is 5 L/min to ensure flushing of CO$_2$ from the mask).
- Advantages
  - A face mask is easy to apply and may be more comfortable than a nasal cannula.
- Disadvantages
  - Flow rates of 5 L/min or lower can result in rebreathing of CO$_2$.
  - This device is poorly tolerated by clients who have anxiety or claustrophobia.
  - Eating, drinking, and talking are impaired.
  - Use caution with clients who have a high risk of aspiration or airway obstruction.
- Nursing Interventions
  - Check for proper fit to ensure a secure seal over the nose and mouth.
  - Ensure that clients wear a nasal cannula during meals.
  - Monitor skin and provide skin care to area covered by the mouth.

○ Partial rebreather mask (covers the client's nose and mouth)

- FiO$_2$ – 60% to 75% at flow rates of 6 to 11 L/min
- Advantages
  - The mask has a reservoir bag with no flaps, which allows the client to rebreathe up to 1/3 of exhaled air together with room air.
- Disadvantages
  - Complete deflation of the reservoir bag during inspiration causes CO$_2$ buildup.
  - The FiO$_2$ varies with the client's breathing pattern.

- This device is poorly tolerated by clients who have anxiety or claustrophobia.
- Eating, drinking, and talking are impaired.
- Use with caution for clients who have a high risk of aspiration or airway obstruction.

- Nursing Interventions
  - Keep the reservoir bag from deflating by adjusting the oxygen flow rate to keep it inflated.
  - Use with caution for clients at high risk of aspiration or airway obstruction.
  - The FiO_2 varies with the client's breathing pattern.
  - Check for proper fit to ensure a secure seal over the nose and mouth.
  - Ensure that clients use a nasal cannula during meals.
  - Make sure the reservoir does not twist or kink.

- Nonrebreather mask (covers the client's nose and mouth)
  - FIO_2 – 80% to 95% at flow rates of 10 to 15 L/min to keep the reservoir bag $^2/_3$ full during inspiration and expiration
  - Advantages
    - Delivers the highest O_2 concentration possible (except for intubation).
    - A one-way valve situated between the mask and reservoir allows clients to inhale maximum O_2 from the reservoir bag. The two exhalation ports have flaps covering them that prevent room air from entering the mask.
  - Disadvantages
    - The valve and flap on the mask must be intact and functional during each breath.
    - Poorly tolerated by clients who have anxiety or claustrophobia.
    - Eating, drinking, and talking are impaired.
  - Nursing Interventions
    - Check the valve and flap hourly.
    - Check for proper fit to ensure a secure seal over the nose and mouth.
    - Use with caution for clients who have a high risk of aspiration or airway obstruction.
    - Ensure that clients use a nasal cannula during meals.

- High-flow oxygen delivery systems deliver precise amounts of oxygen when properly fitted.
  - Venturi mask (covers the client's nose and mouth)
    - FIO_2 – 24% to 55% at flow rates of 4 to 10 L/min via different sized adaptors

- Monitor oxygenation status with pulse oximetry and ABGs.
- Apply the oxygen delivery device prescribed.
- Check the fit of the mask to ensure a secure seal over the client's nose and mouth.
- Promote good oral hygiene and provide as needed.
- Promote turning, coughing, deep breathing, use of incentive spirometer, and suctioning.
- Promote rest and decrease environmental stimuli.
- Provide emotional support for clients who appear anxious.
- Monitor nutritional status; provide supplements as prescribed.
- Monitor the client's skin integrity; provide moisture and pressure-relief devices as indicated.
- Monitor and document the client's response to oxygen therapy.
- Maintain oxygen flow as prescribed.
- Discontinue supplemental oxygen gradually.
  - Interventions
    - Monitor for signs and symptoms of respiratory depression such as decreased respiratory rate and decreased level of consciousness; notify the provider if these findings are present.
    - For respiratory distress:
      - Position the client for maximum ventilation (Fowler's or semi-Fowler's position).
      - Complete a focused respiratory assessment.
      - Promote deep breathing and use supplemental oxygen as prescribed.
      - Stay with the client and provide emotional support to decrease anxiety.
      - Promote airway clearance by encouraging coughing and oral/oropharyngeal suctioning if necessary.
- Complications and Hazards of Oxygen Therapy
  - Oxygen toxicity
    - Oxygen toxicity can result from high concentrations of oxygen (typically above 50%), long durations of oxygen therapy (typically more than 24 to 48 hr), and the client's degree of lung disease.
    - Signs and symptoms include a nonproductive cough, substernal chest pain, nasal stuffiness, dyspnea, nausea, vomiting, fatigue, headache, sore throat, and hypoventilation.

- Nursing Actions
  - Use the lowest level of oxygen necessary to maintain an adequate SaO_2.
  - Monitor the ABGs and notify the provider if PaO_2 levels are outside of the expected reference range.
  - Use an oxygen mask with continuous positive airway pressure (CPAP), bi-level positive airway pressure (BiPAP), or positive end expiratory pressure (PEEP) as prescribed while the client is on a mechanical ventilator to help decrease the amount of needed oxygen.

○ Oxygen-induced hypoventilation

- Oxygen-induced hypoventilation can develop in clients who have COPD and chronic hypoxemia and hypercarbia. Clients who have COPD rely on low levels of arterial oxygen as their primary drive for breathing. Providing supplemental oxygen at high levels can decrease or eliminate their respiratory drive.

- Nursing Actions
  - Monitor the client's respiratory rate and pattern, level of consciousness, and PaO_2 levels.
  - Provide oxygen therapy at the lowest flow that corrects hypoxemia (usually 1 to 3 L/min).
  - If the client tolerates it, use a Venturi mask to deliver precise oxygen levels.
  - Notify the provider of impending respiratory depression, such as a decreased respiratory rate and a decreased level of consciousness.

○ Combustion

- Oxygen is combustible.

- Nursing Actions
  - Post "No Smoking" or "Oxygen in Use" signs to alert others of a fire hazard.
  - Know where the closest fire extinguisher is located.
  - Educate clients and others about the fire hazard of smoking during oxygen use.
  - Have clients wear a cotton gown, because synthetic or wool fabrics can generate static electricity.
  - Ensure that all electric devices (razors, hearing aids, radios) are working well.
  - Ensure electric machinery (monitors, suction machines) are well-grounded.
  - Do not use volatile, flammable materials (alcohol or acetone) near clients who are receiving oxygen.

- Nursing Actions
  - Preparation of the Client
    - Explain the procedure to clients.
    - Establish a method for communication, such as asking yes/no questions, providing writing materials, using a dry-erase board and/or a picture communication board, or lip-reading.
  - Ongoing care
    - Maintain a patent airway.
      - Check the position and placement of tube.
      - Document the tube placement in centimeters at the client's teeth or lips.
      - Use two staff members for repositioning and resecuring the tube.
      - Apply protective barriers (soft wrist restraints) according to hospital protocol to prevent self-extubation.
      - Use caution when moving clients.
      - Suction oral and tracheal secretions to maintain tube patency.
      - Support ventilator tubing to prevent mucosal erosion and displacement.
    - Check respiratory status every 1 to 2 hr – Breath sounds, respiratory effort, and spontaneous breaths
    - Monitor and document ventilator settings hourly.
      - Rate, FiO$_2$, and tidal volume
      - Mode of ventilation
      - Use of adjuncts (PEEP, CPAP)
      - Plateau or peak inspiratory pressure (PIP)
      - Alarm settings
    - Monitor the ventilator alarms, which signal if the client is not receiving the correct ventilation.
      - Never turn off the ventilator alarms.
      - There are three types of ventilator alarms – Volume, pressure, and apnea alarms
        - Volume (low pressure) alarms indicate a low exhaled volume due to a disconnection, cuff leak, and/or tube displacement.
        - Pressure (high pressure) alarms indicate excess secretions, client biting the tubing, kinks in the tubing, client coughing, pulmonary edema, bronchospasm, and/or pneumothorax.
        - Apnea alarms indicate that the ventilator does not detect spontaneous respiration in a preset time period.

- Maintain adequate (but not excessive) volume in the cuff of the endotracheal tube.

  □ Assess the cuff pressure at least every 8 hr. Maintain the cuff pressure below 20 mm Hg to reduce the risk of tracheal necrosis.

  □ Assess for an air leak around the cuff (client speaking, air hissing, or decreasing SaO_2). Inadequate cuff pressure can result in inadequate oxygenation and/or accidental extubation.

- Administer medications as prescribed.

  □ Analgesics – Morphine and fentanyl (Sublimaze)

  □ Sedatives – Propofol (Diprivan), diazepam (Valium), lorazepam (Ativan), midazolam (Versed), and haloperidol (Haldol)

    ▸ Clients receiving mechanical ventilation may require sedation or paralytic agents to prevent competition between extrinsic and intrinsic breathing and the resulting effects of hyperventilation.

  □ Neuromuscular blocking agents – Pancuronium bromide (Pavulon), atracurium (Tracrium), and vecuronium (Norcuron)

  □ Ulcer-preventing agents – Famotidine (Pepcid) or lansoprazole (Prevacid)

  □ Antibiotics for established infections

- Reposition the oral endotracheal tube every 24 hr or according to protocol. Check for skin breakdown.

  □ Older adult clients have fragile skin and are more prone to skin and mucous membrane breakdown. Older adult clients have decreased oral secretions. They require frequent, gentle skin and oral care.

- Provide adequate nutrition.

  □ Check gastrointestinal functioning every 8 hr.

  □ Monitor bowel habits.

  □ Administer enteral feedings as prescribed.

- Continually monitor clients during the weaning process and watch for signs of weaning intolerance.

  □ Respiratory rate greater than 30/min or less than 8/min

  □ Blood pressure or heart rate changes more than 20% of baseline

  □ SaO_2 less than 90%

  □ Dysrhythmias, elevated ST segment

  □ Significant decrease in tidal volume

  □ Labored respirations, increased use of accessory muscles, and diaphoresis

  □ Restlessness, anxiety, and decreased level of consciousness

- Suction the oropharynx and trachea prior to extubation.

UNIT 3	NURSING CARE OF CLIENTS WITH RESPIRATORY DISORDERS
Section:	Diagnostic and Therapeutic Procedures

Chapter 18 Airway Management

Overview

- Maintenance of a patent airway is critical when providing care to clients, and suctioning and tracheostomy care are procedures that nurses must be knowledgeable about to ensure a patent airway.

- Whenever possible, clients should be encouraged to cough. Coughing is more effective than artificial suctioning at moving secretions into the upper trachea or laryngopharynx.

- Airway suctioning involves the use of a suction machine and catheter to remove secretions from the airway.

- A tracheotomy is a sterile surgical incision made into the trachea for the purpose of establishing an airway. A tracheostomy is the stoma/opening that results from a tracheotomy and the insertion and maintenance of a tracheostomy tube.

Suctioning

- Suctioning can be accomplished orally, nasally, or endotracheally.

- Indications

  - Diagnoses

    - Hypoxemia

  - Client presentation

    - Early signs of hypoxemia (restlessness, tachypnea, tachycardia), decreased SaO_2 levels, adventitious breath sounds, visualization of secretions, cyanosis, and absence of spontaneous cough.

- Client Outcomes

  - The client will maintain a patent airway.

  - The client will maintain a SaO_2 between 95% and 100%.

- Measures for all types of suctioning

  - Use medical aseptic technique to suction the mouth (oropharyngeal).

  - Use surgical aseptic technique for all other types of suctioning.

○ Preprocedure

- Nursing Actions

  □ Perform hand hygiene, provide privacy, and explain the procedure to clients.

  □ Don the required personal protective equipment.

  □ Assist clients to Fowler's or high-Fowler's position for suctioning if possible.

  □ Encourage clients to breathe deeply and cough in an attempt to clear the secretions without artificial suctioning.

  □ Obtain baseline breath sounds and vital signs, including SaO_2 by pulse oximeter. SaO_2 may be monitored continually during the procedure.

  □ Check that the suction equipment is working properly.

- Client Education

  □ Explain the procedure to clients whether conscious or not.

○ Intraprocedure

- Nursing Actions

  □ Open the sterile suction package.

  □ Place a sterile drape or towel on the client's chest.

  □ Set up the container, touching only the outside.

  □ Pour approximately 100 mL of sterile water or 0.9% sodium chloride (NaCl) into the container.

  □ Don sterile gloves.

    ▸ The clean/nondominant hand should hold the connecting tube; this glove protects the nurse.

    ▸ The sterile/dominant hand should hold the sterile catheter; this glove protects clients.

  □ Connect the suction catheter to the wall unit's tubing.

  □ Set suction pressure to no more than 120 mm Hg.

  □ Test the suction setup by aspirating sterile water/0.9% NaCl solution from the cup. If the unit is operating properly, continue with the procedure.

  □ Limit each suction attempt to no longer than 10 to 15 seconds to avoid hypoxemia and the vagal response. Limit suctioning to two to three attempts.

  □ Once suctioning is complete, clear the suction tubing by aspirating sterile water 0.9% NaCl solution.

- ○ Postprocedure
  - ■ Nursing Actions
    - □ Document data (vital signs, SpO_2; breath sound, how clients tolerated the procedure; and the color, consistency, and amount of secretions).
- Oropharyngeal suctioning
  - ○ Preprocedure
    - ■ Nursing Actions
      - □ Obtain baseline breath sounds and vital signs, including SaO_2 by pulse oximeter.
      - □ Use a Yankauer or tonsil-tipped rigid suction catheter for oropharyngeal suctioning.
  - ○ Intraprocedure
    - ■ Nursing Actions
      - □ Insert the catheter into the client's mouth.
      - □ Apply suction and move the catheter around the mouth, gumline, and pharynx.
      - □ Clear the catheter and tubing.
      - □ Repeat as needed.
      - □ Monitor the client's SaO_2 level.
  - ○ Postprocedure
    - ■ Nursing Actions
      - □ Replace the oxygen mask if applicable.
      - □ Store the catheter in a clean, dry place for reuse.
      - □ Allow clients to perform suctioning if possible.
      - □ Document the client's response.
- Nasopharyngeal and nasotracheal suctioning
  - ○ Preprocedure
    - ■ Nursing Actions
      - □ Perform suctioning with a flexible catheter.
      - □ Catheter size is based upon the diameter of the client's nostrils and the thickness of the secretions.

- □ Hyperoxygenate clients during equipment preparation with 100% FiO_2.

- □ Lubricate the distal 6 to 8 cm (2 to 3 in) of the suction catheter with a water-soluble lubricant.

- □ Remove the oxygen delivery device with the nondominant hand if applicable.

- ○ Intraprocedure

  - ■ Nursing Actions

    - □ Insert the catheter into the nares during inhalation.

    - □ Do not apply suction while inserting the catheter.

    - □ Follow the natural course of the nares and slightly slant the catheter downward as it is advanced.

    - □ Advance the catheter the approximate distance from the nose tip to the base of the earlobe.

    - □ Apply suction intermittently by covering and releasing the suction port with the thumb for 10 to 15 seconds.

    - □ Apply suction only while withdrawing the catheter and rotating it with the thumb and forefinger.

    - □ Clear the catheter and tubing.

    - □ Allow clients time for recovery (20 to 30 seconds) between sessions. Hyperoxygenate clients before each suctioning pass.

    - □ Repeat as necessary.

- ○ Postprocedure

  - ■ Nursing Actions

    - □ Document the client's response.

    - □ Do not reuse the suction catheter.

- ● Endotracheal Suctioning (ETS)

  - ○ Preprocedure

    - ■ Nursing Actions

      - □ Perform ETS through a tracheostomy or endotracheal tube.

      - □ Ask for assistance if necessary.

      - □ Obtain a suction catheter with an outer diameter of no more than one-half the size of the internal diameter of the endotracheal tube.

      - □ Hyperoxygenate clients using a bag-valve mask (BVM) or specialized ventilator function with a FiO_2 of 100%.

      - □ Apply a face shield and sterile gloves.

- ○ Intraprocedure
  - ■ Nursing Actions
    - □ Insert the catheter into the lumen of the airway. First remove the BVM or ventilator from the tracheostomy or endotracheal tube if indicated. Advance the catheter until resistance is met. The catheter should reach the level of the carina (location of bifurcation into the main stem bronchi).
    - □ Pull the catheter back 1 cm (0.5 inches) prior to applying suction to prevent mucosal damage.
    - □ Apply suction intermittently by covering and releasing the suction port with the thumb for 10 to 15 seconds.
    - □ Apply suction only while withdrawing the catheter and rotating it with the thumb and forefinger.
    - □ Reattach the BVM or ventilator and supply clients with 100% inspired oxygen.
    - □ Clear the catheter and tubing.
    - □ Allow time for client recovery between sessions.
    - □ Repeat as necessary.
- ○ Postprocedure
  - ■ Nursing Actions
    - □ Document the client's response.
- Complications
  - ○ Hypoxemia
    - ■ A decrease in SaO_2 or cyanosis may occur during suctioning, indicating worsening hypoxemia.
    - ■ Nursing Actions
      - □ To reduce the risk of hypoxemia:
        - ▸ Limit each suction attempt to no longer than 10 to 15 seconds.
        - ▸ Limit suctioning to two to three attempts.
        - ▸ Allow clients time for recovery 20 to 30 seconds between sessions.
        - ▸ Hyperoxygenate clients before each suctioning pass.
        - ▸ Decrease suctioning times for older adult clients.
      - □ If clients shows signs or symptoms of hypoxemia, stop the procedure.
  - ○ Anxiety
    - ■ Clients undergoing suctioning may become anxious during the procedure.

Ⓖ

■ Nursing Actions

□ Explain the procedure to all clients prior to suctioning.

□ Provide reassurance before, during, and after the procedure.

□ Maintain a calm manner.

Artificial Airways and Tracheotomy Care

- A tracheotomy is a sterile surgical incision into the trachea through the skin and muscles made for the purpose of establishing an airway.

- A tracheotomy may be performed as an emergency procedure or as a scheduled surgical procedure; it may be temporary or permanent.

- Artificial airways can be placed in the mouth (orotracheal tube), the nose (nasotracheal tube), or through a tracheostomy.

- A tracheostomy is the stoma/opening that results from a tracheotomy to provide and secure a patent airway.

  ○ Tracheostomy tubes vary in composition (plastic or metal), number of parts, size (long versus short), and shape (50 to 90° angles).

  ○ There is no standard tracheostomy sizing system; however, the diameter of the tracheostomy tube must be smaller than the trachea.

  ○ The outside cannula has a flange or neck plate that sits against the skin of the neck and has holes on each side for attaching ties around the client's neck to stabilize the tracheostomy tube.

- Advantages of a tracheostomy for long-term therapy instead of an endotracheal tube

  ○ Less risk of long-term damage to the airway

  ○ Increased client comfort because no tube is present in the mouth

  ○ Decreased incidence of pressure ulcers in the oral cavity and upper airway

  ○ Ability for clients to eat, because the tube enters lower in the airway

  ○ Ability for clients to talk

- Air flow in and out of a tracheostomy without air leakage (a cuffed tracheostomy tube) bypasses the vocal cords resulting in an inability to produce sound or speech.

- Uncuffed and fenestrated tubes that are in place or capped allow clients to speak. Clients with a cuffed tube, who can be off mechanical ventilation and breathe around the tube, can use a special valve to allow for speech. The cuff is deflated and the valve occludes the opening.

- Swallowing is possible with a tracheostomy tube in place; however, laryngeal elevation is affected and it is important to identify the client's risk for aspiration prior to intake.

Ⓜ **View Media Supplement:** Tracheal Suctioning (Image)

UNIT 3	NURSING CARE OF CLIENTS WITH RESPIRATORY DISORDERS

Section: Respiratory Systems Disorders

Chapter 19   Asthma

 Overview

- Asthma is a chronic inflammatory disorder of the airways that results in intermittent and reversible airflow obstruction of the bronchioles.

    ○ The obstruction occurs either by inflammation or airway hyperresponsiveness.

    ○ Asthma can occur at any age.

    ○ The cause of asthma is unknown; however, it may have a genetic component.

- Manifestations of asthma

    ○ Mucosal edema

    ○ Bronchoconstriction

    ○ Excessive mucus production

 View Media Supplement: Normal and Asthmatic Lung Changes (Image)

- Asthma diagnoses are based on symptoms and classified into one of the following four categories:

    ○ Mild intermittent – Symptoms occur less than twice a week.

    ○ Mild persistent – Symptoms arise more than twice a week but not daily.

    ○ Moderate persistent – Daily symptoms occur in conjunction with exacerbations twice a week.

    ○ Severe persistent – Symptoms occur continually, along with frequent exacerbations that limit the client's physical activity and quality of life.

Data Collection

- Risk Factors

  - Older adult clients have decreased pulmonary reserves due to physiologic lung changes that occur with the aging process.

    - Older adult clients are more susceptible to infections.

    - The sensitivity of beta-adrenergic receptors decreases with age. As the beta receptors age and lose sensitivity, they are less able to respond to agonists, which can result in bronchospasms.

- Subjective Data

  - Dyspnea

  - Chest tightness

  - Anxiety and/or stress

- Objective Data

  - Physical assessment findings

    - Coughing

    - Wheezing

    - Diminished lung sounds

    - Mucus production

    - Use of accessory muscles

    - Poor oxygen saturation (low SaO_2)

    - Barrel chest or increased chest diameter

  - Obtain the client's history regarding current and previous asthma exacerbations.

    - Onset and duration

    - Precipitating factors (stress, exercise, exposure to irritant)

    - Changes in medication regimen

    - Medications that relieve symptoms

    - Other medications taken

    - Self-care methods used to relieve symptoms

- ○ Laboratory Tests
  - ■ ABGs
    - □ Hypoxemia (decreased PaO_2 less than 80 mm Hg)
    - □ Hypocarbia (decreased $PaCO_2$ less than 35 mm Hg – Early in attack)
    - □ Hypercarbia (increased $PaCO_2$ greater than 45 mm Hg – Later in attack)
  - ■ Sputum cultures
    - □ Bacteria can indicate infection.
- ○ Diagnostic procedures
  - ■ Pulmonary function tests (PFTs) are the most accurate tests for diagnosing asthma and its severity.
    - □ Forced vital capacity (FVC) is the volume of air exhaled from full inhalation to full exhalation.
    - □ Forced expiratory volume in the first second (FEV1) is the volume of air blown out as hard and fast as possible during the first second of the most forceful exhalation after the greatest full inhalation.
    - □ Peak expiratory rate flow (PERF) is the fastest airflow rate reached during exhalation.
    - □ A decrease in FEV1 or PERF by 15% to 20% below the expected value is common in clients who have asthma. An increase in these values by 12% following the administration of bronchodilators is diagnostic for asthma.
  - ■ Periodic chest x-rays are used to monitor changes in the client's chest structure.

Collaborative Care

- • Nursing Care
  - ○ Position clients to maximize ventilation (high-Fowler's = 90°).
  - ○ Monitor respiratory status including watching for shortness of breath, dyspnea, and audible wheezing. An absence of wheezing may indicate severe constriction of the alveoli.
  - ○ Administer oxygen therapy as prescribed.
  - ○ Monitor clients receiving IV therapy.
  - ○ Maintain a calm and reassuring demeanor.
  - ○ Provide rest periods for older adult clients who have dyspnea. Design room and walkways with opportunities for rest. Incorporate rest into ADLs.
  - ○ Encourage prompt medical attention for infections and appropriate vaccinations.
  - ○ Administer medications as prescribed.

- Medications

  o Bronchodilators (inhalers)

    ▪ Short-acting beta$_2$ agonists, such as albuterol (Proventil, Ventolin), provide rapid relief of acute symptoms and prevent exercise-induced asthma.

    ▪ Anticholinergic medications, such as ipratropium (Atrovent), block the parasympathetic nervous system. This allows for the sympathetic nervous system effects of increased bronchodilation and decreased pulmonary secretions.

    ▪ Methylxanthines, such as theophylline (Theo-Dur), require close monitoring of serum medication levels due to a narrow therapeutic range.

    ▪ Nursing Considerations

      □ Instruct clients in proper use of MDI, DPA, or nebulizer.

      □ Albuterol – Watch clients for tremors and tachycardia.

      □ Theophylline – Monitor the client's serum levels for toxicity. Side effects will include tachycardia, nausea, and diarrhea.

      □ Ipratropium – Observe clients for dry mouth.

    (M) **View Media Supplement:** Nebulizer (Image)

    ▪ Client Education

      □ Instruct clients to use a bronchodilator inhaler 5 min prior to using an anti-inflammatory inhaler to promote bronchodilation and increased absorption of medication.

      □ Ipratropium – Advise clients to suck on hard candies to help relieve dry mouth.

      □ Teach clients to monitor heart rate.

      □ Increase water/fluid intake to decrease dry mouth and throat irritation.

  o Anti-inflammatory agents

    ▪ These are used to decrease airway inflammation, and they include:

      □ Corticosteroids, such as fluticasone (Flovent) and prednisone (Deltasone)

      □ Leukotriene antagonists, such as montelukast (Singulair), mast cell stabilizers, such as cromolyn sodium (Intal), and monoclonal antibodies, such as omalizumab (Xolair)

    ▪ Nursing Considerations

      □ Watch clients for decreased immune function.

      □ Monitor for hyperglycemia.

      □ Advise clients to report black, tarry stools.

      □ Observe clients for fluid retention and weight gain. This can be common.

      □ Monitor the client's throat and mouth for aphthous lesions (cold sores).

- Client Education
  - Encourage clients to drink plenty of fluids to promote hydration.
  - Encourage clients to take prednisone with food.
  - Instruct children to rinse mouth or gargle with warm saltwater after the use of an inhaler.
  - Instruct children and their families to watch for redness, sores, or white patches in the mouth, and report them to the provider.
- Combination agents (bronchodilator and anti-inflammatory)
  - Ipratropium and albuterol (Combivent)
  - Fluticasone and salmeterol (Advair Diskus)

- Interdisciplinary Care
  - Request respiratory services for inhalers and breathing treatments for airway management.
  - Request nutritional services for weight loss or gain related to medications or diagnosis.
  - Consider rehabilitation care for clients who have prolonged weakness and need assistance with increasing level of activity.

- Care After Discharge
  - Client education
    - If clients smoke, promote smoking cessation.
    - Advise clients to use protective equipment (mask) and ensure proper ventilation while working in environments that contain carcinogens or particles in the air.
    - Encourage influenza and pneumonia vaccinations for all clients who have asthma and especially for the older adults.
    - Teach clients how to recognize and avoid triggering agents, such as:
      - Environmental factors, such as changes in temperature (especially warm to cold) and humidity
      - Air pollutants
      - Strong odors (perfume)
      - Seasonal allergens (grass, tree, and weed pollens) and perennial allergens (mold, feathers, dust, roaches, animal dander, foods treated with sulfites)
      - Stress and emotional distress
      - Medications (aspirin, NSAIDS, beta-blockers, cholinergics)
      - Enzymes, including those in laundry detergents
      - Chemicals (household cleaners)
      - Sinusitis with postnasal drip
      - Viral respiratory tract infection

- Instruct clients how to properly self-administer medications (nebulizers and inhalers).

> (M) **View Media Supplement:** Asthmatic Breathing Metered-Dose Inhaler (Video)

- Educate clients regarding infection prevention techniques.

- Encourage regular exercise as part of asthma therapy. Remind clients to use medication prior to activity if necessary.

  □ Promotes ventilation and perfusion.

  □ Maintains cardiac health.

  □ Enhances skeletal muscle strength.

- Client Outcomes

  o The client will maintain adequate gas exchange.

  o The client will prevent acute attacks.

  o The client will have relief of symptoms.

  o The client will adhere to the medication regimen.

Complications

- Respiratory failure

  o Persistent hypoxemia related to asthma can lead to respiratory failure.

  o Nursing Actions

    - Monitor oxygenation levels and acid-base balance.

    - Assist with intubation and mechanical ventilation as indicated.

- Status asthmaticus

  o This is a life-threatening episode of airway obstruction that is often unresponsive to common treatment. It involves extreme wheezing, labored breathing, use of accessory muscles, and distended neck veins, and creates a risk for cardiac and/or respiratory arrest.

  o Nursing actions

    - Assist with emergency intubation.

    - Administer humidified oxygen.

    - Monitor IV access, ABGs and serum electrolytes.

    - Other therapies may include:

      □ Bronchodilators, epinephrine, and systemic steroid therapy.

    - Prepare clients for admission for continued management.

(A) APPLICATION EXERCISES

1. A nurse is reinforcing discharge teaching with a client who has a new prescription for prednisone (Deltasone) for asthma. Which of the following client statements indicates a need for further teaching?

    A. "I will drink plenty of fluids while taking this medication."

    B. "I will tell the doctor if I have black, tarry stools."

    C. "I will take my medication on an empty stomach."

    D. "I will monitor my mouth for cold sores"

2. A nurse is reinforcing healthy habits with a client who has asthma. Which of the following would be appropriate to include? (Select all that apply.)

    _____ Quit smoking.

    _____ Wear a mask around irritants.

    _____ Stay indoors.

    _____ Get a flu shot yearly.

    _____ Exercise regularly.

3. Two hours after arriving on the medical-surgical unit, the client develops dyspnea. SaO_2 is 91%, and the client is exhibiting audible wheezing and use of accessory muscles. Which of the following medications should the nurse expect to administer?

    A. Antibiotic

    B. Beta-blocker

    C. Antiviral

    D. $Beta_2$ agonist

4. A nurse collects data from a client for possible side effects of corticosteroid therapy for asthma. Which of the findings below are consistent with side-effects of corticosteroids?

    A. Hyperglycemia

    B. Frequent brown stools

    C. Weight loss

    D. Pink oral mucosa

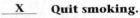

APPLICATION EXERCISES ANSWER KEY

1. A nurse is reinforcing discharge teaching with a client who has a new prescription for prednisone (Deltasone) for asthma. Which of the following client statements indicates a need for further teaching?

    A. "I will drink plenty of fluids while taking this medication."

    B. "I will tell the doctor if I have black, tarry stools."

    C. **"I will take my medication on an empty stomach."**

    D. "I will monitor my mouth for cold sores"

    The third statement, "I will take my medication on an empty stomach," indicates a need for further teaching. Prednisone can cause an upset stomach and gastric irritation, so it should be taken with food. The other options are all correct statements regarding this medication.

    NCLEX® Connection: Pharmacological Therapies, Adverse Effects/Contraindications/Side Effects/Interactions

2. A nurse is reinforcing healthy habits with a client who has asthma. Which of the following would be appropriate to include? (Select all that apply.)

__X__	**Quit smoking.**
__X__	**Wear a mask around irritants.**
_____	Stay indoors.
__X__	**Get a flu shot yearly.**
__X__	**Exercise regularly.**

    Quitting smoking, wearing a mask when working around irritants, and getting a flu shot will decrease the number and severity of asthma attacks. Instead of staying inside, it is better if the client understands what triggers the attacks. Clients with asthma should exercise regularly to promote cardiac health and muscle strength.

    NCLEX® Connection: Health Promotion and Maintenance, Health Promotion/Disease Prevention

PN ADULT MEDICAL SURGICAL NURSING

3. Two hours after arriving on the medical-surgical unit, the client develops dyspnea. SaO_2 is 91%, and the client is exhibiting audible wheezing and use of accessory muscles. Which of the following medications should the nurse expect to administer?

   A. Antibiotic

   B. Beta-blocker

   C. Antiviral

   D. Beta$_2$ agonist

   The nurse should expect to administer a beta$_2$ agonist. Beta$_2$ agonists are used for relief of acute symptoms. An antibiotic, antiviral, and beta blocker would not be indicated for this condition.

   Ⓝ NCLEX® Connection: Pharmacological Therapies, Expected Actions/Outcomes

4. A nurse collects data from a client for possible side effects of corticosteroid therapy for asthma. Which of the findings below are consistent with side-effects of corticosteroids?

   A. Hyperglycemia

   B. Frequent brown stools

   C. Weight loss

   D. Pink oral mucosa

   Hyperglycemia is a side effect of anti-inflammatory drugs. Other side effects include, black tarry stools, weight gain, fluid retention, and mouth sores. Brown stools and pink oral mucosa are expected findings. Weight gain, instead of weight loss, is a side effect of corticosteroid therapy.

   Ⓝ NCLEX® Connection: Pharmacological Therapies, Adverse Effects/Contraindications/Side Effects/Interactions

UNIT 3	NURSING CARE OF CLIENTS WITH RESPIRATORY DISORDERS
Section:	Respiratory Systems Disorders
Chapter 20	Chronic Obstructive Pulmonary Disease (COPD)

Overview

- Chronic obstructive pulmonary disease (COPD) encompasses two diseases – emphysema and chronic bronchitis. Most clients who have emphysema also have chronic bronchitis. COPD is irreversible.

- Emphysema is characterized by the loss of lung elasticity and hyperinflation of lung tissue. Emphysema causes destruction of the alveoli, leading to a decreased surface area for gas exchange, carbon dioxide retention, and respiratory acidosis.

- Chronic bronchitis is an inflammation of the bronchi and bronchioles due to chronic exposure to irritants.

- COPD typically affects middle age to older adults.

Data Collection

- Risk Factors

  o Advanced age

  o Cigarette smoking is the primary risk factor for the development of COPD.

  o Second-hand smoke

  o Alpha$_1$-antitrypsin (AAT) deficiency

  o Exposure to air pollution

- Subjective Data

  o Chronic dyspnea

- Objective Data

  o Physical Assessment Findings

    ■ Dyspnea upon exertion

    ■ Productive cough that is most severe upon rising in the morning

    ■ Respiratory acidosis and compensatory metabolic alkalosis

    ■ Crackles and wheezes

- Rapid and shallow respirations
- Use of accessory muscles
- Barrel chest or increased chest diameter (with emphysema)

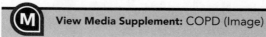
View Media Supplement: COPD (Image)

- Hyperresonance on percussion due to "trapped air" (with emphysema)
- Irregular breathing pattern
- Thin extremities and enlarged neck muscles
- Dependent edema secondary to right-sided heart failure
- Clubbing of fingers and toes
- Pallor and cyanosis of nail beds and mucous membranes (late stages of the disease)
- Decreased oxygen saturation levels (expected reference range is 95% to 100%)
- In clients who have dark-colored skin or in older adults, oxygen saturation levels can be slightly lower.

- Laboratory tests
  - An increased hematocrit level is due to low oxygenation levels.
  - Use sputum cultures and WBC counts to diagnose acute respiratory infections.
- Diagnostic procedures
  - Pulmonary function tests
    - These tests are used for diagnosis, as well as determining the effectiveness of therapy.
    - Comparisons of forced expiratory volume (FEV) to forced vital capacity (FVC) are used to classify COPD as mild to very severe.
    - As COPD advances, the FEV to FVC ratio decreases. The expected reference range is 100%. For mild COPD, the FEV/FVC ratio is decreased to less than 70%. As the disease progresses to moderate and severe, the ratio decreases to less than 50%.
  - Chest x-ray
    - Reveals hyperinflation of alveoli and flattened diaphragm in the late stages of emphysema.
    - It is often not useful for the diagnosis of early or moderate disease.

View Media Supplement: X-ray of Lungs with Emphysema (Image)

- Arterial blood gases (ABGs)
  - Hypoxemia (decreased PaO_2 less than 80 mm Hg)
  - Hypercarbia (increased $PaCO_2$ greater than 45 mm Hg)
  - Respiratory acidosis, metabolic alkalosis compensation
- Pulse oximetry
  - Clients who have COPD usually have oxygen levels less than the expected reference range of 95% to 100%
- AAT (alpha$_1$ antitrypsin) levels used to assess for AAT deficiency
  - A deficiency in a special enzyme produced by the liver that helps regulate other enzymes (that help breakdown pollutants) from attacking lung tissue.

Collaborative Care

- Nursing Care
  - Position clients to maximize ventilation (high-Fowler's is 90°).
  - Encourage effective coughing, or suction to remove secretions.
  - Encourage deep breathing and use of an incentive spirometer.
  - Administer breathing treatments and medications as prescribed.
  - Administer oxygen as prescribed.
    - Clients who have COPD may need 2 to 4 L/min of oxygen via nasal cannula or up to 40% via Venturi mask.
    - Often clients with COPD usually have chronically increased $PaCO_2$ (hypercarbia) and hypoxia which is their stimulus to breath. Therefore, these clients should only receive 1 to 2 L/min of oxygen via nasal cannula. It is important to recognize that low arterial levels of oxygen serve as the primary drive for breathing.
  - Monitor for skin breakdown around the nose and mouth from the oxygen device.
  - Promote adequate nutrition. Encourage soft, high-calorie foods to conserve energy.
  - Encourage clients to consume 2 to 3 L/day of fluid from food and beverage sources.
  - Monitor current weight and note any changes.
  - Instruct clients to practice breathing techniques to control dyspneic episodes.
    - For diaphragmatic, or abdominal, breathing, instruct clients to:
      - Take breaths deep from the diaphragm.
      - Lie on back with knees bent.
      - Rest hand over abdomen to create resistance.
      - If the client's hand rises and lowers upon inhalation and exhalation, the breathing is being performed correctly.

- For pursed-lip breathing, instruct clients to:
    □ Form the mouth as if preparing to whistle.
    □ Take a breath in through the nose and out through the lips/mouth.
    □ Not puff the cheeks.
    □ Take breaths deep and slow.
  ○ Incentive spirometry
    - This is used to monitor and promote optimal lung expansion.
    - Nursing Actions
        □ Show clients how to use the incentive spirometry machine.
    - Client Education
        □ Instruct clients to keep a tight mouth seal around mouthpiece and to inhale and hold breath for 3 to 5 seconds. As clients exhale, the needle of the spirometry machine will rise. This promotes lung expansion.
  ○ Determine the client's physical limitations and structure activity to include periods of rest.
  ○ Provide rest periods for older adult clients who have dyspnea. Design the room and walkways with opportunities for relaxation.
  ○ Provide support to clients and their families.
    - Talk about disease and lifestyle changes, including home care services such as portable oxygen.
  ○ Encourage verbalization of feelings.
- Medications
  ○ Bronchodilators (inhalers)
    - Short-acting beta$_2$ agonists, such as albuterol (Proventil, Ventolin) provide rapid relief.
    - Cholinergic antagonists (anticholinergic medications), such as ipratropium (Atrovent), block the parasympathetic nervous system. This allows for the sympathetic nervous system effects of increased bronchodilation and decreased pulmonary secretions.
    - Methylxanthines, such as theophylline (Theo-Dur), relax smooth muscles of the bronchi. These medications require close monitoring of serum medication levels due to narrow therapeutic ranges.
    - Nursing Considerations
        □ Watch clients for tremors and tachycardia when taking albuterol.
        □ Observe clients for dry mouth when taking ipratropium.
        □ Monitor the client's serum levels for toxicity when taking theophylline. Side effects will include tachycardia, nausea, and diarrhea.

- Client Education
  - Encourage clients to suck on hard candies to help moisten dry mouth while taking ipratropium.
  - Anti-inflammatory agents
    - These medications decrease airway inflammation.
    - If corticosteroids, such as fluticasone (Flovent) and prednisone (Deltasone), are given systemically, monitor for side effects (immunosuppression, fluid retention, hyperglycemia, hypokalemia, poor wound-healing).
    - Leukotriene antagonists, such as montelukast (Singulair); mast cell stabilizers, such as cromolyn sodium (Intal); and monoclonal antibodies, such as omalizumab (Xolair), can be used.
    - Nursing Considerations
      - Watch clients for a decrease in immunity function.
      - Monitor clients for hyperglycemia.
      - Advise clients to report black, tarry stools.
      - Observe clients for fluid retention and weight gain. This is common.
      - Check the client's throat and mouth for aphthous lesions (cold sores).
    - Client Education
      - Encourage clients to drink adequate fluids to promote hydration.
      - Encourage clients to take glucocorticoids (Prednisone) with food.
- Interdisciplinary Care
  - Request referral for respiratory services to assist with inhalers, breathing treatments, and suctioning for airway management.
  - Request a referral for nutritional services to assist with weight loss or gain related to medications or diagnosis. Clients may also need assistance with food preparation and delivery.
  - Request a referral for rehabilitative care if clients have prolonged weakness and need assistance with increasing level of activity.
  - Request a referral for a home health aide for assistance with ADLs. May also need assistance with obtaining home oxygen.
- Therapeutic Procedures
  - Chest physiotherapy uses percussion and vibration to mobilize secretions.
  - Raising the foot of the bed slightly higher than the head can facilitate optimal drainage and removal of secretions by gravity.

- Care after Discharge
  - Client education
    - Promote smoking cessation.
    - Instruct clients to use protective equipment, such as a mask, and ensure proper ventilation while working in environments that contain carcinogens or particles in the air.
    - Recommend influenza and pneumonia immunizations, especially for the older adult client.
    - Encourage clients to eat high-calorie foods to promote energy.
    - Encourage rest periods as needed.
    - Remind clients to perform frequent hand hygiene to prevent infection.
    - Reinforce the importance of taking medications (inhalers, oral medications) as prescribed.
    - Reinforce to clients to use oxygen as prescribed. Inform other caregivers not to smoke around the oxygen due to flammability.
    - Provide support to the clients and their families.
- Client Outcomes
  - The client will maintain adequate gas exchange.
  - The client will be able to keep a patent airway.
  - The client will remain free from infection.
  - The client will be able to stay within 10% of ideal body weight.

Complications

- Respiratory infection
  - Respiratory infections result from increased mucus production and poor oxygenation levels.
  - Nursing Actions
    - Administer oxygen therapy.
    - Monitor oxygenation levels.
    - Administer antibiotics and other medications as prescribed.
- Right-sided heart failure (cor pulmonale)
  - Air trapping, airway collapse, and stiff alveoli lead to increased pulmonary pressures.
  - Blood flow through the lung tissue is difficult. This increased workload leads to enlargement and thickening of the right atrium and ventricle.

- o Manifestations include:
    - Low oxygenation levels
    - Cyanotic lips
    - Enlarged and tender liver
    - Distended neck veins
    - Dependent edema
- o Nursing actions
    - Monitor respiratory status and administer oxygen therapy.
    - Monitor heart rate and rhythm.
    - Administer medications as prescribed.
    - Monitor clients receiving IV fluids and diuretics to maintain fluid balance.

Ⓐ **APPLICATION EXERCISES**

Scenario: A nurse is reinforcing discharge teaching to a client who has COPD. The client will be using oxygen at home.

1. Prior to discharge, the nurse monitors the client for signs of cor pulmonale. Which of the following are findings of cor pulmonale? (Select all that apply.)

   _____ Cyanotic lips

   _____ Enlarged liver

   _____ Tachypnea

   _____ Distended neck veins

   _____ Normal sinus rhythm

   _____ Insatiable appetite

2. During discharge teaching, which of the following is most important for the nurse to reinforce?

   A. Smoking cessation

   B. Equipment maintenance

   C. Incorporating rest into ADLs

   D. Anxiety management

3. The client is concerned about leaving the house while on continuous oxygen. Which of the following statements should the nurse make?

   A. "There are portable oxygen delivery systems that you can take with you."

   B. "When you go out you can remove the oxygen, just make sure you place it back on when you get home."

   C. "You probably will not be able to go out as much as you used to."

   D. "Home health services will come to you so you will not need to go out."

---

4. A nurse is collecting data from a client newly admitted with COPD. Which of the following findings should the nurse expect to find? (Select all that apply.)

   _____ Crackles and wheezes heard upon auscultation

   _____ Shortness of breath upon exertion

   _____ A nonproductive cough, especially upon rising in the morning

   _____ Clubbing of fingers and toes

   _____ Rapid and shallow breathing

   _____ Oxygen saturation of 95%

(A) APPLICATION EXERCISES ANSWER KEY

Scenario: A nurse is reinforcing discharge teaching to a client who has COPD. The client will be using oxygen at home.

1. Prior to discharge, the nurse monitors the client for signs of cor pulmonale. Which of the following are findings of cor pulmonale? (Select all that apply.)

    _X_ **Cyanotic lips**
    _X_ **Enlarged liver**
    _X_ **Tachypnea**
    _X_ **Distended neck veins**
    _____ Normal sinus rhythm
    _____ Insatiable appetite

    Cyanotic lips, enlarged liver, tachypnea, and distended neck veins are signs of cor pulmonale. Clients with cor pulmonale are more likely to have cardiac dysrhythmias and anorexia.

    (N) NCLEX® Connection: Physiological Adaptation, Basic Pathophysiology

2. During discharge teaching, which of the following is most important for the nurse to reinforce?

    A. Smoking cessation
    B. Equipment maintenance
    C. Incorporating rest into ADLs
    D. Anxiety management

    Keeping the client free from injury and harm is the first priority. Oxygen enhances combustion; therefore, all flames, including lit cigarettes and candles, should be kept away from oxygen flow. Equipment maintenance, incorporating rest into ADLs, and anxiety management are all important topics to reinforce but they are not the priority.

    (N) NCLEX® Connection: Physiological Adaptation, Illness Management

3. The client is concerned about leaving the house while on continuous oxygen. Which of the following statements should the nurse make?

   A. **"There are portable oxygen delivery systems that you can take with you."**
   B. "When you go out you can remove the oxygen, just make sure you place it back on when you get home."
   C. "You probably will not be able to go out as much as you used to."
   D. "Home health services will come to you so you will not need to go out."

   The client should be informed that there are portable oxygen systems that he can use to leave the house. This should allay his anxiety. The other responses are not appropriate options for the client.

   Ⓝ NCLEX® Connection: Physiological Adaptation, Alterations in Body Systems

---

4. A nurse is collecting data from a client newly admitted with COPD. Which of the following findings should the nurse expect to find? (Select all that apply.)

__X__	**Crackles and wheezes heard upon auscultation**
__X__	**Shortness of breath upon exertion**
_____	A nonproductive cough, especially upon rising in the morning
__X__	**Clubbing of fingers and toes**
__X__	**Rapid and shallow breathing**
_____	Oxygen saturation of 95%

   Crackles and wheezes heard upon auscultation, shortness of breath upon exertion, clubbing of the fingers and toes, as well as rapid and shallow breathing, are all expected clinical findings that the nurse should expect to find when collecting data from a client with COPD. A client with COPD may have a productive cough upon rising in the morning along with oxygen saturation below the expected reference range of 95% to 100%.

   Ⓝ NCLEX® Connection: Physiological Adaptation, Alterations in Body Systems

UNIT 3	NURSING CARE OF CLIENTS WITH RESPIRATORY DISORDERS
Section:	Respiratory Systems Disorders
Chapter 21	Pneumonia

Ⓞ Overview

- Pneumonia is an inflammatory process in the lungs that produces excess fluid. Pneumonia is triggered by infectious organisms or by the aspiration of an irritant, such as fluid or a foreign object.

- The inflammatory process in the lung parenchyma results in edema and exudate that fills the alveoli.

- Pneumonia can be a primary disease or a complication of another disease or condition. It affects people of all ages, but the young, older adult clients, and clients who are immunocompromised are more susceptible. Immobility can be a contributing factor in the development of pneumonia.

- There are two types of pneumonia. Community acquired pneumonia (CAP) is the most common type and often occurs as a complication of influenza. Hospital acquired pneumonia (HAP) has a higher mortality rate and is more likely to be resistant to antibiotics. It usually takes 24 to 48 hr from the time clients are exposed to acquire HAP.

Ⓖ - Older adult clients are more susceptible to infections and have decreased pulmonary reserves due to normal lung changes, including decreased lung elasticity and thickening alveoli.

Data Collection

- Risk Factors

Ⓖ
    o Advanced age

    o Recent exposure to viral or influenza infections

    o No history of pneumonococcal vaccination

    o Tobacco use

    o Substance abuse (alcohol, cocaine)

    o Chronic lung disease (asthma, emphysema)

    o Conditions that increase the risk of aspiration (dysphagia)

    o Mechanical ventilation (ventilator acquired pneumonia)

- ○ Impaired ability to mobilize secretions (decreased level of consciousness, immobility, recent abdominal or thoracic surgery)
- ○ Immunocompromised status
- ○ Inactivity and immobility
- Subjective Data
  - ○ Anxiety
  - ○ Fatigue
  - ○ Weakness
  - ○ Chest discomfort
  - ○ Confusion from hypoxia is the most common manifestation of pneumonia in older adult clients.
- Objective Data
  - ○ Physical assessment findings
    - Fever
    - Chills
    - Flushed face
    - Diaphoresis
    - Shortness of breath or difficulty breathing
    - Tachypnea
    - Pleuritic chest pain (sharp)
    - Sputum production (yellow-tinged)
    - Crackles and wheezes
    - Coughing
    - Dull chest percussion over areas of consolidation
    - Decreased oxygen saturation levels (expected reference range is 95% to 100%)
    - Fever, cough, and yellow-tinged sputum are often absent in clients who have pneumonia.
  - ○ Laboratory Tests
    - CBC
      - □ Elevated WBC count (may not be present in older adult clients)

- Sputum culture and sensitivity
    - Obtain specimen before starting antibiotic therapy.
    - Obtain specimen by suctioning if clients are unable to cough.
    - Older adult clients have a weak cough reflex and decreased muscle strength. Therefore, older adult clients have trouble expectorating, which can lead to difficulty in breathing and make specimen retrieval more difficult.
- ABGs
    - Hypoxemia (decreased PaO_2 less than 80 mm Hg)
- Diagnostic procedures
    - Chest x-ray
        - A chest x-ray will show consolidation (solidification, density) of lung tissue.
        - A chest x-ray is an important diagnostic tool because the early signs and symptoms of pneumonia are often vague in older adult clients.

 View Media Supplement: Pneumonia (Image)

    - Pulse Oximetry
        - Clients who have pneumonia usually have oximetry levels less than the expected reference range of 95% to 100%.

Collaborative Care

- Nursing Care
    - Position clients to maximize ventilation (high-Fowler's = 90%).
    - Encourage coughing or suction to remove secretions.
    - Administer breathing treatments and medications as prescribed.
    - Administer oxygen therapy as prescribed.
    - Monitor for skin breakdown around the nose and mouth from the oxygen device.
    - Encourage deep breathing with an incentive spirometer to prevent alveolar collapse.
    - Determine the client's physical limitations and structure activity to include periods of rest.
    - Promote adequate nutrition. Encourage soft, high-calorie foods to conserve energy.
    - Encourage fluid intake of 2 to 3 L/day from food and beverage sources to promote hydration and thinning of secretions, unless contraindicated due to another condition.
    - Provide rest periods for older adult clients who have dyspnea.
    - Reassure clients who are experiencing respiratory distress.

- Medications
  - Antibiotics
    - Antibiotics are given to destroy infectious pathogens, and commonly used antibiotics include penicillins and cephalosporins.
    - Antibiotics are often initially given via intermittent IV bolus and then switched to an oral form as the client's condition improves.
    - It is important to obtain any culture specimens prior to giving the first dose of an antibiotic. Once the specimen has been obtained, the antibiotics can be given while waiting for the results of the ordered culture.
    - Nursing Considerations
      - Observe clients taking cephalosporins for frequent stools.
      - Monitor the client's kidney function, especially older adults who are taking penicillins and cephalosporins.
    - Client Education
      - Encourage clients to take penicillins and cephalosporins with food. Some penicillins should be taken 1 hr before meals or 2 hr after.
  - Bronchodilators
    - Bronchodilators are given to reduce bronchospasms and reduce irritation.
      - Short-acting beta$_2$ agonists, such as albuterol, provide rapid relief.
      - Cholinergic antagonists (anticholinergic medications), such as ipratropium (Atrovent), block the parasympathetic nervous system, allowing for increased bronchodilation and decreased pulmonary secretions.
      - Methylxanthines, such as theophylline (Theo-Dur), require close monitoring of serum medication levels due to the narrow therapeutic range.
    - Nursing Considerations
      - Watch for tremors and tachycardia for clients taking albuterol.
      - Observe for dry mouth for clients taking ipratropium.
      - Monitor serum medication levels for toxicity for clients taking theophylline. Side effects will include tachycardia, nausea, and diarrhea.
    - Client Education
      - Encourage clients to suck on hard candies to help moisten dry mouth while taking ipratropium.
  - Anti-inflammatories
    - Anti-inflammatories decrease airway inflammation.
    - Glucocorticosteroids, such as fluticasone (Flovent) and prednisone (Deltasone), can be prescribed to help with inflammation. Monitor for immunosuppression, fluid retention, hyperglycemia, hypokalemia, and poor wound-healing.

- Nursing Considerations
  - Monitor clients for decreased immune function.
  - Monitor clients for hyperglycemia.
  - Advise clients to report black, tarry stools.
  - Observe clients for fluid retention and weight gain. This can be common.
  - Monitor the client's throat and mouth for aphthous lesions (cold sores).
- Client Education
  - Encourage clients to drink adequate fluids to promote hydration.
  - Encourage clients to take glucocorticosteroids with food.

- Interdisciplinary Care
  - Recognize the need for a referral for respiratory services to assist with inhalers, breathing treatments, and suctioning for airway management.
  - Recognize the need for a referral for nutritional assistance with clients' weight loss or gain related to medications or diagnosis.
  - Recognize the need for a referral for rehabilitation if clients have prolonged weakness and need assistance with increasing level of activity.

- Care after Discharge
  - Client education
    - Reinforce to clients the importance of continuing medications for treatment of pneumonia.
    - Encourage rest periods as needed.
    - Encourage clients to maintain hand hygiene to prevent infection.
    - Encourage clients to avoid crowded areas to reduce the risk of infection.
    - Remind clients that treatment of and recovery from pneumonia can take time.
    - Encourage immunizations for influenza and pneumonia.
    - Promote smoking cessation if clients smoke.
  - Client outcomes
    - The client is able to maintain adequate gas exchange.
    - The client is able to maintain a patent airway.
    - The client remains free from infection.

UNIT 3	NURSING CARE OF CLIENTS WITH RESPIRATORY DISORDERS
Section:	Respiratory Systems Disorders

Chapter 22   Tuberculosis

Overview

- Tuberculosis (TB) is an infectious disease caused by *Mycobacterium tuberculosis* (a non-moving, slow-growing, acid-fast rod).

- TB is transmitted through aerosolization (airborne route).

- Once inside the lung, the body encases the TB bacillus with collagen and other cells. This may appear as a Ghon tubercle (primary lesion) on a chest x-ray.

- Only a small percentage of people infected with TB actually develop an active form of the infection. The TB bacillus may lie dormant for many years before producing the disease.

- TB primarily affects the lungs but can spread to any organ in the blood.

- The risk of transmission decreases after 2 to 3 weeks of antibiotic therapy.

- Individuals who have been exposed to TB but have not developed the disease may have latent TB. This means that the mycobacterium tuberculosis is in the body, but the body has been able to fight off the infection. If not treated, it can lie dormant for several years and then become active as the individual becomes older or immunocompromised.

Data Collection

- Risk Factors

    o   Frequent and close contact with an untreated individual

    o   Lower socioeconomic status and homelessness

    o   Immunocompromised status (HIV, chemotherapy)

    o   Poorly ventilated, crowded environments (prisons, long-term care facilities)

    o   Advanced age

    o   Recent travel outside of the United States to areas where TB is endemic

    o   Substance abuse including drugs and alcohol

    o   Health care occupation that involves performance of high-risk activities (respiratory treatments, suctioning, coughing procedures)

- Subjective Data

  - Persistent cough

  - Purulent sputum, possibly blood-streaked

  - Fatigue and lethargy

  - Weight loss and anorexia

  - Night sweats and low-grade fever in the afternoon

- Objective Data

  - Physical assessment findings

    - Older adult clients often present with atypical symptoms of the disease (altered mentation or unusual behavior, fever, anorexia, weight loss).

    - Dullness heard with percussion of lungs

    - Adventitious breath sounds include bronchial breath sounds and crackles

  - Laboratory tests

    - QuantiFERON-TB Gold

      □ Blood test that detects release of interferon-gamma (IFN-g) in fresh heparinized whole blood from sensitized people

      □ Diagnostic for infection, whether it is active or latent

  - Diagnostic procedures

    - Mantoux test (should be read in 48 to 72 hr)

      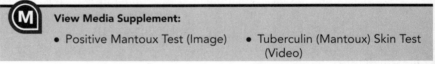

      View Media Supplement:
      - Positive Mantoux Test (Image)
      - Tuberculin (Mantoux) Skin Test (Video)

      □ An intradermal injection of an extract of the tubercle bacillus is made.

      □ An induration (palpable, raised, hardened area) of 10 mm or greater in diameter indicates a positive skin test.

      □ An induration of 5 mm is considered a positive test for immunocompromised clients.

      □ A positive Mantoux test indicates that clients have developed an immune response to TB. A client's TB test will be positive within 2 to 10 weeks of exposure to the infection. It does not confirm that active disease is present. Clients who have been treated for TB may retain a positive reaction.

      □ Individuals who have latent TB may have a positive Mantoux test and may receive treatment to prevent development of an active form of the disease.

      □ Clients who have received a Bacillus Calmette-Guerin vaccine within the past 10 years may have a false-positive Mantoux test. These clients will need a chest x-ray to evaluate the presence of active TB infection.

□ Client Education

▸ Reinforce to clients the importance of returning for a reading of the injection site by a health care provider within 48 to 72 hr.

- A chest x-ray may be ordered to detect active lesions in the lungs.

- Acid-fast bacilli smear and culture

□ A positive acid-fast test suggests an active infection.

□ The diagnosis is confirmed by a positive culture for *Mycobacterium tuberculosis*.

□ Nursing Actions

▸ Three early morning sputum samples are obtained.

▸ Wear personal protective equipment when obtaining specimens.

▸ Obtain samples in a negative airflow room.

Collaborative Care

- Nursing Care

  ○ Prevent infection transmission.

  - Wear an N95 or HEPA respirator when caring for clients who are hospitalized with TB.

 View Media Supplement: N95 Mask (Image)

  - Place clients in a negative airflow room and implement airborne precautions.

  - Use barrier protection when the risk of hand or clothing contamination exists.

  - Have clients wear a mask if transportation to another department is necessary. Clients should be transported using the shortest and least busy route.

  - Teach clients to cough and expectorate sputum into tissues that are disposed of by clients into provided sacks.

  ○ Administer medications as prescribed.

  ○ Promote adequate nutrition.

  - Encourage fluid intake and a well-balanced diet for adequate caloric intake.

  - Encourage foods that are rich in protein, iron, and vitamin C.

  ○ Provide emotional support.

- Medications

  ○ Due to the resistance that is developing against the anti-tuberculin medications, combination therapy of up to four medications at a time is presently recommended.

  ○ The current four-medication regimen includes isoniazid (Nydrazid), rifampin (Rifadin), pyrazinamide (PZA), and ethambutol hydrochloride (Myambutol).

- o Isoniazid

  - Isoniazid, commonly referred to as INH, is bactericidal and inhibits growth of mycobacteria by preventing synthesis of mycolic acid in the cell wall.

  - Nursing considerations

    - Monitor for hepatotoxicity and neurotoxicity, such as tingling of the hands and feet.

    - Administer vitamin B_6 (pyridoxine) to prevent neurotoxicity from isoniazid

  - Client education

    - Instruct clients to take medication on an empty stomach.

    - Advise clients not to drink alcohol while taking isoniazid, because it may increase the risk for hepatotoxicity.

- o Rifampin

  - Rifampin, commonly referred to as RIF, is a bacteriostatic and bactericidal antibiotic that inhibits DNA-dependent RNA polymerase activity in susceptible cells.

  - Nursing considerations

    - Observe for hepatotoxicity.

  - Client education

    - Inform clients that urine and other secretions will be orange.

    - Advise clients to report yellowing of the skin, pain or swelling of joints, loss of appetite, or malaise immediately.

    - Inform clients that this medication may interfere with the efficacy of oral contraceptives.

- o Pyrazinamide

  - Pyrazinamide, commonly referred to as PZA, is a bacteriostatic and bactericidal, and its exact mechanism of action is unknown.

  - Nursing considerations

    - Observe for hepatotoxicity.

  - Client education

    - Instruct clients to drink a glass of water with each dose and increase fluids during the day.

    - Advise clients to report yellowing of the skin, pain or swelling of joints, loss of appetite, or malaise immediately.

    - Advise clients to avoid using alcohol while taking pyrazinamide.

- o Ethambutol

  - Ethambutol, commonly referred to as EMB, is a bacteriostatic and works by suppressing RNA synthesis, subsequently inhibiting protein synthesis.

- Nursing considerations
  - Obtain baseline visual acuity tests.
  - Determine color discrimination ability.
- Client education
  - Instruct clients to report changes in vision immediately.

○ Streptomycin

- Streptomycin is an aminoglycoside antibiotic. It potentiates the efficacy of macrophages during phagocytosis. It is administered either IM or IV.
- Nursing considerations
  - Recognize that due to its high level of toxicity, this medication should only be used in clients who have multi-drug resistance TB.
  - Monitor hearing function to detect ototoxicity.
  - Report significant changes in urine output and renal function studies.
  - Administer IM or assist with intermittent IV bolus administration.
- Client education
  - Advise clients to consume at least 2 to 3 L of fluid from food and beverage sources daily.
  - Advise clients to notify the provider if hearing declines.

- Interdisciplinary Care
  - ○ Request a referral for social services if clients need assistance in obtaining prescribed medications.
  - ○ Request a referral to a community clinic as necessary for follow-up appointments to monitor medication regimen and status of disease.
  - ○ Request a referral to a nutritionist for specialized needs.

- Care After Discharge
  - ○ Client education
    - Inform family members of the need to be tested for TB.
    - Educate clients to continue medication therapy for its full duration of 6 to 12 months. Emphasize that failure to take the medications may lead to a resistant strain of TB.
    - Instruct clients to continue with follow-up care for 1 full year.
    - Inform clients that sputum samples are needed every 2 to 4 weeks to monitor therapy effectiveness. Clients are no longer considered infectious after three negative sputum cultures.
    - Encourage proper hand hygiene.

- Inform clients that contaminated tissues should be disposed of in plastic bags.

- Advise clients with active TB to wear masks when in public places.

  o Client outcomes

- The client will adhere with the medication regimen.

- The client's sputum will test negative for TB.

Complications

- Miliary TB

  o The organism invades the blood stream and can spread to multiple body organs with complications including:

    - Headaches, neck stiffness, and drowsiness (can be life-threatening)

    - Pericarditis

      □ Dyspnea, swollen neck veins, pleuritic pain, and hypotension due to an accumulation of fluid in pericardial sac that inhibits the heart's ability to pump effectively

  o Nursing actions

    - Treatment is the same as for pulmonary TB.

Ⓐ APPLICATION EXERCISES

1. A home health nurse is caring for an older adult client who has active tuberculosis (TB). She lives at home with her husband who has tested negative for TB. She is prescribed the following medication regimen: Isoniazid (INH) 250 mg PO daily, Rifampin (RIF) 500 mg PO daily, Pyrazinamide (PZA) 750 mg PO daily, Ethambutol 1 g PO daily. Which of the following statements indicates her understanding of appropriate home care measures? (Select all that apply.)

   _____ "I can substitute one medication for another since they all fight the infection."

   _____ "I need to wash my hands each time I cough or sneeze."

   _____ "I will increase my intake of citrus fruits, red meat, and whole grains."

   _____ "I am glad that I don't have to collect any more sputum specimens."

   _____ "I will remember to wear a mask when I am in a public place."

2. A client recently diagnosed with TB is prescribed the medication ethambutol (EMB). Which of the following instructions should the nurse reinforce to the client?

   A. "Your urine may turn a dark orange."

   B. "The sclera's color may change to yellow."

   C. "Watch for any changes in vision."

   D. "Take a small daily dose of vitamin B_6."

3. A client with possible TB is admitted to the unit. The client complains of night sweats, coughing up sputum that is streaked with blood, and weight loss. The priority nursing action is to

   A. start airborne precautions.

   B. obtain height and weight.

   C. collect sputum for culturing.

   D. encourage fluid intake.

Ⓐ APPLICATION EXERCISES ANSWER KEY

1. A home health nurse is caring for an older adult client who has active tuberculosis (TB). She lives at home with her husband who has tested negative for TB. She is prescribed the following medication regimen: Isoniazid (INH) 250 mg PO daily, Rifampin (RIF) 500 mg PO daily, Pyrazinamide (PZA) 750 mg PO daily, Ethambutol 1 g PO daily. Which of the following statements indicates her understanding of appropriate home care measures? (Select all that apply.)

   _____ "I can substitute one medication for another since they all fight the infection."

   __X__ **"I need to wash my hands each time I cough or sneeze."**

   __X__ **"I will increase my intake of citrus fruits, red meat, and whole grains."**

   _____ "I am glad that I don't have to collect any more sputum specimens."

   __X__ **"I will remember to wear a mask when I am in a public place."**

   The correct statements demonstrate understanding by the client on how to prevent transmission of infection and promote nutrition. All of the medications should be taken until the provider discontinues one and sputum collection should be continued to monitor response of the disease to drug therapy.

   Ⓝ NCLEX® Connection: Physiological Adaptation, Alterations in Body Systems

2. A client recently diagnosed with TB is prescribed the medication ethambutol (EMB). Which of the following instructions should the nurse reinforce to the client?

   A. "Your urine may turn a dark orange."

   B. "The sclera's color may change to yellow."

   C. **"Watch for any changes in vision."**

   D. "Take a small daily dose of vitamin B$_6$."

   Clients taking ethambutol will need to watch for changes in vision due to optic neuritis, such as blurred vision, altered color discrimination, and constriction of visual fields. Clients receiving isoniazid should take B$_6$ every day and observe for signs of hepatotoxicity. Clients receiving rifampin should expect their urine to turn a dark orange to brown; however, if the sclera turns yellow, this could indicate liver damage and should be reported to the provider.

   Ⓝ NCLEX® Connection: Pharmacological Therapies, Adverse Effects/Contraindications/Side Effects/Interactions

3. A client with possible TB is admitted to the unit. The client complains of night sweats, coughing up sputum that is streaked with blood, and weight loss. The priority nursing action is to

A. start airborne precautions.

B. obtain height and weight.

C. collect sputum for culturing.

D. encourage fluid intake.

The greatest risk is the spread of the infection to others, and based on the Centers for Disease Control and Prevention guidelines, airborne precautions for the client should be initiated first. Obtaining the client's baseline height and weight will provide information to compare future data with; obtaining a sputum specimen is necessary for diagnosis; and encouraging fluid intake will help maintain hydration. These actions are all important but are not the priority.

NCLEX® Connection: Safety and Infection Control, Standard/Transmission-Based/Other Precautions/Surgical Asepsis

UNIT 3	NURSING CARE OF CLIENTS WITH RESPIRATORY DISORDERS
Section:	Respiratory Systems Disorders

Chapter 23 Respiratory Cancers

(O) Overview

- Cancers of the respiratory system include laryngeal cancer and lung cancer. Exposure to smoke, both first and secondhand, is a major risk factor. Treatment includes surgery, radiation and/or chemotherapy.

LARYNGEAL CANCER

(O) Overview

- Men are three times more likely to be affected than women, and most cancers occur after 60 years of age.

- Most laryngeal cancers are slow-growing squamous cell carcinomas.

- Treatment includes laryngectomy, radiation, and/or chemotherapy.

Data Collection

- Risk Factors

  o Tobacco and alcohol use are the primary risk factors. Their effects are synergistic when used in combination.

  o Poor oral hygiene

  o Chronic exposure to harmful chemicals (asbestos, metals, wood, paint fumes, tar products) also increases risk.

- Subjective Data

  o Persistent or recurrent hoarseness or sore throat

  o Lump in throat, mouth, or neck

  o Dysphagia

  o Persistent, unilateral ear pain

  o Weight loss and anorexia

  o Foul breath

- Objective Data
  - Physical assessment findings
    - Hard, immobile lymph nodes in the neck (if metastasis has occurred)
    - Hoarse, raspy voice
    - Dyspnea (if tumor is in an advanced stage)
  - Laboratory tests
    - Tumor mapping may be done by taking multiple biopsy samples.
    - Mapping verifies where the tumor is located, its margins, and type.
    - Staging is done using this information.
  - Diagnostic procedures
    - X-rays of skull, sinuses, neck, and chest; CT scan; magnetic resonance imaging (MRI) scan; single photon emission computed tomography and positron emission tomography scans
      - These help to determine the extent and exact location of the tumor and level of soft tissue invasion.
    - Indirect and direct laryngoscopy
      - An indirect laryngoscopy is initially done to see if the tumor can be visualized. Clients are awake and a topical anesthetic is applied to the tongue and throat. Visualization is done using a laryngeal mirror or fiberoptic laryngoscope.
      - Direct laryngoscopy is used to visualize the tumor more closely and to obtain biopsy, which will definitively determine cell type and staging.
      - Nursing Actions
        - Prepare clients for the procedure as appropriate (informed consent, NPO).
        - Monitor clients and maintain clients' safety following the procedure (vital signs, return of gag reflex). A small amount of bloody sputum is normal.
      - Client Education
        - Inform clients that after the topical anesthetic is applied, they may feel like they cannot swallow. Encourage clients to relax and spit out secretions if they cannot be swallowed.

Collaborative Care

- Nursing Care

  o Maintain a patent airway.

    - Suction the client's mouth, throat, and airway as needed. Use aseptic technique when suctioning the airway.

    - Position clients upright to facilitate ventilation.

  o Administer medications as prescribed.

    - Crush pills to aid in swallowing.

    - Obtain elixirs when possible.

  o Provide pain relief.

    - Administer analgesics as prescribed.

    - Consider alternative/adjunctive pain relief methods, such as a humidifier, cough and throat lozenges, and salt water or antiseptic/anesthetic gargles or throat sprays.

  o Provide oral care.

  o Provide emotional support.

- Interdisciplinary Care

  o Request a referral for speech therapy to discuss communication options.

  o Suggest clients and their families attend a support group.

  o Request a referral for social services if outpatient radiation or chemotherapy is ordered.

- Surgical Interventions

  o Laryngectomy

    - May be a partial (removal of one or part of one vocal cord) or total laryngectomy (removal of both vocal cords)

      □ If the cancer is advanced, all or part of the epiglottis may need to be removed.

    - Temporary tracheostomies may be established for clients who require only a partial laryngectomy. Permanent tracheal stomas are created for clients who have undergone total laryngectomies.

    - A laryngectomy tube is inserted into the stoma immediately after the surgery. This prevents contractures from forming while the stoma is healing. Care is the same as caring for any other type of tracheostomy tube.

View Media Supplement: Laryngectomy (Image)

- Nursing Actions
  - Preoperative care
    - Provide preoperative teaching.
    - Determine the preferred alternate form of communication (dry-erase board, pen and paper, alphabet board, picture board).
    - Inform clients about care of the airway, including tracheostomy care and suctioning techniques.
    - Discuss pain control methods that will be used postoperatively.
    - Determine the client's anxiety level and provide psychological support.
  - Postoperative care
    - Elevate the head of the bed.
    - Monitor airway patency, vital signs and signs of bleeding.
    - Provide frequent suctioning, but suction gently to prevent trauma to fragile tissue. Allow clients to perform oral suctioning.
    - Place the call light within easy reach of clients.
    - Monitor the client's pain level and administer analgesics as prescribed.
    - Cleanse and dress wounds as prescribed.
    - Initiate nutritional intake as ordered. Nasogastric feedings are usually provided for the first few days until the surgical site has had a chance to heal.
    - If a nodal neck dissection ("radical neck") is done, monitor for eleventh cranial nerve damage, which may be evident as shoulder drop.

- Client Education
  - Inform clients undergoing total laryngectomies that they will lose their natural voice.
  - Tracheoesophageal fistula, esophageal speech, and electrolarynx devices are methods of speech communication that may be explored and developed following a total laryngectomy. These will allow clients to speak, but the quality of the client's speech will always sound different.

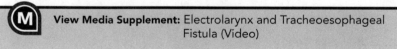

View Media Supplement: Electrolarynx and Tracheoesophageal Fistula (Video)

  ○ A cordectomy or hemilaryngectomy (excision of one vocal cord) may be performed.

- Nursing Actions

  □ An epiglottidectomy (excision of epiglottis) involves the removal of the epiglottis, leaving the trachea open to swallowed fluids.

  □ If clients had all or part of the epiglottis removed, reinforce to clients how to swallow without aspirating. Instruct clients to tuck the chin under when swallowing to prevent aspiration. Arching the tongue in the back of the mouth when swallowing may also be effective.

- Care After Discharge

  o Client education

    - Instruct clients about the importance of smoking cessation if applicable. Provide nicotine replacement as prescribed.

    - Instruct clients about appropriate techniques for stoma care and suctioning.

    - Instruct clients to:

      □ Use saline and cotton-tipped swabs to cleanse the stoma.

      □ Use a humidifier and/or saline atomizer to moisten the environment and stoma frequently during the day.

      □ Wear a buttoned cotton shirt or a stoma covering (crocheted bib, scarf or bandana) to keep dust and other particles out of the lungs.

      □ Wear a shower shield over the stoma when taking a shower.

      □ Report any signs of incisional or lung infection (fever, purulent drainage, redness, four odor, swelling).

      □ Consume a diet high in protein and calories.

      □ Avoid water sports. All other activities are allowed, but lifting may be more difficult because clients will be unable to perform the Valsalva maneuver with an open airway.

- Client Outcomes

  o The client will maintain a patent airway.

  o The client will be able to swallow food and fluids without choking.

  o The client will relearn how to speak using an alternate method of vocalization.

Complications

- Airway obstruction

  o Following a laryngectomy, clients may have copious amounts of secretions. If secretions are not removed, mucous plugs may form and can occlude a client's airway.

- o Nursing actions

  - ▪ Monitor respiratory status (SaO_2, breath sounds).

  - ▪ Maintain humidity in the form of aerosolized oxygen or room air. Supplement with a saline atomizer as needed to keep secretions thin.

  - ▪ Suction clients when needed and be sure to oxygenate prior to suctioning.

  - ▪ Encourage deep breathing and coughing to aid in secretion removal.

- Aspiration

  - o Clients who have had one vocal cord or the epiglottis removed are at an increased risk for aspiration.

  - o Aspiration may lead to the development of pneumonia.

  - o Clients who have had total laryngectomies (removal of both vocal cords) will not be able to aspirate due to the surgical separation of the trachea from the esophagus.

  - o Nursing actions

    - ▪ Maintain clients in an upright position. Have clients duck their chin down when swallowing.

    - ▪ Use thickened liquids.

    - ▪ Cut food into small pieces, and instruct clients to chew well before swallowing. Mechanical soft/pureed diets may be better tolerated than full liquid or soft diets.

    - ▪ Provide foods that can be formed into a bolus before swallowing (meats, bread).

    - ▪ Notify the provider if aspiration is suspected. Place clients on NPO status until swallowing ability can be determined.

  - o Client education

    - ▪ Have clients follow previously described methods of swallowing.

    - ▪ Instruct clients to notify the provider if symptoms of aspiration or pneumonia develop (fever, shortness of breath, fatigue).

LUNG CANCER

Overview

- Lung cancer most commonly occurs between the ages of 45 and 70.

- Prognosis of lung cancer is poor because it is often diagnosed in an advanced stage, when metastasis has occurred. Palliative care or treatment geared toward relieving symptoms is often the focus at the advanced stage.

- Bronchogenic carcinomas (arising from the bronchial epithelium) account for 90% of primary lung cancers.

- Histologic cell type determines lung cancer classification. Categories include:

  o Non-small cell lung cancer (NSCLC)

    ▪ Most lung cancers are from this category.

    ▪ They include squamous, adeno, and large cell carcinomas.

  o Small cell lung cancer (SCLC)

    ▪ Fast-growing

    ▪ Almost always associated with a history of cigarette smoking

- Staging of lung cancer is defined with the TMN system.

  o T = Tumor

  o N = Nodes

  o M = Metastasis

- Chemotherapy is the primary choice of treatment for lung cancers. It is often used in combination with radiation and/or surgery.

Data Collection

- Risk Factors

  o Cigarette smoking (both first and secondhand smoke)

  o Radiation exposure

  o Chronic exposure to inhaled environmental irritants (air pollution, asbestos, other talc dusts)

  o Older adult clients have decreased pulmonary reserves due to normal lung changes, including decreased lung elasticity and thickening alveoli. This contributes to impaired gas exchange.

  o Structural changes in the skeletal system decrease diaphragmatic expansion, thereby restricting ventilation.

- Subjective Data

  o Determine the client's history regarding use of tobacco products (cigarettes, cigars, pipes, and chewing tobacco).

  o Determine the pack-year history, which is the number of packs of cigarettes smoked per day times the number of years smoked.

  o Determine amount of exposure to secondhand smoke.

  o Chronic cough

  o Chronic dyspnea

- Objective Data
  - Clients who have lung cancer may experience few symptoms early in the disease. Monitor for signs and symptoms that often appear late in the disease.
    - Persistent cough, with or without hemoptysis (rust-colored or blood-tinged sputum)
    - Hoarseness
    - Dyspnea
    - Unilateral wheezing (if the airway is obstructed)
    - Chest wall pain
    - Chest wall masses
    - Muffled heart sounds
    - Fatigue, weight loss, or anorexia
    - Fever
    - Clubbing of fingers
  - Diagnostic procedures
    - Chest x-ray and CT scan
      - Provides initial identification of the tumor
    - Fiberoptic bronchoscopy
      - Can provide direct visibility of the tumor
      - Allows for specimen and biopsy collection
      - Nursing actions
        - Prepare clients for the procedure as appropriate (informed consent, NPO), monitor clients, and maintain client safety following the procedure (vital signs, return of gag reflex, sedatives, and supplemental oxygen as needed).
      - Client Education
        - Inform clients to have nothing to eat or drink after the procedure until the gag reflex returns.
        - Inform clients that the throat may be sore after the procedure.

Collaborative Care

- Nursing Care
  - Monitor nutritional status, weight loss, and anorexia.
    - Promote adequate nutrition to provide needed calories for increased work of breathing and prevention of infection.
    - Encourage intake of soft, high-calorie foods.
    - Encourage fluids to promote adequate hydration.

- ○ Maintain a patent airway and suction as needed.

- ○ Position clients in Fowler's position to maximize ventilation.

- ○ Determine the client's physical limitations and provide periods of rest.

- ○ Provide emotional support to clients and their families. Encourage verbalization of feelings about the disease.

- ○ Discuss the topic of death and dying with clients (if cancer is terminal), and encourage clients to express feelings.

- • Medications

  - ○ Chemotherapy agents

    - □ Chemotherapy is the treatment of choice for lung cancer. The purpose of these medications is to destroy cancer cells, as well as healthy cells, to prevent DNA formation. Platinum compounds such as cisplatin (Platinol AQ) are commonly used.

    - ■ Nursing considerations

      - □ Watch clients for a decrease in immune function.

      - □ Observe clients for nausea and vomiting.

      - □ Monitor clients for fatigue and shortness of breath.

      - □ Observe the client's throat and mouth for aphthous (cold sore) lesions.

    - ■ Client education

      - □ Encourage clients to inform the nurse if nausea and vomiting persist.

      - □ Encourage clients to use frequent oral hygiene and use a soft-bristled toothbrush. Advise clients to avoid alcohol-based mouthwashes.

      - □ Inform clients that hair loss (alopecia) occurs 7 to 10 days after treatment begins. Encourage clients to select a hairpiece before treatment starts.

  - ○ Opioid agonists (pain medication)

    - □ Morphine sulfate (MS Contin), oxycodone (OxyContin), and fentanyl (Duragesic) are opioid agents used to treat moderate to severe pain.

    - □ Use cautiously with clients who have asthma or emphysema due to the risk of respiratory depression.

    - ■ Nursing considerations

      - □ Check the client's pain level every 4 hr.

      - □ Remind clients receiving the fentanyl patch that the initial patch takes several hours to take effect. A short-acting pain medication will be administered for breakthrough pain.

      - □ Watch clients for signs of respiratory depression, especially in older adult clients. If respirations are 12/min or less, stop the medication and notify the health care provider immediately.

- ☐ Observe clients for nausea and vomiting.
- ☐ Encourage fluid intake and activity related to a decrease in gastric motility.
- ☐ Administer bronchodilators and corticosteroids to help decrease inflammation and to dry secretions.
  - ■ Client education
    - ☐ Encourage clients to suck on hard candies to help with dry mouth.
    - ☐ Encourage clients to drink adequate fluids to help prevent constipation.
    - ☐ Advise clients to increase fiber intake to help with constipation.
    - ☐ Advise clients to notify the nurse if nausea and vomiting persists.
    - ☐ Advise clients to avoid driving while taking the medication

- Interdisciplinary Care
  - ○ Request a referral for respiratory services to assist with inhalers, breathing treatments, and suctioning for airway management.
  - ○ Request a referral for nutritional services to assist with weight loss related to medications or diagnosis.
  - ○ Request a referral for rehabilitation care if clients have prolonged weakness and need assistance with increasing the level of activity.
  - ○ Recommend clients attend a support group.
  - ○ Request a referral for hospice care if indicated.

- Therapeutic Procedures
  - ■ Palliative care
    - ☐ Includes medication, radiation, and laser therapy; thoracentesis; pain management; and hospice referral and care

- Surgical Interventions
  - ○ The goal of surgery is to remove all tumor cells, including involved lymph nodes.
    - ■ Often involves removal of a lung (pneumonectomy), lobe (lobectomy), segment (segmentectomy), or peripheral lung tissue (wedge resection)
  - ○ Nursing actions
    - ■ Provide preoperative care.
  - ○ Client education
    - ■ Reinforce to clients about the surgical procedure and chest tube placement.
    - ■ Relieve client anxiety and encourage verbalization of feelings.

- Care After Discharge
  - Client education
    - Encourage clients to take rest periods as needed.
    - Encourage clients to eat high-calorie foods to promote energy.
    - Encourage clients to perform hand hygiene to prevent infection.
    - Encourage clients to avoid crowded areas to reduce the risk of infection.
    - Promote smoking cessation if clients smoke.
    - Discuss the topic of death and dying (if the cancer is terminal) with clients, and encourage clients to express their feelings.
- Client Outcomes
  - The client will be able to keep a patent airway.
  - The client will remain free from pain.
  - The client will remain free from infection.
  - The client will be able to stay within 10% of ideal body weight.

Complications

- Superior vena cava syndrome
  - Superior vena cava syndrome results from pressure placed on the vena cava by a tumor. It is a medical emergency.
  - Nursing actions
    - Monitor for signs.
      - Early signs include facial edema, edema in neck, nosebleeds, peripheral edema, and dyspnea.
      - Late signs include mental status changes, cyanosis, hemorrhage, and hypotension.
    - Notify the provider immediately.
    - Radiation and stent placement provide temporary relief. Prepare clients for the procedure (informed consent, NPO if possible, client transport).
    - Monitor the client's status (vital signs, oxygenation) during and after the procedure.
- Metastasis
  - Metastasis to the bones can cause bone pain and increase the risk of pathologic fractures.
  - Metastasis to the central nervous system can lead to changes in mentation, lethargy, and bowel and bladder malfunction.

- ○ Nursing Actions
  - Encourage clients to ambulate carefully.
  - Reorient clients as needed.
  - Provide pain management.

Ⓐ APPLICATION EXERCISES

Scenario: A nurse is admitting a client whose main symptom is hoarseness which has persisted for more than 2 months. The client reports that he has had difficulty swallowing due to the feeling that he has a lump in his throat. A CT scan reveals a subglottic lesion with lymph node enlargement on the right side of the neck. A direct laryngoscopy reveals a lesion involving both vocal cords, and biopsies confirm the presence of malignancy. The client is diagnosed with laryngeal cancer and is admitted for a total laryngectomy with a right radical neck dissection.

1. The client asks the nurse if he will be able to speak after surgery. Which of the following is an appropriate response by the nurse?

   A. "There is a good chance that you will be able to speak in your natural voice once you heal."

   B. "You will have to use a written form of communication, like a white erase board, the rest of your life."

   C. "You will not be able to speak again with your natural voice, but there are options for re-establishing speech."

   D. "The primary concern at this time is to remove the cancer, so you shouldn't worry about your voice at this time."

2. The client returns from surgery and has a tracheostomy tube in a permanent stoma and an NG tube. Which statement by the client's partner reveals the need for further reinforcement of teaching?

   A. "The NG tube will provide nourishment until his throat heals."

   B. "In 3 to 5 days the NG tube will be taken out."

   C. "He can no longer communicate using his vocal cords."

   D. "Once the NG tube comes out he can begin eating normally again."

3. The nurse is reinforcing discharge instructions. Which of the following client statements about stoma care indicates a need for clarification?

   A. "I need to avoid water sports but other sports are alright."

   B. "I can take a shower, but I need to cover the stoma with a plastic shield."

   C. "I should wear clothing that does not touch the stoma."

   D. "I have to concentrate on eating foods high in protein and calories."

4. Which of the following clients are at an increased risk for the development of laryngeal cancer? (Select all that apply.) A client who

   _____ paints houses for a living.

   _____ uses chewing tobacco.

   _____ is less than 50 years old.

   _____ smokes only cigars, not cigarettes.

   _____ lives with a spouse who smokes cigarettes.

   _____ is female.

5. A nurse is caring for a client who is in the emergency department and is reporting dyspnea and rust colored sputum that has persisted for nearly 3 weeks. Lung cancer is suspected, and diagnostic tests are ordered. A CT scan reveals the presence of a mass at the base of the bronchial tree. The client is expected to undergo a bronchoscopy. The client asks, "What is a bronchoscopy?" An appropriate response by the nurse is to reinforce that, "A bronchoscopy is when

   A. a needle is inserted between two ribs and a piece of the tumor is aspirated, and then sent to the lab."

   B. a set of x-rays is taken that provides a three-dimensional picture of the lungs and the tumor."

   C. sectional pictures of the lungs and tumor are taken utilizing magnetic fields to outline the tumor."

   D. a flexible tube is inserted through your mouth and into the lungs to see the tumor and obtain a biopsy."

6. A nurse is caring for a client in the emergency department who has advanced lung cancer. The client reports dyspnea on exertion and at rest, and her family states that she has become disoriented over the last 72 hr. A chest x-ray reveals a baseball-sized mediastinal tumor. Vital signs are: heart rate 104 beats/min, blood pressure 88/42 mm Hg, respiratory rate 38/min, temperature 37.9° C (100.2° F). The client's SaO_2 is 89% on room air. Which of the following interventions should the nurse implement first?

   A. Notify the provider.

   B. Obtain prescribed CT scan.

   C. Administer oxygen.

   D. Provide family support.

Ⓐ APPLICATION EXERCISES ANSWER KEY

Scenario: A nurse is admitting a client whose main symptom is hoarseness which has persisted for more than 2 months. The client reports that he has had difficulty swallowing due to the feeling that he has a lump in his throat. A CT scan reveals a subglottic lesion with lymph node enlargement on the right side of the neck. A direct laryngoscopy reveals a lesion involving both vocal cords, and biopsies confirm the presence of malignancy. The client is diagnosed with laryngeal cancer and is admitted for a total laryngectomy with a right radical neck dissection.

1. The client asks the nurse if he will be able to speak after surgery. Which of the following is an appropriate response by the nurse?

    A. "There is a good chance that you will be able to speak in your natural voice once you heal."

    B. "You will have to use a written form of communication, like a white erase board, the rest of your life."

    C. "You will not be able to speak again with your natural voice, but there are options for re-establishing speech."

    D. "The primary concern at this time is to remove the cancer, so you shouldn't worry about your voice at this time."

    There are several methods and devices, such as an electrolarynx and esophageal speech, which can be used to help the client re-establish communication. If these options are not satisfactory, establishment of a tracheoesophageal fistula may be done along with the insertion of a prosthesis that can simulate sounds previously made by the vocal cords.

 NCLEX® Connection: Physiological Adaptation, Alterations in Body Systems

2. The client returns from surgery and has a tracheostomy tube in a permanent stoma and an NG tube. Which statement by the client's partner reveals the need for further reinforcement of teaching?

    A. "The NG tube will provide nourishment until his throat heals."

    B. "In 3 to 5 days the NG tube will be taken out."

    C. "He can no longer communicate using his vocal cords."

    D. "Once the NG tube comes out he can begin eating normally again."

    The NG tube will be left in for 7 to 10 days in order to allow the incisions in the throat to heal. The NG tube will provide nutrition during this time. After the throat has healed, the client can eat normally again, and aspiration will be impossible since the airway and esophagus have been completely separated. Communication using the vocal cords will also be impossible since they have been removed as a part of a total laryngectomy.

Ⓝ NCLEX® Connection: Reduction of Risk Potential, Therapeutic Procedures

3. The nurse is reinforcing discharge instructions. Which of the following client statements about stoma care indicates a need for clarification?

    A. "I need to avoid water sports but other sports are alright."

    B. "I can take a shower, but I need to cover the stoma with a plastic shield."

    C. "I should wear clothing that does not touch the stoma."

    D. "I have to concentrate on eating foods high in protein and calories."

Clothing to cover the stoma is recommended in order to keep dust and other particles out of the lungs. The client needs to avoid water sports to prevent the incision from getting wet. The client needs to keep the incision site dry and intact. This prevents infection of the incision. The client may shower but needs to cover the stoma with a plastic shield and avoid direct contact with the water. It is important that the client consume foods high in protein and calories. Additional calories need to be provided for the client's increased effort to breathe. The client needs high protein to prevent infection.

(N) NCLEX® Connection: Physiological Adaptations, Alterations in Body Systems

4. Which of the following clients are at an increased risk for the development of laryngeal cancer? (Select all that apply.) A client who

    __X__   **paints houses for a living.**

    __X__   **uses chewing tobacco.**

    _____   is less than 50 years old.

    __X__   **smokes only cigars, not cigarettes.**

    __X__   **lives with a spouse who smokes cigarettes.**

    _____   is female.

Clients who use alcohol or tobacco in any form, or are exposed to harmful chemicals, including secondhand smoke, are at risk for laryngeal cancer. Men are at greater risk than women and the cancer generally shows up after 60 years.

(N) NCLEX® Connection: Health Promotion and Maintenance, Health Promotion/Disease Prevention

5. A nurse is caring for a client who is in the emergency department and is reporting dyspnea and rust colored sputum that has persisted for nearly 3 weeks. Lung cancer is suspected, and diagnostic tests are ordered. A CT scan reveals the presence of a mass at the base of the bronchial tree. The client is expected to undergo a bronchoscopy. The client asks, "What is a bronchoscopy?" An appropriate response by the nurse is to reinforce that, "A bronchoscopy is when

    A. a needle is inserted between two ribs and a piece of the tumor is aspirated, and then sent to the lab."

    B. a set of x-rays is taken that provides a three-dimensional picture of the lungs and the tumor."

    C. sectional pictures of the lungs and tumor are taken utilizing magnetic fields to outline the tumor."

    D. a flexible tube is inserted through your mouth and into the lungs to see the tumor and obtain a biopsy."

A bronchoscopy is a diagnostic test that is performed by inserting a flexible tube through the mouth and into the lungs in order to visualize and biopsy a tumor. Option A describes a needle biopsy, option B describes a CT scan, and option C describes an MRI.

(N) NCLEX® Connection: Reduction of Risk Potential, Diagnostic Tests

6. A nurse is caring for a client in the emergency department who has advanced lung cancer. The client reports dyspnea on exertion and at rest, and her family states that she has become disoriented over the last 72 hr. A chest x-ray reveals a baseball-sized mediastinal tumor. Vital signs are: heart rate 104 beats/min, blood pressure 88/42 mm Hg, respiratory rate 38/min, temperature 37.9° C (100.2° F). The client's SaO_2 is 89% on room air. Which of the following interventions should the nurse implement first?

    A. Notify the provider.

    B. Obtain prescribed CT scan.

    C. Administer oxygen.

    D. Provide family support.

The client is experiencing superior vena cava syndrome, which is a medical emergency. According to the "airway, breathing, circulation" approach to client care, administering oxygen is the most important intervention for the nurse to take. Notifying the provider, obtaining a CT scan, and providing family support are all interventions.

(N) NCLEX® Connection: Physiological Adaptation, Medical Emergencies

UNIT 3	NURSING CARE OF CLIENTS WITH RESPIRATORY DISORDERS
Section:	Respiratory Systems Disorders
Chapter 24	Respiratory Emergencies

Overview

- Respiratory emergencies place clients at risk for decreased cardiac output. Respiratory emergencies include pulmonary embolism, spontaneous and tension pneumothorax, hemothorax, acute respiratory failure and respiratory distress syndrome.

PULMONARY EMBOLISM

Overview

- A pulmonary embolism (PE) occurs when a substance (solid, gaseous, or liquid) enters venous circulation and forms a blockage in the pulmonary vasculature.

- Emboli originating from deep vein thrombosis (DVT) are the most common cause. Tumors, bone marrow, amniotic fluid, and foreign matter can also become emboli.

 View Media Supplement: Pulmonary Embolism (Image)

- Increased hypoxia to pulmonary tissue and impaired blood flow can result from a large embolus. A PE is a medical emergency.

Data Collection

- Risk Factors

  - Long-term immobility

  - Oral contraceptive use and estrogen therapy

  - Pregnancy

  - Tobacco use

  - Hypercoagulability (elevated platelet count)

  - Obesity

  - Surgery (especially orthopedic surgery of the lower extremities or pelvis)

  - Heart failure or chronic atrial fibrillation

- o Autoimmune hemolytic anemia (sickle cell)

- o Long bone fractures

(G)

- o Advanced age

- o Older adult clients have decreased pulmonary reserves due to normal lung changes, including decreased lung elasticity and thickening alveoli. Older adult clients can decompensate more quickly.

- o Certain pathological conditions and procedures that predispose clients to DVT formation (peripheral vascular disease, hypertension, hip and knee orthoplasty) are more prevalent in older adults.

- o Many older adult clients experience decreased physical activity levels, thus predisposing them to DVT formation and pulmonary emboli.

- Subjective Data

  - o Anxiety

  - o Feelings of impending doom

  - o Pressure in chest

  - o Pain upon inspiration

  - o Dyspnea and air hunger

  - o Cough

- Objective Data

  - o Physical assessment findings

    - Pleurisy

    - Tachycardia

    - Hypotension

    - Tachypnea

    - Adventitious breath sounds (crackles) and cough

    - Heart murmur in S_3 and S_4

    - Diaphoresis

    - Decreased oxygen saturation levels (the expected reference range is 95% to 100%) – low SaO_2

    - Petechiae (red dots under the skin) and cyanosis

    - Pleural effusion (fluid in the lungs)

    - Low-grade fever

- ○ Laboratory tests
  - ▪ ABG analysis
    - □ $PaCO_2$ levels are low (the expected reference range is 35 to 45 mm Hg) due to initial hyperventilation (respiratory alkalosis).
    - □ As hypoxemia progresses, respiratory acidosis occurs.
  - ▪ CBC analysis
    - □ D-dimer
      - ‣ Is elevated above expected reference range in response to clot formation and release of fibrin degradation products (the expected reference range is 0.43 to 2.33 mcg/mL).
- ○ Diagnostic procedures
  - ▪ Chest x-ray and computed tomography (CT) scan
    - □ These provide initial identification of a PE. A CT scan is most commonly used. A chest x-ray can show a large PE.
  - ▪ Ventilation and perfusion scan (V/Q scan)
    - □ Images show the circulation of air and blood in the lungs and can detect a PE.
  - ▪ Pulmonary angiography
    - □ This is the most thorough test to detect a PE, but it is invasive and costly. A catheter is inserted into the vena cava to visually see a PE.
    - □ Pulmonary angiography is a higher risk procedure than a V/Q scan.
    - □ Nursing actions
      - ‣ Verify that informed consent has been obtained.
      - ‣ Monitor the client's status (vital signs, SaO_2, anxiety, bleeding with angiography) after the procedure.

Collaborative Care

- • Nursing Care
  - ○ Administer oxygen therapy as prescribed to relieve hypoxemia and dyspnea.
    - ▪ Position clients to maximize ventilation (high-Fowler's = 90%)
  - ○ Monitor clients receiving IV fluids.
  - ○ Administer medications as prescribed.
  - ○ Provide emotional support and comfort to control client anxiety.
  - ○ Monitor changes in level of consciousness and mental status.

- Medications
  - Anticoagulants – Enoxaparin (Lovenox), heparin, and warfarin (Coumadin)
    - Anticoagulants are used to prevent clots from getting larger or other clots from forming.
    - Nursing considerations
      - Check for contraindications (active bleeding, peptic ulcer disease, history of stroke, recent trauma).
      - Monitor bleeding times – Prothrombin time (PT) and international normalized ratio (INR) for warfarin, partial thromboplastin time (aPTT) for heparin, and complete blood count (CBC)
      - Monitor for side effects of anticoagulants (thrombocytopenia, anemia, hemorrhage).
  - Thrombolytic therapy – Alteplase (Activase) and streptokinase (Streptase)
    - Used to dissolve blood clots and restore pulmonary blood flow
    - Similar side effects and contraindications as anticoagulants
    - Nursing considerations
      - Check for contraindications (known bleeding disorders, uncontrolled hypertension, active bleeding, peptic ulcer disease, history of stroke, recent trauma or surgery, pregnancy).
      - Monitor for evidence of bleeding, thrombocytopenia, and anemia.
- Interdisciplinary Care
  - Request a referral for respiratory services for oxygen therapy, breathing treatments, and ABGs.
    - If clients are homebound, set up home care services to perform weekly blood draws.
    - Request a referral for social services to supply portable oxygen for clients who have severe dyspnea.
- Surgical Interventions
  - Embolectomy
    - Surgical removal of embolus
    - Nursing actions
      - Prepare clients for the procedure (NPO status, informed consent).
      - Monitor postoperatively (vital signs, SaO_2, incision drainage, pain management).

- ○ Vena cava filter
  - □ Insertion of a filter in the vena cava to prevent further emboli from reaching the pulmonary vasculature
  - ■ Nursing actions
    - □ Prepare clients for the procedure (NPO status, informed consent).
    - □ Monitor postoperatively (vital signs, SaO₂, incision drainage, pain management).

- Care After Discharge
  - ○ Client education
    - ■ Promote smoking cessation if clients smoke.
    - ■ Encourage clients to avoid long periods of immobility.
    - ■ Encourage physical activity such as walking.
    - ■ Encourage clients to wear compression stockings to promote circulation.
    - ■ Encourage clients to avoid crossing their legs.
    - ■ Advise clients to adhere to a schedule for monitoring PT and INR, follow instructions regarding medication dosage adjustments (for clients on warfarin), and adhere with the need for weekly blood draws.
    - ■ Remind clients of the increased risk for bruising and bleeding.
      - □ Instruct clients to avoid taking aspirin products, unless specified by health care provider.
      - □ Encourage clients to check mouth and skin daily for bleeding and bruising.
      - □ Encourage clients to use electric shavers and soft-bristled toothbrushes.

- Client Outcomes
  - ○ The client will adhere with anticoagulant therapy.
  - ○ The client will maintain adequate gas exchange.
  - ○ The client will be free from severe bleeding incidences.
  - ○ The client will be pain-free.
  - ○ The client will maintain an appropriate weight for height and body frame.

Complications

- Hemorrhage
  - ○ Receiving anticoagulant therapy increases the risk for bleeding.

- o Nursing Actions
  - Check for oozing, bleeding, or bruising from injection and surgical sites.
  - Monitor for internal bleeding (measure abdominal girth and abdominal or flank pain).
  - Monitor cardiovascular status (blood pressure, heart rate and rhythm).
  - Monitor CBC (hemoglobin, hematocrit, platelets) and bleeding times (PT, aPTT, INR).
  - Provide care for clients receiving IV fluids and blood products.
  - Test stools, urine, and vomit for occult blood.

PNEUMOTHORAX AND HEMOTHORAX

Overview

- A pneumothorax is the presence of air or gas in the pleural space that causes lung collapse.

- A tension pneumothorax occurs when air enters the pleural space during inspiration through a one-way valve and is not able to exit upon expiration. The trapped air causes pressure on the heart and the lung. As a result, the increase in pressure compresses blood vessels and limits venous return, leading to a decrease in cardiac output. Death can be a result if not treated immediately.

  - o As a result of a tension pneumothorax, air and pressure continue to rise in the pleural cavity, which cause a mediastinal shift.

- A hemothorax is an accumulation of blood in the pleural space.

- A spontaneous pneumothorax can occur when there has been no trauma. A small bleb on the lung ruptures and air enters the pleural space.

Data Collection

- Risk Factors

  - o Blunt chest trauma

  - o Penetrating chest wounds

  - o Closed/occluded chest tube

  - o Older adult clients have decreased pulmonary reserves due to normal lung changes, including decreased lung elasticity and thickening alveoli.

  - o Older adult clients are more susceptible to infections.

- Subjective Data

  - o Anxiety

  - o Pleuritic pain

- Objective Data
  - Physical assessment findings
    - Signs of respiratory distress (tachypnea, tachycardia, hypoxia, cyanosis, dyspnea, and use of accessory muscles)
    - Tracheal deviation to the unaffected side (tension pneumothorax)
    - Reduced or absent breath sounds on the affected side
    - Asymmetrical chest wall movement
    - Hyperresonance on percussion due to trapped air (pneumothorax)
    - Dull percussion (hemothorax)
    - Subcutaneous emphysema (air accumulating in subcutaneous tissue)
  - Laboratory tests
    - ABGs
      - Hypoxemia (PaO_2 less than 80 mm Hg)
  - Diagnostic procedures
    - Chest x-ray
      - Used to confirm pneumothorax or hemothorax

View Media Supplement:
- Pneumothorax (Image)
- Hemothorax (Image)

    - Thoracentesis may be used to confirm hemothorax.
      - Thoracentesis is the surgical perforation of the chest wall and pleural space with a large-bore needle.
      - Nursing actions
        - Verify that informed consent has been obtained.
        - Make sure clients understand the importance of remaining still during the procedure.
        - Assist with client positioning and specimen transport. Monitor the client's status (vital signs, SaO_2, injection site). Assist the client to the edge of the bed and to lean over a bedside table.
        - Inform clients they will feel discomfort when the local anesthetic solution is injected, and when the needle is inserted into the lung, some pressure may be felt, but no pain.

Collaborative Care

- Nursing Care

  o Administer oxygen therapy.

  o Check ABGs, SaO$_2$, CBC, and chest x-ray results.

  o Position clients to maximize ventilation (high-Fowler's = 90%).

  o Provide emotional support to clients and their families.

  o Monitor chest tube drainage.

  o Administer medications as prescribed.

  o Encourage prompt medical attention when signs of infection occur.

- Medications

  o Benzodiazepines

    ▪ Lorazepam (Ativan) or midazolam (Versed) may be used to decrease the client's anxiety.

    ▪ Nursing considerations

      □ Monitor the client's vital signs (benzodiazepines may cause hypotension and respiratory distress).

    ▪ Client education

      □ Remind clients that medications may cause drowsiness.

  o Opioid agonists

      □ Morphine sulfate and fentanyl (Duragesic) are opioid agents used to treat moderate to severe pain.

    ▪ Nursing considerations

      □ Use cautiously with clients who have asthma or emphysema, due to the risk of respiratory depression.

      □ Check the client's pain level every 4 hr.

      □ Remind clients who are receiving the fentanyl patch that the initial patch takes several hours to take effect. A short-acting pain medication will be administered for breakthrough pain.

      □ Watch clients, especially older adults, for signs of respiratory depression. If respirations are 12/min or less, stop the medication and notify the provider immediately.

      □ Monitor the client's vital signs closely for signs of hypotension and decreased respirations.

    ▪ Client education

      □ Remind clients that medication may cause drowsiness.

- Interdisciplinary Care

  o Request a referral for respiratory services to assist with inhalers, breathing treatments, suctioning for airway management and chest tube management.

  o Request a referral for social services and home health care to assist with ADLs and home portable oxygen.

  o Request a referral for rehabilitation care if clients have prolonged weakness and need assistance with an increasing level of activity.

- Surgical Interventions

  o Chest tube insertion

    ▪ Chest tubes are inserted in the pleural space to drain fluid, blood, or air; re-establish a negative pressure; facilitate lung expansion; and restore normal intrapleural pressure.

    ▪ Nursing actions

      □ Verify informed consent, gather supplies, monitor the client's status (vital signs, SaO_2, chest tube drainage), report abnormalities to the health care provider, and administer pain medications.

      □ Continually monitor vital signs and the client's response to the procedure.

      □ Monitor chest tube placement and function.

- Care After Discharge

  o Client education

    ▪ Encourage clients to take rest periods as needed.

    ▪ Remind clients to use proper hand hygiene to prevent infection.

    ▪ Encourage immunizations for influenza as well as pneumonia.

    ▪ Remind clients that recovery from a pneumothorax/hemothorax may be lengthy.

    ▪ Encourage smoking cessation if clients currently smoke.

    ▪ Stress the importance of follow-up care and instruct clients to report the following to the provider:

      □ Upper respiratory infection

      □ Fever

      □ Cough

      □ Difficulty breathing

      □ Sharp chest pain

- Client Outcomes

  o The client will maintain a patent airway.

  o The client will maintain adequate gas exchange.

- o   The client will remain free from pain.

- o   The client will remain free from infection.

- o   The client will remain free from anxiety.

- o   The client will gradually increase exercise and activity to previous levels.

Complications

- Decreased cardiac output

  - o   The amount of blood pumped by the heart is decreased.

  - o   This is a result of intrathoracic pressures rising.

  - o   Hypotension develops.

  - o   Nursing actions

    - Assist with care of clients receiving IV fluids and blood products.

    - Monitor heart rate and rhythm.

    - Monitor intake and output (chest tube drainage).

RESPIRATORY FAILURE

Overview

- Acute respiratory failure (ARF)

  - o   ARF is caused by failure to adequately ventilate and/or oxygenate.

  - o   Ventilatory failure is due to a mechanical abnormality of the lungs or chest wall, impaired muscle function (the diaphragm), or a malfunction in the respiratory control center of the brain.

  - o   Oxygenation failure can result from a lack of perfusion to the pulmonary capillary bed (a pulmonary embolism) or a condition that alters the gas exchange medium (pulmonary edema, pneumonia).

  - o   Both inadequate ventilation and oxygenation can occur in individuals with diseased lungs (asthma, emphysema). Diseased lung tissue can cause oxygenation failure and increased work of breathing, eventually resulting in respiratory muscle fatigue and ventilatory failure.

- Acute respiratory distress syndrome (ARDS)

  - o   ARDS is a state of acute respiratory failure with a high mortality rate.

  - o   A systemic inflammatory response injures the alveolar-capillary membrane. It becomes permeable to large molecules, and the lung space is filled with fluid.

  - o   A reduction in surfactant weakens the alveoli, which causes collapse or filling of fluid, leading to worsening edema.

- Severe acute respiratory syndrome (SARS)

  - SARS is the result of a viral infection from a mutated strain of the corona viruses, a group of viruses that also cause the common cold.

  - The virus invades the pulmonary tissue, which leads to an inflammatory response.

  - The virus is spread easily through airborne droplets from sneezing, coughing, or talking.

Data Collection

- Risk Factors

  - ARF

  - Ventilatory failure

    - COPD

    - Pulmonary embolism and pneumothorax

    - ARDS

    - Asthma

    - Pulmonary edema

    - Fibrosis of lung tissue

    - Neuromuscular disorders, (multiple sclerosis, Guillain-Barré syndrome), spinal cord injuries, and cerebrovascular accident that impair the client's rate and depth of respiration

    - Elevated intracranial pressure (closed-head injuries, cerebral edema, hemorrhagic stroke)

  - Oxygenation failure

    - Pneumonia

    - Hypoventilation

    - Hypovolemic shock

    - Pulmonary edema

    - Low hemoglobin

    - Low concentrations of oxygen (carbon monoxide poisoning, high altitude, smoke inhalation)

  - ARDS

    - May result from localized lung damage or from the effects of other systemic problems:

      - Aspiration

      - Pulmonary emboli (fat, amniotic fluid)

      - Pneumonia and other pulmonary infections

- □ Sepsis
- □ Near-drowning accident
- □ Trauma
- □ Damage to the CNS
- □ Smoke or toxic gas inhalation
- □ Drug ingestion/overdose (heroin, opioids, salicylates)
- ○ SARS
  - Exposure to an infected individual
  - Immunocompromised individuals (chemotherapy, AIDS)
- ○ Subjective data
  - Shortness of breath
  - Dyspnea with or without exertion
  - Orthopnea (difficulty breathing while laying flat)
- ○ Objective data
  - Physical assessment findings
    - □ Dyspnea
    - □ Rapid, shallow breathing
    - □ Cyanotic, mottled, dusky skin
    - □ Tachycardia
    - □ Hypotension
    - □ Substernal or suprasternal retractions
    - □ Decreased SaO_2 (less than 90%), may be despite administration of 100% oxygen
    - □ Adventitious breath sounds (wheezing, rales)
    - □ Cardiac arrhythmias
    - □ Confusion
    - □ Lethargy
- ○ Laboratory tests
  - ABG sample
  - Room air, PaO_2 less than 60 mm Hg, SaO_2 less than 90%
  - $PaCO_2$ greater than 50 mm Hg and pH less than 7.30 (hypoxemia, hypercarbia)
  - Sputum culture (used to rule out or diagnose an infection)
  - CBC (elevated WBC count may indicate infection or inflammation)

- Diagnostic procedures
  - Chest x-ray
    - Results may include:
      - Pulmonary edema (ARF, ARDS)
      - Cardiomegaly (ARF)
      - Diffuse infiltrates and white-out or ground-glass appearance (ARDS)
      - Infiltrates (SARS)
    - Nursing actions
      - Assist with client positioning before and after the x-ray.
      - Interpret and communicate the results to the appropriate personnel in a timely manner.
  - Electrocardiogram (ECG)
    - Used to rule out cardiac involvement

Collaborative Care

- Nursing Care

  - Maintain a patent airway and monitor respiratory status every hour as needed.

  - Continually monitor vital signs, including SaO_2.

  - Suction clients as needed. Oxygenate before suctioning secretions to prevent further hypoxemia.

  - Observe and document sputum color, amount, and consistency.

  - Mechanical ventilation is often required. Use positive-end expiratory pressure (PEEP) to prevent alveolar collapse during expiration. Follow facility protocol for monitoring and documenting ventilator settings.

  - Monitor for pneumothorax (a high PEEP may cause the lungs to collapse).

  - Obtain ABGs as prescribed and following each ventilator setting adjustment.

  - Maintain continuous ECG monitoring for changes that may indicate increased hypoxemia, especially when repositioning and applying suction.

  - Position clients to facilitate ventilation and perfusion.

  - Prevent infection
    - Perform frequent hand hygiene.
    - Use appropriate suctioning technique.
    - Provide oral care every 2 hr and as needed.
    - Wear protective clothing (gown, gloves, mask) when appropriate.

- o Promote nutrition
  - Monitor bowel sounds and elimination patterns.
  - Obtain daily weights.
  - Record urine output.
  - Administer enteral feedings as prescribed.
  - Elevate the head of the bed 30° to 45°.
    - □ Confirm nasogastric (NG) tube placement prior to feeding.
- o Provide emotional support to clients and their families.
  - Encourage verbalization of feelings.
  - Provide alternative communication means (dry-erase board, pen and paper).
- Medications

PHARMACOLOGIC AGENTS	ACTIONS	NURSING CONSIDERATIONS
Benzodiazepines • Lorazepam (Ativan) • Midazolam (Versed)	• Reduces anxiety and resistance to ventilation and decreases oxygen consumption	• Monitor respirations on clients who are not ventilated. • Monitor blood pressure and SaO_2. • Use cautiously in conjunction with opioid narcotics.
General anesthesia • Propofol (Diprivan)	• Used to induce and maintain anesthesia • May be used to sedate clients who are to be placed on mechanical ventilation	• Contraindicated for clients with hyperlipidemia and egg allergies. • Monitor clients who are intubated and receiving mechanical ventilation. • Monitor ECG, blood pressure, and sedation levels.
Opioid analgesics • Morphine sulfate • Fentanyl citrate (Sublimaze)	• Provides pain management	• Monitor respirations on clients who are not ventilated. • Monitor blood pressure, heart rate, and SaO_2. • Monitor ABGs (hypercapnia can result from depressed respirations). • Use cautiously in conjunction with hypnotic sedatives. • Check the client's pain level and response to medication. • Document the client's pain level. • Have naloxone hydrochloride (Narcan) and resuscitation equipment available for severe respiratory depression in clients who are not receiving ventilation.

PHARMACOLOGIC AGENTS	ACTIONS	NURSING CONSIDERATIONS
Neuromuscular blocking agents • Vecuronium (Norcuron)	• Facilitate ventilation and decrease oxygen consumption • Often used with painful ventilatory modes (inverse ratio ventilation and PEEP)	• Given only to clients that are intubated and ventilated. • Monitor ECG, blood pressure, and muscle strength. • Give pain medication and sedatives with neuromuscular blocking agents. • Neuromuscular blocking agents do not sedate or relieve pain (clients may be awake and frightened). • Have neostigmine methylsulfate (Prostigmin) and atropine sulfate (Atropair) available to reverse the effects of the neuromuscular blocking agent. • Have resuscitation equipment available. • Reassure clients that paralysis is medication-induced. • Explain all procedures to clients.
Corticosteroids • Cortisone acetate (Cortistan) • Methylprednisolone sodium succinate (Solu-Medrol) • Dexamethasone sodium phosphate (Decadron)	• Reduce WBC migration, decrease inflammation, and help stabilize the alveolar-capillary membrane during ARDS	• Discontinue the medication gradually. • Administer with an anti-ulcer medication to prevent peptic ulcer formation. • Monitor weight and blood pressure. • Monitor glucose and electrolytes. • Advise clients to take oral doses with food and avoid stopping the medication suddenly.
Antibiotics sensitive to cultured organism(s) • Vancomycin (Vancocin)	• Treats identified organisms	• Culture sputum prior to administration of first dose. • Monitor for a hypersensitivity reaction. • Advise client to take oral doses with food and finish the prescribed dose.

- Interdisciplinary Care
  - Respiratory therapy
    - The respiratory therapist typically manages the ventilator, adjusts the settings, and provides chest physical therapy to improve ventilation and chest expansion.
    - The respiratory therapist may also suction the endotracheal tube and administer inhalation medications, such as bronchodilators.
  - Physical therapy
    - Indicated for extended ventilatory support and rehabilitation

- o Nutritional therapy
  - Enteral or parenteral feeding
  - Nutritional support following extubation
- Therapeutic Procedures
  - o Intubation and mechanical ventilation
    - Artificial airway insertion with mechanical ventilation
    - Nursing actions
      - □ Monitor ECG, SaO$_2$, breath sounds, and color.
      - □ Sedate as needed.
      - □ Provide reassurance to calm clients.
      - □ Have suction equipment, manual resuscitation bag, and facemask available at all times.
      - □ Suction secretions as needed.
      - □ Preintubation
        - ▸ Oxygenate with 100% oxygen.
        - ▸ Assist ventilation with manual resuscitation bag and facemask.
        - ▸ Have emergency resuscitation equipment readily available.
      - □ Postintubation
        - ▸ Check bilateral breath sounds, symmetrical chest movement, and chest x-ray to confirm placement of the endotracheal tube.
        - ▸ Secure the endotracheal tube per institutional guidelines.
        - ▸ Periodically check the balloon cuff for air leaks.
      - □ PEEP
        - ▸ Positive pressure is applied at the end of expiration to keep the alveoli expanded.
        - ▸ PEEP is added to the ventilator setting to increase oxygenation and improve lung expansion.
    - Client education
      - □ Explain all procedures to clients.
      - □ Reassure and calm clients.
      - □ Explain to clients and their families that clients will be unable to speak while the endotracheal tube is in place.

- o Kinetic therapy
  - A special kinetic bed that rotates laterally and alters client positioning to reduce atelectasis and improve ventilation.
  - Nursing actions
    - □ Begin slowly and gradually increase the degree of rotation as tolerated.
    - □ Monitor ECG, SaO_2, breath sounds, and blood pressure.
    - □ Stop rotation if clients become distressed.
    - □ Provide routine skin care to prevent breakdown.
    - □ Sedate as needed.
  - Client education
    - □ Explain all procedures to clients.
- Client Outcomes
  - o The client will be able to breathe independently with no respiratory assistance.
  - o The client will be able to maintain an SaO_2 greater than 90% on room air.
  - o The client will be free of infection.
  - o The client will maintain optimal physical and mental functioning.

Complications

- o Aspiration pneumonia
  - Nursing actions
    - □ Check the cuff on the endotracheal tube for leaks.
    - □ Check suction contents for gastric secretions.
    - □ Verify NG tube placement.
- o Infection
  - Nursing actions
    - □ Prevent infection by using proper hand hygiene and suctioning technique.
    - □ Monitor color, amount, and consistency of secretions.
- o Blocked endotracheal tube
  - The high-pressure alarm on the ventilator may indicate a blocked endotracheal tube.
  - Nursing Actions
    - □ Suction secretions to relieve a mucous plug or insert an oral airway to prevent biting on the tube.

- o Immobilization
  - ▪ Can result in muscle atrophy, pneumonia, and pressure sores
  - ▪ Nursing Actions
    - □ Reposition and suction every 2 hr.
    - □ Provide routine skin care.
    - □ Implement range-of-motion exercises to prevent muscle atrophy.

APPLICATION EXERCISES

1. Which of the following clients are at risk for a pulmonary embolism (PE)? (Select all that apply.) A client who

    _____ is taking birth control pills.

    _____ is postmenopausal.

    _____ has a fractured femur.

    _____ smokes one pipe daily.

    _____ is a marathon runner.

    _____ has chronic atrial fibrillation.

2. A nurse is caring for a middle adult female client who is admitted to the coronary care unit with acute dyspnea and diaphoresis. The client states that she is anxious because she feels like she can't get enough air. Vital signs are: heart rate 117 beats/min, respiratory rate 38/min, temperature 38.4° C (101.2° F), and blood pressure 100/54 mm Hg. Which of the following is the priority nursing action?

    A. Administer oxygen therapy to the client.

    B. Obtain an ABG sample from the client.

    C. Maintain the client on bed rest.

    D. Transfer the client for a CT scan.

3. A nurse is assisting with the care of a client who has a pulmonary embolus and is to start a prescription for heparin by continuous IV infusion. Which of the following client statements poses an immediate concern for the nurse?

    A. "I am allergic to morphine."

    B. "I take antacids several times a day."

    C. "I had a blood clot in my leg several years ago."

    D. "It hurts to take a deep breath."

4. A young adult male client is admitted to the medical unit with a gunshot wound to the chest. Vital signs are: blood pressure 108/55 mm Hg, heart rate 124 beats/min, respiratory rate 36/min, temperature 38.6° C (101.4° F), and SaO_2 95% on 15 L/min by a nonrebreather mask. He reports dyspnea and pain. The nurse reassesses the client 30 min later. Which of the data should be reported to the charge nurse? (Select all that apply.)

    _____ SaO_2 of 90%

    _____ Tracheal deviation

    _____ Blood pressure 104/54 mm Hg

    _____ Heart rate 142 beats/min

    _____ Hemoptysis

5. Which of the following clients are at risk for the development of acute respiratory distress syndrome (ARDS)? (Select all that apply.) A client

_____ who received 2 min of CPR following a near-drowning.

_____ with coronary artery bypass grafts and two chest tubes.

_____ with a hemoglobin level of 14.5 mg/dL.

_____ with pancreatitis.

_____ with dysphagia.

_____ with a sinus infection.

6. In reviewing the plan of care for a client who has severe acute respiratory syndrome (SARS), which of the following is an appropriate action? (Select all that apply.)

_____ Antibiotics

_____ Supplemental oxygen

_____ Antiviral medications

_____ Bronchodilators

_____ Mechanical ventilation

7. An older adult client with postoperative pain has been prescribed morphine. Which of the following nursing actions should be the highest priority?

A. Monitor level of consciousness.

B. Take blood pressure.

C. Check respiratory rate.

D. Encourage fluid intake.

APPLICATION EXERCISES ANSWER KEY

1. Which of the following clients are at risk for a pulmonary embolism (PE)? (Select all that apply.) A client who

   __X__ **is taking birth control pills.**

   _____ is postmenopausal.

   __X__ **has a fractured femur.**

   __X__ **smokes one pipe daily.**

   _____ is a marathon runner.

   __X__ **has chronic atrial fibrillation.**

   Estrogen use and smoking can cause hypercoagulability, which increases the risk of a blood clot. A client with turbulent blood flow in the heart, such as with a dysrhythmia, is also at increased risk of a blood clot. A bone fracture, particularly in a long bone such as the femur, increases the risk of fat emboli. A client who is postmenopausal and a client who is a marathon runner are not at risk for developing a PE.

 NCLEX® Connection: Reduction of Risk Potential, Potential for Alterations in Body Systems

2. A nurse is caring for a middle adult female client who is admitted to the coronary care unit with acute dyspnea and diaphoresis. The client states that she is anxious because she feels like she can't get enough air. Vital signs are: heart rate 117 beats/min, respiratory rate 38/min, temperature 38.4° C (101.2° F), and blood pressure 100/54 mm Hg. Which of the following is the priority nursing action?

   A. Administer oxygen therapy to the client.

   B. Obtain an ABG sample from the client.

   C. Maintain the client on bed rest.

   D. Transfer the client for a CT scan.

   According to the ABC priority-setting framework, administering oxygen therapy to the client is the highest priority at this time. Obtaining an ABG sample, maintaining the client on bed rest, and transferring the client for a CT scan are part of this priority, but not the highest priority at this time.

   NCLEX® Connection: Physiological Adaptation, Medical Emergencies

3. A nurse is assisting with the care of a client who has a pulmonary embolus and is to start a prescription for heparin by continuous IV infusion. Which of the following client statements poses an immediate concern for the nurse?

    A. "I am allergic to morphine."

    B. "I take antacids several times a day."

    C. "I had a blood clot in my leg several years ago."

    D. "It hurts to take a deep breath."

    Option B indicates that this client may have peptic ulcer disease. The nurse should collect further data since this can place the client at an increased risk for hemorrhage once the heparin drip is started. Heparin is not contraindicated in clients who are allergic to morphine, a previous history of a blood clot may indicate the client's high risk for pulmonary embolism, and pain in the chest is an expected finding in a client with a pulmonary embolus.

    Ⓝ NCLEX® Connection: Pharmacological Therapies, Adverse Effects/Contraindications/Side Effects/Interactions

4. A young adult male client is admitted to the medical unit with a gunshot wound to the chest. Vital signs are: blood pressure 108/55 mm Hg, heart rate 124 beats/min, respiratory rate 36/min, temperature 38.6° C (101.4° F), and SaO₂ 95% on 15 L/min by a nonrebreather mask. He reports dyspnea and pain. The nurse reassesses the client 30 min later. Which of the data should be reported to the charge nurse? (Select all that apply.)

__X__	**SaO₂ of 90%**
__X__	**Tracheal deviation**
_____	Blood pressure 104/54 mm Hg
__X__	**Heart rate 142 beats/min**
__X__	**Hemoptysis**

    An SaO₂ of 90%, tracheal deviation, heart rate of 142/min, and hemoptysis, are all signs that indicate the client's condition is worsening and needs to be reported to the charge nurse. A blood pressure of 104/54 mm Hg is not a clinical finding that the client's condition is worsening.

    Ⓝ NCLEX® Connection: Physiological Adaptation, Medical Emergencies

5. Which of the following clients are at risk for the development of acute respiratory distress syndrome (ARDS)? (Select all that apply.) A client

　　__X__　**who received 2 min of CPR following a near-drowning.**

　　__X__　**with coronary artery bypass grafts and two chest tubes.**

　　_____　with a hemoglobin level of 14.5 mg/dL.

　　__X__　**with pancreatitis.**

　　__X__　**with dysphagia.**

　　_____　with a sinus infection.

Clients that are at risk for developing ARDS include anyone with a lung injury such as from aspiration (near-drowning or dysphagia), pancreatitis or post-coronary artery bypass graft. A hemoglobin of 14.5 is within the expected reference range, and a sinus infection does not put a client at risk for ARDS.

 NCLEX® Connection: Reduction of Risk Potential, Potential for Alterations in Body Systems

6. In reviewing the plan of care for a client who has severe acute respiratory syndrome (SARS), which of the following is an appropriate action? (Select all that apply.)

　　_____　Antibiotics

　　__X__　**Supplemental oxygen**

　　_____　Antiviral medications

　　__X__　**Bronchodilators**

　　__X__　**Mechanical ventilation**

SARS is caused by one of the corona viruses. Treatment involves supplemental oxygen, bronchodilators, and mechanical ventilation. Antibiotics may be indicated for a secondary infection, but not for SARS. There are no effective antiviral medications to treat the corona virus at this time.

 NCLEX® Connection: Physiological Adaptation, Medical Emergencies

7. An older adult client with postoperative pain has been prescribed morphine. Which of the following nursing actions should be the highest priority?

A. Monitor level of consciousness.

B. Take blood pressure.

C. Check respiratory rate.

D. Encourage fluid intake.

The most serious side effect of morphine is respiratory depression. Using the ABC priority-setting framework, respiratory status is the highest priority. Therefore, the highest priority action is for the nurse to check the client's respiratory rate. A baseline respiratory rate should be documented prior to the first dose and if the respiratory rate falls to less than 12 breaths per minute, the morphine should be withheld and the provider notified. The client's level of consciousness, blood pressure, and fluid intake are all important, but not the priority.

 NCLEX® Connection: Physiological Adaptation, Medical Emergencies

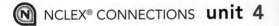

UNIT 4: NURSING CARE OF CLIENTS WITH CARDIOVASCULAR DISORDERS

- Diagnostic and Therapeutic Procedures
- Cardiac Disorders
- Vascular Disorders

NCLEX® CONNECTIONS

When reviewing the chapters in this section, keep in mind the relevant sections of the NCLEX® outline, in particular:

CLIENT NEEDS: HEALTH PROMOTION AND MAINTENANCE

Relevant topics/tasks include:
- Data Collection Techniques
  - Collect data for health history.
- Health Promotion/Disease Prevention
  - Gather data on client health history and risk for disease.
- Lifestyle Choices
  - Identify client lifestyle practices that may have an impact on health.

CLIENT NEEDS: BASIC CARE AND COMFORT

Relevant topics/tasks include:
- Mobility/Immobility
  - Identify signs and symptoms of venous insufficiency and intervene to promote venous return.
- Nutrition and Oral Hydration
  - Monitor impact of disease/illness on client nutritional status.
- Personal Hygiene
  - Reinforce teaching to client on required adaptations for performing activities of daily living (ADLs).

CLIENT NEEDS: PHARMACOLOGICAL THERAPIES

Relevant topics/tasks include:
- Adverse Effects/Contraindications/Side Effects/Interactions
  - Monitor anticipated interactions among client prescribed medications and fluids.
- Dosage Calculation
  - Use clinical decision making when calculating doses.
- Pharmacological Pain Management
  - Monitor and document client response to pharmacological interventions.

UNIT 4	NURSING CARE OF CLIENTS WITH CARDIOVASCULAR DISORDERS
Section:	Diagnostic and Therapeutic Procedures

Chapter 25   Cardiovascular Diagnostic Procedures

Overview

- Cardiovascular diagnostic procedures evaluate the functioning of the heart by monitoring for enzymes in the blood; using ultrasound to visualize the heart; determining the heart's response to exercise; and using catheters to determine blood volume, perfusion, fluid status, how the heart is pumping, and degree of artery blockage.

- Cardiovascular diagnostic procedures that nurses should be familiar with include:

  o Cardiac enzymes (cardiac markers) and lipid profile

  o Echocardiogram

  o Stress testing (exercise electrocardiography)

  o Angiography

Cardiac Enzymes (Cardiac Markers) and Lipid Profile

- Cardiac enzymes are released into the bloodstream when the heart muscle suffers ischemia. A lipid profile provides information regarding cholesterol levels and is used for early detection of heart disease.

- Cardiac enzymes are a specific marker in diagnosing an MI.

- Indications

  o Angina

  o MI

  o Heart disease

  o Hyperlipidemia

- Interpretation of Findings

CARDIAC ENZYME	EXPECTED REFERENCE RANGE	ELEVATED LEVELS FIRST DETECTABLE FOLLOWING MYOCARDIAL INJURY	EXPECTED DURATION OF ELEVATED LEVELS
Creatine kinase MB isoenzyme (CK-MB) – more sensitive to myocardium	0% of total CK (30 to 170 units/L)	4 to 6 hr	3 days
Troponin T	< 0.2 ng/L	3 to 5 hr	14 to 21 days
Troponin I	< 0.03 ng/L	3 hr	7 to 10 days
Myoglobin	< 90 mcg/L	2 hr	24 hr

TEST	EXPECTED REFERENCE RANGE	PURPOSE
Cholesterol (total)	< 200 mg/dL	Screening test for heart disease
HDL	Greater than 40 mg/dL	"Good" cholesterol produced by the liver
LDL	< 130 mg/dL	"Bad" cholesterol can be up to 70% of total cholesterol
Triglycerides	< 150 mg/dL	Evaluating test for atherosclerosis

- Preprocedure

  - Nursing actions

    - Explain the reason for the test to clients.

- Intraprocedure

  - A blood specimen is drawn from the client via venipuncture.

- Postprocedure

  - Laboratory findings will be discussed with clients by the provider, and choice of treatment will be determined.

Echocardiogram

- An echocardiogram is an ultrasound of the heart. The test is used to diagnose valve disorders and cardiomyopathy.

- Indications

  - Cardiomyopathy

  - Heart failure

- o Angina

- o MI

- Interpretation of Findings

  - o An echocardiogram can be used to determine blood flow insufficiency, cardiac tissue damage, and valve disorders. This test can also be used to measure the size and depth of the heart, ejection fraction and cardiac output.

- Preprocedure

  - o Nursing actions

    - Explain the reason for the test to clients. The test is pain-free and takes up to 1 hr.

- Intraprocedure

  - o Nursing actions

    - Position clients on left side with the head of the bed elevated 15° to 20° and instruct them to remain still.

- Postprocedure

  - o Nursing actions

    - Inform clients that the results of the test and a plan for follow-up care will be provided by the provider. There are no specific postprocedure instructions that need to be followed.

Stress Testing (Exercise Electrocardiography)

- The cardiac muscle is exercised by clients walking on a treadmill. This provides information regarding the workload of the heart. Once the client's heart rate reaches a certain rate, the test is discontinued.

- A pharmacological stress test may be used for clients who are disabled or unable to be physically challenged. A medication such as adenosine (Adenocard), is given to stress the heart instead of walking on the treadmill.

- Indications

  - o Angina

  - o Heart failure

  - o MI

  - o Dysrhythmia

- Interpretation of Findings

  - o During the stress test, the client's heart will increase due to the workload of the heart. This is an expected finding for this test. Abnormal findings can include arrhythmias while the test is being completed, signs of coronary artery disease such as angina, and shortness of breath.

- Preprocedure

  o Nursing actions

    ▪ Verify that informed consent has been obtained.

    ▪ Explain to clients that they will be walking on a treadmill, and comfortable shoes and clothing are recommended.

    ▪ Clients are instructed to fast 2 to 4 hr before the procedure according to agency policy, and to avoid tobacco, alcohol, and caffeine before the test.

- Intraprocedure

  o Nursing Actions

    ▪ Remind clients that once the heart reaches a certain rate, the test will be discontinued.

- Postprocedure

  o Nursing Actions

    ▪ Clients are monitored by ECG and their blood pressure is checked frequently until they are stable.

    ▪ Monitor ECG and vital signs.

    ▪ The provider will discuss findings with client.

Angiography

- A coronary angiogram, also called a cardiac catheterization, is an invasive diagnostic procedure used to evaluate the presence and degree of coronary artery blockage.

  o Angiography can also be done on the lower extremities to determine blood flow and areas of blockage.

  o Angiography involves the insertion of a catheter into a femoral (sometimes a brachial) vessel and threading it into the right or left side of the heart. Coronary artery narrowings and/or occlusions are identified by the injection of contrast media under fluoroscopy.

 View Media Supplement: Cardiac Catheterization (Image)

- Indications

  o Unstable angina and ECG changes (T wave inversion, ST segment elevation, depression)

  o Confirm and determine location and extent of heart disease.

- Interpretation of Findings

  o Angiography can be performed to view the coronary arteries. This allows the provider to see if narrowing of the coronary arteries has occurred or if plaque has accumulated. These findings can be related to heart disease or a myocardial infarction.

- Preprocedure

  o Nursing actions

    ▪ Verify that the consent form is signed.

    ▪ Maintain clients on NPO status for at least 8 hr (risk for aspiration when lying flat for the procedure).

    ▪ Check for iodine/shellfish allergy (contrast media).

    ▪ Administer premedications as prescribed [methylprednisone (Solu-Medrol), diphenhydramine (Benadryl and a mild sedative)].

    ▪ Shave and antiseptically prepare the catheterization site according to agency policy

  o Client education

    ▪ Instruct clients that they can be awake and sedated during procedure. A local anesthetic should be used. A small incision is made, often in the groin to insert the catheter. Clients can feel warm and flushed when the dye is inserted. After the procedure, clients must keep the affected leg straight. Pressure (a sandbag) can be placed on the incision to prevent bleeding.

- Postprocedure

  o Nursing actions

    ▪ Check vital signs every 15 min x 4, every 30 min x 2, every hour x 4, and then every 4 hr (follow hospital protocol).

    ▪ Check the groin site at the same intervals for:

      □ Bleeding and hematoma formation

      □ Thrombosis; document pedal pulse, color, temperature

    ▪ Maintain bed rest in prescribed position (supine or head of the bed to be elevated 30° to 45° with extremity straight for prescribed time.

      □ A vascular closure device may be used to hasten hemostasis following catheter removal.

    ▪ Assist with continuous cardiac monitoring for dysrhythmias (reperfusion following angioplasty can cause dysrhythmias).

    ▪ Administer medications as prescribed to prevent clot formation and restenosis.

      □ Aspirin

      □ Clopidogrel (Plavix), ticlopidine (Ticlid)

      □ Heparin

- □ Low molecular weight heparin (Enoxaparin, Lovenox)
- □ GP IIb/IIIa inhibitors, such as eptifibatide (Integrilin)
- ■ Administer anxiolytics (Ativan) and analgesia (morphine) as needed.
- ■ Monitor urine output and monitor IV fluids for hydration.
  - □ Monitor pressure dressing after sheath removal.
- ○ Client education
  - ■ Instruct clients to:
    - □ Avoid strenuous exercise for the prescribed period of time.
    - □ Immediately report bleeding from the insertion site, chest pain, shortness of breath, and changes in the color or temperature of the extremity.
    - □ Restrict lifting (less than 10 lb) for the prescribed period of time.
  - ■ Clients with stent placement will receive anticoagulation therapy for 6 to 8 weeks. Instruct clients to:
    - □ Take the medication at the same time each day.
    - □ Have regular laboratory tests to determine therapeutic levels.
    - □ Avoid activities that could cause bleeding (use soft toothbrush, wear shoes when out of bed).
  - ■ Encourage clients to follow lifestyle guidelines (manage weight, consume a low-fat/low-sodium diet, get regular exercise, stop smoking, decrease alcohol intake).
- ● Complications
  - ○ Cardiac tamponade
    - ■ Cardiac tamponade can result from fluid accumulation in the pericardial sac.
      - □ Signs include hypotension, jugular venous distention, muffled heart sounds, and paradoxical pulse (variance of 10 mm Hg or more in systolic blood pressure between expiration and inspiration).
      - □ Hemodynamic monitoring will reveal intracardiac and pulmonary artery pressures similar and elevated (plateau pressures).
    - ■ Nursing actions
      - □ Notify the provider immediately.
      - □ Administer IV fluids to combat hypotension as prescribed.
  - ○ Hematoma formation
    - ■ Blood clots may form near the insertion site.
    - ■ Nursing actions
      - □ Check the groin at prescribed intervals and as needed.
      - □ Hold pressure for uncontrolled oozing/bleeding.

▫ Monitor peripheral circulation.

▫ Notify the provider.

○ Restenosis of treated vessel

■ Clot reformation in the coronary artery can occur immediately or several weeks after procedure.

■ Nursing actions

▫ Check ECG patterns and check for occurrence of chest pain.

▫ Notify the provider immediately.

▫ Prepare clients for return to the cardiac catheterization laboratory.

(A) APPLICATION EXERCISES

1. A nurse is caring for a client following an angiography. The nurse informs the client he should lie still for 6 hr because he is at risk for which of the following?

    A. Urinary retention

    B. Infection

    C. Respiratory depression

    D. Bleeding

2. A nurse is instructing a client who is scheduled for an echocardiogram. Which of the following should the nurse include in the client's teaching?

    A. "You may experience some discomfort during this test."

    B. "This test will require up to 2 hours to complete."

    C. "You will need to lie flat during the test."

    D. "This test allows us to see a picture of the inside of your heart."

3. A client in a provider's office tells a nurse, "My cholesterol is 198 mg/dL, but my doctor says my bad cholesterol is too high." Which of the following responses should the nurse give?

    A. "This means that your LDL is too high."

    B. "This means that your HDL is too high."

    C. "This means that your triglycerides are too high."

    D. "This means that your cholesterol (total) is too high."

Ⓐ APPLICATION EXERCISES ANSWER KEY

1. A nurse is caring for a client following an angiography. The nurse informs the client he should lie still for 6 hr because he is at risk for which of the following?

   A. Urinary retention

   B. Infection

   C. Respiratory depression

   D. Bleeding

   Following angiography, the client should lie still for 6 hr due to the increased risk for bleeding. Urinary retention, infection, and respiratory depression are risks unrelated to the client lying still.

   Ⓝ NCLEX® Connection: Reduction of Risk Potential, Potential for Complications of Diagnostic Tests/Treatments/Procedures

2. A nurse is instructing a client who is scheduled for an echocardiogram. Which of the following should the nurse include in the client's teaching?

   A. "You may experience some discomfort during this test."

   B. "This test will require up to 2 hours to complete."

   C. "You will need to lie flat during the test."

   D. "This test allows us to see a picture of the inside of your heart."

   An echocardiogram is an ultrasound of the heart and allows the provider to detect structural defects of the client's heart. This test can be used to detect valve disorders as well as cardiomyopathy. This test is pain-free and takes up to an hour to complete. During the test, clients are required to lie still and be on their left side.

   Ⓝ NCLEX® Connection: Reduction of Risk Potential, Diagnostic Tests

3. A client in a provider's office tells a nurse, "My cholesterol is 198 mg/dL, but my doctor says my bad cholesterol is too high." Which of the following responses should the nurse give?

   A. "This means that your LDL is too high."

   B. "This means that your HDL is too high."

   C. "This means that your triglycerides are too high."

   D. "This means that your cholesterol (total) is too high."

   The LDL is the bad cholesterol and can be up to 70% of the total cholesterol. This value should be less than 130 mg/dL. HDL is the good cholesterol produced by the liver. This value should be greater than 40 mg/dL. Triglycerides are used to detect atherosclerosis. This level should be less than 150 mg/dL. Cholesterol (total) is the total value of cholesterol and is the screening test for heart disease. This value should be less than 200 mg/dL.

   Ⓝ NCLEX® Connection: Reduction of Risk Potential, Diagnostic Tests

UNIT 4	NURSING CARE OF CLIENTS WITH CARDIOVASCULAR DISORDERS
Section:	Diagnostic and Therapeutic Procedures

Chapter 26   Electrocardiography and Dysrhythmia Monitoring

 Overview

- Cardiac electrical activity can be monitored by using an ECG. The heart's electrical activity can be monitored by a standard 12-lead ECG (resting ECG), ambulatory ECG (Holter monitoring), continuous cardiac monitoring, or by telemetry.

> **(M)** **View Media Supplement:** ECG Strip (Image)

- Cardiac dysrhythmias are heartbeat disturbances (beat formation, beat conduction, or myocardial response to beat).

- Nurses should be familiar with cardioversion and defibrillation procedures for treating dysrhythmias.

Electrocardiography

- Electrocardiography uses an electrocardiograph to record the electrical activity of the heart over time. The electrocardiograph is connected by wires (leads) to skin electrodes placed on the chest and limbs of a client.

  o Continuous cardiac monitoring requires clients to be in close proximity to the monitoring system.

  o Telemetry allows clients to ambulate while maintaining proximity to the monitoring system.

- Indications

  o Diagnoses

    ▪ Bradycardia

    ▪ Heart block

    ▪ Atrial fibrillation

    ▪ Supraventricular tachycardia

    ▪ Ventricular tachycardia

- Ventricular fibrillation
- Myocardial Infarction (size and extent)
- Client presentation
  - Cardiovascular disease
  - Myocardial infarction
  - Hypoxia
  - Acid-base imbalances
  - Electrolyte disturbances
  - Chronic renal failure, liver, or lung disease
  - Pericarditis
  - Drug or alcohol abuse
  - Hypovolemia
  - Shock

- Interpretation of Findings
  - An electrocardiography can identify dysrhythmias, heart ischemia, cardiac injury, chamber enlargement, or conduction abnormalities.

- Preprocedure
  - Nursing actions
    - Prepare clients for a 12-lead ECG by:
      - Positioning clients in a supine position with chest exposed.
      - Washing the client's skin to remove oils.
      - Attaching one electrode to each of the client's extremities by applying electrodes to flat surfaces above the wrists and ankles and the other six electrodes to the chest, avoiding chest hair. (Chest hair may need to be shaved on male clients).

 View Media Supplement: 12-lead ECG (Image)

- Intraprocedure
  - Nursing actions
    - Instruct clients to remain still and breathe normally while the 12-lead ECG is performed.
    - Monitor clients for signs and symptoms of dysrhythmia (chest pain, decreased level of consciousness, and shortness of breath) and hypoxia.

- Postprocedure

  - Nursing actions

    - Remove leads from client, print ECG report, and notify the provider.

    - Apply a Holter monitor if clients are on a telemetry unit and/or need continuous cardiac monitoring.

    - Continue to monitor clients for symptoms of dysrhythmia (chest pain, decreased level of consciousness, and shortness of breath) and hypoxia.

    - Dysrhythmia treatment is based on the client's symptoms and the cardiac rhythm, which can require cardioversion or defibrillation after an ECG has been completed and a diagnosis has been found.

Dysrhythmias

- Dysrhythmias are classified by the:

  - Site of origin – sinoatrial (SA) node, atria, atrioventricular node, or ventricle.

    - Electrophysiological study determines the area of the heart causing the dysrhythmia. Ablation of the area is possible.

  - Effect on the rate and rhythm of the heart – bradycardia, tachycardia, heart block, premature beat, flutter, fibrillation, or asystole.

- Dysrhythmias can be benign or life-threatening.

- The life-threatening effects of dysrhythmias are generally related to decreased cardiac output and ineffective tissue perfusion.

- Ⓖ Dysrhythmias can present atypically in older adult clients.

- Risks for heart disease, hypertension, dysrhythmias, and atherosclerosis increase with age.

- Assist with the care of clients experiencing dysrhythmias

DYSRHYTHMIA	MEDICATION	ELECTRICAL MANAGEMENT
Bradycardia (any rhythm less than 60/min) Treat if clients are symptomatic	Atropine and isoproterenol	Pacemaker
Atrial fibrillation, supraventricular tachycardia, or ventricular tachycardia with pulse	Amiodarone (Cordarone), adenosine, and verapamil (Calan)	Synchronized cardioversion
Ventricular tachycardia without pulse or ventricular fibrillation	Amiodarone, lidocaine, and epinephrine	Defibrillation

Cardioversion and Defibrillation

- Cardioversion is the delivery of a synchronized, direct countershock to the heart.

- Defibrillation is the delivery of an asynchronous countershock to the heart. Defibrillation stops all electrical activity of the heart, allowing the SA node to take over and re-establish a perfusing rhythm. The earlier it is performed, the greater the chance of survival.

- Indications

  - Cardioversion – elective treatment of atrial dysrhythmias, supraventricular tachycardia, and ventricular tachycardia with a pulse. Cardioversion is the treatment of choice for clients who are symptomatic.

  - Defibrillation – ventricular fibrillation or pulseless ventricular tachycardia.

- Client Outcome

  - The client's heart will return to a normal rhythm.

- Preprocedure

  - Clients who have atrial fibrillation of unknown duration must receive adequate anticoagulation prior to cardioversion therapy to prevent dislodgement of thrombi into the bloodstream. An anesthesiologist may administer a short acting anesthetic IV bolus for sedation.

  - Nursing actions

    - Prepare clients for cardioversion, if prescribed.

    - Explain the procedure to clients and verify consent.

    - Administer oxygen.

    - Document preprocedure rhythm.

    - Have emergency equipment available.

- Postprocedure

  - Nursing actions

    - After cardioversion or defibrillation, check the client's vital signs, check airway patency, and obtain an ECG.

    - Provide clients and their families with reassurance and emotional support.

  - Client education

    - Teach clients and families how to check pulse rate.

    - Advise clients to report palpitations or irregularities.

Ⓐ APPLICATION EXERCISES

1. A nurse is assisting a charge nurse who is caring for a client who reports feeling lightheaded. Assessment of his vital signs reveals: heart rate 144/min and irregular, blood pressure 84/49mm Hg, and SaO_2 95%. An ECG reveals atrial fibrillation with a rapid ventricular response. Synchronized cardioversion is performed at 50 joules. Which of the following observations should the nurse include in her documentation? (Select all that apply.)

   _____ The client reports feeling lightheaded.

   _____ The client's ECG reveals atrial fibrillation with a rapid ventricular response.

   _____ The client's vital signs are within the expected reference range.

   _____ The client is synchronized with cardioversion at 50 joules.

   _____ The client's oxygen saturation is 95%.

2. Two hours after the client's cardioversion, he develops ventricular fibrillation. Which of the following actions should the nurse take first?

3. Which of the following clients is at risk for the development of dysrhythmias? (Select all that apply.)

   _____ A client who has ABG results of: pH 7.26, PaO_2 75 mm Hg, $PaCO_2$ 58 mm Hg, HCO_3^- 32 mEq/L

   _____ A client who has a serum potassium level of 4.3 mEq/L

   _____ A client who has an SaO_2 of 96%

   _____ A client who has COPD

   _____ A client who is 3 hr postmyocardial infarction

Ⓐ APPLICATION EXERCISES ANSWER KEY

1. A nurse is assisting a charge nurse who is caring for a client who reports feeling lightheaded. Assessment of his vital signs reveals: heart rate 144/min and irregular, blood pressure 84/49mm Hg, and SaO$_2$ 95%. An ECG reveals atrial fibrillation with a rapid ventricular response. Synchronized cardioversion is performed at 50 joules. Which of the following observations should the nurse include in her documentation? (Select all that apply.)

   __X__ **The client reports feeling lightheaded.**
   __X__ **The client's ECG reveals atrial fibrillation with a rapid ventricular response.**
   _____ The client's vital signs are within the expected reference range.
   __X__ **The client is synchronized with cardioversion at 50 joules.**
   __X__ **The client's oxygen saturation is 95%.**

   The client feeling lightheaded, an ECG revealing atrial fibrillation with rapid ventricular response, a client synchronized with cardioversion at 50 joules, and a client with an oxygen saturation 95% would all be included in the nurse's documentation. The client's vital signs are not within the expected reference range.

Ⓝ NCLEX® Connection: Reduction of Risk Potential, Therapeutic Procedures

2. Two hours after the client's cardioversion, he develops ventricular fibrillation. Which of the following actions should the nurse take first?

   When a client has a lethal rhythm such as ventricular fibrillation, the first intervention is defibrillation.

Ⓝ NCLEX® Connection: Reduction for Risk Potential, Potential for Alterations in Body Systems

3. Which of the following clients is at risk for the development of dysrhythmias? (Select all that apply.)

   __X__ **A client who has ABG results of: pH 7.26, PaO$_2$ 75 mm Hg, PaCO$_2$ 58 mm Hg, HCO$_3$- 32 mEq/L**
   _____ A client who has a serum potassium level of 4.3 mEq/L
   _____ A client who has an SaO$_2$ of 96%
   __X__ **A client who has COPD**
   __X__ **A client who is 3 hr postmyocardial infarction**

   These ABG results, COPD, and recent myocardial infarction are risk factors for developing a dysrhythmia. A potassium level of 4.3 mEq/L (expected reference range) and an oxygen saturation of 96% (expected reference range) do not increase the risk for developing dysrhythmias.

Ⓝ NCLEX® Connection: Reduction of Risk Potential, Potential for Alterations in Body Systems

UNIT 4	NURSING CARE OF CLIENTS WITH CARDIOVASCULAR DISORDERS
Section:	Diagnostic and Therapeutic Procedures
Chapter 27	Invasive Cardiac Procedures

 Overview

- Invasive cardiovascular procedures are methods used to maintain an acceptable cardiac rhythm or improve blood flow for arteries and veins that have become occluded.

- Invasive cardiovascular procedures are indicated if symptoms persist after non-invasive interventions have been tried, such as diet, exercise, and medications.

- Invasive cardiovascular procedures that nurses should be knowledgeable about include:

  o Pacemaker insertion and care

  o Angioplasty

  o Coronary artery bypass grafts

  o Peripheral bypass grafts

PACEMAKERS

Overview

- An artificial pacemaker is a battery-operated device that electrically stimulates the heart when the natural pacemaker of the heart fails to maintain an acceptable rhythm.

View Media Supplement: Pacemaker (Image)

- Pacemakers may be temporary or permanent.

- Pacemakers are composed of two parts:

  o The pulse generator houses the energy source (battery) and the control center.

  o The electrodes are wires that attach to the myocardial muscle on one side and connect to the pulse generator on the other.

- Nurses should be familiar with the various types of pacemakers, how they function, and the care involved with their placement/insertion.

(G)   • Conduction of electrical impulses through the sinoatrial node may be slowed with aging, causing bradycardia and conduction defects.

Types of Pacemakers

- Temporary Pacemakers (the energy source is provided by an external battery pack)

  ○ External (transcutaneous)

    ■ Pacing energy is delivered transcutaneously through the thoracic musculature to the heart via two electrode patches placed on the skin.

    ■ It requires large amounts of electricity, which can be painful for a client.

    ■ It is only used in emergency resuscitation of a client who does not have pacing wires inserted.

  ○ Epicardial

    ■ Pacemaker leads are attached directly to the heart during open heart surgery. Wires run externally through the chest incision and may be attached to an external impulse generator if needed.

    ■ It is commonly used during and immediately following open heart surgery.

  ○ Endocardial (transvenous)

    ■ Pacing wires are threaded through a large central vein (subclavian, jugular, or femoral) and lodged into the wall of the right ventricle (ventricular pacing), right atrium (atrial pacing), or both chambers (dual chamber pacing).

- Permanent Pacemakers (contain an internal pacing unit)

  ○ Indicated for chronic or recurrent dysrhythmias due to sinus or atrioventricular (AV) node malfunction

  ○ Can be programmed to pace the atria, ventricles, or both (AV sequential pacing)

  ○ Pacemaker modes

    ■ Fixed rate (asynchronous) – fires at a constant rate without regard for the heart's electrical activity

    ■ Demand mode (synchronous) – detects the heart's electrical impulses and fires at a preset rate only if the heart's intrinsic rate is below a certain level

    ■ Antidysrhythmic function – can overpace a tachydysrhythmia or deliver an electrical shock

Pacemaker Placement

- Indications
  - Diagnoses
    - Symptomatic bradycardia
    - Complete heart block
    - Sick sinus syndrome
    - Sinus arrest
    - Asystole
    - Atrial tachydysrhythmias
    - Ventricular tachydysrhythmias
  - Client presentation
    - Symptoms
      - Dizziness
      - Palpitations
      - Chest pain or pressure
      - Anxiousness
      - Fatigue
      - Nausea
      - Breathing difficulties
    - Signs
      - Bradycardia
      - Tachycardia
      - Abnormal ECG
      - Dyspnea, tachypnea
      - Restlessness
      - Distended jugular vein
      - Vomiting
      - Hypotension
      - Diaphoresis
      - Decreased cardiac output

- Client Outcomes

  - The client will be able to tolerate activities of daily living free of cardiac symptoms.

  - The client will use strategies to reduce stress and improve cardiac health.

  - The client will recognize cardiac symptoms and seek medical attention immediately when needed.

- Preprocedure

  - Nursing actions

    - Determine the client's knowledge of the procedure and need for pacemaker (if nonemergent situation).

    - Verify informed consent.

  - Client education

    - Reinforce to clients about the type of pacemaker that is to be inserted and information about the procedure.

      □ Temporary pacemaker

        ▸ Explain that wires and a pacemaker box will be on the client's chest after the procedure.

        ▸ Instruct clients not to touch the dials on the pacemaker box.

        ▸ The wires and box will need to be kept dry. Clients will not be able to shower.

      □ Permanent pacemaker

        ▸ Explain that a small incision will be made using a local anesthetic and IV sedation.

        ▸ The pacemaker may be reprogrammed externally after the procedure.

- Postprocedure

  - Nursing actions

    - Document the time and date of insertion, model (permanent pacemaker), settings, rhythm strip, presence of adequate pulse and blood pressure, and client response.

    - Continually monitor heart rate and rhythm.

    - Obtain chest x-ray as prescribed to assess lead placement and for pneumothorax, hemothorax, or pleural effusion.

    - Provide analgesia as prescribed.

    - Minimize shoulder movement initially and provide a sling (if prescribed) to allow leads to anchor.

- Maintain the client's safety.
  - □ Ensure that all electrical equipment has grounded connections.
  - □ Remove any electrical equipment that is damaged.
  - □ For a temporary pacemaker:
    - ▸ Wear gloves when handling pacemaker leads.
    - ▸ Insulate pacemaker terminals and leads with nonconductive material when not in use (rubber gloves).
    - ▸ Keep spare generator, leads, and batteries at the client's bedside.
    - ▸ Secure the pacemaker battery pack. Take care when moving clients and ensure that there is enough wire slack.
  - □ For a permanent pacemaker:
    - ▸ Provide clients with a pacemaker identification card including the manufacturer's name, model number, mode of function, rate parameters, and expected battery life.
- Check clients for hiccups, which may indicate that the generator is pacing the diaphragm.
  - ○ Client education
    - Temporary pacemakers are only used in a controlled facility-like environment with telemetry for continuous ECG monitoring. If needed, a permanent pacemaker is inserted before discharge to home.
    - Permanent pacemaker discharge teaching
      - □ Instruct clients to carry a pacemaker identification card at all times.
      - □ Reinforce to clients that batteries last 10 years on average.
      - □ Tell clients to wear a sling when out of bed, if prescribed.
      - □ Reinforce to clients not to raise the arm on the surgical side above the shoulder for 1 to 2 weeks.
      - □ Reinforce to clients to take pulse daily at the same time.
      - □ Reinforce to clients to set the rate of the pacemaker. Notify the provider if the heart rate is less than 5 beats below the pacer rate.
      - □ Instruct clients to report signs of dizziness, fainting, fatigue, weakness, chest pain, hiccupping, or palpitations.
      - □ For clients with pacer-defibrillators, inform clients and their families that anyone touching the client when the device delivers a shock will feel a slight electrical impulse but that the impulse will not harm the person.
      - □ Inform clients of activity restrictions as prescribed, including no contact sports or heavy lifting for 2 months.
      - □ Inform clients that they can resume sexual activity as desired, avoiding positions that put stress on the incision site.

- □ Inform clients that household appliances should not affect pacemaker function unless held directly over pacer generator. This includes garage door openers, burglar alarms, microwave ovens, and antitheft devices.

- □ Instruct clients to inform airport security agents that airport security detectors will be set off. Inform clients that this should not affect pacemaker functioning.

- □ Instruct clients to inform other providers and dentists about the pacemaker. Some tests, such as magnetic resonance imaging and therapeutic diathermy (heat therapy), may be contraindicated.

- Complications

  - ○ Pacemaker insertion complications

    - ■ Infection or hematoma

      - □ The insertion site can develop an infection or hematoma.

      - □ Nursing actions

        - ‣ Monitor the incision site for redness, pain, drainage, or swelling.

        - ‣ Treat an infection with antibiotics as prescribed.

        - ‣ Monitor coagulation and CBC.

    - ■ Pneumothorax or hemothorax

      - □ Trauma during the procedure can cause a pneumothorax or hemothorax.

      - □ Nursing actions

        - ‣ Monitor the client's breath sounds and chest movement.

        - ‣ Monitor oxygen saturation.

        - ‣ Obtain a chest x-ray after the procedure.

    - ■ Arrhythmias

      - □ Irritation of a ventricle from a pacing electrode may cause ectopic beats, such as premature ventricular contractions.

      - □ Nursing actions

        - ‣ Monitor ECG and blood pressure.

        - ‣ Assist with emergency care of clients.

  - ○ Pacemaker complications

    - ■ Failure to capture

      - □ The pacemaker initiates a stimulus, but depolarization of the myocardium does not happen.

        - ‣ An ECG shows pacing spikes without the expected P wave or QRS complex.

- ▸ Failure to capture causes include dislodgement of the electrode, MI or ischemia, antidysrhythmic medications, electrolyte imbalances (hypokalemia, hyperkalemia), and too low of a voltage (mA).
- ▸ Treatment depends on the cause. A dislodged electrode may reattach by turning clients onto the left side. The provider may need to increase the voltage delivered if the voltage is too low to capture.

- ■ Failure to sense
  - ▢ The pacemaker fails to sense the heart's intrinsic electrical activity, resulting in the delivery of an unnecessary stimulus.
    - ▸ An ECG shows pacemaker spikes at intervals different from the programmed interval.
    - ▸ Discharge of an impulse during the T wave can lead to life-threatening ventricular dysrhythmias.
    - ▸ Treatment involves decreasing the amplitude at which the pacemaker recognizes intrinsic electrical activity (mV).

- ■ Failure to pace (no output)
  - ▢ Failure to pace may be caused by a broken lead wire.
    - ▸ Treatment involves replacing the battery or lead.

- ■ Oversensing
  - ▢ The pacemaker is oversensitive and sensing excessive electrical activity.
    - ▸ The provider may need to increase the voltage delivered (mA) to reduce sensitivity.

- ■ Stimulation of chest wall or diaphragm
  - ▢ The pacemaker's electrical charge may stimulate the client's chest wall or diaphragm.
    - ▸ Stimulation is indicated by muscle twitching or hiccups.
    - ▸ It is often caused by lead wire perforation with high electrical current.
    - ▸ Stimulation can lead to cardiac tamponade.
  - ▢ Nursing actions
    - ▸ Monitor clients for signs of cardiac tamponade such as dyspnea, chest pain, hypotension, and distended neck veins.
  - ▢ Client education
    - ▸ Instruct clients to notify the provider with symptoms of chest muscle twitching or hiccups. The pacemaker wires may need to be repositioned.

- **Microshock**
  - □ A small electrical current is sent through unattached external pacemaker wires and may cause cardiac arrhythmias or ventricular fibrillation. This may occur with pacemaker wires that are not attached to a pacemaker generator.
  - □ Nursing actions
    - ▸ Cover wires with nonconductive insulation (rubber gloves) and nonconductive tape.
    - ▸ Made sure all equipment is grounded with a three-pronged plug. Contact the engineering department for all ungrounded or unsafe electrical equipment (frayed wires).
    - ▸ Wear rubber gloves when handling pacing wires. Static electricity may be transmitted to the pacing wires from hands, causing serious arrhythmias.
  - □ Client education
    - ▸ Instruct clients not to touch the pacemaker wires. If wires are exposed, clients should alert a provider to secure them.
    - ▸ Tell clients not to plug in or unplug electrical items. Advise clients not to use an electric razor or blow dryer.

ANGIOPLASTY

 Overview

- Percutaneous transluminal coronary angioplasty (PTCA) involves inflating a balloon to dilate the arterial lumen and the adhering plaque, thus widening the arterial lumen. A stent (mesh-wire device) is often placed to prevent restenosis of the artery.

> **ⓜ View Media Supplement:** Stent Placement (Animation)

- Indications
  - ○ PTCA can be performed on an elective basis to treat coronary artery disease when there is greater than 50% occlusion of one to two coronary arteries. The area of occlusion is confined, not scattered, and easy to access (proximal).
  - ○ PTCA may reduce ischemia during the occurrence of an acute MI, and it is most effective if it is done within 90 min of chest pain.
  - ○ PTCA with stent placement, to prevent artery reocclusion, may be used to dilate the left main coronary artery, which supplies blood flow to a large area of the heart.

- o Client Presentation
  - Subjective Data
    - □ Chest pain may occur with or without exertion. Pain may radiate to the jaw, left arm, through the back, or to the shoulder. Symptoms may increase in cold weather or with exercise. Other symptoms may include dyspnea, nausea, fatigue, and diaphoresis.
  - Objective Data
    - □ ECG changes may include ST elevation, depression, or nonspecific ST changes. Other signs may include bradycardia, tachycardia, hypotension, elevated blood pressure, vomiting, and mental disorientation.
- Client Outcomes
  - o The client will be able to perform activities of daily living free of pain or shortness of breath.
  - o The client will use strategies to reduce stress and modify lifestyle habits.
- Preprocedure
  - o Nursing Actions
    - Verify informed consent.
    - Maintain clients on NPO status for at least 8 hr if possible (risk for aspiration when lying flat for the procedure).
    - Determine that clients and their families understand the procedure.
    - Check clients for an iodine/shellfish allergy. (Use contrast dye instead of contrast media for consistency.)
    - Administer premedications as prescribed (antiplatelet medications, antianxiety agents).
    - Perform surgical preparation and shaving of the catheterization site.
    - Insert an indwelling urinary catheter if ordered.
  - o Client Education
    - Instruct clients that they may be awake and sedated for the procedure. A local anesthetic should be used. A small incision is made - often in the groin - to insert the catheter. Clients may feel warmth and flushed when the dye is inserted. After the procedure, clients will be asked to keep the affected leg straight. Pressure (a sandbag) may be placed on the incision to prevent bleeding.
- Postprocedure
  - o Nursing Actions
    - Monitor the client's vital signs every 15 min x 4, every 30 min x 2, every hour x 4, and then every 4 hr (or per facility protocol).

- Check the groin site at the same intervals for:
  - □ Bleeding and hematoma formation.
  - □ Thrombosis – document pedal pulse, color, and temperature.
- Maintain clients on bed rest in a supine position with leg straight for a prescribed time.
- Conduct continuous cardiac monitoring for dysrhythmias (reperfusion following angioplasty may cause dysrhythmias).
- Monitor clients receiving:
  - □ Antiplatelet or thrombolytic agents to prevent clot formation and restenosis.
  - □ Aspirin.
  - □ Clopidogrel (Plavix), tirofiban (Aggrastat).
  - □ Heparin.
  - □ Low molecular weight heparin enoxaparin (Lovenox).
  - □ Glycoprotein (GP IIb/IIIa) inhibitors (antiplatelet), such as eptifibatide (Integrilin).
  - □ Diltiazem (Cardizem) by IV bolus to prevent coronary vasospasm.
  - □ Anxiolytics for sedation.
  - □ Analgesics for pain.
- Monitor urine output and IV fluids for hydration.
  - □ Contrast dye acts as an osmotic diuretic.
- Monitor clients for signs and symptoms of hypokalemia.
- Assist with sheath removal from the insertion site (artery or vein).
  - □ The catheter sheath is a short hollow tube placed inside the artery or vein at the insertion site. It is used as a guide for the balloon catheter. After the angioplasty, the catheter sheath may be left in for access, so that the angioplasty may be repeated, if needed (for restenosis or perforation).
  - □ Apply pressure to arterial/venous sites for the prescribed period of time (varies depending upon the method used for vessel closure).
  - □ Observe for vagal response (hypotension, bradycardia) from compression of vagus nerve.
  - □ Apply a pressure dressing.

- o Client Education
  - Instruct clients to:
    - □ Avoid strenuous exercise for the prescribed period of time.
    - □ Immediately report bleeding from the insertion site, chest pain, shortness of breath, and changes in the color or temperature of the extremity.
    - □ Restrict lifting (less than 10 lb) for the prescribed period of time.
  - Clients with stent placement will receive anticoagulation therapy for 6 to 8 weeks (Clopidogrel may be needed for as long as 6 to 9 months). Instruct clients to:
    - □ Take the medication at the same time each day.
    - □ Have regular laboratory tests to determine therapeutic levels.
    - □ Avoid activities that could cause bleeding (use a soft toothbrush, wear shoes when out of bed).
  - Encourage clients to follow lifestyle guidelines (manage weight, consume a low-fat/low-cholesterol diet, exercise regularly, stop smoking, and decrease alcohol intake).
- Complications
  - o Hematoma formation
    - A blood clot may form near the insertion site.
    - Nursing Actions
      - □ Monitor for sensation, color, and peripheral pulses in the extremity distal to the insertion site.
      - □ Check the groin for signs of a hematoma at prescribed intervals and as needed.
      - □ Hold pressure for uncontrolled oozing/bleeding.
      - □ Notify the provider.
  - o Embolism
    - Plaque or a clot could become dislodged.
    - Nursing Actions
      - □ Monitor clients for chest pain during and after the procedure.
      - □ Monitor the client's vital signs and SaO_2.
  - o Restenosis of treated vessel
    - Clot reformation in the coronary artery may occur immediately or several weeks after the procedure.

- ■ Nursing Actions
  - □ Monitor ECG patterns and for the occurrence of chest pain.
  - □ Notify the provider immediately.
  - □ Prepare clients for return to the cardiac catheterization laboratory.
- ■ Client Education
  - □ Advise clients to notify the provider of cardiac symptoms and to take all medications as prescribed.

CORONARY ARTERY BYPASS GRAFTS

Overview

- Coronary artery bypass grafting (CABG) is an invasive surgical procedure that aims to restore vascularization of the myocardium.

> **View Media Supplement:** Bypass Graft (Image)

  - ○ Performed to bypass an obstruction in one or more of the coronary arteries, CABG does not alter the atherosclerotic process, but improves the quality of life for clients restricted by painful coronary artery disease.
  - ○ Older adult clients are more likely to experience transient neurological changes, toxic effects from cardiac medications, and dysrhythmias.
- Indications
  - ○ Diagnoses
    - ■ Over 50% blockage of the left main coronary artery with anginal episodes (blockage inaccessible to angioplasty and stenting)
    - ■ Significant two-vessel or triple-vessel disease
    - ■ Coronary artery disease nonresponsive to medical management
    - ■ Heart valve disease
    - ■ Ischemia with heart failure
    - ■ Coronary vessels unsuitable for PTCA
  - ○ Client Presentation
    - ■ Subjective Data
      - □ Chest pain may occur with or without exertion. Pain may radiate to the jaw, left arm, through the back, or to the shoulder. Symptoms may increase in cold weather or with exercise. Other symptoms may include dyspnea, nausea, fatigue, and diaphoresis.

- Objective Data
  - ECG changes may include ST elevation, depression, or nonspecific ST changes. Other signs may include bradycardia, tachycardia, hypotension, elevated blood pressure, vomiting, and mental disorientation.

- Client Outcomes
  - The client will be able to perform activities of daily living free of pain or shortness of breath.
  - The client will use strategies to reduce stress and modify lifestyle habits.

- Preprocedure
  - Nursing Actions
    - A CABG may be an elective procedure or done as an emergency. When planned, preparation begins before clients come to the facility for the procedure.
    - Verify that clients have signed the informed consent form.
    - Confirm that recent chest x-ray, ECG, and blood work results are available if needed.
    - Administer preoperative medications as prescribed.
      - Anxiolytics, such as lorazepam (Ativan) and diazepam (Valium)
      - Prophylactic antibiotics
      - Anticholinergics, such as scopolamine, to reduce secretions
    - Provide safe transport of clients to the operating suite. Monitor heart rate and rhythm, oxygenation, and other vital indicators.
  - Client Education
    - Provide instruction to clients and their families about the procedure and the postsurgical environment.
      - Inform clients of the importance of coughing and deep breathing and splinting the incision after the procedure to prevent complications.
      - Instruct clients to report any pain to the nursing staff. The majority of pain stems from the harvest site for the vein.
      - Inform clients and their families to expect the following postoperatively:
        - Endotracheal tube and mechanical ventilator for airway management for several hours following surgery
        - Inability to talk while the endotracheal tube is in place
        - Sternal incision and possible leg incision
        - One to 2 chest tubes
        - Indwelling urinary catheter
        - Pacemaker wires
        - Hemodynamic monitoring devices (pulmonary artery catheter, arterial line)

- □ Instruct clients to alter or discontinue regular medications as prescribed by the provider.
    - ▸ Medications frequently discontinued for CABG
        - ▷ Diuretics 2 to 3 days before surgery
        - ▷ Aspirin and other anticoagulants 1 week before surgery
    - ▸ Medications often continued for CABG
        - ▷ Potassium supplements
        - ▷ Scheduled antidysrhythmics, such as amiodarone (Cordarone)
        - ▷ Scheduled antihypertensives, such as metoprolol (Lopressor), a beta-blocker, and diltiazem (Cardizem), a calcium-channel blocker
        - ▷ Insulin (clients who have diabetes mellitus and are insulin-dependent usually receive half the regular insulin dose)
- Postprocedure
    - ○ Nursing Actions
        - ■ Provide postoperative care to prevent complications - usually in a specialty postoperative unit. Clients will receive mechanical ventilation for 3 to 6 hr.
    - ○ Client Education
        - ■ Instruct clients to monitor and report signs of infection such as fever, incisional drainage, and redness.
        - ■ Instruct clients to adhere to the pharmacological regimen.
        - ■ Instruct clients who have diabetes mellitus to closely monitor blood glucose levels.
        - ■ Encourage clients to consume a heart-healthy diet (low-fat, low-cholesterol, high-fiber, and low-salt).
        - ■ Encourage physical activity. Consult the cardiac rehabilitation program or a physical therapist to devise a specific program.
        - ■ Instruct clients to remain home during the first week after surgery and to resume normal activities slowly.
            - □ Week 2 – possible return to work part time, increase in social activities
            - □ Week 3 – lifting of up to 15 lb, avoidance of heavier lifting for 6 to 8 weeks
        - ■ Inform clients that they can resume sexual activity based on the advice of the provider.
            - □ Walking 1 block or climbing 2 flights of stairs symptom-free generally indicates that it is safe for clients to resume normal sexual activity.
        - ■ Encourage clients to verbalize their feelings.

- Complications

    o Pulmonary complications

        ▪ Atelectasis is a primary complication of a CABG. Other complications include pneumonia and pulmonary edema.

        ▪ Nursing Actions

            □ Turn clients every 2 hr and advance them out of bed as soon as possible.

            □ Monitor breath sounds, SaO_2, ABGs, pulmonary artery pressures, cardiac output, and urine output, and obtain a chest x-ray as indicated.

        ▪ Client Education

            □ Encourage coughing, deep breathing, and use of an incentive spirometer. Explain to clients that increasing activity reduces postoperative complications.

Peripheral Bypass Grafts

- Bypass graft surgery aims to restore adequate blood flow to the areas affected by peripheral artery disease.

    o A peripheral bypass graft involves suturing graft material or autogenous saphenous veins proximal and distal to an occluded area of an artery. This procedure improves blood supply to the area normally served by the blocked artery.

    o If bypass surgery fails to restore circulation, clients may need to undergo amputation of the limb.

- Indications

    o Acute circulatory compromise in limb

    o Severe pain at rest that interferes with ability to work

    o Client Presentation

        ▪ Subjective Data

            □ Numbness or burning pain to the lower extremity with exercise, and may stop with rest (intermittent claudication)

            □ Numbness or burning pain to the lower extremity at rest, and may wake client at night; pain may be relieved by lowering the extremity below heart

        ▪ Objective Data

            □ Decreased or absent pulses to feet. Dry, hairless, shiny skin on calves. Muscles may atrophy with advanced disease. Skin may be cold and dark colored. Feet and toes may be mottled and dusky, and toenails may be thick. Skin may become reddened (rubor) when extremity is dropped to a dependent position. Ulcers or lesions may be noted on toes (arterial ulcers) or ankles (venous ulcers).

- Client Outcomes

  o The client will have increased circulation in the extremity/foot.

  o The client will be pain free, and the foot will be intact without ulcerations or lesions.

  o The client will follow a recommended diet, exercise, and maintain foot care.

- Preprocedure

  o Nursing Actions

    ▪ Determine the client/family's understanding of the procedure.

    ▪ Verify that clients have signed the informed consent form.

    ▪ Check clients for allergies.

    ▪ Document the client's baseline vital signs and peripheral pulses.

    ▪ Administer prophylactic antibiotic therapy to clients as prescribed.

    ▪ Instruct clients to maintain NPO status for at least 8 hr prior to surgery.

  o Client Education

    ▪ Include information about postoperative pain management and teach clients deep breathing/ incentive spirometer exercises.

    ▪ Advise clients not to cross their legs.

    ▪ Clients may have an arterial line inserted for blood work and blood pressure monitoring.

    ▪ Explain to clients that pedal pulses will be checked frequently.

- Postprocedure

  o Nursing Actions

    ▪ Provide postoperative care to prevent complications.

  o Client Education

    ▪ Reinforce activity restrictions.

    ▪ Remind clients to avoid crossing their legs.

    ▪ Advise clients to avoid risk factors for atherosclerosis (smoking, sedentary life style, uncontrolled diabetes mellitus).

    ▪ Reinforce to clients techniques of foot inspection and care. Encourage clients to:

      □ Keep feet dry and clean.

      □ Avoid extreme temperatures.

      □ Use lotion.

      □ Avoid constraining garments.

      □ Wear clean, white, cotton socks and always wear shoes.

- Complications
  - Graft occlusion
    - The graft may occlude due to reduced blood flow and clot formation.
    - Nursing Actions
      - Notify the provider immediately for any noted changes in pedal pulse, extremity color, or temperature.
      - Prepare clients for thrombectomy or thrombolytic therapy.
      - Monitor for bleeding with thrombolytics.
      - Monitor coagulation studies.
      - Monitor for anaphylaxis.
  - Compartment syndrome
    - Pressure from tissue swelling or bleeding within a compartment or a restricted space causes reduced blood flow to the area. Untreated, the affected tissue will become necrotic and die.
    - Nursing Actions
      - Check for worsening pain, swelling, and tense or taut skin.
      - Report abnormal findings to the provider immediately.
      - Prepare clients for a fasciotomy to relieve compartmental pressure.
  - Infection
    - Infection of the surgical site may result in the loss of the graft and increased ischemia.
    - Nursing Actions
      - Monitor the wound for increased redness, swelling, and drainage.
      - Monitor WBC count and temperature.
      - Collect specimens (wound or blood cultures).
      - Administer antibiotic therapy.
    - Client Education
      - Advise clients to notify the provider of decreased sensation, increased ischemic pain, redness, or swelling at the incisional site or in the affected limb.

(A) APPLICATION EXERCISES

1. A nurse is caring for a client who has just received a temporary venous pacemaker. The pacemaker is set as a VVI pacemaker at a rate of 70/min. Which of the following findings should the nurse recognize as a concern?

   A. Observed pacing spike followed by a QRS complex

   B. Twitching of intercostal muscle

   C. Heart rate 72/min

   D. Blood pressure 110/64 mm Hg

2. A nurse is reinforcing teaching to a client who has received a permanent pacemaker. Which of the following statements made by the client indicates a need for further teaching?

   A. "I will call my doctor if I experience hiccups or muscle twitching."

   B. "I will take my pulse every morning when I awake."

   C. "I will stand across the room when using my microwave."

   D. "I will notify my dentist about my pacemaker."

3. A nurse is caring for a client who has had a peripheral bypass graft. Which of the following findings should the nurse recognize as a complication related to this procedure?

   A. Trace of bloody drainage on first dressing change

   B. Capillary refill of affected limb of 6 seconds

   C. Throbbing pain of affected limb that is decreased with administration of morphine

   D. Pulse of 2+ in the affected limb

(A) APPLICATION EXERCISES ANSWER KEY

1. A nurse is caring for a client who has just received a temporary venous pacemaker. The pacemaker is set as a VVI pacemaker at a rate of 70/min. Which of the following findings should the nurse recognize as a concern?

   A. Observed pacing spike followed by a QRS complex

   B. Twitching of intercostal muscle

   C. Heart rate 72/min

   D. Blood pressure 110/64 mm Hg

   Twitching of intercostal muscle may be a sign of lead wire perforation and stimulation of the diaphragm. A pacing spike followed by a QRS complex, heart rate 72/min, and blood pressure 110/64mm Hg are expected findings.

   (N) **NCLEX® Connection: Reduction of Risk Potential, Potential for Complications of Diagnostic Tests/Treatments/Procedures**

2. A nurse is reinforcing teaching to a client who has received a permanent pacemaker. Which of the following statements made by the client indicates a need for further teaching?

   A. "I will call my doctor if I experience hiccups or muscle twitching."

   B. "I will take my pulse every morning when I awake."

   C. "I will stand across the room when using my microwave."

   D. "I will notify my dentist about my pacemaker."

   Household appliances should not affect the pacemaker function unless held directly over pacer generator. This includes garage door openers, burglar alarms, microwave ovens, and antitheft devices. This indicates that the client does not understand the teaching and needs additional information. It is important for the client to notify the provider if he experiences hiccups or muscle twitching. This could be an indication that the pacemaker is pacing the diaphragm. The client should take his pulse every day at the same time. This indicates whether the pacemaker is functioning properly. The client should inform his dentist that he has had a pacemaker implanted. The dentist needs this information in case the client needs x-rays of the teeth.

   (N) **NCLEX® Connection: Reduction of Risk Potential, Therapeutic Procedures**

3. A nurse is caring for a client who has had a peripheral bypass graft. Which of the following findings should the nurse recognize as a complication related to this procedure?

    A. Trace of bloody drainage on first dressing change

    B. Capillary refill of affected limb of 6 seconds

    C. Throbbing pain of affected limb that is decreased with administration of morphine

    D. Pulse of 2+ in the affected limb

Capillary refill greater than 3 seconds and a limb that appears mottled indicate decreased circulation and may indicate graft occlusion. The provider should be notified immediately. A trace of bloody drainage on the first dressing change is an expected finding with this surgery. Throbbing pain that is decreased with morphine is a desired effect of this medication. A pulse of 2+ in the affected limb is a strong and desired pulse after this type of surgery.

NCLEX® Connection: Reduction of Risk Potential, Potential for Complications of Diagnostic Tests/Treatments/Procedures

UNIT 4	NURSING CARE OF CLIENTS WITH CARDIOVASCULAR DISORDERS
Section:	Cardiac Disorders
Chapter 28	Angina and Myocardial Infarction

 Overview

- The continuum from angina to myocardial infarction (MI) is termed acute coronary syndrome. Symptoms of acute coronary syndrome are due to an imbalance between myocardial oxygen supply and demand.

   View Media Supplement: Myocardial Infarction (Image)

- Angina pectoris is a warning sign of an impending acute MI.

- Women and older adults do not always experience symptoms typically associated with angina or MI.

- The majority of deaths from an MI occur within 1 hr of symptom onset.

- When blood flow to the heart is compromised, ischemia causes chest pain. Anginal pain is often described as a tight squeezing, heavy pressure, or constricting feeling in the chest. The pain can radiate to the jaw, neck, or arm.

   View Media Supplement: Anginal Pain (Image)

- There are three types of angina:

  ○ Stable angina (exertional angina) occurs with exercise or emotional stress and is relieved by rest or nitroglycerin (Nitrostat).

  ○ Unstable angina (preinfarction angina) occurs with exercise or emotional stress, but it increases in occurrence, severity, and duration over time. It may be poorly relieved by rest or nitroglycerin.

  ○ Variant angina (Prinzmetal's angina) is due to a coronary artery spasm, often occurring during periods of rest.

- An abrupt interruption of oxygen to the heart muscle produces myocardial ischemia. Ischemia can lead to tissue necrosis (infarction) if blood supply and oxygen are not restored. Ischemia is reversible, while an infarction results in permanent damage.

- Ischemic injury to cardiac muscle results in the release of cardiac enzymes into the bloodstream, providing specific markers of MI.

- MIs are classified based on:

  - The affected area of the heart (anterior, anterolateral).

  - The depth of involvement (transmural versus nontransmural).

  - The ECG changes produced (Q wave, non-Q wave). Non-Q-wave MIs are more common in older adults, women, and clients who have diabetes mellitus.

ANGINA	MYOCARDIAL INFARCTION
Precipitated by exertion or stress	Can occur without cause, often in the morning after rest
Relieved by rest or nitroglycerin	Relieved only by opioids
Symptoms usually last less than 15 min	Symptoms usually last greater than 30 min
Not associated with nausea, epigastric distress, dyspnea, anxiety, diaphoresis	Associated with nausea, epigastric distress, dyspnea, anxiety, diaphoresis

Data Collection

- Risk Factors

  - Male gender or postmenopausal women

  - Hypertension

  - Tobacco use

  - Hyperlipidemia

  - Metabolic disorders (diabetes mellitus, hyperthyroidism)

  - Methamphetamine or cocaine use

  - Stress (occupational, physical exercise, and sexual activity)

  - The incidence of cardiac disease increases with age, especially in the presence of hypertension, diabetes mellitus, hypercholesterolemia, elevated homocysteine, and highly sensitive C-reactive protein.

- Subjective Data

  - Women and older adults may not experience typical symptoms associated with angina or an MI.

  - Anxiety, feeling of impending doom

  - Chest pain (substernal or precordial)

    - Pain can radiate down the shoulder or arm or may present in the form of jaw pain.

    - Pain may be described as a crushing or aching pressure, tightness, or burning sensation.

- o Nausea

- o Dizziness

- o Shortness of breath

- Objective Data

  - o Physical Assessment Findings

    - Pallor and cool, clammy skin

    - Tachycardia and/or heart palpitations

    - Diaphoresis

    - Vomiting

    - Decreased level of consciousness

  - o Laboratory Tests

    - Cardiac enzymes released with cardiac muscle injury:

      - □ Myoglobin – Levels no longer evident after 24 hr

      - □ Creatine kinase-MB – Levels no longer evident after 3 days

      - □ Troponin I – Levels no longer evident after 7 days

      - □ Troponin T – Levels no longer evident after 14 to 21 days

  - o Diagnostic Procedures

    - Electrocardiograms (ECG)

      - □ Electrocardiography uses an electrocardiograph to record the electrical activity of the heart over time. The electrocardiograph is connected by wires (leads) to skin electrodes placed on various areas of the body.

      - □ Nursing Actions

        - ▸ Position clients in a supine position with the chest exposed.

        - ▸ Wash the client's skin to remove oils.

        - ▸ Attach one electrode to each extremity by applying electrodes to flat surfaces above the wrists and ankles and the other six electrodes to the chest, avoiding chest hair. (On male clients, chest hair may need to be shaved.)

        - ▸ Check for changes on serial ECGs.

        - ▸ Angina – ST depression and/or T-wave inversion (ischemia)

        - ▸ MI – T-wave inversion (ischemia), ST-segment elevation (injury), and an abnormal Q wave (necrosis)

    - Thallium scans

      - □ Assess for ischemia or necrosis. Radioisotopes cannot reach areas with decreased or absent perfusion and they appear as "cold spots."

□ Nursing Actions

▸ Instruct clients to avoid smoking and consuming caffeinated beverages 4 hr prior to the procedure.

■ Cardiac catheterization

□ A coronary angiogram, also called a cardiac catheterization, is an invasive diagnostic procedure used to evaluate the presence and degree of coronary artery blockage.

Collaborative Care

- Nursing Care

  o Monitor:

    ■ Vital signs every 15 min until stable, then every hour

    ■ Serial ECG, continuous cardiac monitoring

    ■ Location, severity, quality, and duration of pain

    ■ Hourly urine output – greater than 30 mL/hr indicates renal perfusion

    ■ Laboratory data (cardiac enzymes, electrolytes, ABGs)

  o Administer oxygen (2 to 4 L via nasal cannula)

  o Assist with administration of IV fluids.

  o Promote energy conservation (cluster nursing interventions).

- Medications

  o Vasodilators

    ■ Nitroglycerin (Nitrostat) prevents coronary artery vasospasm and reduces preload and afterload, decreasing myocardial oxygen demand.

    ■ Nursing Considerations

      □ Administer to treat angina and help control blood pressure.

      □ Monitor for orthostatic hypotension.

    ■ Client Education

      □ Client education regarding response to chest pain:

        ▸ Instruct clients to:

          ▷ Stop activity.

          ▷ Take a dose of rapid-acting nitroglycerin immediately.

          ▷ Wait 5 min.

          ▷ Call 9-1-1, or be driven to an emergency department if pain is unrelieved.

          ▷ Take another dose.

▷ Wait 5 min.

▷ Take another dose if pain unrelieved.

□ Remind clients that a headache is a common side effect of this medication.

□ Encourage clients to change positions slowly.

o Analgesics

■ Morphine sulfate is an opioid analgesic used to treat moderate to severe pain.

■ Use cautiously with clients who have asthma or emphysema due to the risk of respiratory depression.

■ Nursing Considerations

□ Assist with client receiving morphine sulfate via IV bolus. Check the client's pain level every 5 to 15 min.

□ Watch clients for signs of respiratory depression, especially older adults. If the respirations are 12/min or less notify the provider immediately.

□ Observe clients for nausea and vomiting.

■ Client Education

□ If nausea and vomiting persist, advise clients to notify a nurse.

o Beta-blockers

■ Metoprolol tartrate (Lopressor) has antidysrhythmic and antihypertensive properties that decrease the imbalance between myocardial oxygen supply and demand by reducing afterload.

■ Nursing Considerations

□ Hold the medication if the client's apical pulse is less than 60/min and notify the provider.

□ Use with caution in clients who have heart failure.

■ Client Education

□ Remind clients to notify the provider immediately if shortness of breath, edema, weight gain, or cough occurs.

o Thrombolytic agents

■ Streptokinase (Streptase) and alteplase (Activase) are used to break up blood clots.

■ Thrombolytic agents have similar side effects and contraindications as anticoagulants.

■ For best results give within 6 hr of infarction.

o Antiplatelet agents

■ Aspirin (Ecotrin) and clopidogrel (Plavix) prevent platelets from forming together, which can produce arterial clotting.

- ■ Nursing Considerations
    - ☐ Use cautiously with clients who have a history of GI ulcers.
- ■ Client Education
    - ☐ Remind clients of the risk for bruising and bleeding while on this medication.
    - ☐ Encourage clients to use aspirin tablets with enteric coating and to take with food.
- ○ Anticoagulants
    - ■ Heparin and enoxaparin (Lovenox) are used to prevent clots from becoming larger or other clots from forming.
    - ■ Nursing Considerations
        - ☐ Check for contraindications (active bleeding, peptic ulcer disease, history of CVA, or recent trauma).
        - ☐ Monitor bleeding times – PT, aPTT, INR, and CBC.
        - ☐ Monitor for side effects of anticoagulants (thrombocytopenia, anemia, and hemorrhage).
    - ■ Client Education
        - ☐ Remind clients of the risk for bruising and bleeding while on this medication.
- ○ Glycoprotein IIB/IIIA inhibitors
    - ■ Eptifibatide (Integrilin) is used to prevent the binding of fibrogen, in turn blocking platelet aggregation. In combination with aspirin therapy, IIB/IIA inhibitors are standard therapy.
    - ■ Nursing Considerations
        - ☐ Monitor clients for bleeding.
    - ■ Client Education
        - ☐ Instruct clients to report signs of bleeding during medication therapy.
- • Interdisciplinary Care
    - ○ Request a referral for cardiac rehabilitation care if clients have prolonged weakness and need assistance with increasing level of activity.
    - ○ Request a referral for nutritional services for diet modification to promote low-sodium and low-saturated fat food choices.

- Surgical Interventions

  o Angioplasty

    - Percutaneous transluminal coronary angioplasty (PTCA) involves inflating a balloon to dilate the arterial lumen and the adhering plaque, thus widening the arterial lumen. A stent (mesh-wire device) is often placed to prevent restenosis of the artery.

    - Nursing Actions

      □ Verify that the consent form is signed.

      □ Ensure that clients are kept NPO 8 hr prior to the procedure.

      □ Check for iodine/shellfish allergy (contrast media).

  o Bypass graft

    - Coronary artery bypass graft (CABG) surgery restores myocardial tissue perfusion by the addition of grafts bypassing the obstructed coronary arteries. It is the most common form of cardiac surgery.

    - Nursing Actions

      □ A CABG can be an elective procedure or done in an emergency. When planned, preparation begins before clients come to the hospital for the procedure.

      □ Verify that the informed consent is signed.

      □ Confirm recent chest x-ray, ECG, and blood work results are available or needed.

- Care after Discharge

  o Client Education

    - Encourage clients to maintain an exercise routine to remain physically active. Clients should consult with a provider before starting any exercise regimen.

    - Remind clients to adhere to follow-up appointments to have their cholesterol level and blood pressure checked regularly.

    - Encourage clients to consume a diet low in saturated fats and sodium.

    - If clients are smokers promote smoking cessation.

    - Instruct clients to monitor and report signs of infection, such as fever, incisional drainage, and redness.

    - Reinforce to clients to avoid straining, strenuous exercise, or emotional stress when possible.

- Client Outcomes

  o The client will be free of pain.

  o The client will be able to maintain exercise routine.

UNIT 4	NURSING CARE OF CLIENTS WITH CARDIOVASCULAR DISORDERS
Section:	Cardiac Disorders
Chapter 29	Heart Failure

 Overview

- Heart failure (pump failure) occurs when the heart muscle is unable to pump effectively, resulting in inadequate cardiac output, myocardial hypertrophy, and pulmonary/systemic congestion. The heart is unable to maintain adequate circulation to meet tissue needs.

- Heart failure is the result of an acute or chronic cardiopulmonary problem, such as systemic hypertension, myocardial infarction (MI), pulmonary hypertension, dysrhythmias, valvular heart disease, pericarditis, and cardiomyopathy.

- The severity of heart failure is graded on the New York Heart Association's functional classification scale indicating how little or how much activity it takes to make clients symptomatic (chest pain, shortness of breath).

    ○ Class I: Clients exhibit no symptoms with activity.

    ○ Class II: Clients have symptoms with ordinary exertion.

    ○ Class III: Clients display symptoms with minimal exertion.

    ○ Class IV: Clients have symptoms at rest.

- Low-output heart failure can initially occur on either the left or right side of the heart.

    ○ Left-sided heart (ventricular) failure results in inadequate left ventricle (cardiac) output and consequently in inadequate tissue perfusion.

    ○ Right-sided heart (ventricular) failure results in inadequate right ventricle output and systemic venous congestion (peripheral edema).

Data Collection

- Risk Factors

    ○ Left-sided heart (ventricular) failure

        ■ Hypertension

        ■ Coronary artery disease, angina, MI

        ■ Valvular disease (mitral and aortic)

- ○ Right-sided heart (ventricular) failure
  - ■ Left-sided heart (ventricular) failure
  - ■ Right ventricular MI
  - ■ Pulmonary problems (COPD, ARDS)
- Subjective and Objective Data
  - ○ Left-sided failure
    - ■ Dyspnea, orthopnea (shortness of breath while lying down), nocturnal dyspnea
    - ■ Fatigue
    - ■ Displaced apical pulse (hypertrophy)
    - ■ S_3 heart sound (gallop)
    - ■ Pulmonary congestion (dyspnea, cough, bibasilar crackles)
    - ■ Frothy sputum (can be blood-tinged)
    - ■ Altered mental status
    - ■ Symptoms of organ failure, such as oliguria (decrease in urine output)
  - ○ Right-sided failure
    - ■ Jugular vein distention
    - ■ Ascending dependent edema (legs, ankles, sacrum)
    - ■ Abdominal distention, ascites
    - ■ Fatigue, weakness
    - ■ Nausea and anorexia
    - ■ Polyuria at rest (nocturnal)
    - ■ Liver enlargement (hepatomegaly) and tenderness
    - ■ Weight gain
  - ○ Laboratory Tests
    - ■ Human B-type natriuretic peptides (hBNP): Elevated in heart failure. Used to differentiate dyspnea related to heart failure versus respiratory problem and to monitor the need for and the effectiveness of aggressive heart failure intervention.
      - □ A level below 100 pg/mL indicates no heart failure.
      - □ Levels between 100 to 300 pg/mL suggest heart failure is present.
      - □ A level above 300 pg/mL indicates mild heart failure.
      - □ A level above 600 pg/mL indicates moderate heart failure.
      - □ A level above 900 pg/mL indicates severe heart failure.

- o Diagnostic Procedures
  - ■ Hemodynamic monitoring
    - □ Heart failure generally results in increased central venous pressure (CVP), increased right arterial pressure, increased pulmonary wedge pressure (PAWP), increased pulmonary artery pressure (PAP), and decreased cardiac output (CO).
  - ■ Ultrasound
    - □ An ultrasound (also called cardiac ultrasound or echocardiogram), 2-D (2-dimensional), or 3-D (3-dimensional), is used to measure both systolic and diastolic function of the heart.
      - ▸ Left ventricular ejection fraction (LVEF): The volume of blood pumped from the left ventricle into the arteries upon each beat. Normal is 55% to 70%.
      - ▸ Right ventricular ejection fraction (RVEF): The volume of blood pumped from the right ventricle to the lungs upon each beat. Normal is 45% to 60%.
  - ■ A chest x-ray can reveal cardiomegaly and pleural effusions.
  - ■ Electrocardiogram (ECG), cardiac enzymes, electrolytes, and ABGs are used to assess factors contributing to heart failure and/or the impact of heart failure.

Collaborative Care

- • Nursing Care
  - o Monitor daily weight and I&O.
  - o Administer oxygen as prescribed.
  - o Position clients to maximize ventilation (high-Fowler's position).
  - o Check ABGs, electrolytes (especially potassium if on diuretics), SaO_2, and chest x-ray results.
  - o Encourage bed rest until clients are stable.
  - o Encourage energy conservation by assisting with care and ADLs.
  - o Maintain dietary restrictions as prescribed (restricted fluid intake, restricted sodium intake).
  - o Provide emotional support to clients and their families.
- • Medications
  - o Diuretics
    - ■ Diuretics are used to decrease preload.
      - □ Loop diuretics, such as furosemide (Lasix), bumetanide (Bumex)
      - □ Thiazide diuretics, such as hydrochlorothiazide (Hydrodiuril)
      - □ Potassium-sparing diuretics, such as spironolactone (Aldactone)

- Nursing Considerations
  - Administer potassium supplements for clients taking loop and thiazide diuretics to prevent.
- Client Education
  - Teach clients taking loop or thiazide diuretics to ingest foods and drinks that are high in potassium to counter the effects of hypokalemia.

○ Afterload-reducing agents
- Afterload-reducing agents help the heart pump more easily by altering the resistance to contraction. These include:
  - Angiotensin-converting enzyme (ACE) inhibitors, such as enalapril (Vasotec), captopril (Capoten)
  - Angiotensin receptor II blockers, such as losartan (Cozaar)
- These are contraindicated for clients who have renal deficiency.
- Nursing Considerations
  - Monitor clients taking ACE inhibitors for hypotension following the initial dose. Monitor clients for 2 hr following first dose.
    - ACE inhibitors can cause angioedema (swelling of the tongue and throat).
    - Monitor for increased levels in potassium.
    - ACE inhibitors can cause a decreased sense of taste or rash on the skin.
- Client Education
  - Inform clients to monitor and notify the provider for dry cough, rash, altered taste sensation, or swelling of the tongue and pharynx. Medication should be discontinued.

○ Inotropic agents
- Inotropic agents, such as digoxin (Lanoxin), are used to increase contractility and thereby improve cardiac output.
- Nursing Considerations
  - For a client taking digoxin, take the apical heart rate for 1 min. Hold the medication if apical pulse is less than 60/min and notify the provider.
  - Observe clients for toxicity such as bradycardia, anorexia, nausea, vomiting fatigue, muscle weakness, and vision changes (blurred vision, diplopia, yellow-green or white halos around objects).

- Client Education
  - Reinforce to clients who are self-administering digoxin to:
    - Count pulse for 1 min before taking the medication. If the pulse rate is irregular or the pulse rate is outside of the limitations set by the provider (usually less than 60/min or greater than 100/min), instruct clients to hold the dose and to contact the provider.
    - Take the digoxin dose at the same time each day.
    - Do not take digoxin at the same time as antacids. Separate the two medications by at least 2 hr.
    - Report signs of toxicity, including fatigue, muscle weakness, confusion, and loss of appetite.
    - Regularly have digoxin and potassium levels checked.
- Vasodilators
  - Nitroglycerine (Nitrostat) and isosorbide mononitrate (Imdur) prevent coronary artery vasospasm and reduce preload and afterload, decreasing myocardial oxygen demand.
  - Nursing Considerations
    - Administer vasodilators to treat angina and help control blood pressure.
    - Use cautiously with other antihypertensive mediations.
    - Monitor for orthostatic hypotension.
  - Client Education
    - Remind clients that a headache is a common side effect of this medication.
    - Encourage clients to change slowly.
- Human B-type natriuretic peptides (hBNP)
  - hBNPs, such as nesiritide (Natrecor), are used to treat acute heart failure by causing natriuresis (loss of sodium and vasodilation).
  - Nursing Considerations
    - hBNPs can cause hypotension, as well as a number of cardiac effects that include, ventricular tachycardia and bradycardia.
    - BNP levels will increase while on this medication.
    - Monitor ECG and blood pressure.
  - Client Education
    - Remind clients to change positions slowly.

- ○ Anticoagulants

  - ▪ Anticoagulants, such as warfarin (Coumadin), can be prescribed if clients have a history of thrombus formation.

  - ▪ Nursing Considerations

    - ☐ Check for contraindications (active bleeding, peptic ulcer disease, history of cerebrovascular accident, recent trauma).

    - ☐ Monitor bleeding times – PT, aPTT, INR, and CBC.

  - ▪ Client Education

    - ☐ Remind clients of the risk for bruising and bleeding while on this medication.

    - ☐ Remind clients to have blood monitored routinely to check bleeding times.

- • Interdisciplinary Care

  - ○ Request a referral for respiratory services to assist with inhalers, breathing treatments, and suctioning for airway management.

  - ○ Request a referral for cardiac rehabilitation services if clients have prolonged weakness and need assistance with increasing level of activity.

  - ○ Request a referral for nutritional services for diet modification to promote low-sodium and low-saturated fat food choices.

- • Surgical Interventions

  - ○ Ventricular assist device (VAD)

    - ☐ A VAD is a mechanical pump that assists a heart that is too weak to pump blood through the body. A VAD is used in clients who are eligible for heart transplants or who have severe end-stage heart failure and are not candidates for heart transplants. Heart transplantation is the treatment of choice for clients who have severe dilated cardiomyopathy.

    - ▪ Nursing Actions

      - ☐ Prepare clients for the procedure (NPO status and informed consent).

      - ☐ Monitor postoperatively (vital signs, SaO_2, incision drainage, and pain management).

  - ○ Heart Transplantation

    - ▪ Heart transplantation is a possible option for clients who have end-stage heart failure. Immunosuppressant therapy is required posttransplantation to prevent rejection.

- Nursing Actions
    - Prepare clients for the procedure (NPO status and informed consent).
    - Monitor postoperatively (vital signs, SaO_2, incision drainage, and pain management).
- Client Education
    - Take medications as prescribed.
    - Take diuretics in the early morning and early afternoon.
    - Maintain fluid and sodium restriction – A dietary consult can be useful.
    - Increase dietary intake of potassium (cantaloupe or bananas) if clients are taking potassium-losing diuretics, such as loop and thiazide diuretics.
    - Check weight daily at the same time and notify the provider for a weight gain of 2 lb in 24 hr or 5 lb in 1 week.
    - Schedule regular follow-up visits with the provider.
    - Get vaccinations (pneumococcal and yearly influenza vaccines).

- Care After Discharge
    - Client Education
        - Encourage clients to maintain an exercise routine to remain physically active and consult with the provider before starting any exercise regimen.
        - Recommend clients consume a diet low in sodium, along with fluid restrictions and consult with the provider regarding diet specifications.
        - Promote smoking cessation.
        - Instruct clients to follow medication regimen and follow up with the provider as needed.

- Client Outcomes
    - The client will have adequate gas exchange.
    - The client will have a decrease in anxiety.
    - The client will maintain fluid balance.
    - The client will improve tolerance to activity.
    - The client will have an increase in cardiac output.

Complications

- Cardiomyopathy

 View Media Supplement: Cardiomyopathy (Image)

  - Cardiomyopathy is an impaired cardiac function leading to heart failure. Blood circulation is impaired to the lungs or body when the cardiac pump is compromised. Of the three types (dilated cardiomyopathy, hypertrophic cardiomyopathy, restrictive cardiomyopathy), dilated cardiomyopathy is the most common.
    - Dilated – Decreased contractility and increased ventricular filling pressures
    - This can be a result of:
      - Coronary artery disease
      - Infection or inflammation of the heart muscle
      - Various cancer treatments
      - Prolonged alcohol abuse
  - Data Collection
    - Subjective and Objective Data
      - Fatigue, weakness
      - Heart failure (left with dilated type, right with restrictive type)
      - Dysrhythmias (heart block)
      - S_3 gallop
      - Cardiomegaly (enlarged heart)
  - Nursing Actions
    - Monitor clients for increased fatigue, weakness, and dysrhythmias.
    - Notify provider of findings.
    - Provide quiet, calm environment and promote rest.
  - Client Education
    - Reinforce to clients about measures to improve tolerance to activity, such as alternating periods of activity with periods of rest.

- Acute pulmonary edema
  - Acute pulmonary edema is a life-threatening medical emergency.
  - Nursing Actions
    - Administer prescribed medications to improve cardiac output.
    - Symptoms include anxiety, tachycardia, acute respiratory distress, dyspnea at rest change in level of consciousness, and an ascending fluid level within the lungs (crackles, cough productive of frothy, blood-tinged sputum).

UNIT 4	NURSING CARE OF CLIENTS WITH CARDIOVASCULAR DISORDERS
Section:	Cardiac Disorders
Chapter 30	Valvular Heart Disease and Inflammatory Disorders

Overview

- Valvular heart disease and inflammatory conditions of the heart (pericarditis, myocarditis, rheumatic endocarditis, infective endocarditis) may result in dysfunction that impacts clients' ability to meet tissue and oxygen demands.

VALVULAR HEART DISEASE

Overview

- Valvular heart disease describes an abnormality or dysfunction of any of the heart's four valves: the mitral and aortic valves (left side) and the tricuspid and pulmonic valves (right side).

 View Media Supplement: Normal Blood Flow in a Heart and Altered Blood Flow (Image)

- Valvular heart disease is classified as:

  ○ Stenosis – Narrowed opening that impedes blood moving forward.

  ○ Insufficiency – Improper closure – Some blood flows backwards (regurgitation).

- Valvular heart disease can have congenital or acquired causes.

  ○ Congenital valvular heart disease can affect all four valves and cause either stenosis or insufficiency.

  ○ Acquired valvular heart disease is classified as one of three types:

    ▪ Degenerative disease – Due to damage over time from mechanical stress. The most common cause is hypertension.

    ▪ Rheumatic disease – Gradual fibrotic changes, calcification of valve cusps. The mitral valve is most commonly affected.

    ▪ Infective endocarditis – Infectious organisms destroy the valve. Streptococcal infections are a common cause.

Data Collection

- Risk Factors

  - Hypertension

  - Rheumatic fever (mitral stenosis and insufficiency)

  - Infective endocarditis

  - Congenital malformations

  - Female gender

  - Marfan syndrome (connective tissue disorder that affects the heart and other areas of the body)

  - In older adult clients, the predominant causes of valvular heart disease are degenerative calcification, papillary muscle dysfunction, and infective endocarditis.

  - A murmur is heard with turbulent blood flow. The location of the murmur and timing (diastolic versus systolic) help determine the valve involved. Murmurs are graded on a scale of I (very faint) to VI (extremely loud).

- Subjective and Objective Data

LEFT-SIDED VALVE DAMAGE RESULTS IN DYSPNEA, FATIGUE, INCREASED PULMONARY ARTERY PRESSURE, AND DECREASED CARDIAC OUTPUT.			
MITRAL STENOSIS	**MITRAL INSUFFICIENCY**	**AORTIC STENOSIS**	**AORTIC INSUFFICIENCY**
• Palpitations • Hemoptysis • Hoarseness • Dysphagia • Jugular vein distention • Orthopnea • Cough • Diastolic murmur • Atrial fibrillation	• Proximal nocturnal • Dyspnea • Orthopnea • Palpitations • S_3 and/or S_4 sounds • Crackles in lungs • Possible diminished lung sounds • Systolic murmur • Atrial fibrillation	• Angina • Syncope • Decreased SVR • S_3 and/or S_4 sounds • Systolic murmur • Narrowed pulse pressure	• Angina • S_3 sounds • Diastolic murmur • Widened pulse pressure

RIGHT-SIDED VALVE DAMAGE RESULTS IN DYSPNEA, FATIGUE, INCREASED RIGHT ATRIAL PRESSURE, PERIPHERAL EDEMA, JUGULAR VEIN DISTENTION, AND HEPATOMEGALY.			
TRICUSPID STENOSIS	**TRICUSPID INSUFFICIENCY**	**PULMONIC STENOSIS**	**PULMONIC INSUFFICIENCY**
• Atrial dysrhythmias • Diastolic murmur • Decreased cardiac output	• Conduction delays • Supraventricular tachycardia • Systolic murmur	• Cyanosis • Systolic murmur	• Diastolic murmur

- o Diagnostic Procedures
  - Chest x-ray
    - □ A chest x-ray shows chamber enlargement, pulmonary congestion, and valve calcification.
  - 12-lead electrocardiogram (ECG)
    - □ An ECG shows chamber hypertrophy.
  - Echocardiogram
    - □ An echocardiogram shows chamber size, hypertrophy, specific valve dysfunction, ejection function, and amount of regurgitant flow.
  - Exercise tolerance testing/stress echocardiography
    - □ A stress echocardiography is used to assess the impact of the valve problem on cardiac functioning during stress.
  - Radionuclide studies
    - □ Radionuclide studies determine ejection fraction during activity and rest.
  - Angiography
    - □ Angiography reveals chamber pressures, ejection fraction, regurgitation, and pressure gradients.

Collaborative Care

- • Nursing Care
  - o Monitor current weight and note any recent changes.
  - o Monitor heart rate and rhythm. Check for murmurs.
  - o Administer oxygen and medications as prescribed.
  - o Maintain fluid and sodium restriction.
  - o Assist clients to conserve energy.
- • Medications
  - o Diuretics
    - Diuretics are used to decrease preload.
      - □ Loop diuretics, such as furosemide (Lasix), bumetanide (Bumex)
      - □ Thiazide diuretics, such as hydrochlorothiazide (Hydrodiuril)
      - □ Potassium-sparing diuretics, such as spironolactone (Aldactone)
    - Nursing Considerations
      - □ Monitor for hypokalemia with loop and thiazide diuretics. Administer a potassium supplement as needed.

- Client Education
  - Reinforce to clients who are taking loop or thiazide diuretics to ingest foods and drinks that are high in potassium to counter hypokalemia effect.
- Afterload-reducing agents
  - Afterload-reducing agents help the heart pump more easily by altering the resistance to contraction.
    - Angiotensin-converting enzyme (ACE) inhibitors, such as enalapril (Vasotec), captopril (Capoten)
    - Beta-blockers
    - Calcium-channel blockers
  - Nursing Considerations
    - Monitor clients taking ACE inhibitors for initial dose hypotension.
- Inotropic agents
  - Inotropic agents, such as digoxin (Lanoxin), are used to increase contractility and thereby improve cardiac output.
  - Client Education
    - Reinforce to clients who are self-administering digoxin to:
      - Count pulse for 1 min before taking the medication. If the pulse rate is irregular or the pulse rate is outside of the limitations set by the provider (usually less than 60/min or greater than 100/min), clients should hold the dose and contact the provider.
      - Take the dose of digoxin at the same time every day.
      - Do not take digoxin at the same time as antacids. Separate the two medications by at least 2 hr.
      - Report signs of toxicity, including fatigue, muscle weakness, confusion, visual changes, and loss of appetite.
- Anticoagulants
  - Anticoagulation therapy is used for clients who have a mechanical valve replacement, atrial fibrillation, or severe left ventricle dysfunction.
- Interdisciplinary Care
  - Request a referral for respiratory services to assist with inhalers, breathing treatments, and suctioning for airway management.
  - Request a referral for nutritional services for weight loss or gain related to medications or diagnosis.
  - Request a referral for rehabilitative care if clients have prolonged weakness and need assistance with increasing level of activity.

- Surgical Interventions

  - Percutaneous balloon valvuloplasty

    - This procedure can open aortic or mitral valves affected by stenosis. A catheter is inserted through the femoral artery and advanced to the heart. A balloon is inflated at the stenotic lesion to open the fused commissures and improve leaflet mobility.

  - Miscellaneous surgical management

    - Surgeries used in the treatment of valvular disorders include valve repair, chordae tendineae reconstruction, commissurotomy (relieve stenosis on leaflets), annuloplasty ring insertion (correct dilatation of valve annulus), and prosthetic valve replacement.

      - Prosthetic valves can be mechanical or tissue. Mechanical valves last longer but require anticoagulation. Tissue valves last 10 to 15 years.

      - Medical management is appropriate for many older adult clients; surgery is indicated when symptoms interfere with ADLs. The goal of surgery can be to improve the quality of life rather than to prolong life.

      - Nursing Actions

      - Postsurgery care is similar to coronary artery bypass surgery (care for sternal incision, activity limited for 6 weeks, report fever).

- Care after Discharge

  - Client Education

    - Remind clients of the need for prophylactic antibiotics prior to dental work, surgery, or other invasive procedures.

    - Encourage clients to follow the prescribed exercise program.

    - Encourage clients to consume a diet low in sodium and follow fluid restrictions prescribed by provider to prevent heart failure. Reinforce energy conservation to clients.

- Client Outcomes

  - The client will maintain the prescribed medication treatment regimen.

  - The client will maintain an unrestricted activity level without shortness of breath or chest pain.

  - The client will be free from anxiety.

  - The client will remain free from infection.

  - The client will be able to maintain within 10% of the ideal body weight.

Complications

- Heart Failure

  - Heart failure is the inability of the heart to maintain adequate circulation to meet tissue needs for oxygen and nutrients. Ineffective valves result in heart failure.

  - Nursing Actions

    - Monitor client's cardiac status.

INFLAMMATORY DISORDERS

Overview

- Inflammation related to the heart is an extended inflammatory response that often leads to the destruction of healthy tissue. This primarily includes the layers of the heart.

- Inflammatory disorders related to the cardiovascular system that nurses should be familiar with include:

  - Pericarditis

  - Myocarditis

  - Rheumatic endocarditis

  - Infective endocarditis (previously called bacterial endocarditis)

Health Promotion and Disease Prevention

- Early treatment of streptococcal infections can prevent rheumatic fever.

- Prophylactic treatments (including antibiotics for clients who have cardiac defects) can prevent infective endocarditis.

- Influenza and pneumonia vaccinations are important for all clients in order to decrease the incidence of myocarditis, especially in older adults.

Data Collection

- Risk Factors

  - Congenital heart defect/cardiac anomalies

  - Immunosuppression

  - Rheumatic endocarditis

  - School-age children who have long duration of streptococcus infection

  - Malnutrition

  - Overcrowding

  - Lower socioeconomic status

- Subjective and Objective Data

INFLAMMATORY DISORDER	DESCRIPTION OF DISEASE PROCESS	RELEVANT INFORMATION
Pericarditis	This is an inflammation of the pericardium.	• This commonly follows a respiratory infection. • Pericarditis can be due to a myocardial infarction. • Findings include chest pressure/pain, friction rub auscultated in the lungs, shortness of breath, and pain relieved when sitting and leaning forward.
Myocarditis	This is an inflammation of the myocardium.	• This can be due to a viral or fungal infection. • Myocarditis can be due to a systemic disease (Crohn's disease). • Findings include tachycardia, murmur, friction rub auscultated in the lungs, cardiomegaly, and dysrhythmias.
Rheumatic endocarditis	This is an infection of the endocardium due to streptococcal bacteria.	• This is followed by an upper respiratory infection. • Rheumatic endocarditis produces lesions in the heart. • This occurs with half of the clients who have rheumatic fever. • Findings include fever, chest pain, joint pain, tachycardia, shortness of breath, rash on trunk and extremities, friction rub, murmur, and muscle spasms.
Infective endocarditis	This is also known as bacterial endocarditis, and is an infection of the endocardium due to streptococcal or staphylococcal bacteria.	• This is most common in IV drug users or clients who have cardiac malformations. • Findings include fever, flu-like symptoms, murmur, petechiae (on the trunk and mucous membranes), positive blood cultures, and splinter hemorrhages (red streaks under the nail beds).

- ○ Laboratory Tests

  - ■ Blood cultures can be drawn to detect a bacterial infection.

  - ■ An elevated WBC count can be indicative of a bacterial infection.

  - ■ Cardiac enzymes can be elevated with pericarditis.

  - ■ Throat cultures can be taken to detect a streptococcal infection, which can lead to rheumatic fever.

- ○ Diagnostic Procedures

  - ■ ECG can detect a murmur or heart block, which is indicative of rheumatic fever.

Collaborative Care

- Nursing Care

  o Monitor vital signs (watch for fever).

  o Auscultate heart sounds (listen for murmur).

  o Check breath sounds in all lung fields (listen for friction rub).

  o Check ABGs, SaO_2, and chest x-ray results.

  o Administer oxygen as prescribed.

  o Monitor ECG and notify the provider of changes.

  o Obtain throat cultures to identify bacteria to treat with antibiotics.

  o Administer antibiotics, antipyretics, and analgesics as prescribed.

  o Encourage bed rest.

- Medications

TYPE	PURPOSE	NURSING CONSIDERATIONS	CLIENT EDUCATION
Medication: Penicillin			
Antibiotic	This is given to treat an infection.	• Monitor for skin rash and hives. • Monitor electrolyte and kidney levels.	• Instruct clients to report signs of skin rash or hives. • Inform clients that the medication may cause gastrointestinal (GI) distress.
Medication: Ibuprofen (Advil)			
NSAID (non-steroidal anti-inflammatory drug)	This is given to treat fever and inflammation.	• Do not use in clients who have peptic ulcer disease. • Watch for signs of GI distress. • Monitor platelets, and liver and kidney levels.	• Instruct clients to take the medication with food. • Inform clients that the medication may cause GI distress. • Instruct clients to avoid alcohol consumption while taking the medication.

TYPE	PURPOSE	NURSING CONSIDERATIONS	CLIENT EDUCATION
Medication: Prednisone (Deltasone)			
Glucocorticosteroid	This is given to treat inflammation.	• Use in low doses. • Monitor blood pressure. • Monitor electrolytes and blood sugar levels. • Clients may heal slowly on this medication.	• Instruct clients to take the medication with food. • Instruct clients to avoid stopping the medication abruptly. • Instruct clients to report signs of an unexpected weight gain.
Medication: Amphotericin B (Amphocin)			
Antifungal	This is given to treat fungus.	• Monitor liver and kidney levels.	• Inform clients that the medication may cause GI distress.
Medication: Diazepam (Valium)			
Benzodiazepine	This is given to treat anxiety.	• Start in low doses, and monitor for sleepiness and lightheadedness. • Monitor the client's liver function.	• Instruct clients to take the medication as prescribed. • Instruct clients to avoid alcohol consumption while taking the medication. • Instruct clients to avoid stopping the medication abruptly.

- Interdisciplinary Care
  - Cardiology services may be consulted to manage cardiac dysfunction.
  - Request a referral for physical therapy to increase the client's level of activity once prescribed.
  - Request a referral for home health care to assist with IV administration of antibiotics.
- Surgical Interventions
  - Pericarditis
    - Pericardiocentesis
      - A needle is inserted into the pericardium to aspirate pericardial fluid. This can be done in the emergency department or a procedure room.
    - Nursing Actions
      - Pericardial fluid can be sent to the laboratory for culture and sensitivity.
      - Monitor for reoccurrence of cardiac tamponade.

- o Infective endocarditis
  - □ Valve debridement, draining of abscess, and repairing congenital shunts are procedures involved with infective endocarditis.
  - ■ Nursing Actions
    - □ Monitor for signs of bleeding, infection, and cardiac output.

- Care after Discharge
  - o Client Education
    - ■ Encourage clients to take rest periods as needed.
    - ■ Encourage clients to wash hands and practice good oral hygiene to prevent infection.
    - ■ Encourage clients to avoid crowded areas to reduce the risk of infection.
    - ■ Educate clients about the importance of taking medications as prescribed.
    - ■ Promote smoking cessation.

- Client Outcomes
  - o The client will be free from infection.
  - o The client will be free from pain.
  - o The client will take medications as prescribed.

Complications

- Cardiac tamponade
  - o Pericardial tamponade
    - ■ Cardiac tamponade can result from fluid accumulation in the pericardial sac.
      - □ Signs include hypotension, muffled heart sounds, jugular venous distention, and paradoxical pulse (variance of 10 mm Hg or more in systolic blood pressure between expiration and inspiration).
    - ■ Nursing Actions
      - □ Notify the provider immediately.
      - □ Obtain a chest x-ray or echocardiogram to confirm the diagnosis.
      - □ Prepare clients for pericardiocentesis (informed consent, gather materials, administer medications as appropriate).

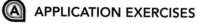 **APPLICATION EXERCISES**

1. A nurse is assisting with the care of a client who is postoperative following a mitral valve replacement 12 hr ago. The nurse should monitor which of the following? (Select all that apply.)

   _____ Vital signs

   _____ Cardiac rhythm

   _____ Oxygen saturation

   _____ Bowel sounds

   _____ Heart and lung sounds

2. A nurse is reinforcing discharge education with a client following tissue valve replacement. Which of the following should the nurse include in the education?

   A. Inform the client the prosthetic valve should last up to 7 years.

   B. Reinforce to the client that antibiotics are recommended prior to dental work.

   C. Instruct the client that activity should be limited for 4 weeks.

   D. Encourage the client to restrict foods that contain sodium.

3. A nurse is caring for a client who has a history of mitral insufficiency. Which of the following findings should the nurse expect? (Select all that apply.)

   _____ Crackles in lung bases

   _____ Petechiae

   _____ Jugular vein distention

   _____ Pulmonary congestion

   _____ Splenomegaly

   _____ Orthopnea

4. A nurse is caring for a client who has aortic insufficiency. Which of the following findings should the nurse anticipate?

   A. Palpitations

   B. Angina

   C. Atrial fibrillation

   D. Narrowed pulse pressure

5. Which of the following clients has the greatest risk of acquiring rheumatic endocarditis?

   A. An older adult who has chronic obstructive pulmonary disease

   B. A child who has an upper respiratory streptococcus infection

   C. A middle age adult who has Lupus

   D. A young adult who is 6 months pregnant

APPLICATION EXERCISES ANSWER KEY

1. A nurse is assisting with the care of a client who is postoperative following a mitral valve replacement 12 hr ago. The nurse should monitor which of the following? (Select all that apply.)

X	**Vital signs**
X	**Cardiac rhythm**
X	**Oxygen saturation**
	Bowel sounds
X	**Heart and lung sounds**

    Vital signs, cardiac rhythm, oxygen saturation, heart and lung sounds, and hemodynamics are all indicated for immediate assessment. Bowel sounds are not indicated in the immediate postoperative period because the client is postoperative and has been NPO.

     NCLEX® Connection: Reduction of Risk Potential, Potential for Alterations in Body Systems

2. A nurse is reinforcing discharge education with a client following tissue valve replacement. Which of the following should the nurse include in the education?

    A. Inform the client the prosthetic valve should last up to 7 years.

    B. Reinforce to the client that antibiotics are recommended prior to dental work.

    C. Instruct the client that activity should be limited for 4 weeks.

    D. Encourage the client to restrict foods that contain sodium.

    The nurse should teach the client that antibiotics are recommended prior to dental work or surgery to decrease the risk of infection. The client's prosthetic valve should last up to 10 to 15 years. The client's activity should be limited for up to 6 weeks. The client should be encouraged to adhere to a diet low in sodium, but does not need to restrict all sodium intake.

    NCLEX® Connection: Reduction of Risk Potential, Potential for Complications from Surgical Procedures and Health Alterations

3. A nurse is caring for a client who has a history of mitral insufficiency. Which of the following findings should the nurse expect? (Select all that apply.)

X	**Crackles in lung bases**
	Petechiae
X	**Jugular vein distention**
X	**Pulmonary congestion**
	Splenomegaly
X	**Orthopnea**

Findings of mitral valve insufficiency initially results in crackles in the lungs, dyspnea, orthopnea, and pulmonary congestion. Clients with mitral valve insufficiency can also exhibit jugular vein distention that can occur with left ventricular failure due to progressive mitral insufficiency. Petechiae can occur with endocarditis. Hepatomegaly, not splenomegaly, can occur with heart failure associated with mitral insufficiency.

 NCLEX® Connection: Reduction of Risk Potential, Alterations in Body Systems

4. A nurse is caring for a client who has aortic insufficiency. Which of the following findings should the nurse anticipate?

A. Palpitations

B. Angina

C. Atrial fibrillation

D. Narrowed pulse pressure

Angina is found in clients who have aortic insufficiency. Palpitations and atrial fibrillation are findings that can occur with mitral insufficiency. A narrowed pulse pressure is a finding that can occur with aortic stenosis.

 NCLEX® Connection: Reduction of Risk Potential, Potential for Alterations in Body Systems

5. Which of the following clients has the greatest risk of acquiring rheumatic endocarditis?

A. An older adult who has chronic obstructive pulmonary disease

B. A child who has an upper respiratory streptococcus infection

C. A middle age adult who has Lupus

D. A young adult who is 6 months pregnant

A child who has an upper respiratory streptococcus infection is at greatest risk for acquiring rheumatic endocarditis. Rheumatic endocarditis develops due to an upper respiratory infection most commonly caused by the bacteria streptococcus. An older adult who has chronic obstructive pulmonary disease is at risk, but not the highest. A middle age adult who has Lupus would still be at risk, but not the highest. A young adult who is 6 months pregnant is at risk, but not the highest.

 NCLEX® Connection: Physiological Adaptation, Basic Pathophysiology

UNIT 4	NURSING CARE OF CLIENTS WITH CARDIOVASCULAR DISORDERS
Section:	Vascular Disorders
Chapter 31	Peripheral Vascular Disease

Overview

- Peripheral vascular diseases include peripheral arterial disease (PAD) and peripheral venous disorders, both of which interfere with normal blood flow.

PERIPHERAL ARTERIAL DISEASE (PAD)

Overview

- PAD results from atherosclerosis that usually occurs in the arteries of the lower extremities and is characterized by inadequate flow of blood. Tissue damage occurs below the arterial obstruction.

- Atherosclerosis is caused by a gradual thickening of the intima and media of the arteries, ultimately resulting in the progressive narrowing of the vessel lumen. Plaques may form on the walls of the arteries, making them rough and fragile.

- Progressive stiffening of the arteries and narrowing of the lumen decreases the blood supply to affected tissues and increases resistance to blood flow.

- Atherosclerosis is actually a type of arteriosclerosis, which means "hardening of the arteries," and alludes to the loss of elasticity of arteries over time, due to thickening of their walls.

- Buerger's disease, subclavian steal syndrome, thoracic outlet syndrome, Raynaud's disease and Raynaud's phenomenon, and popliteal entrapment are examples of PADs.

Data Collection

- Risk Factors

  o Hypertension

  o Hyperlipidemia

  o Diabetes mellitus

  o Cigarette smoking

  o Obesity

- ○ Sedentary lifestyle
- ○ Familial predisposition
- ○ Age

  - Older adult clients have a higher incidence of PAD (rate of occurrence is increased in men over 45 and in women who are postmenopausal) and have a higher mortality rate from complications than younger individuals.

- Subjective Data

  - ○ Burning, cramping, and pain in the legs during exercise (intermittent claudication)
  - ○ Numbness or burning pain primarily in the feet when in bed
  - ○ Placing legs at rest in a dependent position relieves pain.

- Objective Data

  - ○ Physical Assessment Findings
    - Bruit over femoral and aortic arteries

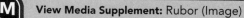

View Media Supplement: Bruit (Audio)

    - Decreased capillary refill of toes (greater than 3 seconds)
    - Decreased or nonpalpable pulses
    - Loss of hair on lower calf, ankle, and foot
    - Dry, scaly, mottled skin
    - Thick toenails
    - Cold and cyanotic extremity
    - Pallor of extremity with elevation
    - Dependent rubor

View Media Supplement: Rubor (Image)

    - Muscle atrophy
    - Ulcers and possible gangrene of toes
  - ○ Diagnostic Procedures
    - Arteriography
      - Arteriography of the lower extremities involves arterial injection of contrast medium to visualize areas of decreased arterial flow on an x-ray.
      - It is usually done only to determine isolated areas of occlusion that can be treated during the procedure with percutaneous transluminal angioplasty and possible stent placement.

- □ Nursing Actions
  - ▸ Monitor clients for bleeding and hemorrhage.
  - ▸ Palpate pedal pulses to check for postprocedure occlusions.
- ■ Exercise tolerance testing
  - □ A stress test is done with or without the use of a treadmill (medications such as dipyridamole (Persantine) and adenosine (Adenocard) may be given to mimic the effects of exercise in clients who cannot tolerate a treadmill) with measurement of pulse volumes and blood pressures prior to and following the onset of symptoms or 5 min of exercise. Delays in return to normal pressures and pulse waveforms indicate arterial disease. This test evaluates claudication during exercise.
- ■ Plethysmography
  - □ Plethysmography is used to determine the variations of blood passing through an artery, thus identifying abnormal arterial flow in the affected limb.
  - □ Blood pressure cuffs are attached to the client's upper extremities and a lower extremity and attached to the plethysmograph machine. This test records variations in peripheral pulses between the upper and lower extremity.
  - □ A decrease in pulse pressure of the lower extremity indicates a possible blockage in the leg.
- ■ Segmental systolic blood pressure measurements
  - □ A Doppler probe takes various blood pressure measurements (thigh, calf, ankle, brachial) for comparison. In the absence of peripheral arterial disease, pressures in the lower extremities are higher than those of the upper extremities.
  - □ With arterial disease, the pressures in the thigh, calf, and ankle are lower.

Collaborative Care

- • Nursing Care
  - o Monitor skin every 8 hr.
  - o Provide skin care with warm water, mild soap, and moisturizing lotions.
  - o Provide a warm environment for clients, and offer socks and blankets.
  - o Encourage frequent position changes.
  - o Do not use the knee-gatch or pillows under the knees.
  - o Have client avoid 90° hip flexion.
  - o Keep linens from applying pressure to extremities by using a foot cradle.
  - o Monitor pain level and treat accordingly.

- ○ Instruct clients to avoid crossing their legs.
- ○ Tell clients to refrain from wearing restrictive garments.
- Medications
  - ○ Antiplatelet medications – Aspirin, clopidogrel (Plavix), Pentoxifylline (Trental)
    - ☐ Antiplatelet medications reduce blood viscosity by decreasing blood fibrinogen levels, enhancing erythrocyte flexibility, and increasing blood flow in the extremities. Medications, such as aspirin and clopidogrel (Plavix), may be prescribed. Pentoxifylline (Trental) specifically treats intermittent claudication experienced by clients who have PAD.
    - ■ Nursing Considerations
      - ☐ Give medication with meals.
    - ■ Client Education
      - ☐ Inform clients that the medication's effects might not be apparent for several weeks.
      - ☐ Advise clients to monitor for signs of bleeding such as abdominal pain, coffee ground emesis, or black, tarry stools.
- Therapeutic Procedures
  - ○ Percutaneous transluminal angioplasty
    - ■ Invasive intra-arterial procedure uses a balloon and stent to open and help maintain the patency of the vessel.
    - ■ Use for candidates who are not suitable for surgery or in cases where amputation is inevitable.
  - ○ Laser-assisted angioplasty
    - ■ Laser-assisted angioplasty is an invasive procedure where a laser probe is advanced through a cannula to the site of stenosis.
    - ■ The laser vaporizes atherosclerotic plaque and open the artery.
    - ■ Nursing Actions
      - ☐ Monitor puncture site for bleeding.
      - ☐ Closely monitor the client's vital signs, peripheral pulses, and capillary refill.
      - ☐ If prescribed, keep clients on bed rest with limb straight for 6 to 8 hr before ambulation.
    - ■ Client Education
      - ☐ Inform clients of the need for antiplatelet therapy for 1 to 3 months.

- Surgical Interventions

  o Arterial revascularization surgery is used with clients who have severe claudication and/or limb pain at rest, or with clients who are at risk for losing a limb due to poor arterial circulation.

    ▪ Bypass grafts reroute the circulation around the arterial occlusion.

    ▪ Grafts can be harvested from clients (autologous) or made from synthetic materials.

  o Nursing Actions

    □ Mark the pedal or dorsalis pulse and note strength.

    □ Compare pulse, color, temperature, and capillary refill with the contralateral leg on a scheduled basis using a Doppler.

    □ Look for warmth, redness, and possibly edema of the affected limb as a result of increased blood flow.

    □ Monitor clients for pain. Pain may be severe due to the re-establishment of blood flow to the extremity.

    □ Monitor the client's blood pressure for hypotension or hypertension. Hypotension may result in an increased risk of clotting or graft collapse, while hypertension increases the risk for bleeding from sutures.

    □ Instruct clients to limit bending of the hip and knee to decrease the risk of clot formation.

- Care After Discharge

  o Client Education

    ▪ Instruct clients to avoid crossing their legs or raising legs above the level of the heart.

    ▪ Encourage clients to sit with legs in dependent position to allow gravity to facilitate arterial blood flow to the lower extremities.

    ▪ Instruct clients to wear loose clothing.

    ▪ Instruct clients on wound care if revascularization surgery was done.

    ▪ Discourage smoking and exposure to cold temperatures.

    ▪ Instruct clients about foot care (keep feet clean and dry, wash with mild soap and warm water, pat skin dry, especially between the toes, apply moisturizing lotions and powder if desired, wear good-fitting shoes and a clean pair of cotton socks each day, never go barefoot, cut toenails straight across or have the podiatrist cut nails).

- Client Outcomes

  o The client's extremity distal to the repaired occlusion will be warm, pink, and have a 2+ pulse.

  o The client will report being able to walk without pain in the affected leg.

  o Encourage clients to exercise to build up collateral circulation.

- ○ Initiate exercise gradually and increase slowly.

- ○ Instruct clients to walk until the point of pain, stop and rest for 3 min, and then walk a little farther.

- ○ Walk at least 8 times per day.

- ○ Tell clients to never apply direct heat to the affected extremity, as sensitivity is decreased and they may inadvertently burn themselves.

- ○ Instruct clients to avoid exposure to cold (causes vasoconstriction and decreased arterial flow).

- ○ Instruct clients to avoid stress, caffeine, and nicotine, which also cause vasoconstriction.

Complications

- • Graft Occlusion

    - ■ Graft occlusion may occur within the first 24 hr following arterial revascularization surgery.

    - ○ Nursing Actions

        - ■ Promptly notify the surgeon of signs and symptoms of occlusion, such as absent or reduced pedal pulses, increased pain, change in extremity color, or temperature.

        - ■ Be prepared to assist with treatment, which may include an emergency thrombectomy (removal of a clot), local intra-arterial thrombolytic therapy with an agent such as tissue plasminogen activator, infusion of a platelet inhibitor, or a combination of the above. With these treatments, closely monitor clients for manifestations of bleeding.

- • Compartment Syndrome

    - ■ Compartment syndrome is considered a medical emergency. Tissue pressure within a confined body space can restrict blood flow and the resulting ischemia can lead to irreversible tissue damage.

View Media Supplement: Compartment Syndrome (Image)

- ○ Nursing Actions

    - ■ Monitor for signs and symptoms of compartment syndrome (tingling, numbness, worsening pain, edema, pain on passive movement, unequal pulses). Immediately report symptoms to the provider.

    - ■ Loosen dressings.

    - ■ Prepare to assist with fasciotomy (surgical opening into the tissues), which may be necessary to prevent further injury and to save the limb.

View Media Supplement: Fasciotomy (Image)

PERIPHERAL VENOUS DISORDERS

 Overview

- Peripheral venous disorders interfere with adequate return of blood flow from the extremities.

- There are superficial and deep veins in the lower extremities that have valves that prevent backflow of blood as it returns to the heart. The action of the skeletal muscles of the lower extremities during walking and other activities also promotes venous return.

- Peripheral venous disorders include:

  o Phlebitis, which refers to a vein inflammation

  o Thrombophlebitis refers to a thrombus that is associated with inflammation. Deep vein thrombophlebitis (deep vein thrombosis) is a blood clot believed to form as a result of venous stasis, endothelial injury, or hypercoagulability. Thrombus formation can lead to a pulmonary embolism, a life-threatening complication.

  o Venous insufficiency occurs secondary to incompetent valves in the deeper veins of the lower extremities, which allows pooling of blood and dilation of the veins. The veins' inability to carry fluid and wastes from the lower extremities precipitates the development of swelling, venous stasis ulcers, and in advanced cases, cellulitis.

  o Varicose veins are enlarged, twisted, and superficial veins that may occur in any part of the body; however, they are commonly observed in the lower extremities and in the esophagus.

 View Media Supplements:
  - Thrombophlebitis (Image)
  - Deep Vein Thrombosis (Image)
  - Varicose Veins (Image)

Data Collection

- Risk Factors

  o Deep vein thrombophlebitis

    ▪ Hip surgery, total knee arthroplasty, open prostate surgery

    ▪ Heart failure

    ▪ Immobility

    ▪ Pregnancy

    ▪ Oral contraceptives

  o Venous insufficiency

    ▪ Sitting or standing in one position for a long period of time

    ▪ Obesity

    ▪ Pregnancy

    ▪ Thrombophlebitis

- ▸ Ensure that protamine sulfate, the antidote for heparin, is available if needed for excessive bleeding.
- ▸ Monitor for hazards and side effects associated with anticoagulant therapy.
- ▪ Low-molecular weight heparin is given subcutaneously and is based on a client's weight. Use enoxaparin (Lovenox) for the prevention and treatment of deep vein thrombosis. It is usually given in the facility, but the twice daily injections can be given in the home setting if adequate medical support is available.
  - ☐ Nursing Actions
    - ▸ Ensure that protamine sulfate, the antidote for heparin, is available if needed for excessive bleeding.
  - ☐ Client Education
    - ▸ Instruct clients to observe for signs of bleeding.
    - ▸ Instruct clients on bleeding precautions that should be taken (Use an electric instead of a bladed razor, and brush teeth with a soft toothbrush.).
- ▪ Warfarin (Coumadin) inhibits synthesis of the four vitamin K-dependent clotting factors. The therapeutic effect takes 3 to 4 days to develop, so it is usually begun while clients are still on heparin, prior to discharge.
  - ☐ Nursing Actions
    - ▸ Monitor clients for bleeding.
    - ▸ Monitor the client's PT and INR.
    - ▸ Ensure that vitamin K (the antidote for warfarin) is available in case of excessive bleeding.
    - ▸ Instruct clients to observe for signs of bleeding.
    - ▸ Instruct clients on bleeding precautions.
  - ○ Deep vein thrombosis – Thrombolytic therapy
    - ▪ Thrombolytic therapy dissolves clots that have already developed. Therapy must be started within 5 days after the development of the clot for the therapy to be effective. Alteplase (Activase), a thrombolytic agent, and platelet inhibitors such as abciximab (ReoPro), and eptifibatide (Integrilin), can be effective in dissolving a clot or preventing new clots during the first 24 hr.
- ● Interdisciplinary Care
  - ○ Venous insufficiency
    - ▪ Care of venous stasis ulcers requires long-term management.
    - ▪ Consultation with a dietitian and wound care specialist will facilitate the healing process.

- Therapeutic Procedures

  - Varicose veins – Sclerotherapy

    - A sclerosing irritating chemical solution is injected into the varicose vein to produce localized inflammation, which will, over time, close the lumen of the vessel. For larger vessels, an incision and drainage of the trapped blood in a sclerosed vein may need to be performed 2 to 3 weeks after the injection. Pressure dressings are applied for approximately 1 week after each procedure to keep the vessel free of blood.

    - Client Education

      □ Instruct clients to wear elastic stockings for prescribed time.

      □ Instruct clients to take a mild analgesic, such as acetaminophen, for discomfort.

- Surgical Interventions

  - Varicose veins – Vein stripping

    □ Vein stripping is the removal of large varicose veins that cannot be treated with less-invasive procedures.

    - Nursing Actions

      □ Preoperatively

        ▸ Assist the provider with vein marking.

        ▸ Evaluate the client's pulses as baseline for postoperative comparison.

      □ Postoperatively

        ▸ Maintain elastic bandages on the client's legs.

        ▸ Monitor the client's groin and leg for bleeding through the elastic bandages.

        ▸ Monitor the client's extremity for edema, warmth, color, and pulses.

        ▸ Elevate the client's legs above the level of the heart.

        ▸ Encourage clients to engage in range-of-motion exercises of the legs.

        ▸ Instruct clients to elevate legs when sitting, and to avoid dangling them over the side of the bed.

    - Client Education

      □ Emphasize the importance of wearing elastic stockings after bandage removal.

  - Varicose veins – Endovenous laser treatment

    - This type of treatment uses a laser fiber that is inserted into the vessel proximal to the area to be treated and then threaded to the involved area where heat from the laser is used to close the dilated vein.

  - Varicose veins – Application of radio frequency energy

    - This type of treatment uses a small catheter with a radiofrequency electrode, instead of a laser, that is inserted into the vessel proximal to the area to be treated that scars and closes a dilated vein.

- Care After Discharge
  - Client Education
    - Venous Insufficiency
      - Instruct clients to avoid crossing legs and wearing constrictive clothing or stockings.
      - Instruct clients to put on elastic compression stockings when they wake up and before getting out of bed.
- Client Outcomes
  - The client's lower extremities will be warm, pink, and free of pain.

Complications

- Ulcer Formation
  - Venous stasis ulcers often form over the medial malleolus. Venous ulcers are chronic, hard to heal, and often recur. They can lead to amputation and/or death.

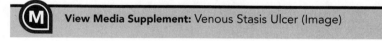
View Media Supplement: Venous Stasis Ulcer (Image)

  - Clients who also have neuropathy may not feel as much discomfort from the ulcer.
  - Nursing Actions
    - Apply oxygen-permeable polyethylene films to superficial ulcers.
    - Apply occlusive, hydrocolloid dressings on deeper ulcers to promote granulation tissue and reepithelialization.
    - Leave a dressing on for 3 to 5 days.
    - Apply prescribed topical enzymatic agents to debride the ulcer, eliminate necrotic tissue, and promote healing.
    - Administer systemic antibiotics as prescribed.
  - Client Education
    - Recommend to clients a diet high in zinc, protein, and vitamins A and C.

- Pulmonary Embolism

  A pulmonary embolism occurs when a thrombus is dislodged, becomes an embolus, and lodges in a pulmonary vessel. This can lead to obstruction of pulmonary blood flow, decreased systemic oxygenation, pulmonary tissue hypoxia, and possible death.

  o Nursing Actions

    ▪ Monitor for symptoms, which include sudden onset dyspnea, pleuritic chest pain, restlessness and apprehension, feelings of impending doom, cough, and hemoptysis.

    ▪ Monitor for signs, which include tachypnea, crackles, pleural friction rub, tachycardia, S_3 or S_4 heart sounds, diaphoresis, a low-grade fever, petechiae over chest and axillae, and decreased arterial oxygen saturation.

    ▪ Notify the provider immediately, reassure clients, and assist them to a position of comfort with the head of the bed elevated.

Data Collection

- Risk Factors
  - Essential hypertension
    - Positive family history
    - Excessive sodium intake
    - Physical inactivity
    - Obesity
    - High alcohol consumption
    - African American
    - Smoking
    - Hyperlipidemia
    - Stress
  - Secondary hypertension
    - Renal disease
    - Cushing's disease (excessive glucocorticoid secretion)
    - Primary aldosteronism (causes hypertension and hypokalemia)
    - Pheochromocytoma (excessive catecholamine release)
    - Brain tumors, encephalitis
    - Medications such as estrogen, steroids, sympathomimetics
- Subjective Data
  - Clients who have hypertension can experience few or no symptoms. Nurses should monitor for:
    - Headaches, particularly in the morning
    - Dizziness
    - Fainting
    - Retinal changes, visual disturbances
    - Nocturia
- Objective Data
  - Physical Assessment Findings
    - When a blood pressure reading is elevated, it should be taken in both arms and with clients sitting and standing.

- There are several levels of hypertension, as defined by the Joint National Committee on Prevention, Detection, Evaluation, and Treatment of High Blood Pressure.

  □ Prehypertension – Systolic 120 mm Hg to 139 mm Hg; diastolic 80 mm Hg to 89 mm Hg

  □ Stage I hypertension – Systolic 140 mm Hg to 159 mm Hg; diastolic 90 mm Hg to 99 mm Hg

  □ Stage II hypertension – Systolic greater than or equal to 160 mm Hg; diastolic greater than or equal to 100 mm Hg

- Laboratory Tests

  - No laboratory tests exist to diagnose hypertension; however, several laboratory tests can identify the causes of secondary hypertension and target organ damage.

    □ BUN, creatinine – Elevation indicative of renal disease

    □ Elevated serum corticoids to detect Cushing's disease

    □ Blood glucose and cholesterol studies can identify contributing factors related to blood vessel changes.

- Diagnostic Procedures

  - An ECG is used to evaluate cardiac function.

    □ Tall R-waves are often seen with left-ventricular hypertrophy.

  - A chest x-ray may show cardiomegaly.

Collaborative Care

- Nursing Care

  - Discuss factors with clients that increase the risk of hypertension and how they can be managed.

- Medications

  - Clients who are taking antihypertensives should be instructed to change positions slowly, be careful when getting out of bed, driving, and climbing stairs until the medication's effects are fully known.

  - Diuretics

    - Thiazide diuretics, such as hydrochlorothiazide (Hydrodiuril), inhibit water and sodium reabsorption, and increase potassium excretion.

    - Other diuretics may be used to treat hypertension not responsive to the thiazide diuretics.

      □ Loop diuretics, such as furosemide (Lasix), decrease sodium reabsorption and increase potassium excretion.

      □ Potassium-sparing diuretics, such as spironolactone (Aldactone), affect the distal tubule and prevent reabsorption of sodium in exchange for potassium.

- Nursing Considerations
  - Monitor the client's potassium levels and watch for muscle weakness, irregular pulse, and dehydration. Thiazide and loop diuretics can cause hypokalemia, and potassium-sparing diuretics can cause hyperkalemia.
- Client Education
  - Encourage clients to keep all appointments with the provider to monitor efficacy of pharmacologic treatment and possible electrolyte imbalance (hyponatremia, hyperkalemia).
  - If clients are taking a potassium-depleting diuretic, encourage consumption of potassium-rich foods, such as bananas.
- Calcium-channel blockers
  - Verapamil hydrochloride (Calan), amlodipine (Norvasc), and diltiazem (Cardizem) alter the movement of calcium ions through the cell membrane, causing vasodilation and lowering blood pressure.
  - Nursing Considerations
    - Monitor the client's blood pressure and pulse for hypotension and change in heart rate.
  - Client Education
    - Remind clients to change position slowly.
    - Encourage clients taking verapamil hydrochloride to increase intake of foods that are high in fiber to prevent constipation.
    - Reinforce to clients how to take their pulse and to call the provider if the pulse is irregular or lower than the established rate.
    - Instruct clients to avoid grapefruit juice, which potentiates the medication's effects, increases hypotensive effects, and increases the risk of medication toxicity.
- Angiotensin-converting enzyme (ACE) inhibitors
  - ACE inhibitors, such as captopril (Capoten) and lisinopril (Zestril), prevent the conversion of angiotensin I to angiotensin II, which prevents vasoconstriction.
  - Nursing Considerations
    - Monitor the client's blood pressure and pulse for hypotension.
    - Monitor clients for signs of heart failure, such as edema.
  - Client Education
    - Reinforce to clients to report a cough immediately, as the medication should be discontinued.
    - Reinforce to clients to report signs of heart failure (edema).

○ Angiotensin-II receptor antagonists

- Also called angiotensin-receptor blockers (ARBs), these medications, such as candesartan (Atacand), losartan (Cozaar), and telmisartan (Micardis), are a good option for clients taking ACE inhibitors who report cough and those who have hyperkalemia. Also, ARBs do not require a dosage adjustment for older adult clients.

- Nursing Considerations

  □ Monitor clients for signs of angioedema or heart failure. Angioedema is a serious, but uncommon adverse effect, and heart failure can result from taking this medication.

- Client Education

  □ Encourage clients to change positions slowly.

  □ Instruct clients to report signs of angioedema (swollen lips or face) or heart failure (edema).

○ Aldosterone-receptor antagonists

- Aldosterone-receptor antagonists, such as eplerenone (Inspra), block aldosterone action. The blocking effect of eplerenone on aldosterone receptors promotes the retention of potassium and excretion of sodium and water.

- Nursing Considerations

  □ Monitor the client's renal function, triglycerides, sodium, and potassium levels. The risk of adverse effects increases with deteriorating renal function. Hypertriglyceridemia, hyponatremia, and hyperkalemia can occur as the dose increases.

    ▸ Monitor the client's potassium levels every 2 weeks for the first few months and every 2 months thereafter. Do not give clients potassium supplements or potassium-sparing diuretics.

- Client Education

  □ Inform clients about potential medication and herbal interactions. Grapefruit juice and St. John's wort can increase adverse effects.

  □ Instruct clients not to take salt substitutes with potassium or other foods that are rich in potassium.

○ Beta blockers

- Beta blockers, such as metoprolol (Lopressor) and atenolol (Tenormin), are indicated for clients who have unstable angina or MI. They decrease cardiac output and block the release of renin, subsequently decreasing vasoconstriction of the peripheral vasculature.

- Nursing Considerations

  □ Monitor the client's blood pressure and pulse.

  □ Monitor the client's blood glucose level as these medications can mask hypoglycemia in clients who have diabetes mellitus.

- Client Education
  - Reinforce to clients that these medications may cause fatigue, weakness, depression, and sexual dysfunction.
  - Advise clients not to suddenly stop taking the medication without consulting with the provider. Stopping suddenly can cause rebound hypertension.
  - Reinforce to clients who have diabetes to monitor for signs and symptoms of hypoglycemia.
- Central-alpha agonists
  - Central-alpha agonists, such as clonidine (Catapres), reduce peripheral vascular resistance and decrease blood pressure by inhibiting the reuptake of norepinephrine.
  - Nursing Considerations
    - Monitor the client's blood pressure and pulse.
    - This medication is not indicated for first-line management of hypertension.
  - Client Education
    - Teach clients that side effects include sedation, orthostatic hypotension, and impotence.
- Alpha-adrenergic Antagonists
  - Alpha-adrenergic antagonists, such as prazosin (Minipress), reduce blood pressure by causing vasodilation.
  - Nursing Considerations
    - Start treatment with a low dose of the medication.
    - Give clients the first dose at night and monitor blood pressure for 2 hr after initiation of treatment.
  - Client Education
    - Advise clients to rise slowly to prevent postural hypotension. Tell clients to use caution when driving until the effects of the medication are known.
- Care After Discharge
  - Client Education
    - Remind clients and their families of the importance of adhering to the medication regimen, even if clients are asymptomatic.
    - Provide verbal and written education to clients regarding medications and their side effects.
    - Ensure that clients have the resources necessary to pay for and obtain prescribed antihypertensive medication.
    - Encourage clients to schedule regular provider appointments to monitor hypertension and cardiovascular status.

- Encourage clients to report symptoms or side effects, as they may be indicative of additional problems. Medications can often be changed to alleviate side effects.

(G)

- Inform older adult clients that they are more likely to experience medication interactions and orthostatic hypotension.

- Treatment involves clients making lifestyle changes.

- Sodium restriction

  □ Monitor potassium with salt substitute use.

  □ Follow prescribed sodium restriction (between 500 to 3,000 mg/day).

- Weight reduction

  □ Consume a diet low in fat, saturated fat, and cholesterol.

  □ Control alcohol intake (2 oz of liquor, 8 oz of wine, 24 oz of beer per day).

  □ Clients should maintain a body mass index of less than 30.

- Exercise

  □ Begin slowly and gradually advance the program with the guidance of the provider and physical therapist.

  □ Exercise at least three times a week in a manner that provides aerobic benefits.

- Smoking cessation

  □ Smoking is not directly linked to hypertension, but it should be avoided due to its high association with the development of cardiovascular diseases.

- Stress reduction

  □ Encourage clients to use stress-management techniques during times of stress.

  □ Encourage clients to try yoga, massage, hypnosis, or other forms of relaxation.

- Client Outcomes

  o The client's blood pressure will be maintained with a systolic pressure less than 140 and a diastolic pressure less than 90.

  o The client will be able to verbalize proper administration of medications and side effects that should be reported to the provider.

  o The client will not report side effects such as postural hypotension, dizziness, weakness, or fatigue.

Complications

- Hypertensive Crisis

  o Hypertensive crisis often occurs when clients do not follow the medication therapy regimen.

○ Nursing Actions

▪ Recognize signs and symptoms

□ Severe headache

□ Extremely high blood pressure (generally, systolic blood pressure greater than 240 mm Hg, diastolic greater than 120 mm Hg)

□ Blurred vision, dizziness, and disorientation

□ Epistaxis

▪ Monitor clients receiving IV antihypertensive therapies, such as nitroprusside (Nipride), nicardipine (Cardene IV), and labetalol (Normodyne).

▪ Monitor the client's neurological status by checking pupils, level of consciousness, and muscle strength frequently to monitor for cerebrovascular change.

Ⓐ APPLICATION EXERCISES

Scenario: A nurse is caring for an older adult client in a medical clinic who has been newly diagnosed with hypertension.

1. The client is prescribed captopril (Capoten). Which of the following should the nurse instruct the client to monitor and report to the provider?

    A. Dry cough

    B. Urinary retention

    C. Headache

    D. Diarrhea

2. The nurse is reinforcing teaching regarding lifestyle changes that the client should make. What should the nurse include in the teaching?

3. The nurse is now providing discharge instruction. The provider has prescribed a 2 g sodium diet. Which of the following food selections made by the client indicates a need for further teaching?

    A. 8 oz of low-fat milk

    B. Frozen vegetables

    C. Two graham crackers

    D. A can of tomato juice

Ⓐ **APPLICATION EXERCISES ANSWER KEY**

Scenario: A nurse is caring for an older adult client in a medical clinic who has been newly diagnosed with hypertension.

1. The client is prescribed captopril (Capoten). Which of the following should the nurse instruct the client to monitor and report to the provider?

   A. Dry cough
   B. Urinary retention
   C. Headache
   D. Diarrhea

   Dry cough is an adverse effect of captopril that results from a buildup of bradykinin, which can lead to fatal angioedema. Urinary retention, headache, and diarrhea are not adverse effects of captopril.

Ⓝ **NCLEX® Connection: Pharmacological Therapies, Adverse Effects/Contraindications/Side Effects/Interactions**

2. The nurse is reinforcing teaching regarding lifestyle changes that the client should make. What should the nurse include in the teaching?

   The client should follow a sodium-restricted diet as prescribed by the provider. The client should limit salt substitutes due to the risk of hyperkalemia. The client should consume a diet low in fat, saturated fat, and cholesterol. The client should limit alcohol intake (2 oz of liquor, 8 oz of wine, 24 oz of beer per day) and maintain a body mass index of less than 30. The client should exercise at least three times a week in a manner that provides aerobic benefits, and use stress-management techniques during times of stress.

Ⓝ **NCLEX® Connection: Health Promotion and Maintenance, Health Promotion/Disease Prevention**

3. The nurse is now providing discharge instruction. The provider has prescribed a 2 g sodium diet. Which of the following food selections made by the client indicates a need for further teaching?

   A. 8 oz of low-fat milk
   B. Frozen vegetables
   C. Two graham crackers
   D. A can of tomato juice

   A can of tomato juice contains 330 mg of sodium and would indicate that the client needs further teaching. An 8 oz glass of low-fat milk, frozen vegetables, and two graham crackers are low in sodium and are appropriate food choices for this client.

Ⓝ **NCLEX® Connection: Health Promotion and Maintenance, Health Promotion/Disease Prevention**

UNIT 4 NURSING CARE OF CLIENTS WITH CARDIOVASCULAR DISORDERS

Section: Vascular Disorders

Chapter 33 Aneurysms

 Overview

- A weakness in a section of a dilated artery that causes a widening or ballooning in the wall of the blood vessel is called an aneurysm.

- Aneurysms can occur in two forms. They can be saccular (only affecting one side of the artery), or they can be fusiform (involving the complete circumference of the artery).

- Seventy-five percent of aneurysms are abdominal aortic aneurysms.

 View Media Supplement: Common Aneurysm Sites (Image)

- Aortic dissection can occur when blood accumulates within the aortic wall (hematoma) following a tear in the lining of the aorta (usually due to hypertension).

Data Collection

- Risk Factors

  o Atherosclerosis

  o Uncontrolled hypertension

  o Tobacco use

   o Older age

- Subjective and Objective Data

  o Initially, clients are often asymptomatic.

  o Abdominal aortic aneurysm (most commonly related to atherosclerosis)

  ▪ Constant gnawing feeling in abdomen; flank or back pain

  ▪ Pulsating abdominal mass

  ▪ Bruit

  ▪ Elevated blood pressure (unless in cardiac tamponade or rupture of aneurysm)

- Aortic dissections (often associated with Marfan's syndrome)
    - Sudden onset of "tearing," "ripping," and "stabbing" abdominal or back pain
    - Hypovolemic shock
        - Diaphoresis, nausea, vomiting, faintness, apprehension
        - Decreased or absent peripheral pulses
        - Neurological deficits
        - Hypotension and tachycardia (initial)
- Thoracic aortic aneurysm
    - Hoarseness, shortness of breath, and difficulty swallowing
    - Severe back pain
    - May also result in hypovolemic shock
- Diagnostic procedures
    - X-ray
        - X-rays can reveal the classic "eggshell" appearance of an aneurysm.
    - Computed tomography (CT) and ultrasonography
        - CT scans and ultrasonography are used to assess the size and location of aneurysms and are often repeated at periodic intervals to monitor the progression of an aneurysm.

Collaborative Care

- Nursing Care
    - Take the client's vital signs every 15 min until stable, then every hour (Watch for increased blood pressure.).
    - Check the onset, quality, duration, and severity of the client's pain.
    - Check the client's temperature, circulation, and function of all extremities.
    - Continuously monitor the client's cardiac rhythm.
    - Monitor ABGs, SaO_2, electrolytes, and CBC laboratory values.
    - Monitor the client's hourly urine output – Greater than 30 mL/hr indicates adequate renal perfusion.
    - Administer oxygen as prescribed.
    - Administer medications as prescribed.
        - Note – All aneurysms can be life-threatening and need medical attention.

- Medications

  o The priority intervention is to reduce systolic blood pressure between 100 and 120 mm Hg during an emergency, and to maintain a systolic blood pressure at or less than 130 to 140 mm Hg.

    ■ Monitor clients receiving antihypertensive agents as prescribed. Often more than one is prescribed (beta blockers and calcium blockers).

- Interdisciplinary Care

  o Cardiology services may be consulted to manage and treat hypertension.

  o Radiology should be consulted for diagnostic studies to determine an aneurysm.

  o Vascular services may be consulted for surgical intervention.

  o Request a referral for cardiac rehabilitation services for clients experiencing prolonged weakness and assistance in increasing the client's level of activity.

  o Request a referral for nutritional services to assist clients with food choices that are low in fat and cholesterol.

- Surgical Interventions

  o Abdominal aortic aneurysm (AAA) resection

    ■ An AAA resection involves the excision of the aneurysm and the placement of a synthetic graft. Risks include significant blood loss and the consequences of reduced cardiac output and tissue ischemia (graft occlusion, MI, renal failure, respiratory distress, paralytic ileus).

    ■ Nursing Actions

      □ Provide postoperative interventions to prevent complications.

      □ Avoid flexion of the graft (keep the head of the bed below 45°).

      □ Monitor and maintain normal blood pressure for clients. Prolonged hypotension can cause thrombi to form within the graft, and severe hypertension can cause leakage or rupture at the arterial anastomosis suture line.

      □ Maintain a warm environment to prevent temperature-induced vasoconstriction.

      □ Monitor the client's urinary output (report less than 50 mL/hr), daily weights, BUN, and serum creatinine to detect for signs of altered renal perfusion and renal failure (secondary to surgical clamping of aorta).

      □ Report any signs of graft occlusion or rupture immediately (changes in pulses, coolness or weakness of extremities below graft, white or blue extremities or flanks, severe pain, abdominal distention, decreased urine output).

- Client Education
  - Reinforce to clients regarding postoperative activity restrictions (avoid lifting more than 15 lb, strenuous activity).
  - Ensure adequate nutrition – Specifically a diet high in protein, vitamin C, vitamin A, and zinc – to promote healing.
- Percutaneous aneurysm repair
  - Percutaneous insertion of endothelial stent grafts for aneurysm repair avoids abdominal incision and shortens the postoperative period (can be used to repair a thoracic aortic aneurysm).
  - Nursing Actions
    - Nursing care after the procedure is similar to care following an arteriogram or cardiac catheterization (pedal pulse checks).
  - Client Education
    - Reinforce to clients regarding postoperative activity restrictions (avoidance of lifting more than 15 lb, strenuous activity).
- Thoracic aortic aneurysm repair
  - Procedure similar to thoracic surgery, such as open heart. The course of action depends on the location of the aneurysm. Cardiopulmonary bypass is commonly used for this procedure.
  - Nursing Actions
    - Provide postoperative care to prevent complications.
  - Client Education
    - Provide client teaching regarding postoperative activity restrictions (avoid lifting more than 15 lb, strenuous activity) and introduce cardiac rehabilitation information.
- Care After Discharge
  - Client Education
    - Reinforce to clients the importance of monitoring and controlling blood pressure.
    - Reinforce to clients the importance of following through on scheduled tests to monitor size (nonsurgical client).
    - Promote smoking cessation if clients smoke.
    - Encourage clients to consume a low-fat, low-cholesterol diet and participate in regular activity.
    - Explain symptoms of aneurysm rupture that need to be promptly reported (abdominal fullness or pain, chest or back pain, shortness of breath, difficulty swallowing, hoarseness).
    - Inform clients about weight restrictions and activities that should be avoided, how to care for the incision, and the signs and symptoms of infection (surgical client).

- Client Outcomes

  o The client will be free of pain.

  o The client will have blood pressure within the expected reference range.

  o The client will be free from infection.

Complications

- Rupture

  o Aneurysm rupture is a life-threatening emergency. A ruptured aneurysm may result in massive hemorrhage causing shock and death.

  o It requires simultaneous resuscitation and immediate surgical repair.

- Thrombus formation

  o A thrombus may form inside the aneurysm. Emboli may be dislodged, blocking arteries distal to the aneurysm, which causes ischemia and shuts down other body systems.

  o Check circulation distal to aneurysm, including pulses and color and temperature of the lower extremities. Monitor the client's urine output.

(A) APPLICATION EXERCISES

Scenario: A nurse is admitting a 72-year-old male client who has an abdominal aortic aneurysm and is scheduled for surgery in 2 days.

1. Which of the following data the nurse collects supports the diagnosis? (Select all that apply.)

    _____ Elevated blood pressure

    _____ Palpable abdominal pulsations

    _____ Bruit heard on auscultation

    _____ Client reports presence of back pain

    _____ Client describes difficulty swallowing

2. Which of the following becomes the priority medication the nurse should anticipate administering to this client?

    A. Acetaminophen (Tylenol)

    B. Propranolol (Inderal)

    C. Warfarin (Coumadin)

    D. Alprazolam (Xanax)

3. The nurse is talking with the client's wife who says, "I know my husband had high blood pressure, but are there other reasons why this happened to him?" Which of the following is an appropriate response by the nurse?

    A. "The walls of blood vessels become thick and are not as flexible due to the aging process, which can lead to an aneurysm."

    B. "The fact that your husband is tall and thin contributed to this problem."

    C. "There is nothing your husband could have done to prevent the aneurysm."

    D. "This is an inherited disorder so it would be important to know if other family members have had similar problems."

4. The client is being discharged following resection of an abdominal aortic aneurysm and the nurse is reviewing home care instructions with the client. Which of the following client statements indicates the need for reinforcement of the teaching?

    A. "I'm glad to be going home so my wife won't have to take out the garbage."

    B. "I'll take my multivitamin with zinc."

    C. "My wife knows about reducing fats and cholesterol in my diet."

    D. "I will call if I feel short of breath or have difficulty breathing."

Ⓐ APPLICATION EXERCISES ANSWER KEY

Scenario: A nurse is admitting a 72-year-old male client who has an abdominal aortic aneurysm and is scheduled for surgery in 2 days.

1. Which of the following data the nurse collects supports the diagnosis? (Select all that apply.)

   __X__ **Elevated blood pressure**

   __X__ **Palpable abdominal pulsations**

   __X__ **Bruit heard on auscultation**

   __X__ **Client reports presence of back pain**

   _____ Client describes difficulty swallowing

   Most clients are often asymptomatic initially. Elevated blood pressure, a pulsating abdominal mass, bruit noted on auscultation, a gnawing feeling in the abdomen, and flank or back pain can be present. Difficulty swallowing is characteristic of a thoracic aortic aneurysm.

   Ⓝ NCLEX® Connection: Reduction of Risk Potential, Potential for Alterations in Body Systems

2. Which of the following becomes the priority medication the nurse should anticipate administering to this client?

   A. Acetaminophen (Tylenol)

   B. Propranolol (Inderal)

   C. Warfarin (Coumadin)

   D. Alprazolam (Xanax)

   The greatest risk to the client is the risk for aneurysmal rupture, and therefore, treatment of the client's hypertension is the priority. The goal is to maintain a systolic blood pressure at or less than 130 to 140 mm Hg. Typically more than one antihypertensive medication, such as propranolol (Inderal), is prescribed to include beta blockers and calcium channel blockers.

   Ⓝ NCLEX® Connection: Pharmacological Therapies, Expected Actions/Outcomes

3. The nurse is talking with the client's wife who says, "I know my husband had high blood pressure, but are there other reasons why this happened to him?" Which of the following is an appropriate response by the nurse?

    A. "The walls of blood vessels become thick and are not as flexible due to the aging process, which can lead to an aneurysm."

    B. "The fact that your husband is tall and thin contributed to this problem."

    C. "There is nothing your husband could have done to prevent the aneurysm."

    D. "This is an inherited disorder so it would be important to know if other family members have had similar problems."

    Aneurysms are caused by loss of elasticity and stiffening of arteries, which is related to the aging process and uncontrolled hypertension. Other risk factors include atherosclerosis and tobacco use. Being overweight contributes to atherosclerosis, but being tall and thin is not a risk factor. Maintaining a healthy lifestyle, controlling blood pressure, not smoking, and eating a low-fat diet can contribute to improved circulation and prevent aneurysms. Marfan's syndrome is a genetic disorder associated with aortic dissections.

    Ⓝ NCLEX® Connection: Physiological Adaptations, Basic Pathophysiology

4. The client is being discharged following resection of an abdominal aortic aneurysm and the nurse is reviewing home care instructions with the client. Which of the following client statements indicates the need for reinforcement of the teaching?

    A. "I'm glad to be going home so my wife won't have to take out the garbage."

    B. "I'll take my multivitamin with zinc."

    C. "My wife knows about reducing fats and cholesterol in my diet."

    D. "I will call if I feel short of breath or have difficulty breathing."

    Strenuous activity and lifting objects greater than 15 lb are to be avoided. The client should be advised to avoid carrying the garbage. Increasing daily intake of protein, vitamin C, vitamin A, and zinc will promote healing. A low-fat and low-cholesterol diet is recommended. Calling the provider for signs of respiratory or other infections is encouraged.

    Ⓝ NCLEX® Connection: Reduction of Risk Potential, Potential for Complications from Surgical Procedures and Health Alterations

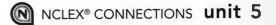

UNIT 5: NURSING CARE OF CLIENTS WITH HEMATOLOGIC DISORDERS

- Diagnostic and Therapeutic Procedures

- Hematologic Disorders

NCLEX® CONNECTIONS

When reviewing the chapters in this section, keep in mind the relevant sections of the NCLEX® outline, in particular:

CLIENT NEEDS: PHARMACOLOGICAL THERAPIES

Relevant topics/tasks include:
- Medication Administration
  - Assist in preparing client for insertion of central line.
  - Monitor client intravenous (IV) site and flow rate.
  - Monitor transfusion of blood product.

CLIENT NEEDS: REDUCTION OF RISK POTENTIAL

Relevant topics/tasks include:
- Laboratory Values
  - Reinforce client teaching on purposes of laboratory tests.

- Complications

  - Transfusion Reactions

TYPE OF REACTION	ONSET	SIGNS AND SYMPTOMS/NURSING INTERVENTIONS
Acute hemolytic	Immediate	• This reaction may be mild or life-threatening (cardiovascular collapse, acute renal failure, disseminated intravascular coagulation, shock, death). • Findings include: Chills, fever, low back pain, tachycardia, flushing, hypotension, chest tightening or pain, tachypnea, nausea, anxiety, and hemoglobinuria.
Febrile	30 min to 6 hr after transfusion	• Findings include: Chills, fever, flushing, headache, and anxiety. • Use WBC filter. • Administer an antipyretic, such as acetaminophen (Tylenol).
Mild allergic	During or up to 24 hr after transfusion	• Findings include: Itching, urticaria, and flushing. • Administer an antihistamine, such as diphenhydramine (Benadryl).
Anaphylactic	Immediate	• Findings include: Wheezing, dyspnea, chest tightness, cyanosis, and hypotension. • Assist with emergency care (Maintain airway; administer oxygen, IV fluids, antihistamines, corticosteroids, and epinephrine.).

- Nursing Actions

  - Stop the transfusion immediately if a reaction is suspected.

  - Maintain an infusion of 0.9% sodium chloride. Initiate the infusion through a separate IV line, so as not to infuse more blood from the transfusion tubing.

  - Save the blood bag with the remaining blood and the blood tubing for testing at the laboratory following agency protocol.

- Client Education

  - Explain to clients the reason that the blood is being discontinued.

- Circulatory overload

  - Clients who have impaired cardiac function can experience circulatory overload as a result of a transfusion.

    - Signs and symptoms include – Dyspnea, chest tightness, tachycardia, tachypnea, headache, hypertension, jugular-vein distention, peripheral edema, orthopnea, sudden anxiety, and crackles in the base of the lungs.

- Nursing Actions
  - □ Administer oxygen, monitor vital signs, slow the infusion rate, and administer diuretics as prescribed.
  - □ Notify the provider immediately.
- Sepsis and septic shock
  - Symptoms include – Fever, nausea, vomiting, abdominal pain, chills, and hypotension.
  - Nursing Actions
    - □ Maintain patent airway and administer oxygen.
    - □ Administer antibiotic therapy as prescribed.
    - □ Obtain samples for blood cultures.
    - □ Assist with emergency care (Use vasopressors, such as dopamine, to combat vasodilation in the late phase.).
    - □ Elevate the client's feet.

- o Inadequate dietary intake
  - ▪ Iron deficiency
  - ▪ Vitamin B_{12} deficiency – Pernicious anemia due to deficiency of intrinsic factor produced by gastric mucosa, which is necessary for absorption of vitamin B_{12}
  - ▪ Folic-acid deficiency
    - □ Women who are pregnant should plan to take an adequate amount of folic acid to prevent neural tube defects (spina bifida) in the newborn.
  - ▪ Pica, or a persistent eating of substances not normally considered food (non-nutritive substances), such as soil or chalk, for at least 1 month, may limit the amount of healthy food choices a client makes
- o Bone-marrow suppression
  - ▪ Exposure to radiation or chemicals (such as insecticides or solvents)
  - ▪ Aplastic anemia results in a decreased number of RBCs as well as decreased platelets and WBCs.
- o Older adult clients are at risk for nutrition-deficient anemias (iron, vitamin B_{12}, folate).
- o Anemia may be misdiagnosed as depression or debilitation in older adult clients.
- o Gastrointestinal bleeding is a common cause of anemia in older adult clients.
- Subjective Data
  - o May be asymptomatic in mild cases
  - o Pallor
  - o Fatigue
  - o Irritability
  - o Numbness and tingling of extremities
  - o Dyspnea on exertion
  - o Sensitivity to cold
  - o Pain and hypoxia with sickle-cell crisis
- Objective Data
  - o Physical Assessment Findings
    - ▪ Shortness of breath/fatigue, especially upon exertion
    - ▪ Tachycardia and palpitations
    - ▪ Dizziness or fainting upon standing or with exertion
    - ▪ Pallor with pale nail beds and mucous membranes
    - ▪ Nail bed deformities
    - ▪ Smooth, sore, bright red tongue (vitamin B_{12} deficiency)

- ○ Laboratory Tests
  - ■ CBC count
    - □ RBCs are the major carriers of Hgb in the blood.
    - □ Hgb transports oxygen and carbon dioxide to and from the cells and can be used as an index of the oxygen-carrying capacity of the blood.
    - □ Hct is the percentage of RBCs in relation to the total blood volume.
  - ■ RBC indices are used to determine the type and cause of most anemias.
    - □ Mean corpuscular volume (MCV) – size of RBCs
      - ▸ Normocytic – Normal size
      - ▸ Microcytic – Small cells
      - ▸ Macrocytic – Large cells
  - ■ Mean corpuscular hemoglobin (MCH) – to determine the amount of Hgb per RBC
    - □ Normochromic – normal amount of Hgb per cell
    - □ Hypochromic – decreased Hgb per cell
  - ■ Mean corpuscular hemoglobin concentration (MCHC) – to indicate Hgb amount relative to the size of the cell

RBC INDICES	CLASSIFICATION	POSSIBLE CAUSES
Normal MCV, MCH, MCHC	Normocytic, normochromic anemia	• Acute blood loss • Sickle-cell disease
Decreased MCV, MCH, MCHC	Microcytic, hypochromic anemia	• Iron-deficiency anemia • Anemia of chronic illness • Chronic blood loss
Increased MCV	Macrocytic anemia	• Vitamin B_{12} deficiency • Folic-acid deficiency

  - ■ Iron studies
    - □ Total iron-binding capacity (TIBC) reflects an indirect measurement of serum transferrin, a protein that binds with iron and transports it for storage.
    - □ Serum ferritin is an indicator of total iron stores in the body.
    - □ Serum iron measures the amount of iron in the blood. Low serum iron and elevated TIBC indicates iron-deficiency anemia.
  - ■ Hgb electrophoresis separates normal Hgb from abnormal. It is used to detect thalassemia and sickle-cell disease.
  - ■ A sickle-cell test evaluates the sickling of RBCs in the presence of decreased oxygen tension.
  - ■ A Schilling test measures vitamin B_{12} absorption with and without intrinsic factor. It is used to differentiate between malabsorption and pernicious anemia.

- o Diagnostic Procedures
  - ■ Bone-marrow examination
    - □ It is used to diagnose aplastic anemia (failure of bone marrow to produce RBCs as well as platelets and WBCs).

Collaborative Care

- • Nursing Care
  - o Encourage clients to increase dietary intake of the deficient nutrient (iron, vitamin B_{12}, folic acid).
  - o Administer medications to clients, as prescribed, at the proper time for optimal absorption, and using an appropriate technique.
  - o Reinforce to clients and their families about the client conserving energy and the risk of dizziness upon standing.
  - o Reinforce to clients about the time frame for resolution.
- • Medications
  - o Iron supplements – ferrous sulfate (Feosol), ferrous fumarate (Feostat), ferrous gluconate (Fergon)
    - ■ Oral iron supplements are used to replenish the client's serum iron and iron stores. Iron is an essential component of Hgb, and subsequently, oxygen transport.
    - ■ Parenteral iron supplements (iron dextran) are only given for severe anemia.
    - ■ Nursing Considerations
      - □ Administer parenteral iron to clients using the Z-track method.
    - ■ Client Education
      - □ Instruct clients to have Hgb checked in 4 to 6 weeks to determine efficacy.
      - □ Instruct clients to take capsules or tablets with citrus or tomato juice (vitamin C) to increase oral iron absorption.
      - □ Instruct clients to take iron supplements between meals to increase absorption, if tolerated.
  - o Erythropoietin – Epoetin alfa (Epogen, Procrit)
    - ■ A hematopoietic growth factor is used to increase production of RBCs
    - ■ Nursing Considerations
      - □ Observe clients for an increase in blood pressure.
      - □ Monitor Hgb and Hct twice a week.
      - □ Monitor clients for cardiovascular event if Hgb increases too rapidly (>1 gm/dL in 2 weeks).

- Client Education
  - Reinforce the importance of having Hgb and Hct evaluated on a twice-a-week basis.

○ Vitamin B$_{12}$ supplementation (cyanocobalamin)

- Vitamin B$_{12}$ is necessary to convert folic acid from its inactive to its active form. All cells rely on folic acid for DNA production.

- Vitamin B$_{12}$ supplementation can be given orally if the deficit is due to inadequate dietary intake. However, if deficiency is due to lack of intrinsic factor being produced by the parietal cells of the stomach or malabsorption syndrome, it must be given parenterally or intranasally to be absorbed.

- Nursing Considerations
  - Give vitamin B$_{12}$ according to the appropriate route related to cause of vitamin B$_{12}$ anemia (parenteral versus oral).
  - Administer parenteral forms of vitamin B$_{12}$ IM or deep subcutaneous to decrease irritation. Do not mix other medications in the syringe.

- Client Education
  - Inform clients who lack intrinsic factor or have an irreversible-malabsorption syndrome that this therapy must be continued for the rest of their lives.
  - Inform clients that vitamin B$_{12}$ injections should occur on a monthly basis.

○ Folic acid supplements

- Folic acid is a water-soluble, B-complex vitamin. It is necessary for the production of new RBCs.

- Nursing Considerations
  - Administer folic acid orally or parenterally.

- Client Education
  - Inform clients that large doses of folic acid will turn the client's urine dark yellow.

- Therapeutic Procedures

  ○ Blood transfusions lead to an immediate improvement in blood-cell counts and client signs and symptoms.

  - Typically only used when clients have significant symptoms of anemia, because of the risk of bloodborne infections.

- Care After Discharge

  ○ Client Education

  - Instruct clients who are iron-deficient, but have elevated cholesterol levels, to integrate iron-rich foods that are not red or organ meats into their diets (iron-fortified cereal and breads, fish and poultry, and dried peas and beans).

- Client Outcomes

    o   The client's Hgb and Hct will return to a value within the normal reference range.

    o   The client will report less fatigue.

Complications

- Heart failure

    o   Heart failure can develop due to the increased demand on the heart to increase oxygen to tissues.

    o   A low Hct decreases the amount of oxygen carried to tissues in the body, which makes the heart work harder and beat faster (tachycardia, palpitations).

    o   Nursing Actions

    ▪   Administer oxygen and monitor the client's pulse oximetry.

    ▪   Monitor the client's cardiac rhythm.

    ▪   Obtain the client's daily weight.

    ▪   Monitor clients receiving a blood transfusion.

    ▪   Give clients cardiac medications as prescribed (diuretics, antidysrhythmics).

    ▪   Give clients antianemia medications as prescribed.

Ⓐ APPLICATION EXERCISES

1. A nurse is reviewing instructions about prenatal vitamins given to a client who is in the first trimester of her pregnancy. Which of the following must be taken in adequate amounts to prevent spina bifida?

   A. Vitamin B_{12}
   B. Folic acid
   C. Calcium
   D. Iron

2. A nurse is caring for a client who has decreased renal function. Which of the following medications should the nurse administer to promote formation of RBCs?

   A. Vitamin B_{12}
   B. Ferrous sulfate (Feosol)
   C. Epoetin alfa (Epogen)
   D. Vitamin C

3. Fill in the following blanks.

   A. When giving parenteral iron, use the _____ for the injection.
   B. Iron is bound to _____ and is necessary to carry oxygen to the tissues.
   C. A smooth, sore, bright red tongue is an indication of _____ deficiency.

4. A nurse is reviewing discharge instructions with a client who received a new prescription for oral iron supplements. Which of the following statements by the client indicates a need for further teaching?

   A. "I can increase orange juice in my diet as well."
   B. "I will be sure to come to the clinic to have my blood checked in about 4 weeks."
   C. "I will take my iron pills with food."
   D. "My stools will turn green-black when I take this medication."

(A) APPLICATION EXERCISES ANSWER KEY

1. A nurse is reviewing instructions about prenatal vitamins given to a client who is in the first trimester of her pregnancy. Which of the following must be taken in adequate amounts to prevent spina bifida?

   A. Vitamin B_{12}

   B. Folic acid

   C. Calcium

   D. Iron

   Folic acid must be taken in adequate amounts to prevent neural tube defects (spina bifida). While it is important to ingest adequate amounts of vitamin B_{12}, calcium, and iron, inadequate intake of these vitamins or minerals will not cause neural tube defects.

   (N) NCLEX® Connection: Basic Care and Comfort, Nutrition and Oral Hydration

2. A nurse is caring for a client who has decreased renal function. Which of the following medications should the nurse administer to promote formation of RBCs?

   A. Vitamin B_{12}

   B. Ferrous sulfate (Feosol)

   C. Epoetin alfa (Epogen)

   D. Vitamin C

   The client who has decreased renal function lacks sufficient erythropoietin, which is necessary to produce RBCs. Administer epoetin alfa, a hematopoietic growth factor to increase production of RBCs. Administer vitamin B_{12} in cases of inadequate dietary iron intake or lack of intrinsic factor. Administer ferrous sulfate if there is inadequate iron intake. Vitamin C consumption increases the absorption of iron.

   (N) NCLEX® Connection: Pharmacological Therapies, Medication Administration

3. Fill in the following blanks.

   A. When giving parenteral iron, use the **Z-track technique or method** for the injection.

   B. Iron is bound to **red blood cells** and is necessary to carry oxygen to the tissues.

   C. A smooth, sore, bright red tongue is an indication of **vitamin B_{12}** deficiency.

   (N) NCLEX® Connection: Physiological Adaptations, Basic Pathophysiology

4. A nurse is reviewing discharge instructions with a client who received a new prescription for oral iron supplements. Which of the following statements by the client indicates a need for further teaching?

    A. "I can increase orange juice in my diet as well."

    B. "I will be sure to come to the clinic to have my blood checked in about 4 weeks."

    C. "I will take my iron pills with food."

    D. "My stools will turn green-black when I take this medication."

Instruct the client to take iron supplements between meals to increase absorption, if tolerated. Instruct the client to increase vitamin C in the diet to promote better absorption of the iron. Adding orange juice is a good source of vitamin C. Instruct the client to have hemoglobin checked in 4 to 6 weeks to determine efficacy of treatment. The client's stool can turn dark green-black after several weeks of taking oral iron.

Ⓝ NCLEX® Connection: Pharmacological Therapies, Medication Administration

UNIT 5	NURSING CARE OF CLIENTS WITH HEMATOLOGIC DISORDERS
Section:	Hematologic Disorders

Chapter 37   Leukemia and Lymphoma

Overview

- Leukemias are cancers of WBCs or of cells that will develop into WBCs.

    - In leukemia, the WBCs are not functional. They invade and destroy bone marrow, and they can metastasize to the liver, spleen, lymph nodes, testes, and brain.

    - Leukemias are divided into acute (acute lymphocytic leukemia and acute myelogenous leukemia) and chronic (chronic lymphocytic leukemia and chronic myelogenous leukemia) and are further classified by the type of WBCs primarily affected.

    - Clients with leukemia are vulnerable to infection and can develop anemia secondary to bone marrow destruction.

- Lymphomas are cancers of lymphocytes (a type of WBC) and lymph nodes (which produce antibodies and fight infection).

    - There are two types of lymphomas – Hodgkin's lymphoma (HL) and non-Hodgkin's lymphoma (NHL).

    - Lymphomas can metastasize to almost any organ.

Data Collection

- Risk Factors

    - Immunologic factors (immunosuppression)

    - Exposure to some chemicals and medications (chemotherapy agents and drugs that suppress bone marrow)

    - Genetic factors (hereditary conditions)

    - Ionizing radiation (radiation therapy, environmental)

        - Older adult clients often have diminished immune function and decreased bone marrow function, which increases their risk of complications of leukemia and lymphoma.

        - Older adult clients also have decreased energy reserves and will tire more easily during treatment. Safety is a concern with ambulation.

- Subjective and Objective Data
  - Acute leukemia
    - Bone pain
    - Joint swelling
    - Enlarged liver and spleen
    - Weight loss
    - Fever
    - Poor wound healing (infected lesions)
    - Signs of anemia (fatigue, pallor, tachycardia, dyspnea on exertion)
    - Signs of bleeding (ecchymoses, hematuria, bleeding gums)
  - HL and NHL
    - Some clients may only experience an enlarged lymph node (usually in the neck with HL).
    - Other possible findings include fever, fatigue, and infections.
  - Laboratory Tests
    - WBC – count often elevated (20,000 to 100,000/mm³) with immature WBCs in leukemia prior to treatment; decreased with treatment
    - Hgb, Hct, and platelets – decreased
    - Bleeding times – increased
  - Diagnostic Procedures
    - Bone marrow aspiration and biopsy
      - Identification of prolific quantities of immature leukemic blast cells and protein markers indicates the specific type of leukemia – lymphoid or myeloid.
      - Nursing Actions
        - Apply pressure to the site for 5 to 10 min.
        - Check vital signs frequently.
        - Apply pressure dressing.
        - Monitor for signs of bleeding and infection for 24 hr.
    - Lymph node biopsy
      - This biopsy involves a tissue sample to diagnose disease. Dye can sometimes be used with this type of biopsy.
      - Hodgkin's lymphoma (HL) – The presence of Reed-Sternberg cells (B-lymphocytes that have become cancerous) is diagnostic for Hodgkin's disease.

Collaborative Care

- Nursing Care

  - Monitor for any signs of infection or bleeding and report immediately.

  - Prevent infection.

    - Frequent, thorough hand hygiene.

    - Place clients in a private room.

    - Screen visitors carefully.

    - Encourage good nutrition (low-bacteria diet- avoid salads, raw fruits, and vegetables) and fluid intake.

    - Monitor WBC counts.

    - Encourage good personal hygiene.

    - Avoid crowds if possible.

  - Prevent injury.

    - Monitor platelet counts.

    - Check clients frequently for obvious and occult signs of bleeding.

    - Protect clients from trauma (avoid injections and venipunctures, apply firm pressure, increase vitamin K intake).

    - Instruct clients on how to avoid trauma (use electric shaver, soft-bristled toothbrush, avoid contact sports).

  - Conserve the client's energy.

    - Encourage rest, good nutrition, and fluid intake.

    - Ensure clients get adequate sleep.

    - Plan activities as appropriate.

- Medications

  - Chemotherapy

    - Chemotherapy is used to treat leukemia and lymphoma. Treatment may also include radiation of the brain and spinal cord.

PHASE	GOAL	PROCEDURE	LENGTH OF TIME
Induction therapy – Places client at high risk for infection and hemorrhage following this phase	To induce remission – Defined as absence of all signs of leukemia including less than 5% blasts in bone marrow	CNS prophylaxis administered as chemotherapy to the CSF (intrathecal) or as radiation to the brain and spinal cord	Lasts 4 to 6 weeks

PHASE	GOAL	PROCEDURE	LENGTH OF TIME
Consolidation or intensification therapy	To eradicate any residual leukemic cells	High doses of chemotherapy frequently administered	Lasts about 6 months
Maintenance therapy	Prevention of relapse	Use of oral chemotherapy	Lasts 2 to 3 years
Reinduction therapy – For clients who relapse	Primary purpose is to place clients back in remission	Combinations of chemotherapy used to achieve remission	Probability of relapse occurring decreases over time

- ■ Client Education
    - ☐ Inform clients of potential side effects of medications and other treatments and actions to take.
    - ☐ Encourage clients to inform the nurse if nausea and vomiting persist. A nutritional consult may be helpful if adequate intake is difficult to assume.
    - ☐ Instruct clients to use frequent oral hygiene and use a soft toothbrush. Avoid alcohol-based mouthwash.
    - ☐ Instruct clients to report signs and symptoms of infection or illness immediately to the provider.
    - ☐ Inform clients that hair loss (alopecia) occurs 7 to 10 days after treatment begins. Encourage the client to select a hairpiece before treatment starts.
- o Colony-stimulating medications such as filgrastim (Neupogen)
    - ■ Stimulate the production of leukocytes
    - ■ Nursing Considerations
        - ☐ Monitor for signs of bone pain. Monitor CBC twice weekly to check leukocyte level. Use cautiously with clients who have bone marrow cancer.
    - ■ Client Education
        - ☐ Encourage clients to inform nurse if bone discomfort occurs.
- • Interdisciplinary Care
    - o Oncology services may be consulted for chemotherapy.
    - o Request a referral for nutritional services to assist with weight loss or gain of clients related to medications or diagnosis.
    - o Request a referral for rehabilitation services to assist clients with prolonged weakness and who need assistance with increasing level of activity.
    - o Request a referral for home health services to assist clients in their home.

- Therapeutic Procedures
  - o Bone marrow transplantation
    - Bone marrow is destroyed or "ablated" using radiation or chemotherapy.
    - Closely matched donor stem cells are infused to replace destroyed cells.
      - □ Autologous cells are the client's own cells that are collected before chemotherapy.
      - □ Syngeneic cells are donated from the client's identical twin.
      - □ Allogeneic cells are obtained from an HLA-matched donor, such as a relative or from umbilical cord blood.
    - Following transplantation, clients are at high risk for infection and bleeding until the transfused stem cells begin producing WBCs again.
- Care after Discharge
  - o Client Education
    - Teach clients and their families to recognize signs of infection, skin breakdown, and nutritional deficiency.
    - Encourage clients to maintain good hygiene.
    - Recommend that clients avoid individuals with colds/infections/viruses.
    - Instruct clients and their families to administer medications and nutritional support at home.
    - Instruct clients and their families in the proper use of vascular access devices.
    - Instruct clients and their families about bleeding precautions and management of active bleeding.
    - Encourage clients to maintain current immunizations for influenza and pneumonia.
- Client Outcomes
  - o Client will be free from infection.
  - o Client will have no signs of bleeding.
  - o Client will have increased level of activity.

Complications

- Pancytopenia – Decrease in white and red blood cells and platelets
  - o Neutropenia secondary to disease and/or treatment, which greatly increases the client's risk for infection
    - An absolute neutrophil count (ANC) less than 2,000/mm³ suggests an increased risk of infection. An ANC of less than 500/mm³ indicates a severe risk of infection.

- Nursing Actions
  - Maintain a hygienic environment and encourage clients to do the same.
  - Monitor clients closely for signs of infection (cough, alterations in breath sounds, urine, or feces). Report temperature greater than 37.8° C (100° F).
  - Administer antimicrobial, antiviral, and antifungal medications as prescribed.
  - Monitor clients receiving blood products (granulocytes).
- Thrombocytopenia secondary to disease and/or treatment, which greatly increases the client's risk for bleeding
  - The greatest risk is at platelet counts less than 50,000/mm³, and spontaneous bleeds can occur at less than 20,000/mm³.
  - Nursing Actions
    - Minimize the risk of trauma (safe environment).
    - Monitor clients receiving blood products (platelets).
    - Administer thrombopoietic growth factor such as oprelvekin (interleukin-11, Neumega).
- Anemia secondary to disease and/or treatment, which greatly increases the client's risk for hypoxemia
  - Nursing Actions
    - Maintain an environment that does not overly tax the client's energy resources/capability.
    - Monitor RBC counts.
    - Provide a diet high in protein and carbohydrates.
    - Administer colony-stimulating factors, such as epoetin alfa (Procrit), as prescribed.
    - Monitor clients receiving blood products (packed RBCs).
- Bone Marrow Transplant Complications
  - Failure of stem cells to engraft
    - If stem cells fail to grow, a bone marrow transplant must be repeated.
  - Graft-versus-host disease
    - Graft rejection
    - Nursing Actions
      - Administer immunosuppressants as prescribed.

- o Phlebitis
  - May occur in the blood vessels of the liver
    - □ May occur up to one month after bone marrow transplant
  - Nursing Actions
    - □ Monitor for jaundice, abdominal pain, and liver enlargement.
    - □ Monitor daily weights and abdominal girth to check for fluid retention.

Ⓐ APPLICATION EXERCISES

Scenario: A nurse is caring for a client who has a new diagnosis of lymphoma and is to begin chemotherapy.

1. The client says he doesn't understand the concept of remission. Which of the following responses by the nurse is appropriate?

    A. "It is the first step in treatment when chemotherapy is given into the spinal column."
    B. "This is the stage when the lymphoma is defined as a chronic condition."
    C. "It involves infusing the client's own cells back into his system to replace destroyed cells."
    D. "It is the absence of signs of the disease, when the bone marrow has minimal blast cells."

2. The client asks the nurse to discuss reasons why he has lymphoma. Describe the possible causes of this disease.

3. Which of the following diagnostic and laboratory tests should the client undergo to confirm a diagnosis of lymphoma? (Select all that apply.)

    _____ Lymph node biopsy
    _____ Hct and Hgb
    _____ WBC count
    _____ Bleeding time
    _____ Bone marrow biopsy

4. The nurse is reviewing dietary instructions with the client. Which of the following foods should be avoided to decrease the risk of infection? (Select all that apply.)

    _____ Fresh spinach salad
    _____ Chicken noodle soup
    _____ Saltine crackers
    _____ Oranges
    _____ Canned tomato juice

APPLICATION EXERCISES ANSWER KEY

Scenario: A nurse is caring for a client who has a new diagnosis of lymphoma and is to begin chemotherapy.

1. The client says he doesn't understand the concept of remission. Which of the following responses by the nurse is appropriate?

    A. "It is the first step in treatment when chemotherapy is given into the spinal column."

    B. "This is the stage when the lymphoma is defined as a chronic condition."

    C. "It involves infusing the client's own cells back into his system to replace destroyed cells."

    D. "It is the absence of signs of the disease, when the bone marrow has minimal blast cells."

    Remission is the goal of treatment. This occurs by returning the client to a state when there is an absence of signs of the disease including less than 5% blasts in the bone marrow. The first step in treatment is the induction phase of therapy. The chronic form of lymphoma is defined as the disease having progressed slowly into its three phases over time. The infusion of a client's own cells into his system to replace destroyed cells is what occurs during bone marrow transplantation.

    NCLEX® Connection: Physiological Adaptations, Basic Pathophysiology

2. The client asks the nurse to discuss reasons why he has lymphoma. Describe the possible causes of this disease.

    The exact cause of lymphoma is unknown. Risk factors include the client having immunologic factors, which do not permit his body to defend itself adequately from the disease. Other possible risk factors include exposure to chemicals and medications that suppress bone marrow activity, hereditary conditions, exposure to radiation, viruses, and environmental factors.

    NCLEX® Connection: Physiological Adaptations, Basic Pathophysiology

3. Which of the following diagnostic and laboratory tests should the client undergo to confirm a diagnosis of lymphoma? (Select all that apply.)

__X__ **Lymph node biopsy**

_____ Hct and Hgb

__X__ **WBC count**

_____ Bleeding time

__X__ **Bone marrow biopsy**

A diagnosis of lymphoma is made based on a lymph node biopsy to determine the specific type of lymphoma. A WBC count identifies alterations in WBCs, which helps to define the type of lymphoma. A bone marrow biopsy identifies the types of cells being produced, which also assists in defining the type of lymphoma. Hgb and bleeding time identify the body's response to the disease process, but do not diagnose lymphoma or leukemia.

 NCLEX® Connection: Reduction of Risk Potential, Diagnostic Tests

4. The nurse is reviewing dietary instructions with the client. Which of the following foods should be avoided to decrease the risk of infection? (Select all that apply.)

__X__ **Fresh spinach salad**

_____ Chicken noodle soup

_____ Saltine crackers

__X__ **Oranges**

_____ Canned tomato juice

The client who has lymphoma is susceptible to infection and should eat foods that are low in bacteria. The client should avoid fresh salads, raw fruits, and vegetables. A fresh spinach salad and oranges are raw foods that should be avoided. Chicken noodle soup, saltine crackers, and canned tomato juice are processed, cooked foods that contain no to minimal bacteria.

 NCLEX® Connection: Basic Care and Comfort, Nutrition and Oral Hydration

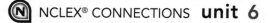

UNIT 6: NURSING CARE OF CLIENTS WITH FLUID AND ELECTROLYTE/ACID-BASE IMBALANCES

- Fluid and Electrolyte Imbalances
- Acid-Base Imbalances

NCLEX® CONNECTIONS

When reviewing the chapters in this section, keep in mind the relevant sections of the NCLEX® outline, in particular:

CLIENT NEEDS: PHYSIOLOGICAL ADAPTATION

Relevant topics/tasks include:
- Basic Pathophysiology
  - Consider general principles of client disease process when providing care.
- Fluid and Electrolyte Imbalances
  - Identify signs and symptoms of client fluid and/or electrolyte imbalances.
- Medical Emergencies
  - Reinforce teaching of emergency intervention explanations to client.

UNIT 6	NURSING CARE OF CLIENTS WITH FLUID AND ELECTROLYTE/ ACID-BASE IMBALANCES
Chapter 38	Fluid and Electrolyte Imbalances

Overview

- Body fluids are distributed between intracellular (ICF) and extracellular (ECF) fluid compartments.

- Fluid can move between compartments (through selectively permeable membranes) by a variety of methods (diffusion, active transport, filtration, osmosis) to maintain homeostasis.

- Electrolytes are minerals (sometimes called salts) that are present in all body fluids. They regulate fluid balance and hormone production, strengthen skeletal structures, and act as catalysts in nerve response, muscle contraction, and the metabolism of nutrients.

- When dissolved in water or another solvent, electrolytes separate into ions and conduct either a positive (cations – magnesium, potassium, sodium, calcium) or negative (anions – phosphate, sulfate, chloride, bicarbonate) electrical current.

- Electrolytes are distributed between ICF and ECF fluid compartments. While laboratory tests can accurately reflect the electrolyte concentrations in plasma, it is not possible to directly measure electrolyte concentrations within cells.

ELECTROLYTE	EXPECTED REFERENCE RANGE
Sodium	136 to 145 mEq/L
Potassium	3.5 to 5.0 mEq/L
Chloride	98 to 106 mEq/L
Calcium	9.0 to 10.5 mg/dL
Magnesium	1.3 to 2.1 mEq/L
Phosphorus	3.5 to 4.5 mg/dL

FLUID IMBALANCES

Overview

- Fluid volume deficits (FVDs) include hypovolemia-isotonic (loss of water and electrolytes from the ECF) and dehydration-osmolar (loss of water with no loss of electrolytes).

- Hemoconcentration occurs with dehydration, resulting in increases in Hct, serum electrolytes, and urine-specific gravity.

- Hypovolemia can lead to hypovolemic shock.

- Fluid volume excesses (FVEs) include hypervolemia-isotonic (water and sodium are retained in abnormally high proportions) and overhydration-osmolar (more water is gained than electrolytes).

- Note – Severe hypervolemia can lead to pulmonary edema and heart failure.

- Note – Compensatory mechanisms include increased release of natriuretic peptides, resulting in increased loss of sodium and water by the kidneys and the decrease in the release of aldosterone.

Data Collection

- Risk Factors

FLUID VOLUME DEFICIT	FLUID VOLUME EXCESS
Causes of Hypovolemia • Abnormal gastrointestinal losses – Vomiting, NG suctioning, diarrhea • Abnormal skin losses – Diaphoresis • Abnormal renal losses – Diuretic therapy, diabetes insipidus, renal disease, adrenal insufficiency, osmotic diuresis • Third spacing – Peritonitis, intestinal obstruction, ascites, burns • Hemorrhage • Altered intake, such as nothing by mouth (NPO)	Causes of Hypervolemia • Chronic stimulus to the kidney to conserve sodium and water (heart failure, cirrhosis, increased glucocorticosteroids) • Abnormal renal function with reduced excretion of sodium and water (renal failure) • Interstitial to plasma fluid shifts (hypertonic fluids, burns) • Age-related changes in cardiovascular and renal function • Excessive sodium intake
Causes of Dehydration • Hyperventilation • Diabetic ketoacidosis • Enteral feeding without sufficient water intake	Causes of Overhydration • Water replacement without electrolyte replacement (strenuous exercise with profuse diaphoresis)

- Subjective and Objective Data

PARAMETER	FLUID VOLUME DEFICIT	FLUID VOLUME EXCESS
Vital signs	Hyperthermia, tachycardia, thready pulse, hypotension, orthostatic hypotension, decreased central venous pressure, tachypneic, hypoxia	Tachycardia, bounding pulse, hypertension, tachypnea, increased central venous pressure
Neuromusculoskeletal	Dizziness, syncope, confusion, weakness, fatigue	Confusion, muscle weakness
Respiratory	Increased rate	Increased rate, shallow respirations, dyspnea, orthopnea, crackles, diminished breath sounds
GI	Thirst, dry furrowed tongue, nausea/vomiting, anorexia, acute weight loss	Weight gain, ascites
Renal	Oliguria (decreased production of urine), concentrated urine	
Other signs	Diminished capillary refill, dry, scaly skin, dry mucous membranes with cracks, poor skin turgor, sunken eyeballs, flattened neck veins	Dependent edema, distended neck veins, cool, pale skin

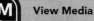

View Media Supplement:

- Crackles (Audio)
- Pitting Edema (Image)

- Laboratory Tests

PARAMETER	FLUID VOLUME DEFICIT	FLUID VOLUME EXCESS
Hct	Increased Hct	Decreased Hct
Serum osmolarity	Increased (hemoconcentration) osmolarity (greater than 300 mOsm/L)	Decreased (hemodilution) osmolarity (less than 270 mOsm/L)
Urine-specific gravity	Increased (concentrated)	Decreased (diluted)
Serum sodium	Increased (hemoconcentration)	Decreased (hemodilution)

Collaborative Care

- Nursing Care

  - Auscultate lung sounds and monitor oxygen saturation.

  - Administer supplemental oxygen as prescribed.

  - Monitor vital signs and heart rhythm.

  - Monitor clients receiving IV fluids as prescribed (isotonic solutions, such as lactated Ringer's, normal saline, blood transfusions).

  - Monitor I&O. Alert the provider for urine output less than 30 mL/hr.

  - Monitor daily weights.

  - Monitor skin (presence of edema).

  - Monitor level of consciousness and maintain client safety.

  - Encourage clients to change positions, slowly rolling from side to side, or standing up.

  - Reposition or have clients change position every 2 hr.

  - Support arms and legs to decrease dependent edema as appropriate.

- Interdisciplinary Care

  - Respiratory services may be consulted for oxygen management.

- Care After Discharge

  - Client Education

    - Fluid volume deficit

      - Encourage clients to drink plenty of liquids to promote hydration.

      - Instruct clients regarding causes of dehydration, such as nausea/vomiting.

      - Encourage clients to increase fluid intake in high altitudes, dry climates and when performing exercise.

      - Encourage clients to avoid drinking fluids that contain alcohol or caffeine. This increases fluid excretion.

    - Fluid volume excess

      - Encourage clients to weigh themselves daily. Notify provider if there is a 1- to 2-lb gain in 24 hr, or a 3-lb gain in a week.

      - Recommend that clients consume a low-sodium diet. Read food labels to check sodium content and keep a record of daily sodium intake.

      - Promote fluid restriction intake. Consult with the provider regarding prescribed restrictions.

- Client Outcomes

  ○ The client will maintain adequate oxygen level.

  ○ The client will be able to maintain adequate hydration.

  ○ The client will be able to tolerate food and liquids.

  ○ The client will be free from anxiety.

  ○ The client will be free from falls/injury.

  ○ The client will adhere to fluid and food instructions.

Complications

- Hypovolemic Shock (fluid volume deficit)

  ○ Vital organ hypoxia/anoxia – Decreased Hgb oxygen saturation and pulse pressure (systolic-diastolic blood pressure)

  ○ Nursing Actions

    ▪ Administer oxygen.

    ▪ Monitor clients receiving fluid replacement with:

      □ Colloids (whole blood, packed RBCs, plasma, synthetic plasma expanders).

      □ Crystalloids (lactated Ringer's, normal saline).

    ▪ Monitor clients receiving emergency care. Clients may receive vasoconstrictors, such as dopamine (Intropin) and norepinephrine (Levophed); coronary vasodilators, such as sodium nitroprusside (Nipride); and/or positive inotropic medications, such as dobutamine (Dobutrex).

- Pulmonary Edema (fluid volume excess)

  ○ Pulmonary edema can be caused by severe fluid overload.

    ▪ Symptoms include anxiety, tachycardia, acute respiratory distress, increased vein distention, dyspnea at rest, change in level of consciousness, and ascending crackles (fluid level within lungs) and cough, productive of frothy pink-tinged sputum.

  ○ Nursing Actions

    ▪ Position clients in high-Fowler's position to maximize ventilation.

    ▪ Administer oxygen.

    ▪ Assist with respiratory support.

    ▪ Monitor clients receiving morphine and diuretic as prescribed.

ELECTROLYTE IMBALANCES

Overview

- Electrolyte imbalances include imbalances of serum sodium, potassium, calcium and magnesium.

SODIUM IMBALANCES

Overview

- Sodium (Na^+) is the major electrolyte found in extracellular fluid.

- Sodium is essential for maintaining acid-base balance, active and passive transport mechanisms, and maintaining irritability and conduction of nerve and muscle tissue.

- The expected reference range for serum sodium levels is between 136 to 145 mEq/L.

Hyponatremia

- o Hyponatremia is a net gain of water or loss of sodium-rich fluids that results in sodium levels less than 136 mEq/L.

- o Water moves from the ECF into the ICF causing cells to swell (cerebral edema).

- o Compensatory mechanisms include the renal excretion of sodium-free water.

- Hypernatremia

- o Hypernatremia is a serum sodium level greater than 145 mEq/L.

- Increased sodium causes hypertonicity of the serum. This causes a shift of water out of the cells, resulting in dehydrated cells.

Data Collection

- Risk factors

HYPONATREMIA	HYPERNATREMIA

• Deficient ECF volume
  ○ Abnormal GI losses – Vomiting, NG suctioning, diarrhea, tap water enemas, gastrointestinal obstructions
  ○ Renal losses – Diuretics, kidney disease, adrenal insufficiency
  ○ Skin losses – Excessive sweating, burns, wound drainage, ascites (as it relates to cirrhosis)
• Increased or normal ECF volume
  ○ Excessive oral water intake
  ○ Syndrome of inappropriate antidiuretic hormone (SIADH) – Excess secretion of antidiuretic hormone (ADH)
• Edematous states – Heart failure, cirrhosis, nephrotic syndrome
• Excessive hypotonic IV fluids
• Inadequate sodium intake (NPO)
	• Water deprivation (NPO)
	• Excessive sodium intake – Dietary sodium intake, hypertonic IV fluids, bicarbonate intake
	• Excessive sodium retention – Renal failure, Cushing's syndrome, aldosteronism, some medications (glucocorticosteroids)
	• Fluid losses – Fever, diaphoresis, burns, respiratory infection, diabetes insipidus, hyperglycemia, watery diarrhea
	• Age-related changes, specifically decreased total body water content and inadequate fluid intake related to an altered thirst mechanism
	• Compensatory mechanisms include increased thirst and production of ADH.

- Subjective Data and Objective Data

PARAMETER	HYPONATREMIA	HYPERNATREMIA
Vital signs	Hypothermia, tachycardia, rapid thready pulse, hypotension, orthostatic hypotension (vital signs can vary based on state of ECF volume)	Hyperthermia, tachycardia, orthostatic hypotension
Neuromusculoskeletal	Headache, confusion, lethargy, muscle weakness to the point of possible respiratory compromise, fatigue, decreased deep-tendon reflexes (DTRs), seizures	Restlessness, irritability, muscle twitching to the point of muscle weakness including respiratory compromise, decreased DTRs to the point of absent DTRs, seizures, coma
GI	Increased motility, hyperactive bowel sounds, abdominal cramping, nausea	Thirst, dry mucous membranes, increased motility, hyperactive bowel sounds, abdominal cramping, nausea
Other signs		Edema, warm flushed skin, oliguria

- Laboratory Tests

PARAMETER	HYPONATREMIA	HYPERNATREMIA
Serum sodium	Decreased – < 136 mEq/L	Increased – > 145 mEq/L
Serum osmolarity	Decreased – < 270 mOsm/L	Increased – > 300 mOsm/L

Collaborative Care

- Nursing Care

  - Auscultate lung sounds and monitor oxygen saturation.

  - Administer supplemental oxygen as prescribed.

  - Monitor vital signs and heart rhythm.

  - Monitor clients receiving IV fluids as prescribed (isotonic solutions, such as lactated Ringer's, normal saline, blood transfusions).

  - Monitor I&O. Alert the provider for urine output less than 30 cc/hr.

  - Monitor daily weights.

  - Monitor skin (presence of edema).

  - Monitor level of consciousness and maintain client safety.

  - Encourage clients to change positions, slowly rolling from side to side, or standing up.

  - Reposition or have clients change position every 2 hr.

  - Report abnormal laboratory findings to the provider.

  - Fluid overload – Restrict water intake as prescribed by the provider.

    - For clients with heart failure and hyponatremia, provide loop diuretics and ACE inhibitors.

  - Monitor clients receiving fluid replacement.

    - Hypertonic oral and IV fluids

    - 3% sodium chloride IV

    - Encourage foods and fluids high in sodium (cheeses, milk, condiments).

    - Restoration of normal ECF volume – Administer isotonic IV therapy (0.9% sodium chloride, lactated Ringer's).

  - Fluid loss:

    - Monitor clients receiving IV fluid replacement that will be based on serum osmolarity and hemodynamic stability.

      - Hypotonic IV fluids (0.45% sodium chloride)

      - Isotonic IV fluids (0.9% sodium chloride)

      ◦ Excess sodium

          ■ Encourage water intake and discourage sodium intake.

          ■ Administer diuretics (loop diuretics) for clients with poor renal excretion.

      ◦ Interdisciplinary Care

          ■ Nephrology may be consulted for electrolyte and fluid replacement.

          ■ Respiratory services may be consulted for oxygen management.

          ■ Request a referral for nutritional services to assist clients with dietary restrictions.

- Care After Discharge

      ◦ Client Education

          ■ Encourage clients to weigh themselves daily and to notify the provider of a 1- to 2-lb gain in 24 hr, or 3 lb gain in a week.

          ■ Instruct clients to follow sodium guidelines, read food labels to check sodium content, and keep a daily record of sodium intake.

- Client Outcomes

      ◦ The client will maintain normal fluid balance as indicated by urinary output, vital signs, and cognitive functioning.

      ◦ The client will adhere to fluid and dietary guidelines.

Complications

- Acute hyponatremia/hypernatremia

      ◦ Complications (coma, seizures, respiratory arrest) can result from acute hyponatremia or hypernatremia if not treated immediately.

      ◦ Nursing Actions

          ■ Maintain an open airway and monitor client's vital signs.

          ■ Implement seizure precautions and take appropriate action if seizures occur.

          ■ Monitor the client's level of consciousness.

POTASSIUM IMBALANCES

Overview

- Potassium (K^+) is the major cation in the intracellular fluid (ICF).

- Potassium plays a vital role in cell metabolism, transmission of nerve impulses, functioning of cardiac, lung, and muscle tissues, and acid-base balance.

- Potassium has a reciprocal action with sodium.

- Expected reference range for serum potassium levels is between 3.5 and 5.0 mEq/L.

- Hypokalemia is the result of an increased loss of potassium from the body or movement of potassium into the cells, resulting in a serum potassium less than 3.5 mEq/L.

- Hyperkalemia is the result of an increased intake of potassium, movement of potassium out of the cells, or inadequate renal excretion resulting in a serum potassium level greater than 5.0 mEq/L.

Data Collection

- Risk Factors

HYPOKALEMIA	HYPERKALEMIA

- Decreased total body potassium
  ○ Abnormal GI losses – Vomiting, NG suctioning, diarrhea, inappropriate laxative use
  ○ Renal losses – Excessive use of diuretics (furosemide [Lasix], corticosteroids)
  ○ Skin losses – Diaphoresis, wound losses
- Insufficient potassium
  ○ Inadequate dietary intake (rare)
  ○ Prolonged administration of nonelectrolyte containing IV solutions (dextrose 5% in water)
- Intracellular shift – Metabolic alkalosis, after correction of acidosis, during periods of tissue repair (burns, trauma, starvation), total parenteral nutrition
- Older adult clients are at greater risk due to increased use of diuretics and laxatives.
	- Increased total body potassium – IV potassium administration, salt substitute
	- Extracellular shift – Decreased insulin, acidosis (diabetic ketoacidosis), tissue catabolism (sepsis, trauma, surgery, fever, MI)
	- Hypertonic states – Uncontrolled diabetes mellitus
	- Decreased excretion of potassium – Renal failure, severe dehydration, potassium-sparing diuretics, angiotensin-converting enzyme inhibitors, NSAIDs, adrenal insufficiency
	- Older adult clients are at a greater risk due to the increased use of salt substitutes, ACE inhibitors, and potassium-sparing diuretics.

- Subjective Data and Objective Data

PARAMETER	HYPOKALEMIA	HYPERKALEMIA
Vital signs	Weak, irregular pulse, hypotension, respiratory distress	Slow, irregular pulse, hypotension
Neuromusculoskeletal	Weakness to the point of respiratory collapse and paralysis, muscle cramping, decreased muscle tone and hypoactive reflexes, paresthesias, mental confusion	Restlessness, irritability, weakness to the point of ascending flaccid paralysis, paresthesias
GI	Decreased motility, abdominal distention, constipation, ileus, nausea, vomiting, anorexia	Nausea, vomiting, increased motility, diarrhea, hyperactive bowel sounds
Other signs	Polyuria (dilute urine)	Oliguria

- Laboratory Tests and Diagnostic Procedures

PARAMETER	HYPOKALEMIA	HYPERKALEMIA
Serum sodium	Decreased (< 3.5 mEq/L)	Increased (> 5.0 mEq/L)
ABGs	Metabolic alkalosis (pH > 7.45)	Metabolic acidosis (pH < 7.35)
ECG	Premature ventricular contractions (PVCs), bradycardia, blocks, ventricular tachycardia, inverted T-waves, and ST depression	Premature ventricular contractions, ventricular fibrillation, peaked T-waves, and widened QRS

Collaborative Care

- Nursing Care

  o Monitor clients as indicated. Report abnormal findings to the provider.

  o Management of hypokalemia

    ▪ Encourage foods high in potassium (avocados, broccoli, dairy products, dried fruit, cantaloupe, bananas).

    ▪ Provide oral potassium supplementation.

  o IV potassium supplementation

    ▪ Never give as an IV bolus (high risk of cardiac arrest).

    ▪ The maximum recommended rate is 5 to 10 mEq/hr.

    ▪ Check for phlebitis (tissue irritant).

    ▪ Monitor clients receiving digoxin (Lanoxin). Hypokalemia increases the risk for digoxin toxicity.

  o Management of hyperkalemia

    ▪ Provide for cardiac protection – Prepare to administer calcium gluconate or calcium chloride.

    ▪ Decrease potassium intake.

    ▪ Stop the infusion of IV potassium.

    ▪ Withhold oral potassium.

    ▪ Provide a potassium-restricted diet (avoid foods high in potassium [avocados, broccoli, dairy products, dried fruit, cantaloupe, bananas]).

  o Promote movement of potassium from ECF to ICF.

    ▪ Monitor clients receiving IV fluids with dextrose and Regular insulin.

    ▪ Monitor clients receiving sodium bicarbonate to reverse acidosis.

  o Medications (to increase potassium excretion)

    ▪ Administer loop diuretics (furosemide [Lasix]) if renal function is adequate.

    ▪ Loop diuretics increase the depletion of potassium from the renal system.

- ■ Nursing Considerations
  - □ Monitor IV access.
- ■ Client Education
  - □ Educate clients on a potassium-restricted diet.
  - □ Instruct clients to hold oral potassium supplements until further advised by the provider.
- ○ Administer cation exchange resins (sodium polystyrene sulfonate [Kayexalate]).
  - ■ Works as a laxative and excretes excess potassium from the body. Can be used on clients with renal problems.
  - ■ Nursing Considerations
    - □ If potassium levels are extremely high, dialysis may be required.
  - ■ Client Education
    - □ Educate clients on a potassium-restricted diet.
    - □ Instruct clients to hold oral potassium supplements until further advised by the provider.

- Interdisciplinary Care
  - ○ Nephrology may be consulted for electrolyte and fluid management.
  - ○ Respiratory services may be consulted for oxygen management.
  - ○ Request a referral for nutritional services to assist clients with dietary restrictions
  - ○ Cardiology may be consulted for dysrhythmias.

- Care After Discharge
  - ○ Client Education
    - ■ Educate clients regarding dietary guidelines (potassium-rich or potassium-restricted foods to consume.) Clients on a potassium-restricted diet should avoid salt substitutes containing potassium.

- Client Outcomes
  - ○ The client will maintain adequate gas exchange.
  - ○ The client will be free from injury.
  - ○ The client will have electrolyte laboratory values within the expected reference range.

- Complications
  - ○ Respiratory Failure
    - ■ Nursing Actions
      - □ Maintain an open airway and monitor the client's vital signs.
      - □ Monitor the client's level of consciousness.

        □   Monitor for hypoxemia and hypercapnia.

        □   Assist with intubation and mechanical ventilation if indicated.

  o Cardiac Arrest

    ■ Nursing Actions

        □   Perform continuous cardiac monitoring.

        □   Treat dysrhythmias.

OTHER ELECTROLYTE IMBALANCES

Overview

Hypocalcemia

- Hypocalcemia is a serum calcium less than 9.0 mg/dL or ionized calcium less than 4.5 mg/dL.

Data Collection

- Risk Factors

  - Malabsorption syndromes (Crohn's disease)

  - Hypoalbuminemia

  - End-stage kidney disease

  - Post thyroidectomy

  - Hypoparathyroidism

  - Inadequate intake of calcium

  - Vitamin D deficiency (becoming more common today) or lack of 25-hydroxy vitamin D related to end-stage kidney disease

  - Pancreatitis

  - Hyperphosphatemia

  - Medications that block parathyroid function, cause hyperphosphatemia, chelate calcium, or prevent absorption of calcium

  - Sepsis

- Subjective and Objective Data

  - Paresthesia of the fingers and lips (early symptom)

  - Muscle twitches/tetany

  - Frequent, painful muscle spasms at rest

  - Hyperactive deep-tendon reflexes

  - Positive Chvostek's sign (tapping on the facial nerve triggering facial twitching)

- o Positive Trousseau's sign (hand/finger spasms with sustained blood pressure cuff inflation)
- o Cardiovascular – Decreased myocardial contractility (decreased heart rate and hypotension)
- o Gastrointestinal – Hyperactive bowel sounds, diarrhea, abdominal cramping
- o Laboratory Tests
  - Calcium level less than 9.0 mg/dL
- o Diagnostic Procedures
  - Electrocardiogram
    - □ ECG changes – Prolonged QT interval

Collaborative Care

- Nursing Care
  - o Administer oral calcium supplements.
  - o Monitor clients receiving IV calcium infusion.
  - o Implement seizure precautions.
  - o Have emergency equipment on standby.
  - o Encourage foods high in calcium including dairy products and dark green vegetables.
- Care After Discharge
  - o Client Education
    - Educate clients about consuming foods high in calcium (yogurt, milk).
    - Teach clients ways to increase calcium intake by reading food labels.
- Client Outcomes
  - o The client will maintain serum calcium levels within the normal range.
  - o The client will be free from injury.
  - o The client will be free from convulsions.

Hypomagnesemia

- Hypomagnesemia is a serum magnesium level less than 1.3 mg/dL.

Data Collection

- Risk Factors
  - o Causes of hypomagnesemia
    - Malnutrition (insufficient magnesium intake)
    - Alcohol ingestion (magnesium excretion)

- Subjective and Objective Data

  o Neuromuscular – Increased nerve impulse transmission (hyperactive deep-tendon reflexes, paresthesias, muscle tetany), positive Chvostek's and Trousseau's signs

  o Gastrointestinal – Hypoactive bowel sounds, constipation, abdominal distention, paralytic ileus.

Collaborative Care

- Nursing Care

  o Discontinue magnesium-losing medications (loop diuretics).

  o Administer oral sulfate following safety protocols. Oral magnesium can cause diarrhea and increase magnesium depletion. Monitor clients closely.

  o Monitor clients receiving IV magnesium sulfate infusion.

  o Encourage foods high in magnesium, including dairy products and dark green vegetables.

  o Oral magnesium can cause diarrhea and increase magnesium depletion. Monitor clients closely.

- Care After Discharge

  o Client Education

    ▪ Educate clients regarding foods that are high in magnesium.

    ▪ Teach clients ways to increase magnesium in diet by reading food labels.

- Client Outcomes

  o The client will be free from injury.

  o The client will be free from seizures.

Ⓐ APPLICATION EXERCISES

1. A nurse is caring for a client who has a potassium level of 5.4 mEq/L. This client is at risk for which of the following?

   A. Dysrhythmias

   B. Constipation

   C. Polyuria

   D. Hypotension

2. A nurse is caring for a client who has an NG tube with suctioning. This client is at risk for which of the following electrolyte imbalances? (Select all that apply.)

   _____ Hyperkalemia

   _____ Hypernatremia

   _____ Hypokalemia

   _____ Hypomagnesemia

   _____ Hyponatremia

3. How does a nurse identify a positive Trousseau's sign?

4. A nurse is caring for a client who has hypokalemia. Which of the following foods should be encouraged in the client's diet? (Select all that apply.)

   _____ Avocados

   _____ Broccoli

   _____ Fish

   _____ Yogurt

   _____ Raisins

5. A nurse is admitting a client who was brought to the emergency department by emergency personnel who administered IV fluids. The laboratory results for the client are: Sodium 136 mEq/L and magnesium 1.0 mEq/L. Which of the following is the likely cause of these results?

   A. History of recent alcohol ingestion

   B. Having been NPO for 4 hr

   C. IV administration of dextrose 5% in water (D₅W) at 75 mL/hr

   D. Administration of a potassium-sparing diuretic

6. Which of the following age-related changes place older adult clients at risk for hypernatremia? (Select all that apply.)

_____ Decreased total body water content

_____ Inadequate water intake

_____ Inadequate intake of calcium

_____ Altered thirst mechanism

_____ Muscle weakness

7. An older adult female at an assisted living facility has become confused and refuses to ambulate due to shortness of breath. Data collection includes the following: temperature 36.8° C (98.4° F), pulse 126/min and bounding, respirations 18/min, blood pressure 156/118 mm Hg, diminished breath sounds in the lung bases with crackles present, oxygen saturation 91%, 2+ edema bilaterally of the ankles, and urine that is cloudy with sediment apparent. The client has refused all solid foods. She is currently receiving oxygen via nasal cannula at 2 L/min. Which of the above data supports a diagnosis of fluid volume excess?

7. An older adult female at an assisted living facility has become confused and refuses to ambulate due to shortness of breath. Data collection includes the following: temperature 36.8° C (98.4° F), pulse 126/min and bounding, respirations 18/min, blood pressure 156/118 mm Hg, diminished breath sounds in the lung bases with crackles present, oxygen saturation 91%, 2+ edema bilaterally of the ankles, and urine that is cloudy with sediment apparent. The client has refused all solid foods. She is currently receiving oxygen via nasal cannula at 2 L/min. Which of the above data supports a diagnosis of fluid volume excess?

    Data that support a diagnosis of fluid volume excess includes: Confusion, shortness of breath, tachycardia, bounding pulse, hypertension, diminished breath sounds with crackles present, and edema of the extremities. The temperature, respiratory rate, oxygen saturation, urine changes, and altered appetite do not support a diagnosis of fluid volume excess.

Ⓝ **NCLEX® Connection: Physiological Adaptations, Fluid and Electrolyte Imbalances**

UNIT 6	NURSING CARE OF CLIENTS WITH FLUID AND ELECTROLYTE/ACID-BASE IMBALANCES
Chapter 39	Acid-Base Imbalances

Overview

- For cells to function optimally, metabolic processes must maintain a steady balance between the acids and bases found in the body.

  ○ Acid-base balance represents homeostasis of hydrogen (H^+) ion concentration in body fluids. Hydrogen shifts between the extracellular and intracellular compartments to compensate for acid-base imbalances.

  ○ Minor changes in hydrogen concentration have major effects on normal cellular function.

- Arterial pH is an indirect measurement of hydrogen ion concentration and is a result of respiratory and renal compensational function. ABGs are most commonly used to evaluate acid-base balance.

  ○ The pH is the expression of the balance between carbon dioxide (CO_2), which is regulated by the lungs, and bicarbonate (HCO_3^-), a base regulated by the kidneys.

    ▪ The greater the concentration of hydrogen, the more acidic the body fluids and the lower the pH.

    ▪ The lower the concentration of hydrogen, the more alkaline the body fluids and the higher the pH.

Maintenance of Acid-Base Balance

- Acid-base balance is maintained by chemical, respiratory, and renal processes.

  ○ Chemical and protein buffers:

    ▪ Are the first line of defense.

    ▪ Either bind or release (H^+) ions as needed.

    ▪ Respond quickly to changes in pH.

- ○ Respiratory buffers:
  - ▪ Are the second line of defense.
  - ▪ Control the level of (H⁺) ions in the blood through the control of CO_2 levels.
  - ▪ When a chemoreceptor senses a change in the level of CO_2, a signal is sent to the brain to alter the rate and depth of respirations.
    - ☐ Hyperventilation = decrease in hydrogen ions
    - ☐ Hypoventilation = increase in hydrogen ions
- ○ Renal buffers
  - ▪ The kidneys are the third line of defense.
  - ▪ This buffering system is much slower to respond, but it is the most effective buffering system with the longest duration.
  - ▪ The kidneys control the movement of bicarbonate in the urine. Bicarbonate can be reabsorbed into the bloodstream or excreted in the urine in response to blood levels of hydrogen.
  - ▪ The kidneys may also produce more bicarbonate when needed.
    - ☐ High hydrogen ions = bicarbonate reabsorption and production
    - ☐ Low hydrogen ions = bicarbonate excretion
- Compensation refers to the process by which the body attempts to correct changes and imbalances in pH levels.
  - ○ Full compensation occurs when the pH level of the blood returns to normal (7.35 to 7.45).
  - ○ If the pH level is not able to normalize, then it is referred to as partial compensation.
- Metabolic alkalosis, metabolic acidosis, respiratory alkalosis, and respiratory acidosis are examples of acid-base imbalances.
- Acid-base imbalances are a result of insufficient compensation. Respiratory and renal function plays a large role in the body's ability to effectively compensate for acid-base alterations. Organ dysfunction negatively affects acid-base compensation.

Data Collection

- Risk Factors/Causes of Acid-Base Imbalances

RESPIRATORY ACIDOSIS – HYPOVENTILATION	RESPIRATORY ALKALOSIS – HYPERVENTILATION
Respiratory acidosis results from: • Respiratory depression from poisons, anesthetics, trauma, or neurological diseases (myasthenia gravis, Guillain-Barré). • Inadequate chest expansion due to muscle weakness, pneumothorax/hemothorax, flail chest, obesity, tumors, or deformities. • Airway obstruction that occurs in laryngospasm, asthma, and some cancers. • Alveolar-capillary blockage secondary to a pulmonary embolus, thrombus, cancer, or pulmonary edema. • Inadequate mechanical ventilation. Respiratory acidosis results in: • Increased CO_2. • Increased H^+ concentration.	Respiratory alkalosis results from: • Hyperventilation due to fear, anxiety, intracerebral trauma, salicylate toxicity, or excessive mechanical ventilation. • Hypoxemia from asphyxiation, high altitudes, shock, or early-stage asthma or pneumonia. Respiratory alkalosis results in: • Decreased CO_2. • Decreased H^+ concentration.
METABOLIC ACIDOSIS	METABOLIC ALKALOSIS

Metabolic acidosis results from:
• Excess production of hydrogen ions.
  o DKA
  o Lactic acidosis
  o Starvation
  o Heavy exercise
  o Seizure activity
  o Fever
  o Hypoxia
  o Intoxication with ethanol or salicylates
• Inadequate elimination of hydrogen ions.
  o Renal failure
• Inadequate production of bicarbonate.
  o Renal failure
  o Pancreatitis
  o Liver failure
  o Dehydration
• Excess elimination of bicarbonate.
  o Diarrhea, ileostomy
Metabolic acidosis results in:
• Decreased HCO_3^-.
• Increased (H+) concentration.
	Metabolic alkalosis results from:
	• Base excess.
	  o Oral ingestion of bases (antacids)
	  o Venous administration of bases (blood transfusions, TPN, or sodium bicarbonate)
	• Acid deficit.
	  o Loss of gastric secretions (through prolonged vomiting, NG suction)
	  o Potassium depletion (due to thiazide diuretics, laxative abuse, Cushing's syndrome)
	Metabolic alkalosis results in:
	• Increased HCO_3^-.
	• Decreased (H+) concentration.

- Subjective and Objective Data

RESPIRATORY ACIDOSIS – HYPOVENTILATION	RESPIRATORY ALKALOSIS – HYPERVENTILATION
• Vital signs – Tachycardia (severe acidosis may lead to bradycardia), tachypnea • Dysrhythmias • Neurological – Anxiety, irritability, confusion, coma • Cardiovascular – Dysrhythmias • Respiratory – Ineffective, shallow, rapid breathing • Skin – Pale or cyanotic	• Vital Signs – Tachypnea • Neurological – Anxiety, tetany, convulsions, tingling, numbness • Cardiovascular – Palpitations, chest pain, dysrhythmias • Respiratory – Rapid, deep respirations
METABOLIC ACIDOSIS	METABOLIC ALKALOSIS
• Vital signs – Bradycardia, weak peripheral pulses, hypotension, tachypnea • Neurological – Muscle weakness, hyporeflexia, flaccid paralysis, fatigue, confusion • Cardiovascular – Dysrhythmias • Respiratory – Rapid, deep respirations (Kussmaul respirations) • Skin – Warm, dry, flushed	• Vital signs – Tachycardia, normotensive or hypotensive • Neurological – Numbness, tingling, tetany, muscle weakness, hyperreflexia, confusion, convulsion • Cardiovascular – Dysrhythmias • Respiratory – Depressed skeletal muscles resulting in ineffective breathing

- ○ Laboratory Tests and Diagnostic Procedures
  - ■ To determine the type of imbalance, follow these steps:
    - □ Step 1: Look at pH.
      - ▸ If less than 7.35, diagnose as acidosis.
      - ▸ If greater than 7.45, diagnose as alkalosis.
    - □ Step 2: Look at $PaCO_2$ and HCO_3^- simultaneously.
      - ▸ Determine which is in the normal range.
      - ▸ Conclude that the other is the indicator of imbalance.
      - ▸ Diagnose less than 35 or greater than 45 $PaCO_2$ as respiratory in origin.
      - ▸ Diagnose less than 22 or greater than 26 HCO_3^- as metabolic in origin.
    - □ Step 3: Combine diagnoses of Steps 1 and 2 to name the type of imbalance.
    - □ Step 4: Evaluate the PaO_2 and the SaO_2.
      - ▸ If the results are below the normal range, the client is hypoxic.

- Step 5: Determine compensation as follows:
  - Uncompensated: The pH will be abnormal and either the HCO_3^- or the $PaCO_2$ will be abnormal.
  - Partially compensated: The pH, HCO_3^-, and $PaCO_2$ will be abnormal.
  - Fully compensated: The pH will be normal, but the $PaCO_2$ and HCO_3^- will both be abnormal. Looking back at the pH will provide a clue as to which system initiated the problem, respiratory or metabolic. If the pH is < 7.40, think "acidosis" and determine which system has the acidosis value. If the pH is > 7.40, think "alkalosis" and determine which system has the alkalosis value.

- The following are the five classic types of ABG results demonstrating balance and imbalance.

STEP 1	STEP 2		STEP 3
If	Determine which is in expected reference range		Combine names
pH	$PaCO_2$	HCO_3^-	Diagnosis
7.35 to 7.45	35 to 45	22 to 26	Homeostasis
Less than 7.35	Greater than 45	22 to 26	Respiratory acidosis
Less than 7.35	35 to 45	Less than 22	Metabolic acidosis
Greater than 7.45	Less than 35	22 to 26	Respiratory alkalosis
Greater than 7.45	35 to 45	Greater than 26	Metabolic alkalosis

Collaborative Care

- Nursing Care

RESPIRATORY ACIDOSIS – HYPOVENTILATION	RESPIRATORY ALKALOSIS – HYPERVENTILATION
- Maintain a patent airway. - Provide oxygen therapy. - Enhance gas exchange – Positioning, breathing techniques, ventilatory support, bronchodilators, and mucolytics	- Provide oxygen therapy. - Promote anxiety reduction techniques. - Promote rebreathing techniques.
METABOLIC ACIDOSIS	METABOLIC ALKALOSIS
- Varies with causes - For DKA, administer insulin. - For GI losses, administer antidiarrheals and provide rehydration. - For low serum bicarbonate administer sodium bicarbonate [1 mEq/kg]).	- Varies with causes - For GI losses, administer antiemetics, fluids, and electrolyte replacements. - For potassium depletion, discontinue causative agent.

- Interdisciplinary Care

  ○ Respiratory services can be consulted for oxygen therapy, breathing treatments, and ABGs.

- Care after Discharge

  ○ Client Education

    ▪ Encourage adherence to the prescribed diet and dialysis regimen for clients who have kidney dysfunction.

    ▪ Encourage clients to weigh themselves daily and notify the provider if there is a 1-to 2-lb gain in 24 hr, or a 3-lb gain in 1 week.

    ▪ Promote smoking cessation.

    ▪ Reinforce to clients to take medication as prescribed. Encourage adherence to the medication regimen for clients who have COPD.

- Client Outcomes

  ○ The client will be free from anxiety.

  ○ The client will maintain an adequate gas exchange.

  ○ The client will have ABG results within the expected reference range.

Complications

- Seizures, Coma, and Respiratory Arrest

  ○ These are potential complications of acid-base imbalances.

  ○ Nursing Actions

    ▪ Implement seizure precautions and perform management interventions if necessary.

    ▪ Assist with emergency care if necessary.

Ⓐ APPLICATION EXERCISES

Scenario: A nurse is caring for an older adult client who is scheduled to be discharged following an admission for pneumonia. The nurse is collecting data first thing in the morning and notes that the client's breathing is shallow and respiratory rate is 30/min. He tells the nurse that he is short of breath and his fingers are tingling. He says he has had anxiety attacks before and now is worried about caring for himself at home. After notifying the provider, the nurse obtains ABGs and the results are: pH 7.48, $PaCO_2$ 28 mm Hg, PaO_2 85 mm Hg, and HCo_3^- 22 mEq/L.

1. What, if any, acid-base imbalance is the client demonstrating?

2. Which findings support this conclusion?

3. The nurse should anticipate taking which of the following actions?

    A. Give oxygen by a rebreathing mask.
    B. Place the client in the supine position.
    C. Maintain NPO status.
    D. Reinforce instructions about home oxygen therapy.

---

4. A nurse is caring for a client who is now on the medical unit following a suicide attempt by overdose of aspirin. This client is at risk for which of the following acid-base imbalances?

    A. Respiratory acidosis
    B. Respiratory alkalosis
    C. Metabolic acidosis
    D. Metabolic alkalosis

UNIT 7: NURSING CARE OF CLIENTS WITH GASTROINTESTINAL DISORDERS

- Diagnostic and Therapeutic Procedures
- Upper Gastrointestinal Disorders
- Lower Gastrointestinal Disorders
- Gallbladder and Pancreas Disorders
- Liver Disorders

NCLEX® CONNECTIONS

When reviewing the chapters in this section, keep in mind the relevant sections of the NCLEX® outline, in particular:

CLIENT NEEDS: BASIC CARE AND COMFORT

Relevant topics/tasks include:
- Elimination
  - Monitor client bowel sounds.
- Non-Pharmacological Comfort Interventions
  - Provide non-pharmacological measures for pain relief.
- Nutrition and Oral Hydration
  - Provide feeding and/or care for client with enteral tubes.

CLIENT NEEDS: PHARMACOLOGICAL THERAPIES

Relevant topics/tasks include:
- Expected Actions/Outcomes
  - Apply knowledge of pathophysiology when addressing client pharmacological agents.
- Medication Administration
  - Identify client need for PRN medications.
- Pharmacological Pain Management
  - Monitor client non-verbal signs of pain/discomfort.

CLIENT NEEDS: REDUCTION OF RISK POTENTIAL

Relevant topics/tasks include:
- Diagnostic Tests
  - Perform diagnostic testing.
- Potential for Alterations in Body Systems
  - Monitor continuous or intermittent suction of nasogastric (NG) tube.
- Therapeutic Procedures
  - Insert nasogastric (NG) tube.

UNIT 7	NURSING CARE OF CLIENTS WITH GASTROINTESTINAL DISORDERS

Section: Diagnostic and Therapeutic Procedures

Chapter 40 Gastrointestinal Diagnostic Procedures

Overview

- Gastrointestinal diagnostic procedures involve the use of scopes and x-rays to visualize parts of the gastrointestinal (GI) system, as well as evaluate GI fluid.

- GI diagnostic procedures that nurses should be knowledgeable about

  - Liver function tests and other blood tests

  - Urine bilinogen

  - Fecal occult blood test (FOBT) and stool samples

  - Endoscopy

  - GI series

Liver Function Tests and Other Blood Tests

- Liver function tests – Aspartate aminotransferase (AST), alanine aminotransferase (ALT), alkaline phosphatase (ALP), bilirubin, and albumin

- Other blood tests that provide information on the functioning of the GI system include – Amylase, lipase, alpha-fetoprotein, and ammonia.

- Indications

  - Suspected liver, pancreatic, or biliary tract disorder

- Interpretation of Findings

BLOOD TEST	NORMAL VALUES	INTERPRETATION OF FINDINGS
Aspartate aminotransferase (AST)	5 to 40 units/L	Increases with hepatitis or cirrhosis
Alanine aminotransferase (ALT)	8 to 20 units/L 3 to 35 IU/L	Increases with hepatitis or cirrhosis
Alkaline phosphatase (ALP)	42 to 128 units/L 30 to 85 IU/L	Increases with liver damage and biliary obstruction
Amylase	56 to 90 IU/L	Increases with pancreatitis

BLOOD TEST	NORMAL VALUES	INTERPRETATION OF FINDINGS
Lipase	0 to 110 units/L	Increases with pancreatitis
Total bilirubin	0.3 to 1.0 mg/dL	Increases with altered liver functioning, bile duct obstruction, or other hepatobiliary disorder
Direct (conjugated) bilirubin	0.1 to 0.4 mg/dL	Increases with altered liver functioning, bile duct obstruction, or other hepatobiliary disorder
Indirect (unconjugated) bilirubin	0.1 to 0.4 mg/dL	Elevations indicate altered liver functioning, bile duct obstruction, or other hepatobiliary disorder
Albumin	3.5 to 5.0 g/dL	Decrease may indicate hepatic disease
Alpha-fetoprotein	< 40 mcg/L	Elevated in liver cancer
Ammonia	15 to 110 mg/dL	Elevated in liver disease

- Preprocedure

    o Explain to clients how blood will be drawn and what information this will provide.

- Postprocedure

    o Let clients know when and how results will be provided.

Urine Bilirubin

- Also known as urobilinogen, this is a urine test done to determine the presence of bilirubin the in urine.

- Indications

    o Suspected liver or biliary tract disorder

- Interpretation of Findings

    o A positive or elevated finding indicates possible liver disorder (cirrhosis, hepatitis) or biliary obstruction.

- Preprocedure

    o Nursing Actions

        ▪ The test may be performed by using a dipstick (urine bilirubin) or a 24-hr urine collection (urobilinogen).

    o Client Education

        ▪ Teach clients how to collect urine and provide proper collection container.

- Postprocedure
    - Nursing Actions
        - Let clients know when and how results will be provided.

Fecal Occult Blood Test and Stool Samples

- A stool sample is collected and tested for blood, ova and parasites (Giardia), and bacteria (*Clostridium difficile*).

- Indications
    - Client Presentation
        - GI bleeding
        - Unexplained diarrhea

- Interpretation of Findings
    - A positive finding for blood is indicative of GI bleeding (ulcer, colitis, cancer).
    - A positive finding for ova and parasites is indicative of a GI parasitic infection.
    - A positive finding for *Clostridium difficile* is indicative of this opportunistic infection, which usually becomes established secondary to use of broad-spectrum antibiotics.

- Preprocedure
    - Nursing Actions
        - Occult blood – Provide clients with cards impregnated with guaiac that can be mailed to provider or with a container for a specimen collection cup. If the cards are used, three samples are usually required.
        - Stool for ova and parasites and bacteria – Provide clients with a specimen collection cup.
    - Client Education
        - Occult blood – Instruct clients about proper collection of a stool sample using a card or sample collection cup. Clients may also need to be instructed about dietary and medication restrictions to follow prior to obtaining samples (red meat, anticoagulants).
        - Stool for ova and parasites and bacteria – Instruct clients about proper collection technique (time frame for submission to laboratory, need for refrigeration).

- Postprocedure
    - Nursing Actions
        - Let the client know when and how the results will be provided.

Endoscopy

- Endoscopic procedures allow direct visualization of body cavities, tissues, and organs through the use of a flexible, lighted tube (endoscope). They are performed for diagnostic and therapeutic purposes.

 View Media Supplement: Endoscope (Image)

  - Endoscopic procedures can be performed in outpatient diagnostic centers, provider offices, and acute-care settings. Endoscopic procedures are primarily performed for diagnostic purposes. However, during an endoscopic procedure, the provider can perform biopsies, remove abnormal tissue, and perform minor surgery, such as cauterizing a bleeding ulcer.

  - During some endoscopic procedures a contrast medium is injected to allow visualization of structures beyond the capabilities of the scope.

  - GI scope procedures

    - Colonoscopy – Allows visualization of the anus, rectum, and colon

    - Esophagogastroduodenoscopy (EGD) – Allows visualization of the oropharynx, esophagus, stomach, and duodenum

    - Endoscopic retrograde cholangiopancreatography (ECRP) – Allows visualization of the liver, gallbladder, bile ducts, and pancreas

    - Sigmoidoscopy – Allows visualization of the anus, rectum, and sigmoid colon

- Indications

  - Potential Diagnoses

    - GI bleeding, ulcerations or inflammation, polyps, malignant tumors

  - Client Presentation

    - Anemia (secondary to bleeding)

    - Abdominal discomfort

    - Abdominal distention or mass

- Interpretation of Findings

  - Findings may indicate a need for medication or surgical removal of a lesion.

- General endoscopic procedures

  - Preprocedure

    - Nursing Actions

      □ Evaluate the client's understanding of the procedure.

      □ Verify that a consent form has been signed for the specific procedure.

      □ Check vital signs and verify the client's allergies.

□ Evaluate baseline laboratory tests and report unexpected or abnormal findings to the provider. Laboratory tests may include CBC, electrolyte panel, BUN, creatinine, PT, aPTT, and liver function studies. A chest x-ray and ECG may also be ordered. ABGs may be measured before and after the procedure to assess oxygenation.

□ Evaluate if the client's medical history increases the risk for complications (age, current health status, cognitive status, support system, recent food or fluid intake, medications).

▸ Ensure that clients followed proper bowel preparation (laxatives, enemas).

▸ Ensure that clients are NPO for at least 6 hr prior to most endoscopic examinations.

- Client Education

□ Provide clients with instructions regarding medication, bowel prep, and food restrictions.

○ Postprocedure

- Nursing Actions

□ Monitor the client's vital signs.

□ Check clients for complications.

- Client Education

□ If a biopsy was done during the procedure, food restrictions may be prescribed.

- Specific Endoscopic Procedures

ANESTHESIA	POSITIONING	PREPARATION	POSTPROCEDURE
Colonoscopy – Involves the use of a flexible fiberoptic colonoscope to visualize the colon. After entering through the anus, the rectum, sigmoid, descending, transverse, and ascending colon can be visualized.			
Moderate sedation – midazolam (Versed) usually given with an opiate analgesic	Left side with knees to chest	• Bowel prep ○ May include laxatives, such as bisacodyl (Dulcolax®) and polyethylene glycol (GoLYTELY®) ○ Clear liquid diet; NPO after midnight • Instruct clients to avoid medications per the provider's order.	• Monitor for rectal bleeding. • Resume normal diet if ordered. • Encourage plenty of fluids. • Monitor vital signs and respiratory status. • Instruct clients that there may be increased flatulence due to air instillation during procedure.

ANESTHESIA	POSITIONING	PREPARATION	POSTPROCEDURE
EGD – Involves insertion of an endoscope through the client's mouth and esophagus, stomach, and duodenum. Allows visualization of these structures.			
Moderate sedation – topical anesthetic	Left side-lying	• NPO 6 to 8 hr; remove dentures prior to procedure.	• Monitor vital signs and respiratory status. • Notify provider of bleeding, abdominal or chest pain, and any evidence of infection. • Withhold fluids until return of gag reflex.
ERCP – Involves insertion of an endoscope through the client's mouth and into the biliary tree via the duodenum. Allows visualization of the biliary ducts and gall bladder.			
Conscious sedation – topical anesthetic	Initially semi-prone with repositioning throughout procedure	• NPO 6 to 8 hr; remove dentures prior to procedure • Explain procedure and need to change positions during procedure.	• Monitor vital signs and respiratory status. • Notify provider of bleeding, abdominal or chest pain, and any evidence of infection. • Withhold fluids until the client's gag reflex returns.
Sigmoidoscopy – Similar to colonoscopy, but scope is shorter, thus allowing visualization of only the anus, rectum, and sigmoid colon.			
None required	On left side	• Bowel prep, which may include laxatives such as, bisacodyl (Dulcolax®) and polyethylene glycol (GoLYTELY®) • Clear liquid diet • NPO after midnight • Instruct clients to avoid medications per the provider's prescription.	• Monitor for rectal bleeding. • Resume normal diet if prescribed. • Encourage plenty of fluids. • Monitor vital signs and respiratory status. • Instruct clients that there may be increased flatulence due to air instillation during procedure.

- Complications

  ○ Oversedation

    ▪ Any endoscopic procedure using moderate sedation places clients at risk for oversedation (difficulty arousing clients, poor respiratory effort, evidence of hypoxemia, tachycardia, and elevated or low blood pressure).

- Nursing Actions
  - Monitor clients for oversedation.
  - Contact charge nurse immediately.
- Client Education
  - Encourage clients to avoid activities requiring alertness.

○ Hemorrhage

  - Signs and symptoms of hemorrhage include bleeding from the site, cool clammy skin, hypotension, tachycardia, dizziness, and tachypnea.
  - Nursing Actions
    - Monitor the client's vital signs after the procedure.
    - Monitor for hemorrhage.
    - Notify the provider immediately if any evidence of bleeding.
  - Client Education
    - Instruct clients to report fever, pain, and bleeding.

○ Aspiration

  - Signs and symptoms of aspiration include dyspnea, tachypnea, adventitious breath sounds, tachycardia, and fever.
  - Nursing Actions
    - Clients should remain NPO until the gag reflex returns.
    - Ensure that clients are awake and alert prior offering any food or fluid.
    - Encourage clients to deep breathe and cough to keep the airway open.
    - The provider should be notified if these symptoms occur.
  - Client Education
    - Have clients report any respiratory congestion or compromise.

Gastrointestinal Series

- GI studies are radiographic studies, done with or without contrast, that help define anatomic or functional abnormalities.

  ○ GI studies provide for imaging of the esophagus, stomach and entire intestinal tract.

  ○ Upper GI imaging is done by having clients drink a radiopaque liquid (barium).

  ○ A barium enema is done by instilling a radiopaque liquid into the client's rectum and colon.

- Indications

  o Potential Diagnoses

    - Gastric ulcers, peristaltic disorders, tumors, varices, and intestinal enlargements or constrictions

  o Client Presentation

    - The client may present with abdominal pain, altered elimination habits (constipation, diarrhea), or GI bleeding.

- Interpretation of Findings

  o Abnormal findings are those that indicate abnormal bowel shape and size, increased motility, or obstruction.

- Preprocedure

  o Nursing Actions

    - Inform clients about medications, food and fluid restrictions (clear liquid and/ or low residue diet, NPO after midnight), and avoiding smoking or chewing gum (increases peristalsis).

    - Inform clients of bowel preparation (laxatives, enemas) so image will not be distorted by feces.

    - Barium enema studies must be scheduled prior to upper GI studies.

    - Check for contraindications to bowel preparation (possible bowel perforation or obstruction, inflammatory disease).

  o Client Education

    - Tell clients to restrict food and fluids for bowel preparation.

    - Inform clients if the small intestine is to be visualized, additional radiographs will be done over the next 24 hr.

- Postprocedure

  o Nursing Actions

    - Monitor the client's elimination of contrast material and administer a laxative if prescribed.

    - Encourage intake of fluids to promote elimination of contrast material.

  o Client Education

    - Instruct clients to monitor elimination of contrast material and to report retention of contrast material (constipation) or diarrhea accompanied by weakness.

    - Discuss the possible need for an over-the-counter medication to prevent constipation resulting from the barium.

APPLICATION EXERCISES

1. A nurse is caring for a client who has been diagnosed with acute pancreatitis. Which of the following laboratory values should subsequently be monitored? (Select all that apply.)

    _____ Total bilirubin

    _____ Amylase

    _____ Aspartate aminotransferase (AST)

    _____ Lipase

    _____ Alanine aminotransferase (ALT)

2. A client is scheduled for a colonoscopy and is given a prescription for polyethylene glycol (GoLYTELY®) for a bowel prep. Which of the following should a nurse reinforce to the client?

    A. Medication taken with this prep will not be absorbed.

    B. Eat a normal diet until the bowel prep has begun.

    C. This solution will usually not begin acting until morning.

    D. Consume at least half of this solution to get the best results.

3. A client has just returned to the unit following an esophagogastroduodenoscopy (EGD). The client's prescriptions include resuming all ADLs and a regular diet and ambulation as desired. Which of the following is the priority nursing action for the nurse to perform at this time?

    A. Determine the presence of a gag reflex prior to giving food or fluids.

    B. Assist the client to the restroom for the first voiding.

    C. Take vital signs and record.

    D. Provide the client with the nursing call light.

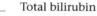 **APPLICATION EXERCISES ANSWER KEY**

1. A nurse is caring for a client who has been diagnosed with acute pancreatitis. Which of the following laboratory values should subsequently be monitored? (Select all that apply.)

    _____ Total bilirubin

    __X__ **Amylase**

    _____ Aspartate aminotransferase (AST)

    __X__ **Lipase**

    _____ Alanine aminotransferase (ALT)

    Amylase and lipase increase in relation to inflammation of the pancreas. Total bilirubin elevates in relation to altered liver functioning, bile duct obstruction, or other hepatobiliary disorders. The AST and ALT elevate in response to hepatitis or cirrhosis.

     NCLEX® Connection: Reduction of Risk Potential, Potential for Complications of Diagnostic Tests/Treatments/Procedures

2. A client is scheduled for a colonoscopy and is given a prescription for polyethylene glycol (GoLYTELY®) for a bowel prep. Which of the following should a nurse reinforce to the client?

    A. Medication taken with this prep will not be absorbed.

    B. Eat a normal diet until the bowel prep has begun.

    C. This solution will usually not begin acting until morning.

    D. Consume at least half of this solution to get the best results.

    Gastrointestinal motility will be increased with the effects of the polyethylene glycol, which will greatly reduce the likelihood of medication absorption. The client should be on a clear liquid diet 12 to 24 hr prior to the colonoscopy. The client should consume the full prescribed amount of polyethylene glycol and its effects are immediate.

    NCLEX® Connection: Reduction of Risk Potential, Potential for Complications of Diagnostic Tests/Treatments/Procedures

3. A client has just returned to the unit following an esophagogastroduodenoscopy (EGD). The client's prescriptions include resuming all ADLs and a regular diet and ambulation as desired. Which of the following is the priority nursing action for the nurse to perform at this time?

A. Determine the presence of a gag reflex prior to giving food or fluids.

B. Assist the client to the restroom for the first voiding.

C. Take vital signs and record.

D. Provide the client with the nursing call light.

Following the ABC priority framework, the priority intervention is airway maintenance. The client's gag reflex should be determined prior to giving any fluids or food. The other interventions are important for the nurse to perform, but are not the highest priority.

 NCLEX® Connection: Reduction of Risk Potential, Potential for Complications of Diagnostic Tests/Treatments/Procedures

UNIT 7	NURSING CARE OF CLIENTS WITH GASTROINTESTINAL DISORDERS
Section:	Diagnostic and Therapeutic Procedures
Chapter 41	Gastrointestinal Therapeutic Procedures

Overview

- Clients undergo gastrointestinal (GI) therapeutic procedures for reasons including treatment of obesity, treatment of gastrointestinal obstructions and other disorders, and the maintenance of nutritional intake.

- GI therapeutic procedures

  - Bariatric surgeries

  - Nasogastric decompression

  - Ostomies

  - Enteral feedings

  - Total parenteral nutrition (TPN)

  - Paracentesis

Bariatric Surgeries

- Bariatric surgeries are done as a treatment for morbid obesity when other weight control methods have failed.

  - Bariatric surgeries reduce the functional size of the stomach.

  - There are several types of procedures that can be done.

    - Stapling a portion of the stomach shut to decrease the functional size of it.

    - Using a band that constricts the functional size of the stomach – can be done laparoscopically.

    - Intestinal bypass that will decrease the length of the functional small intestine to decrease absorption of nutrients.

  - Some procedures combine more than one of these approaches.

  - Many clients will undergo body contouring to remove excess skin after weight is lost.

 View Media Supplement: (Images)
- Stomach Stapling   • Gastric Band   • Intestinal Bypass (Images)

- Indications
  - Diagnoses
    - Long history of morbid obesity
  - Client Presentation
    - BMI > 40
    - BMI > 35 with comorbidities
- Client Outcome
  - The client will experience resolution of obesity-related problems.
- Preprocedure
  - Nursing Actions
    - Identify the client's psychosocial issues related to weight loss.
    - Ensure that clients understand dietary and lifestyle changes that will be required.
    - Arrange for a bariatric bed to be available and mechanical lifting devices to prevent client/staff injury.
- Postprocedure
  - Nursing Actions
    - Provide postoperative care to prevent postoperative complications.
    - Monitor for the development of postoperative complications that are at increased risk due to obesity (atelectasis, thromboemboli, incisional hernia, peritonitis).
    - Apply an abdominal binder to prevent dehiscence.
    - Ambulate clients as soon as possible after surgery. Continue to encourage position changes with use of an over-bed trapeze.
    - Discontinue indwelling urinary catheter as soon as possible to prevent urinary tract infection.
    - Maintain semi-Fowler's position.
    - Facilitate night breathing by using bi-level or continuous positive airway pressure.
    - Apply oxygen via nasal cannula to maintain adequate oxygen saturation.
    - Monitor skin folds for skin breakdown. Prevent breakdown by using absorbent padding between skin folds.
    - Use sequential compression stockings to prevent thrombosis. Administer anticoagulant therapy as prescribed.
    - Monitor abdominal girth daily.
    - Provide six small meals a day when clients can resume intake. Observe for signs of dumping syndrome (cramps, diarrhea, tachycardia, dizziness, and fatigue). The client's first feeding may only consist of 30 mL of liquid.

- ○ Client Education
  - Instruct clients to limit intake of liquids or pureed foods for the first 6 weeks.
  - Instruct clients that meal size should not exceed 1 cup.
  - Recommend that clients walk daily for at least 30 min.
  - Instruct clients to take vitamin and mineral supplements.
- Complications
  - ○ Warn clients that excessive thirst or concentrated urine may be a sign of dehydration and to notify the surgeon.
  - ○ Malabsorption/malnutrition
    - Since bariatric surgeries reduce the size of the stomach or length of the intestinal track, fewer nutrients will be able to be ingested and absorbed.
    - Nursing Actions
      - □ Monitor the client's tolerance of increasing amounts of food and fluids.
      - □ Request a referral for dietary management.
    - Client Education
      - □ Tell clients to eat two servings of protein a day.
      - □ Tell clients to eat only nutrition-dense foods. Avoid empty calories, such as colas and fruity juice drinks.
  - ○ Anastomotic leaks
    - Nursing Actions
      - □ Monitor clients for increasing pain in the back, shoulder or abdomen, agitation, tachycardia and very scant urine output.
      - □ Notify the surgeon immediately.

Nasogastric Decompression

- Nasogastric decompression is a procedure done for clients who have an intestinal obstruction. To perform decompression, insert an NG tube with suction until relief of the obstruction.
- Indications
  - ○ Diagnoses
    - Any disorder that causes a mechanical (tumors, adhesions, fecal impaction) or functional (paralytic ileus) intestinal obstruction

- o Client Presentation
  - Vomiting (begins with stomach contents and continues until fecal material is also being regurgitated)
  - Bowel sounds may be high pitched or hyperactive (mechanical) or absent (paralytic ileus)
  - Intermittent, colicky abdominal pain and distention; hiccups
- Client Outcome
  - o The client will resume normal gastrointestinal function.
- Preprocedure
  - o Nursing Actions
    - Gather necessary equipment and supplies.
  - o Client Education
    - Instruct clients on the purpose of the NG tube and the client's role in its placement.
- Postprocedure
  - o Nursing Actions
    - Check and maintain proper functioning of the tube and suction equipment.
    - Monitor clients for fluid and electrolyte imbalance (metabolic acidosis – low obstruction; alkalosis – high obstruction).
    - Monitor the client's bowel sounds and abdominal girth; return of flatus.
  - o Client Education
    - Instruct clients to maintain NPO status.
- Complications
  - o Strangulated obstruction/intestinal infarction
    - Occurs when a portion of the intestine is twisted or the blood supply is compromised, which may cause ischemia
      - □ Peritonitis and septicemia can result.
      - □ Gangrene of the affected bowel may necessitate removal of a section of the bowel.
    - Nursing Actions
      - □ Monitor clients for an increase in abdominal pain, abdominal rigidity, fever, tachycardia, and hypotension.

Ostomies

- An ostomy is a surgical opening from the inside of the body to the outside. Ostomies can be permanent or temporary and are located in various parts of the body.

  ○ A stoma is an artificial opening from the inside of the body to the outside created during the ostomy surgery.

  ○ The main types of ostomies performed in the abdominal area

    ▪ Ileostomy – a surgical opening into the ileum to drain stool

    ▪ Colostomy – a surgical opening into the large intestine to drain stool

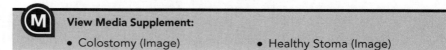

View Media Supplement:
- Colostomy (Image)   • Healthy Stoma (Image)

- Indications

  ○ Diagnoses

    ▪ Crohn's disease requires removal of the entire colon to create an ileostomy.

    ▪ Colon cancer or diverticular disease requires removal of a portion of the bowel to create an colostomy.

- Client Outcomes

  ○ The client will demonstrate ostomy care.

	ILEOSTOMY	TRANSVERSE COLOSTOMY	SIGMOID COLOSTOMY
Normal postoperative output	• Less than 1,000 mL/day • May be bile-colored and liquid	• Small semi-liquid with some mucus 2 to 3 days after surgery • Blood may be present in the first few days after surgery	• Small to moderate amount of mucus with semi-formed stool 4 to 5 days after surgery
Postoperative changes in output	• After several days to weeks, the output will decrease to approximately 500 to 1,000 mL/day • Becomes more paste-like as the small intestine assumes the absorptive function of the large intestine	• After several days to weeks, output will become more stool-like, semi-formed, or formed	• After several days to weeks, output will resemble semi-formed stool
Pattern of output	• Continuous output	• Resumes a pattern similar to the preoperative pattern	• Resumes a pattern similar to the preoperative pattern

- Preprocedure

  o Nursing Actions

    ▪ Determine the client's readiness for the procedure. Determine visual acuity, manual dexterity, cognitive status, cultural influences, and support systems.

  o Client Education

    ▪ Instruct clients and a support person regarding care and management of an ostomy before surgery.

- Postprocedure

  o Nursing Actions

    ▪ Check the type and fit of the ostomy appliance. Monitor for leakage (risk to skin integrity). Base the fit of the ostomy appliance on:

      ▫ The type of ostomy.

      ▫ Location of the ostomy.

      ▫ Visual acuity and manual dexterity of clients.

    ▪ Check peristomal skin integrity and the appearance of the stoma. The stoma should appear pink and moist.

    ▪ Use warm water and soap (per facility policy) to clean the peristomal skin and stoma. Use a towel to pat dry. Avoid soaps with moisturizers or deodorants.

    ▪ Evaluate output from the stoma. The higher up an ostomy is placed in the small intestine, the more liquid and acidic the output will be from the ostomy.

    ▪ Monitor for fluid and electrolyte imbalances, particularly with a new ileostomy.

  o Client Education

    ▫ Instruct clients that foods that can cause odor include fish, eggs, asparagus, garlic, beans, and dark green leafy vegetables.

    ▫ Instruct clients that foods that can cause gas include dark green leafy vegetables, beer, carbonated beverages, dairy products, and corn. Yogurt can be ingested to help decrease gas.

    ▫ Instruct clients that after an ostomy is placed involving the small intestine, they should avoid high-fiber foods for the first 2 months, chew food well, and drink plenty of fluids. Then, they will need to evaluate for any evidence of blockage when slowly adding high-fiber foods.

    ▫ Instruct clients to keep the appliance clean and empty it frequently to decrease odor.

    ▫ Instruct clients to:

      ‣ Empty the ostomy pouch when it's ⅓ to ½ full.

      ‣ Empty the contents prior to removing the pouch to prevent spilling stool.

      ‣ Cut an opening in the wafer of a new appliance that is no more than ⅛ to ¼ inches in diameter.

- ▸ Use a pouch deodorizer or breath mint in the pouch to minimize odor.
- ▸ Avoid aspirin due to ulceration of the stoma.
- Provide opportunities for clients to discuss feelings about the ostomy and concerns about its impact on the client's life. Encourage clients to look at and touch the stoma.
- Recommend that clients participate in a local ostomy support group.
- Complications
  - Stomal Ischemia/necrosis
    - The stomal appearance should normally be pink or red and moist.
      - □ Signs of stomal ischemia are pale pink or bluish/purple in color and dry in appearance.
      - □ If the stoma appears black or purple in color, this indicates a serious impairment of blood flow and requires immediate intervention.
    - Nursing Actions
      - □ Obtain the client's vital signs, pulse oximetry, and current laboratory results. Notify the provider or surgeon of abnormal findings.
    - Client Education
      - □ Teach clients to watch for signs of stomal ischemia/necrosis following discharge.
  - Intestinal obstruction
    - An obstruction can occur for a variety of reasons.
    - Nursing Actions
      - □ Monitor and record output from the stoma.
      - □ Monitor clients for symptoms of obstruction including abdominal pain, hypoactive or absent bowel sounds, distention, nausea, and vomiting. Notify the surgeon of abnormal findings.
    - Client Education
      - □ Reinforce for clients to watch for signs of an intestinal obstruction following discharge.

Enteral Feedings

- Enteral feedings are instituted when a client can no longer take adequate nutrition orally.
- Indications
  - Diagnoses
    - Clients who are intubated
    - Pathologies that cause difficulty swallowing and/or increase risk of aspiration (stroke, advanced Parkinson's disease, and multiple sclerosis)
    - Clients who cannot maintain adequate oral nutritional intake and need supplementation

- ○ Client Presentation

  - Malnutrition

  - Aspiration pneumonia

- Client Outcomes

  - ○ The client will maintain adequate caloric intake to meet nutritional needs and maintain or increase weight.

- Complications

  - ○ Diarrhea

    - Diarrhea occurs secondary to concentration of feeding or its constituents.

    - Nursing Actions

      - □ Slow rate of feeding and notify the provider.

      - □ Confer with the dietitian.

      - □ Provide skin care and protection.

  - ○ Aspiration pneumonia

    - Pneumonia can occur secondary to aspiration of feeding.

    - Nursing Actions

      - □ Stop the feeding.

      - □ Turn clients to their side and suction the airway. Provide oxygen if indicated.

      - □ Monitor the client's vital signs for an elevated temperature.

      - □ Auscultate breath sounds for increased congestion.

      - □ Notify the provider and obtain a chest x-ray if prescribed.

Total Parenteral Nutrition

- Total parenteral nutrition (TPN) is a hypertonic IV solution that provides complete nutrition to a client who does not have a functioning GI tract or needs additional nutritional supplementation (burns). The purpose of TPN administration is to prevent or correct nutritional deficiencies and minimize the adverse effects of malnourishment.

  - ○ TPN administration is usually through a central line, such as a nontunneled triple lumen catheter or a single- or double-lumen peripherally inserted central line (PICC).

  - ○ TPN contains complete nutrition, including calories (through a high concentration – 20% to 50% – of dextrose), lipids/essential fatty acids, protein, electrolytes, vitamins, and trace elements.

  - ○ Partial parenteral nutrition or peripheral parenteral nutrition (PPN) is less hypertonic and intended for short-term use in a large peripheral vein. Usual dextrose concentration is 10% or less. Risks include phlebitis.

- Indications
  - Diagnoses
    - Potential indications for TPN include any condition that:
      - Affects the ability to absorb nutrition.
      - Has a prolonged recovery.
      - Creates a hypermetabolic state.
      - Creates a chronic malnutrition.
    - Specific conditions
      - Chronic pancreatitis
      - Diffuse peritonitis
      - Short bowel syndrome
      - Gastric paresis from diabetes mellitus
      - Severe burns

Paracentesis

- Therapeutically, a paracentesis is performed by inserting a needle or trocar through the abdominal wall into the peritoneal cavity and withdrawing ascitic fluid to relieve abdominal pressure from ascites buildup.
  - Settings for a paracentesis include the provider's office, an outpatient center, or in an acute care setting at the bedside.
- Indications
  - Diagnoses
    - Ascites is an abnormal accumulation of protein-rich fluid in the abdominal cavity most often caused by cirrhosis of the liver.
      - Respiratory distress is the determining factor in the use of a paracentesis to treat ascites. It's also monitored to evaluate the effectiveness of the treatment.
  - Client Presentation
    - Compromised lung expansion
- Client Outcomes
  - The client will be free of respiratory distress as evidenced by regular, even respirations, and the absence of shortness of breath.
  - The client will be free of abdominal discomfort.

- Preprocedure
    - Nursing Actions
        - Determine the client's readiness for the procedure.
        - Have clients void or insert a temporary indwelling urinary catheter.
        - Take the client's baseline vital signs, record weight, and measure abdominal girth.
        - Gather equipment for the procedure.
        - Verify that clients have signed the informed consent forms.
        - Position clients as tolerated. Clients with ascites are typically more comfortable sitting up.
    - Client Education
        - Explain the procedure and its purpose to clients.
        - Instruct clients that they will receive local anesthetics at the needle-insertion site.
        - Explain that there may be pressure or pain with needle insertion.
- Intraprocedure
    - Nursing Actions
        - Monitor the client's vital signs.
        - Adhere to standard precautions.
        - Label laboratory specimens and send to the laboratory.
        - Between 4 and 6 L of fluid is slowly drained from the abdomen by gravity.
- Postprocedure
    - Nursing Actions
        - Maintain pressure at the insertion site for several minutes. Apply a dressing to the site.
        - If the needle-insertion site continues to leak after holding pressure for several minutes, apply dry sterile gauze dressings and change as often as necessary.
        - Take the client's vital signs, record weight, and measure abdominal girth. Document and compare to preprocedure measurements.
        - Continue to monitor the client's vital signs and insertion site per facility protocol.
        - Monitor the client's temperature every 4 hr for a minimum of 48 hr.
        - Check I&O every 4 hr.
        - Assist the client into a position of comfort.
        - Document color, odor, consistency, and amount of fluid removed; location of needle insertion; any evidence of leakage at the insertion site; signs and symptoms of hypovolemia; and changes in mental status.

UNIT 7	NURSING CARE OF CLIENTS WITH GASTROINTESTINAL DISORDERS
Section:	Upper Gastrointestinal Disorders
Chapter 42	Esophageal Disorders

 Overview

- The esophagus is a tube that consists of smooth muscle and leads from the throat to the stomach. Esophageal disorders can affect any part of the esophagus.

View Media Supplement: Esophageal Sphincters (Image)

- There are two sphincters (upper esophageal – UES; lower esophageal – LES) that prevent the reflux of food and fluids back into the mouth or esophagus.

- Contractions of the esophagus propel food and fluids toward the stomach, while the relaxation of the gastroesophageal sphincter allows them to pass into the stomach.

- Esophageal disorders that nurses should be knowledgeable about

  ○ Gastroesophageal Reflux Disease (GERD)

  ○ Esophageal Varices

  ○ Esophageal Cancer

GERD

Overview

- Gastroesophageal reflux disease, or GERD, is a common condition characterized by gastric content and enzyme leakage into the esophagus. These corrosive fluids irritate the esophageal tissue and limit its ability to clear them from the esophagus.

- The primary treatment of GERD is diet and lifestyle changes, advancing into medication use (antacids, H_2 receptor antagonists, proton pump inhibitors), and surgery.

- Untreated GERD leads to inflammation, breakdown, and long-term complications including adenocarcinoma of the esophagus.

Data Collection

- Risk Factors

  - Obesity
  - Older age
  - Sleep apnea
  - NG tube
  - Contributing factors

    - Diet – Excessive ingestion of foods that relax the LES include: fatty and fried foods, chocolate, caffeinated beverages (coffee, peppermint, spicy foods, tomatoes, citrus fruits, alcohol)
    - Distended abdomen from overeating or delayed emptying
    - Increased abdominal pressure resulting from obesity, pregnancy, bending at the waist, ascites or tight clothing at the waist
    - Drugs that relax the LES (theophylline, nitrates, calcium channel blockers, anticholinergics, and diazepam [Valium])
    - Drugs (NSAIDs), or events (stress) that increase gastric acid
    - Debilitation or age-related conditions resulting in weakened LES tone
    - Hiatal hernia (LES displacement into the thorax with delayed esophageal clearance)
    - Lying flat

- Subjective Data

  - Frequent and prolonged substernal heartburn (dyspepsia) and regurgitation (acid reflux) in relationship to eating activities or position
  - Classic symptoms – Dyspepsia after eating an offending food or fluid, and regurgitation
  - Other symptoms – Throat irritation (chronic cough, laryngitis), hypersalivation, eructation, flatulence, bitter taste in mouth, or atypical chest pain from esophageal spasm – chronic GERD can lead to dysphagia
  - GERD may mimic a heart attack due to the substernal pain that can radiate to the jaw and back.

- Objective Data

  - Physical Assessment Findings

    - Tooth erosion
    - Hoarseness

- ○ Diagnostic Procedures
  - ■ Esophagogastroduodenoscopy (EGD) allows visualization of the esophagus, revealing esophagitis or Barrett's epithelium (premalignant cells).
    - □ Nursing Actions – Verify gag response has returned prior to providing oral fluids or food following the procedure.
  - ■ Twenty-four hour ambulatory esophageal pH monitoring is done using a small catheter that is placed through the client's nose and into the distal esophagus. Here, pH readings are taken in relation to food, position, and activity.
    - □ Nursing Actions
      - ▸ Instruct clients to keep a diary of symptoms related to food, position, and activity throughout the day.
  - ■ Esophageal manometry records lower esophageal sphincter pressure.
  - ■ A barium swallow identifies a hiatal hernia, which would contribute to or cause GERD.

Collaborative Care

- • Medications
  - ○ Antacids
    - ■ Antacids (aluminum hydroxide [Mylanta])) neutralize excess acid.
    - ■ Nursing Considerations
      - □ Ensure aluminum is not contraindicated with other prescribed medications (levothyroxine).
    - ■ Client Education
      - □ Instruct clients to take antacids when acid secretion is the highest (1 to 3 hr after eating and at bedtime), and to separate from other medications by at least 1 hr.
  - ○ Histamine$_2$ Receptor Antagonists
    - ■ Histamine$_2$ receptor antagonists (ranitidine [Zantac], famotidine [Pepcid], nizatidine [Axid]) reduce the secretion of acid. The onset is longer than antacids, but the effect has a longer duration.
    - ■ Nursing Considerations
      - □ Use cautiously in clients who are at a high risk for pneumonia (clients with COPD).
    - ■ Client Education
      - □ Encourage adherence to the medication regimen.

- Proton Pump Inhibitors (PPIs)

  - PPIs (pantoprazole [Protonix], omeprazole [Prilosec], esomeprazole [Nexium], and lansoprazole [Prevacid]) reduce gastric acid by inhibiting the cellular pump necessary for secretion.

  - Nursing Considerations

    - Use cautiously in clients at a high risk for pneumonia (clients with COPD).

  - Client Education

    - Suggest clients sprinkle the contents of the sustained-release capsule over food if they are experiencing difficulty swallowing.

- Prokinetics

  - Prokinetic medications (metoclopramide hydrochloride [Reglan]) increase the motility of the esophagus and stomach.

  - Nursing Considerations

    - Monitor clients for extrapyramidal side effects.

  - Client Education

    - Instruct clients to report abnormal, involuntary movement.

- Therapeutic Procedures

  - Stretta Procedure

    - The Stretta procedure uses radiofrequency energy, applied by an endoscope, to the LES muscle. This causes the tissue to contract and tighten.

- Surgical Interventions

  - Fundoplication

    - This surgical option may be indicated for clients who fail to respond to other treatments. The fundus of the stomach is wrapped around and behind the esophagus through a laparoscope to create a physical barrier.

  - Client Education

    - Give clients instructions regarding diet

      - Avoid offending foods.

      - Avoid large meals.

      - Remain upright after eating.

      - Avoid eating before bed.

    - Give clients instructions regarding lifestyle.

      - Avoid tight-fitting clothing around the mid section.

      - Lose weight, if applicable.

- □ Elevate the head of the bed 15.2 to 20.3 cm (6 to 8 in) with blocks. The use of pillows is not recommended, as this rounds the back bringing the stomach contents up closer to the chest.

- □ Sleep on the right side.

- Care After Discharge

  - ○ Client Education

    - ■ Recommend that clients maintain a weight below a BMI of 30.

    - ■ Encourage clients to stop smoking.

    - ■ Recommend that clients drink alcohol in moderation.

- Client Outcomes

  - ○ The client will report less epigastric pain.

  - ○ The client will not experience gastric reflux during sleeping hours.

Complications

- Aspiration of gastric secretion

  - ○ Causes

    - ■ Reflux of gastric fluids into the esophagus can be aspirated into the trachea.

    - ■ Risks associated with aspiration include:

      - □ Asthma exacerbations from inhaled aerosolized acid.

      - □ Frequent upper respiratory, sinus, or ear infections.

      - □ Aspiration pneumonia.

      - □ Barrett's epithelium (premalignant) and esophageal adenocarcinoma.

  - ○ Nursing Actions

    - ■ Determine the cause of GERD with clients and review lifestyle changes that can decrease gastric reflux.

ESOPHAGEAL VARICES

Overview

- Esophageal varices are swollen, fragile blood vessels in the esophagus. As a result of liver damage, blood flow through the liver is restricted and is diverted to other vessels (the vessels of the lower esophagus). The increased blood flow (portal hypertension) causes swelling, and varices result.

View Media Supplement: Varices (Image)

- When esophageal varices hemorrhage, it is often a medical emergency associated with a high mortality rate.

Data Collection

- Risk Factors

  o Portal hypertension is the primary risk factor for the development of esophageal varices. Portal hypertension (elevated blood pressure in veins that carry blood from the intestines to the liver) is caused by impaired circulation of blood through the liver. Collateral circulation is subsequently developed, thus creating varices in the upper stomach and esophagus. Varices are fragile and can bleed very easily.

  o Alcoholic cirrhosis

  o Viral hepatitis

  o Factors that precipitate bleeding are the Valsalva maneuver, lifting heavy objects, coughing, sneezing, and alcohol.

- Subjective Data

  o The client may experience no symptoms until the varices begin to bleed.

- Objective Data

  o Physical Assessment Findings (Bleeding Esophageal Varices)

    ▪ Hematemesis

    ▪ Melena

    ▪ Hypotension

    ▪ Tachycardia

  o Laboratory Tests

    ▪ Liver function tests indicate a liver disorder.

    ▪ Hgb and Hct tests can indicate anemia secondary to occult bleeding or overt bleeding.

  o Diagnostic Procedures

    ▪ Endoscopy

      □ Endoscopic evaluation is the first step in treatment of esophageal varices. Therapeutic interventions can be performed during the endoscopy.

Collaborative Care

- Nursing Care

  o Assist with the care of clients receiving IV fluid replacement.

  o Monitor vital signs.

- Medications
  - Nonselective beta-blockers
    - Nonselective beta-blockers (propranolol [Inderal]) are prescribed to decrease heart rate and consequently reduce hepatic venous pressure.
    - Recommended for prophylactic use and not emergency treatment for hemorrhage.
  - Vasoconstrictors
    - Vasoconstrictors (vasopressin [Desmopressin], octreotide [Sandostatin]), are prescribed to decrease portal inflow.
    - Nursing Considerations
      - Vasopressin is contraindicated for clients with coronary artery disease due to resultant coronary constriction.

- Interdisciplinary Care
  - Alcohol recovery program if varices due to alcohol abuse

- Therapeutic Procedures
  - Endoscopic injection sclerotherapy or variceal band ligation
    - Ligating bands can be placed, and/or injection sclerotherapy can be performed through an endoscopic procedure. Used only for active bleeding and not prophylactically.
  - Transjugular Intrahepatic Portal-Systemic Shunt (TIPS)
    - While clients are under sedation or general anesthesia, a catheter is passed into the liver via the jugular vein in the neck. A stent is then placed between the portal and hepatic veins bypassing the liver. Portal hypertension is subsequently relieved.
  - Esophagogastric Balloon Tamponade
    - An esophagogastric tube with esophageal and gastric balloons is used to compress blood vessels in the esophagus and stomach. Check balloons for leaks prior to insertion. Traction is applied after balloons are inflated to the desired pressure. When the bleeding is stopped, the traction is released and the pressure in the balloons is reduced gradually. Reserved for clients who have unsuccessful TIPS procedures.

- Surgical Interventions
  - Surgery for esophageal varices is considered as a last resort.
  - Bypass procedures
    - Bypass procedures establish a venous shunt that bypasses the liver, decreasing portal hypertension.
    - Nursing Actions (pre, post)
      - Monitor clients for an increase in liver dysfunction or encephalopathy.

- Care After Discharge

  o Encourage clients to avoid alcohol consumption.

- Client Outcomes

  o The client's esophageal varices will stop bleeding.

  o The client will not experience future variceal bleeds.

Complications

- Hypovolemic Shock

  o Hemorrhage from esophageal varices can lead to hypovolemic shock.

  o Nursing Actions

    - Observe clients carefully for signs of hemorrhage and shock.

    - Monitor vital signs, Hgb, and Hct.

    - Assist with the care of clients receiving IV fluid replacement.

ESOPHAGEAL CANCER

Overview

- Esophageal cancer is a fast-growing and metastasizing type of cancer.

- Cancers of the upper esophagus are typically squamous cell and cancers of the lower esophagus are typically adenomas.

- Treatment often involves several weeks of chemotherapy and radiation therapy followed by surgery.

Data Collection

- Risk Factors

  o Smoking

  o Alcohol abuse

  o Nitrites

  o GERD

  o Barrett's esophagus

- Subjective Data

  o Early symptoms are often vague

  o Dysphagia

  o Odynophagia (painful swallowing)

  o Feeling of a lump in the throat

- Objective Data

  o Physical Assessment Findings

    ■ Weight loss

    ■ Halitosis

    ■ Regurgitation

    ■ Hiccups

  o Diagnostic Procedures

    ■ Barium swallow may be done initially to determine cause of dysphagia.

    ■ Esophagogastroduodenoscopy (EGD) is done to visualize tumors and take a biopsy of suspicious tissue.

    ■ CT or positron emission tomography (PET) scans of the chest and abdomen can assess for metastatic disease of the lungs and liver.

    ■ Esophageal ultrasound can determine presence of cancer in mediastinum and lymph nodes.

Collaborative Care

- Nursing Care

  o Weigh clients daily.

  o Support nutrition with a high-caloric diet, semi-soft foods and thickened liquids, and supplements. Record calorie count.

  o Monitor for aspiration during meals. Enteral feedings through a gastrostomy tube may be needed.

  o Keep the client's head elevated at least 30° at all times, and higher after meals.

- Medications

  o Chemotherapy

    ■ Chemotherapy may be given prior to surgery to aid in shrinking the tumor, in place of surgery if the tumor is too extensive, or for palliation. Chemotherapy can make the tumor cells more susceptible to radiation.

- Interdisciplinary Care

    o Dietary consult for appropriate diet

    o Speech therapy consult for swallowing instruction

    o Home health nurse upon discharge from hospital

    o Cancer support groups

- Therapeutic Procedures

    o Radiation

        ▪ Radiation is often given along with chemotherapy or may be given alone. It can be effective in reducing the size of the tumor and making swallowing easier. Esophageal dilation may be needed after treatment in relation to esophageal strictures caused by scarring.

    o Photodynamic therapy (PDT)

        ▪ PDT involves the injection of a photosensitizing agent that is absorbed by all the cells in the body. One to three days later when the agent remains in only the cancer cells, the tumor is exposed to a specific wavelength of light via an endoscope. The cancer cells are subsequently destroyed and tumors are eliminated or reduced in size.

- Surgical Interventions

    o Esophagectomy/esophagogastrostomy

        ▪ Removal of all or part of the esophagus and stomach. Some of the intestine may be used as an anatomic graft for the missing length of the esophagus. A more minimally invasive procedure may be done using a laparoscope, but esophageal cancer is usually too extensive for this type of surgery.

        ▪ Nursing Actions

            □ Provide preoperative teaching and postoperative care.

            □ Maintain clients in a semi-Fowler's position or higher.

            □ Monitor chest tube and drainage.

            □ Maintain NG tube patency and monitor drainage – do not replace NG tube if it comes out.

            □ Do not manipulate or irrigate NG tube unless prescribed by the provider.

            □ Provide enteral feedings if jejunostomy tube was placed.

            □ Keep clients NPO until anastomosis has been determined to be patent (barium swallow).

            □ Monitor for anastomotic leak (fever, saliva seeping through incision).

            □ Provide clients with suction for oral secretions.

            □ Closely observe for aspiration when oral feedings are resumed. Keep clients upright for at least 2 hr after meals.

- Client Education
  - Instruct clients to slowly progress diet beginning with thick liquids and moving to semisolid and well-chewed solid foods.
  - Instruct clients to weigh regularly and increase caloric intake as tolerated to maintain or increase weight.
  - Instruct clients to monitor the incision closely for signs of infection or abnormal drainage (saliva).

Care After Discharge

- Client Education
  - Encourage clients to avoid alcohol consumption and foods containing nitrites.
  - Encourage clients to stop smoking.
  - Encourage clients to get treatment for GERD.
- Client Outcomes
  - The client will be able to ingest a regular diet without aspiration or dysphagia.
  - The client will maintain or gain weight.
  - The client will not develop aspiration pneumonia.

Complications

- Vagotomy syndrome
  - Causes
    - Due to an interruption of the vagal nerve, a syndrome similar to "dumping syndrome" occurs after esophagectomy. This is related to the quick passage of food into the duodenum, which creates an osmotic gradient with large amounts of fluids entering the bowel and manifesting itself as watery diarrhea. It typically occurs 15 to 60 min after a meal.
  - Nursing Actions
    - Observe for postprandial symptoms (diaphoresis, diarrhea, tachycardia, abdominal pain).
    - Request a referral to a dietician to determine what foods to avoid and develop a meal program (six small meals a day that are lactose-free).

Ⓐ APPLICATION EXERCISES

Scenario: A 75-year-old client has been diagnosed with GERD. The client is overweight, has been experiencing dyspepsia, is belching and bloated after meals, has dysphagia, and is experiencing chest pain. She reports taking NSAIDs daily for rheumatoid arthritis, drinks diet cola drinks several times a day, has a history of four full-term deliveries, stress incontinence, takes amlodipine (Norvasc) for high blood pressure, and eats an orange every day for an afternoon snack.

1. What risk factors for GERD does the client have?

2. During client education, which of the following instructions should the nurse reinforce to manage symptoms? (Select all that apply.)

   _____ Eat small frequent meals.

   _____ Chew foods thoroughly.

   _____ Eat a snack every evening.

   _____ Avoid fatty foods.

   _____ Drink a glass of wine just before bedtime.

   _____ Start a weight-loss program.

   _____ Avoid tight-fitting clothing.

   _____ Sleep in a recumbent position with head flat.

   _____ Keep a food diary to see what foods trigger symptoms.

3. Which of the following classifications of medications will help to relieve the symptoms of GERD? (Select all that apply.)

   _____ Antacids

   _____ Histamine$_2$ receptor antagonists

   _____ Opioid analgesics

   _____ Fiber laxatives

   _____ Proton pump inhibitors

4. A client who has esophageal varices is being discharged from the hospital. Which of the following instructions should the nurse reinforce prior to discharge? (Select all that apply.)

   _____ Avoid bearing down during bowel movements.

   _____ Avoid forceful coughing.

   _____ Avoid lifting heavy objects.

   _____ Avoid taking antacids.

   _____ Avoid eating spicy foods.

   _____ Avoid drinking alcoholic beverages.

5. A nurse is assigned a client who is 1 day postoperative an esophagectomy. The client is confused and has been pulling at his NG tube and indwelling urinary catheter. When the nurse enters the room, the NG tube is found on the floor. Which of the following actions should the nurse take?

   A. Obtain a clean NG tube and reinsert.

   B. Make a note in the chart and observe for nausea and vomiting.

   C. Test the client's gag reflex prior to providing ice chips.

   D. Notify the provider regarding accidental removal of the tube.

APPLICATION EXERCISES ANSWER KEY

Scenario: A 75-year-old client has been diagnosed with GERD. The client is overweight, has been experiencing dyspepsia, is belching and bloated after meals, has dysphagia, and is experiencing chest pain. She reports taking NSAIDs daily for rheumatoid arthritis, drinks diet cola drinks several times a day, has a history of four full-term deliveries, stress incontinence, takes amlodipine (Norvasc) for high blood pressure, and eats an orange every day for an afternoon snack.

1. What risk factors for GERD does the client have?

    The client is at risk for GERD because she is an older adult, is overweight, takes NSAIDs regularly, drinks caffeinated beverages several times a day, has been prescribed amlodipine, a calcium channel blocker for high blood pressure, and eats a citrus fruit every afternoon.

    Ⓝ NCLEX® Connection: Physiological Adaptation, Pathophysiology

2. During client education, which of the following instructions should the nurse reinforce to manage symptoms? (Select all that apply.)

__X__	**Eat small frequent meals.**
__X__	**Chew foods thoroughly.**
_____	Eat a snack every evening.
__X__	**Avoid fatty foods.**
_____	Drink a glass of wine just before bedtime.
__X__	**Start a weight-loss program.**
__X__	**Avoid tight-fitting clothing.**
_____	Sleep in a recumbent position with head flat.
__X__	**Keep a food diary to see what foods trigger symptoms.**

    Symptoms of GERD can be minimized by eating small, frequent meals, chewing food thoroughly, avoiding fatty foods, losing weight, wearing clothes that are not tight at the waist, and keeping a food diary to see what additional foods trigger symptoms. Foods should not be eaten prior to bedtime, alcoholic beverages should be avoided, and the client should sleep with the head of the bed elevated and on her right side.

    Ⓝ NCLEX® Connection: Basic Care and Comfort, Nutrition and Oral Hydration

3. Which of the following classifications of medications will help to relieve the symptoms of GERD? (Select all that apply.)

   X   **Antacids**

   X   **Histamine$_2$ receptor antagonists**

   _____   Opioid analgesics

   _____   Fiber laxatives

   X   **Proton pump inhibitors**

Antacids neutralize gastric acid, histamine$_2$ receptor antagonists decrease the secretion of gastric acid, and proton pump inhibitors decrease the production of gastric acid; these are all given to treat GERD. Opioid analgesics and fiber laxatives are not effective in the treatment of symptoms of GERD that result from the reflux of gastrointestinal contents containing acid.

 NCLEX® Connection: Pharmacological Therapies, Expected Actions/Outcomes

4. A client who has esophageal varices is being discharged from the hospital. Which of the following instructions should the nurse reinforce prior to discharge? (Select all that apply.)

   X   **Avoid bearing down during bowel movements.**

   X   **Avoid forceful coughing.**

   X   **Avoid lifting heavy objects.**

   _____   Avoid taking antacids.

   _____   Avoid eating spicy foods.

   X   **Avoid drinking alcoholic beverages.**

The client should be instructed to avoid bearing down during bowel movements, forceful coughing, lifting heavy objects, and drinking alcoholic beverages. Taking antacids and eating spicy foods are not contraindicated.

NCLEX® Connection: Reduction of Risk Potential, Potential for Complications from Surgical Procedures and Health Alterations

5. A nurse is assigned a client who is 1 day postoperative an esophagectomy. The client is confused and has been pulling at his NG tube and indwelling urinary catheter. When the nurse enters the room, the NG tube is found on the floor. Which of the following actions should the nurse take?

   A. Obtain a clean NG tube and reinsert.

   B. Make a note in the chart and observe for nausea and vomiting.

   C. Test the client's gag reflex prior to providing ice chips.

   D. Notify the provider regarding accidental removal of the tube.

   The nurse should immediately notify the provider that the tube was accidentally removed. The occurrence of nausea and vomiting can disrupt the incision site, so waiting to see if they occur could put the client at risk for injury. The NG tube should not be replaced by the nurse due to the risk of interfering with the esophageal incisions. Fluids in any form should not be given until the esophageal incisions have healed.

Ⓝ NCLEX® Connection: Reduction of Risk Potential, Potential for Complications from Surgical Procedures and Health Alterations

UNIT 7	NURSING CARE OF CLIENTS WITH GASTROINTESTINAL DISORDERS

Section: Upper Gastrointestinal Disorders

Chapter 43 Peptic Ulcer Disease

Overview

- A peptic ulcer is an erosion of the mucosal lining of the stomach or duodenum. The mucous membranes can become eroded to the point that the epithelium is exposed to gastric acid and pepsin, and can precipitate bleeding and perforation. Perforation that extends through all the layers of the stomach or duodenum can cause peritonitis. An individual with a peptic ulcer has peptic ulcer disease (PUD).

- There are gastric ulcers, duodenal ulcers, and stress ulcers (these occur after major stress or trauma).

Data Collection

- Risk Factors

  - Causes of peptic ulcers:

    - *Helicobacter pylori (H. pylori)* infection (duodenal)

    - Nonsteroidal anti-inflammatory drug (NSAID) and corticosteroid use

    - Severe stress

    - Hypersecretory states

    - Type O blood

    - Excess alcohol ingestion

    - Chronic pulmonary or renal disease

    - Zollinger-Ellison syndrome (combination of peptic ulcers, hypersecretion of gastric acid, and gastrin secreting tumors)

- Subjective Data

  - Dyspepsia – Heartburn, bloating, nausea, and vomiting, and may be perceived as uncomfortable fullness or hunger

  - Pain

GASTRIC ULCER	DUODENAL ULCER
30 to 60 min after a meal	1.5 to 3 hr after a meal
Rarely occurs at night	Often occurs at night
Exacerbated by ingestion of food	Relieved by ingestion of food or antacid

- Objective Data
  - Physical Assessment Findings
    - Epigastric tenderness upon palpation, and radiates to the back, which may indicate perforation is imminent
    - Bloody emesis (hematemesis) is more likely to occur with a gastric ulcer
    - Bloody stools (melena) are more likely with a duodenal ulcer
    - Weight loss
  - Laboratory Tests
    - *H. pylori* testing:
      - Gastric samples are collected via an endoscopy to test for *H. pylori*.
      - C13 urea breath testing identifies the presence of *H pylori*. After being NPO for 8 hr, the client drinks a radioactive carbon urea solution. Urea breaks down to carbon dioxide and then it is eliminated by the lungs. The client's expired air is measured, and the amount of carbon dioxide will determine if *H pylori* is present.
      - IgG serologic testing documents the presence of *H. pylori* based on antibody assays.
      - Stool sample tests for the presence of the *H. pylori* antigen.
    - Hgb and Hct (decreased values secondary to bleeding)
    - Stool sample for occult blood
  - Diagnostic Procedures
    - Esophagogastroduodenoscopy (EGD)
      - An EGD is the most definitive diagnosis of peptic ulcers and may be repeated to evaluate the effectiveness of treatment. Gastric samples are taken to test for *H. pylori*.
  - Nursing Actions
    - Client Education
      - Instruct clients to avoid taking bismuth, misoprostol, sucralfate, and histamine$_2$ receptor antagonists for a prescribed amount of time prior to testing, because they can interfere with results for *H. pylori* (false negatives).

Collaborative Care

- Nursing Care
  - Monitor for orthostatic changes in vital signs and tachycardia, as these findings are suggestive of gastrointestinal bleeding.
  - Administer saline lavage via an NG tube, if prescribed.
  - Administer medication as prescribed.
  - Decrease environmental stress.
  - Encourage rest periods.
- Medications
  - Antibiotics – Metronidazole (Flagyl), amoxicillin (Amoxil), bismuth (Pepto-Bismol), clarithromycin (Biaxin), tetracycline (Achromycin V)
    - Eliminate *H. pylori* infection
    - Nursing Considerations
      - Clients may require a combination of two to three different antibiotics.
    - Client Education
      - Instruct clients to complete a full course of medication.
  - Histamine$_2$ receptor antagonists – Ranitidine (Zantac), famotidine (Pepcid)
    - Suppress the secretion of gastric acid by selectively blocking H$_2$ receptors in parietal cells lining the stomach.
    - Used in conjunction with antibiotics to treat ulcers caused by *H. pylori*.
    - Nursing Considerations
      - Ranitidine and famotidine can be administered IV for acute situations.
      - Ranitidine can be taken with or without food.
      - Treatment of peptic ulcer disease is usually started as an oral dose twice a day until the ulcer is healed, followed by a maintenance dose usually taken once a day at bedtime.
    - Client Education
      - Instruct clients to notify the provider for any sign of obvious or occult GI bleeding (coffee-ground emesis).
  - Proton pump inhibitors – Pantoprazole (Protonix), esomeprazole (Nexium)
    - Reduce gastric acid secretion by irreversibly inhibiting the enzyme that produces gastric acid.
    - Reduce basal and stimulated acid production.
    - Nursing Considerations
      - There are insignificant side and adverse effects with short-term treatment.

- Client Education
  - Instruct clients not to crush, chew, or break sustained-release capsules.
  - Instruct clients to take omeprazole once a day prior to eating in the morning.
- Antacids – Aluminum carbonate, magnesium hydroxide (Milk of Magnesia)
  - Antacids may be given up to seven times a day – 1 and 3 hr after meals and at bedtime to neutralize gastric acid, which occurs with food ingestion and at bedtime.
  - Nursing Considerations
    - Give 1 to 2 hr apart from other medications to avoid reducing the absorption of other medications.
  - Client Education
    - Encourage adherence by reinforcing the intended effect of the antacid (relief of pain, healing of ulcer).
    - Reinforce to clients to take all medications at least 1 to 2 hr before or after taking an antacid.
- Mucosal protectant – Sucralfate (Carafate)
  - Nursing Considerations
    - Give 1 hr before meals and at bedtime.
    - Monitor for side effects of constipation.

- Interdisciplinary Care
  - Nutrition consult – diet that restricts acid-producing foods (milk products, caffeine, decaffeinated coffee, spicy foods, medications [NSAIDs]).

- Therapeutic Procedures
  - Endoscopic therapies
    - During an esophagogastroduodenoscopy (EGD), areas of bleeding may be treated with epinephrine or laser coagulation.

- Surgical Interventions
  - Gastric Surgery
    - Gastric surgeries
      - Gastrectomy – All or part of the stomach is removed. This surgery may be performed with laparoscopic or open approach.
      - Antrectomy – The antrum portion of the stomach is removed.
      - Gastrojejunostomy (Billroth II procedure) – The lower portion of the stomach is excised and the remaining stomach is anastomosed to the jejunum, and the remaining duodenum is surgically closed.

- □ Vagotomy – The branches of the vagus nerve that supply the stomach are cut to disrupt acid production.

- □ Pyloroplasty – The opening between the stomach and small intestine is enlarged to increase the rate of gastric emptying.

  - ▪ Nursing Actions

    - □ Reinforce pre and postoperative teaching.

    - □ Place clients in a semi-Fowler's position to facilitate respiratory movements.

    - □ Monitor the client's nasogastric output as appropriate, and intervene to avoid abdominal distention (a scant amount of blood is expected in the first 12 to 24 hr). Notify the provider before repositioning or irrigating the NG tube (disruption of sutures).

    - □ Check bowel sounds are diminished or absent with surgery and anesthesia. Monitor for their return (3 to 5 per quadrant/min).

    - □ Follow guidelines for reintroduction of fluids and foods. Healing of sutures is supported by NPO status. Generally, resumption of enteral intake begins with clear liquids and the client's diet is advanced as tolerated. Abdominal distention is avoided.

  - ▪ Client Education

    - □ Educate clients regarding the need for vitamin and mineral supplementation after a gastrectomy, including vitamin B_{12}, vitamin D, calcium, iron, and folate.

- ● Care After Discharge

  - ○ Client Education

    - ▪ Instruct clients to:

    - ▪ Drink alcohol in moderation.

    - ▪ Quit smoking.

    - ▪ Use stress management techniques.

    - ▪ Avoid NSAIDS as indicated.

- ● Client Outcomes

  - ○ The client will experience no further bleeding.

  - ○ The client will be able to verbalize medication regimen and foods that should be avoided.

Complications

- Perforation/Hemorrhage
  - When peptic ulcers perforate or bleed, it is an emergency situation.
    - Perforation presents as severe epigastric pain spreading across the abdomen. The abdomen is rigid, board-like, hyperactive to diminished bowel sounds, and has rebound tenderness. Perforation is a surgical emergency.
    - Gastrointestinal bleeding in the form of hematemesis or melena may cause symptoms of shock (hypotension, tachycardia, dizziness, confusion), and decreased Hgb.
  - Nursing Actions
    - Monitor clients for subtle changes in pain and vital signs that may indicate perforation or bleeding.
    - Report findings to provider.
- Pernicious Anemia
  - Pernicious anemia is due to a deficiency of the intrinsic factor normally secreted by the gastric mucosa.
    - Signs and symptoms include pallor, glossitis, fatigue, and paresthesias.
  - Client Education
    - Inform clients of the need for lifelong vitamin B_{12} injections.
- Dumping Syndrome
  - Dumping syndrome is a complication of gastric surgery that consists of vasomotor symptoms occurring in response to food ingestion. Symptoms result from the rapid emptying of gastric contents into the small intestine. In response to the sudden influx of a hypertonic fluid, the small intestine pulls fluid from the extracellular space to convert the hypertonic fluid to an isotonic fluid. This fluid shift causes a decrease in circulating volume, resulting in vasomotor symptoms (syncope, pallor, palpitations, dizziness, headache).
  - Gastric surgery, especially gastrojejunostomy (Billroth II), poses the greatest risk for dumping syndrome. Following gastric surgery, the reduced stomach has less ability to control the amount and rate of chyme that enters the small intestine after a meal.

- ○ Nursing Actions
  - ■ Monitor for vasomotor symptoms:

	EARLY SYMPTOMS	LATE SYMPTOMS
Onset	Within 30 min after eating	90 min to 3 hr after eating
Cause	Rapid emptying	Excessive insulin release
Symptoms	• Nausea, vomiting, and dizziness • Tachycardia • Palpitations	• Hunger, dizziness, and sweating • Tachycardia and palpitations • Shakiness and feelings of anxiety • Confusion

  - ■ Assist/instruct clients to lie down when vasomotor symptoms occur.
  - ■ Administer medications as prescribed.
    - □ Administration of powdered pectin or octreotide (Sandostatin) subcutaneously may be prescribed if symptoms are severe and not effectively controlled with dietary measures. Pectin slows the absorption of carbohydrates. Octreotide blocks gastric and pancreatic hormones, which can lead to symptoms of dumping syndrome.
    - □ Antispasmodic medications (dicyclomine [Bentyl]).
    - □ Acarbose (Prandase) will slow the absorption of carbohydrates.
    - □ Malnutrition and fluid electrolyte imbalances may occur due to altered absorption. Monitor I&O, laboratory values, and the client's weight.
- ○ Client Education
  - ■ Instruct clients to:
    - □ Lie down after a meal to slow the movement of food within the intestines.
    - □ Limit the amount of fluid ingested at one time.
    - □ Eliminate liquids with meals for 1 hr prior to and following a meal.
    - □ Consume a high-protein, high-fat, low-fiber, and a low to moderate carbohydrate diet.
    - □ Avoid milk, sweets, or sugars (fruit juice, sweetened fruit, milk shakes, honey, syrup, jelly).
    - □ Consume small, frequent meals rather than large meals.

Ⓐ APPLICATION EXERCISES

Scenario: A nurse is caring for a client with peptic ulcer disease.

1. The nurse should expect laboratory results to confirm the presence of which of the following pathogens?

    A. Streptococcus pneumonia

    B. Helicobacter pylori

    C. Respiratory syncytial virus

    D. Bordetella pertussis

2. Match the medication in column A with the intended effect in column B.

_____ Metronidazole (Flagyl)	A. Suppresses the secretion of gastric acid
_____ Ranitidine (Zantac)	B. Mucosal protectant
_____ Pantoprazole (Protonix)	C. Antimicrobial that eliminate *H. pylori* infection
_____ Magnesium hydroxide	D. Reduces gastric acid production
_____ Sucralfate (Carafate)	E. Antacid that neutralize gastric acid

3. For which of the following signs should the nurse monitor? (Select all that apply.)

    _____ Rigid abdomen

    _____ Tachycardia

    _____ Pain in the right shoulder

    _____ Elevated blood pressure

    _____ Circumoral cyanosis

    _____ Rebound tenderness

4. The client experiences a perforation and undergoes a partial gastrectomy. The client reports feeling nauseous, weak, and dizzy with a pounding heart approximately 30 min after eating. The nurse recognizes these symptoms as dumping syndrome and reinforces teaching to prevent its occurrence. Which of the following instructions should the nurse include? (Select all that apply.)

_____ Include foods in meals that are high in protein and fat.

_____ Lie down after each meal.

_____ Eat three moderate-sized meals a day.

_____ Drink at least one glass of water with each meal.

_____ Eat a bedtime snack that contains a milk product.

_____ Increase pectin in the diet.

(A) **APPLICATION EXERCISES ANSWER KEY**

Scenario: A nurse is caring for a client with peptic ulcer disease.

1. The nurse should expect laboratory results to confirm the presence of which of the following pathogens?

    A. Streptococcus pneumonia

    B. *Helicobacter pylori*

    C. Respiratory syncytial virus

    D. Bordetella pertussis

    Helicobacter pylori is a bacterium that has been found to cause the majority of the cases of peptic ulcer disease. Streptococcus pneumoniae is a common pathogen that causes pneumonia and otitis media. Respiratory syncytial virus is a common virus found in children under 5, resulting in upper and lower respiratory infections. Bordetella pertussis is bacteria that results in whooping cough.

(N) NCLEX® Connection: Safety and Infection Control, Standard Precautions/Transmission-Based Precautions/Surgical Asepsis

2. Match the medication in column A with the intended effect in column B.

__C__	Metronidazole (Flagyl)	A. Suppresses the secretion of gastric acid
__A__	Ranitidine (Zantac)	B. Mucosal protectant
__D__	Pantoprazole (Protonix)	C. Antimicrobial that eliminate *H. pylori* infection
__E__	Magnesium hydroxide	D. Reduces gastric acid production
__B__	Sucralfate (Carafate)	E. Antacid that neutralize gastric acid

(N) NCLEX® Connection: Pharmacological Therapies, Expected Actions/Outcomes

3. For which of the following signs should the nurse monitor? (Select all that apply.)

    __X__ **Rigid abdomen**

    __X__ **Tachycardia**

    __X__ **Pain in the right shoulder**

    _____ Elevated blood pressure

    _____ Circumoral cyanosis

    __X__ **Rebound tenderness**

    Signs of gastric perforation, as a result of the release of gastric contents into the abdominal cavity, include a rigid abdomen; rebound tenderness; abdominal pain that radiates into the right shoulder; hematemesis; and blood loss (tachycardia, hypotension, syncope). Signs of perforation do not include circumoral cyanosis.

(N) NCLEX® Connection: Physiological Adaptation, Medical Emergencies

PN ADULT MEDICAL SURGICAL NURSING

4. The client experiences a perforation and undergoes a partial gastrectomy. The client reports feeling nauseous, weak, and dizzy with a pounding heart approximately 30 min after eating. The nurse recognizes these symptoms as dumping syndrome and reinforces teaching to prevent its occurrence. Which of the following instructions should the nurse include? (Select all that apply.)

   X   **Include foods in meals that are high in protein and fat.**

   X   **Lie down after each meal.**

          Eat three moderate-sized meals a day.

          Drink at least one glass of water with each meal.

          Eat a bedtime snack that contains a milk product.

   X   **Increase pectin in the diet.**

Include foods in meals that are high in protein and fat. Lying down after each meal along with the addition of pectin in the diet will delay the absorption of food in the small intestine. Encourage small, frequent meals, rather than large meals; discourage drinking liquids with meals and for 1 hr prior to and following meals; and avoid all milk products.

(N) NCLEX® Connection: Reduction of Risk Potential, Potential for Complications from Surgical Procedures and Health Alterations

UNIT 7	NURSING CARE OF CLIENTS WITH GASTROINTESTINAL DISORDERS
Section:	Upper Gastrointestinal Disorders
Chapter 44	**Acute and Chronic Gastritis**

 Overview

- The stomach is coated with a protective layer of mucous. Cox 1 enzymes produce mucosal prostaglandins that protect the lining of the stomach.

- Gastritis is an inflammation in the lining of the stomach.

- Inflammation is the result of an irritation to the stomach mucosa.

> **(M)** **View Media Supplement:** H. pylori Gastritis (Image)

- Gastritis may be chronic or acute.

- Acute gastritis

  - Sudden onset

  - Short duration

  - Severe acute gastritis may result in gastric bleeding

- Chronic gastritis

  - Slow onset

  - Chronic profuse damage to stomach mucosa may cause parietal cell damage

  - Pernicious anemia

  - Extensive gastric mucosal wall damage may cause erosive gastritis (ulcers) and increase the risk of stomach cancer

Data Collection

- Risk Factors

  - Bacterial infection – *Helicobacter pylori* (*H. pylori*), salmonella, streptococci, staphylococci or *Escherichia coli*

  - Family member with *H. pylori* infection

  - Family history of gastritis

- o Prolonged use of NSAIDS, corticosteroids (stops prostaglandin synthesis)
- o Excessive alcohol use
- o Bile reflux disease
- o Autoimmune diseases (systemic lupus, rheumatoid arthritis)
- o Advanced age
- o Radiation therapy
- o Smoking
- o Caffeine
- o Excessive stress
- o Exposure to contaminated food or water
- Subjective Data
  - o Dyspepsia, general abdominal discomfort, indigestion
  - o Upper abdominal pain or burning may increase or decrease after eating
  - o Nausea
  - o Reduced appetite
  - o Abdominal bloating or distention
  - o Hematemesis (bloody emesis)
  - o Erosive gastritis:
    - Black, tarry stools, coffee-ground emesis
    - Acute abdominal pain
- Objective Data
  - o Physical Assessment Findings
    - Vomiting
    - Weight loss
    - Stools or emesis test positive for occult blood
  - o Laboratory Tests
    - Noninvasive tests
      - □ CBC to check for anemia (In women, Hgb less than 12 g/dL and RBC less than 4.2 cells/mcL; in men, Hgb less than 14 g/dL and RBC less than 4.7 cells/mcL)
      - □ Serum and stool antibody/antigen test for presence of *H. pylori*
      - □ C13 urea breath test – measures *H. pylori*

o Diagnostic Procedures

  ▪ Esophagogastroduodenoscopy

    □ A small flexible scope is inserted through the mouth into the esophagus, stomach, and duodenum to visualize the upper digestive tract. This procedure allows for a biopsy, cauterization, removal of polyps, dilation, or diagnosis.

Collaborative Care

- Nursing Care

  o Monitor fluid intake and urine output.

  o Monitor clients receiving IV fluids as prescribed.

  o Assist clients in identifying foods that may trigger symptoms.

  o Provide small, frequent meals and encourage clients to eat slowly.

  o Provide for frequent rest periods.

  o Monitor for signs of gastric bleeding (coffee-ground emesis, black, tarry stools).

  o Monitor for signs of anemia (tachycardia, hypotension, fatigue, shortness of breath, pallor, feeling lightheaded or dizzy, chest pain).

- Medications

CLASSIFICATION/ACTION	MEDICATIONS	NURSING INTERVENTIONS	CLIENT EDUCATION
• Histamine$_2$ receptor antagonists o Decreases gastric acid output by blocking gastric histamine$_2$ receptors	• Nizatidine (Axid) • Famotidine (Pepcid) • Ranitidine (Zantac)	• Allow 1 hr before or after to give antacid. • Monitor for neutropenia and hypotension.	• Advise clients to take oral dose with meals. • Advise clients to monitor for signs of GI bleed (black stools, coffee-ground emesis).

CLASSIFICATION/ACTION	MEDICATIONS	NURSING INTERVENTIONS	CLIENT EDUCATION

• Antacids
  ○ Increases gastric pH and neutralizes pepsin
  ○ Improves mucosal protection
	• Aluminum hydroxide (Amphojel)
	• Magnesium hydroxide with aluminum hydroxide (Maalox, Mylanta)
		• Do not give to clients with renal failure or renal dysfunction.
		• Monitor clients taking aluminum antacids for aluminum toxicity and constipation. For those taking magnesium antacids, monitor for diarrhea or hypermagnesemia.
			• Advise clients to take on an empty stomach.
			• Advise clients to wait 1 to 2 hr to take other medications.

• Proton pump inhibitor ○ Reduces gastric acid by stopping acid-producing proton pump	• Omeprazole (Prilosec) • Lansoprazole (Prevacid) • Rabeprazole sodium (AcipHex) • Pantoprazole (Protonix) • Esomeprazole (Nexium)	• These can cause nausea, vomiting, and abdominal pain. • Use filter for IV administration.	• Advise clients to allow 30 min before eating and not to crush or chew pills. • It can take up to 4 days for clients to see the effects. • Advise clients to take on an empty stomach.
• Prostaglandins ○ Reduces gastric acid secretion	• Misoprostol (Cytotec)	• This may be given with NSAIDs to prevent gastric mucosal damage. • This may cause abdominal pain and diarrhea.	• Advise clients to use contraceptives. • Advise clients to take with food to reduce gastric effects.
• Anti-ulcer/mucosal barrier ○ Inhibits acid and forms a protective coating over mucosa	• Sucralfate (Carafate)	• Allow 30 min before or after to give antacid.	• Advise clients to take on an empty stomach. • Advise clients to notify the provider of tinnitus.

CLASSIFICATION/ACTION	MEDICATIONS	NURSING INTERVENTIONS	CLIENT EDUCATION
• Antibiotics ○ Eliminates *H. pylori* infection	• clarithromycin (Biaxin) • amoxicillin (Amoxil) • tetracycline (Achromycin V) • metronidazole (Flagyl)	• Monitor for increased abdominal pain and diarrhea. • Monitor electrolytes and hydration if fluid is depleted.	• Advise clients to complete prescribed dosage. • Advise clients to notify the provider of persistent diarrhea.

- Interdisciplinary Care

    ○ A nutritionist may be necessary to assist in the alterations to diet.

    ○ Supportive care may be needed to reduce stress, increase exercise, and stop smoking.

- Therapeutic Procedures

    ○ Upper endoscopy

- Surgical Interventions

    ○ May be needed to treat erosive gastritis unrelieved by nonsurgical interventions

    ○ Vagotomy or highly selective vagotomy

        ■ The vagus nerve is cut where it enters the stomach to decrease gastric acid. A highly selective vagotomy severs only the nerve fibers that control gastric acid secretion. This is often done laparoscopically to reduce postoperative complications.

    ○ Pyloroplasty

        ■ The outlet from the stomach to the duodenum is widened to increase gastric emptying. This is usually done at the same time as the vagotomy.

- Care After Discharge

    ○ Client Education

        ■ Instruct clients to:

            □ Eat small, frequent meals.

            □ Follow the recommended diet.

            □ Report constipation, nausea, vomiting, or bloody stools.

            □ Take prescribed medications as instructed and monitor for adverse reactions.

            □ Keep taking medications unless provider states otherwise.

            □ Avoid alcohol, caffeine, and foods that may cause gastric irritation.

            □ Assist clients in identifying ways to reduce stress.

- Client Outcomes

  o The client will maintain adequate nutritional intake.

  o The client will eat a healthy diet without abdominal distress.

  o The client will be pain free.

  o The client will identify methods to reduce stress.

Complications

- Gastric bleeding

  o Causes

    ■ Severe acute gastritis with deep tissue inflammation extending into the stomach muscle

    ■ In chronic erosive gastritis, bleeding may be slow or profuse as in a perforation of the stomach wall

  o Nursing Actions

    ■ Monitor vital signs and airway.

    ■ Provide care for clients receiving fluid and electrolyte replacement and blood products.

    ■ Monitor CBC and clotting factors.

    ■ May need to insert an NG tube for gastric lavage (irrigate with NS or water to stop active gastric bleed).

    ■ Confirm placement of NG tube prior to fluid instillation to prevent aspiration.

    ■ Monitor NG tube output.

  o Client Education

    ■ Instruct clients to monitor for signs of slow gastric bleeding (coffee-ground emesis, black, tarry stools).

    ■ Instruct clients to seek immediate medical attention with severe abdominal pain or vomiting blood.

    ■ Remind clients to take medications as directed.

- Gastric outlet obstruction

  o Causes

    ■ Severe acute gastritis with deep tissue inflammation extending into the stomach muscle

  o Nursing Actions

    ■ Monitor fluids and electrolytes.

    ■ Continuous vomiting may result in metabolic alkalosis (due to loss of hydrochloric acid) and severe fluid and electrolyte depletion.

- Provide care for clients receiving fluid and electrolyte replacement.
- Prepare clients for a diagnostic endoscopy.
  - ○ Client Education
    - Instruct clients to seek medical attention for continuous vomiting, bloating, and nausea.
- Dehydration
  - ○ Causes
    - Loss of fluid due to vomiting or diarrhea
  - ○ Nursing Actions
    - Monitor fluid intake and urine output.
    - Provide IV fluids if needed.
    - Monitor electrolytes.
  - ○ Client Education
    - Instruct clients to contact a health care provider for vomiting and diarrhea.
- Pernicious anemia
  - ○ Causes
    - Chronic gastritis may damage the parietal cells. This may lead to reduced production of intrinsic factor, which is necessary for the absorption of vitamin B_{12}.
    - Insufficient vitamin B_{12} may lead to pernicious anemia.
  - ○ Nursing Actions
    - Monitor for anemia.
    - Administer vitamin B_{12} injections monthly.
  - ○ Client Education
    - Inform clients of the need for monthly vitamin B_{12} injections, which may be lifelong.

Ⓐ APPLICATION EXERCISES

1. A nurse is caring for a client who is diagnosed with chronic gastritis and is at risk for developing pernicious anemia. To prevent pernicious anemia, the nurse should administer

   A. vitamin C.

   B. vitamin B_{12}.

   C. ferrous sulfate (Feosol).

   D. epoetin alfa (Epogen).

2. A nurse is reinforcing discharge teaching to a client who has been prescribed aluminum hydroxide (Amphojel). The nurse should advise the client to

   A. take the aluminum hydroxide with food.

   B. monitor for diarrhea.

   C. wait 1 to 2 hr before taking other oral medications.

   D. avoid foods high in bulk, such as bran and fresh fruits.

3. A nurse is caring for a client who has acute gastritis. Which of the following actions should the nurse take? (Select all that apply.)

   _____ Monitor I&O.

   _____ Monitor electrolytes.

   _____ Provide large, infrequent meals.

   _____ Administer ibuprofen for pain.

   _____ Weigh client daily.

APPLICATION EXERCISES ANSWER KEY

1. A nurse is caring for a client who is diagnosed with chronic gastritis and is at risk for developing pernicious anemia. To prevent pernicious anemia, the nurse should administer

   A. vitamin C.

   B. vitamin B_{12}.

   C. ferrous sulfate (Feosol).

   D. epoetin alfa (Epogen).

   Parietal cell damage can lead to insufficient production of intrinsic factor, which is necessary for the absorption of vitamin B_{12}. Insufficient vitamin B_{12} can lead to pernicious anemia and should be replaced with B_{12} injections.

    NCLEX® Connection: Physiological Adaptation: Pathophysiology

2. A nurse is reinforcing discharge teaching to a client who has been prescribed aluminum hydroxide (Amphojel). The nurse should advise the client to

   A. take the aluminum hydroxide with food.

   B. monitor for diarrhea.

   C. wait 1 to 2 hr before taking other oral medications.

   D. avoid foods high in bulk, such as bran and fresh fruits.

   The client should be advised not to take oral medications within 1 to 2 hr of an antacid because the antacid may interfere with the absorption of the oral medication. Aluminum hydroxide can cause constipation. The client should be advised to increase dietary bulk.

   NCLEX® Connection: Pharmacological Therapies, Medication Administration

3. A nurse is caring for a client who has acute gastritis. Which of the following actions should the nurse take? (Select all that apply.)

X	**Monitor I&O.**
X	**Monitor electrolytes.**
	Provide large, infrequent meals.
	Administer ibuprofen for pain.
X	**Weigh client daily.**

   Nursing care of a client who has acute gastritis should include monitoring fluid intake and urine output, electrolytes, and daily weight. The client should also consume small, frequent meals. Ibuprofen and other NSAIDs should be avoided to prevent further gastric irritation.

   NCLEX® Connection: Reduction of Risk Potential: Potential for Complications from Surgical Procedures and Health Alterations

UNIT 7	NURSING CARE OF CLIENTS WITH GASTROINTESTINAL DISORDERS

Section: Lower Gastrointestinal Disorders

Chapter 45 Appendicitis

 Overview

- Appendicitis occurs when the vermiform appendix (a small projection of the cecum) becomes trapped with hard material (usually feces) that leads to a bacterial infection. The lumen of the appendix is blocked and edematous, which leads to abdominal pain.

- Appendicitis is not preventable; therefore, early detection is important.

> **(M)** **View Media Supplement:** Appendicitis (Image)

Data Collection

- Risk Factors

  ○ Appendicitis is seen most often in people between the ages of 10 to 30. Peak incidence is among adolescent males and individuals between 20 and 30 years of age.

  ○ Appendicitis is rare in older adult clients.

  ○ In older adults, the symptoms of appendicitis are less pronounced. Clients may delay seeking treatment, which increases the risk of perforation.

- Subjective and Objective Data

  ○ The order in which symptoms occur is important to aid in the diagnosis. With appendicitis, classical abdominal pain occurs first and nausea and vomiting later. Clients report cramping and pain around the umbilicus and in the epigastric area. As the condition progresses, the pain moves to the right lower quadrant (McBurney's point).

  ○ Anorexia, nausea, and vomiting may be reported by clients.

  ○ Rebound tenderness (pain after deep pressure is applied and released) over McBurney's point (located halfway between the umbilicus and anterior iliac spine).

  ○ Pain that is relieved by right hip flexion and increases with coughing and movement may indicate perforation with peritonitis.

  ○ Muscle rigidity, tense positioning, and guarding may indicate perforation with peritonitis.

o Normal to low-grade temperature (higher suggests peritonitis)

o Laboratory Tests

- WBC count and differential – Mild to moderate elevation of 10,000 to 18,000/mm³ with left shift is consistent with appendicitis; greater than 20,000/mm³ may indicate peritonitis.

o Diagnostic Procedures

- An ultrasound of the abdomen may show an enlarged appendix.

- Abdominal computed tomography (CT) may be diagnostic if symptoms are recurrent or prolonged. The CT may show the presence of fecal material in the appendix.

Collaborative Care

- Surgical Interventions

  o Surgical management includes an appendectomy, which can be done using a laparoscope (using several small incisions and an endoscope) or an open approach (requiring a larger abdominal incision).

  - Nursing Actions

    □ Preoperative

    ‣ Maintain nothing by mouth (NPO) status in the anticipation of surgery and to prevent GI stimulation.

    ‣ Monitor clients receiving IV fluids.

    ‣ Encourage semi-Fowler's position to contain abdominal drainage in the lower abdomen.

    ‣ Avoid laxatives/enemas or application of heat to the abdomen, which can predispose the client to perforation.

    □ Postoperative

    ‣ Administer opioid analgesia (usually morphine) as prescribed.

    ‣ Monitor clients receiving IV antibiotics (surgical prophylaxis, perforation).

    ‣ Offer food as tolerated with the return of bowel sounds.

    ‣ For peritonitis, monitor NG tube drainage.

    ‣ For perforation or abscess, monitor surgical drains.

    ‣ Prepare clients for discharge 12 to 24 hr after the surgery.

- Care After Discharge
    - Client Education
        - Reinforce to the client:
            - To provide care to the surgical site.
            - How to recognize the signs and symptoms of wound infection (fever, inflammation, malodorous drainage).
            - Use of postoperative medications (purpose, guidelines, adverse effects).
            - Activity restrictions (lifting, driving, returning to work).
- Client Outcomes
    - The client will remain free of signs and symptoms of infection.
    - The client will report that pain is controlled.
    - The client's fluid and electrolyte status will be restored.
    - The client will return to his regular ADLs.

Complications

- Peritonitis, which is an inflammation of the peritoneum and viscera, can occur due to perforation of the appendix. The peritoneal area, which is normally sterile, becomes contaminated with bacteria and gastric juices from the gastrointestinal tract.
    - When a client has appendicitis, the risk of perforation is greatest 24 hr following the onset of pain.
- Nursing Actions
    - Monitor for:
        - Fever.
        - Tachycardia.
        - Signs of dehydration.
        - Distended or board-like abdomen.
        - Nausea and vomiting.
        - Rebound tenderness.
        - Hiccups.
    - Report elevated WBC ($20,000/mm^3$) and elevated neutrophil count.
    - Monitor clients receiving IV fluids and antibiotics.
    - Maintain intermittent NG suction.
    - Provide oxygen by nasal cannula or mask to maintain adequate oxygenation.
    - Measure I&O.

- o Administer medications to control pain, nausea, and vomiting.

- o Place clients in a side-lying position with knees bent to decrease abdominal tension.

- o Reinforce preoperative teaching if surgery is indicated.

- o Provide postoperative care for laparoscopic procedure.

- **Client Education**

  - o Instruct clients to provide care to the surgical site, which may include drains still in place.

  - o Reinforce to clients how to recognize the signs and symptoms of additional infection.

  - o Reinforce to clients use of postoperative medications (purpose, guidelines, adverse effects).

(A) APPLICATION EXERCISES

Scenario: A nurse is caring for a client who is in skeletal traction for a fractured left femur. The client has been reporting abdominal pain and nausea over the past 24 hr. The nurse is beginning to suspect appendicitis and begins asking more questions about the pain.

1. Which of the following reports should support the nurse's suspicion of appendicitis?

    A. Nausea began prior to the pain.

    B. Pain began in the epigastric area, but has moved to the right lower quadrant.

    C. Pain in right lower quadrant is worse when pressure is applied and less when released.

    D. Pain is less after an episode of diarrhea.

2. The nurse determines that the client is experiencing appendicitis. When preparing the client for surgery, the nurse should anticipate which of the following interventions? (Select all that apply.)

    _____ Administer enema.

    _____ Maintain NPO status.

    _____ Encourage semi-Fowler's position.

    _____ Apply heat to the abdomen.

    _____ Verify informed consent is given.

3. During surgery, the client's appendix has been found to have ruptured. Upon return to the unit, the client has an NG tube connected to low intermittent suction and an IV of 0.9% sodium chloride infusing at 100 mL/hr. In providing postoperative care, the nurse should anticipate assisting with which of the following interventions? (Select all that apply.)

    _____ Frequent monitoring of vital signs

    _____ Administration of IV antibiotics

    _____ Visualization of the incision at least every shift

    _____ Administration of a full-liquid diet

    _____ Administration of opioid analgesics

    _____ Measurement of hourly I&O

    _____ Maintenance of bedrest with frequent repositioning

(A) APPLICATION EXERCISES ANSWER KEY

Scenario: A nurse is caring for a client who is in skeletal traction for a fractured left femur. The client has been reporting abdominal pain and nausea over the past 24 hr. The nurse is beginning to suspect appendicitis and begins asking more questions about the pain.

1. Which of the following reports should support the nurse's suspicion of appendicitis?

    A. Nausea began prior to the pain.

    B. Pain began in the epigastric area, but has moved to the right lower quadrant.

    C. Pain in right lower quadrant is worse when pressure is applied and less when released.

    D. Pain is less after an episode of diarrhea.

    The order of the symptoms associated with appendicitis is important. Usually, pain precedes nausea and vomiting and begins in the periumbilical and epigastric region before moving to the lower right quadrant. During palpation, when pressure is applied, pain is worse when the pressure is released than when applied. Pain is also usually not related to bowel movements.

     NCLEX® Connection: Physiological Adaptation, Pathophysiology

2. The nurse determines that the client is experiencing appendicitis. When preparing the client for surgery, the nurse should anticipate which of the following interventions? (Select all that apply.)

    _____ Administer enema.

    __X__ **Maintain NPO status.**

    __X__ **Encourage semi-Fowler's position.**

    _____ Apply heat to the abdomen.

    __X__ **Verify informed consent is given.**

    The client should be maintained on NPO status and encouraged to maintain semi-Fowler's position to contain any abdominal drainage in the lower abdomen. The nurse should verify that the informed consent form has been signed. Enemas and heat to the abdomen are contraindicated because they can increase the risk of perforation.

    NCLEX® Connection: Reduction of Risk Potential, Potential for Complications from Surgical Procedures and Health Alterations

3. During surgery, the client's appendix has been found to have ruptured. Upon return to the unit, the client has an NG tube connected to low intermittent suction and an IV of 0.9% sodium chloride infusing at 100 mL/hr. In providing postoperative care, the nurse should anticipate assisting with which of the following interventions? (Select all that apply.)

    __X__ **Frequent monitoring of vital signs**

    __X__ **Administration of IV antibiotics**

    __X__ **Visualization of the incision at least every shift**

    _____ Administration of a full-liquid diet

    __X__ **Administration of opioid analgesics**

    __X__ **Measurement of hourly I&O**

    _____ Maintenance of bedrest with frequent repositioning

    Routine postoperative care includes monitoring of the abdominal incision for drainage and signs of infection, administering opioid analgesics as prescribed for pain, and the measurement of I&O for clients with an NG tube and IV infusion. Due to the rupture of the appendix, vital signs should be closely monitored for indications of infection and IV antibiotics will be given. A full-liquid diet is contraindicated for a client with an NG tube connected to suction. Progressive activity with ambulation is encouraged to facilitate peristalsis, promote postoperative recovery, and minimize the effects of immobility.

    NCLEX® Connection: Reduction of Risk Potential, Potential for Complications from Surgical Procedures and Health Alterations

UNIT 7	NURSING CARE OF CLIENTS WITH GASTROINTESTINAL DISORDERS
Section:	Lower Gastrointestinal Disorders
Chapter 46	Intestinal Obstruction

Overview

- Intestinal obstruction can result from mechanical or nonmechanical causes. Mechanical obstruction usually requires surgery.

- Symptoms vary according to location.

  o Higher-level obstructions have colicky, intermittent pain, and profuse vomiting.

  o Lower-level obstructions tend to have vague, diffused, constant pain and significant abdominal distention.

- Bowel sounds will be hyperactive above obstruction and hypoactive below.

- Obstructions of the small intestine are the most common.

- Treatment focuses on maintaining fluid and electrolyte balance, decompressing the bowel, and relief/removal of the obstruction.

Data Collection

- Risk Factors

  o Mechanical obstructions (90% of all obstructions) are the result of:

    ■ Encirclement or compression of intestine by adhesions, tumors, fibrosis (endometriosis), or strictures (Crohn's disease, radiation).

    ■ Twisting (volvulus) or telescoping (intussusception) of bowel segments.

    ■ Hernia (bowel becomes trapped in weakened area of abdominal wall).

    ■ Fecal impactions.

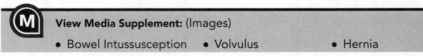

View Media Supplement: (Images)
- Bowel Intussusception • Volvulus • Hernia

  o Postsurgical adhesions are the most common cause of small bowel obstructions.

  o Carcinomas are the most common cause of large intestine obstructions.

- ○ Nonmechanical obstructions (paralytic ileus) are the result of decreased peristalsis secondary to:
  - ■ Neurogenic disorders (manipulation of the bowel during major surgery and spinal fracture).
  - ■ Vascular disorders (vascular insufficiency and mesenteric emboli).
  - ■ Electrolyte imbalances (hypokalemia).
  - ■ Inflammatory responses (peritonitis or sepsis).
  - ■ Diverticulitis and tumors are common causes of obstruction in older adult clients.
  - ■ Older adult clients are at a greater risk for fecal impactions. Bowel regimens can be effective in preventing impactions.
- Subjective and Objective Data
  - ○ Findings vary depending on the location of the obstruction.

SMALL BOWEL AND LARGE INTESTINE OBSTRUCTIONS	SMALL BOWEL OBSTRUCTIONS	LARGE INTESTINE OBSTRUCTIONS
Obstipation – the inability to pass a stool and/or flatus for more than 8 hr despite feeling the need to defecate	Pain is spasmodic and colicky	Pain is diffuse and constant
Abdominal distension	Visible peristaltic waves	Significant abdominal distension
High-pitched bowel sounds before site of obstruction (borborygmi) with hypoactive bowel sounds after, or overall hypoactive; absent bowel sounds later in process	Profuse, (projectile) sudden vomiting with fecal odor; vomiting relieves pain	Infrequent vomiting; clients can have diarrhea around an impaction

- ○ Laboratory tests
  - ■ May reveal signs of dehydration (elevated hemoglobin and hematocrit) and an elevated white blood cell count with bowel strangulation.
  - ■ Metabolic alkalosis with high obstruction of the small bowel, and metabolic acidosis with low obstruction of the large intestine
  - ■ Electrolytes
    - □ Small bowel obstruction — May have severe fluid and electrolyte imbalances
    - □ Large intestine obstruction — Usually has minimal fluid and electrolyte imbalances
- ○ Diagnostic procedures
  - ■ X-ray — Flat plate and upright abdominal x-rays evaluate the presence of free air and gas patterns.
  - ■ Endoscopy helps determine the cause of obstruction.
  - ■ Computed tomography scan helps determine the cause and exact location of the obstruction.

Collaborative Care

- Nursing Care
    - Nonmechanical cause of obstruction
        - Nothing by mouth with bowel rest
        - Check bowel sounds
        - Provide oral care
        - Intravenous fluid and electrolyte replacement (particularly potassium)
        - Pain management once a diagnosis is made
        - Ambulation
    - Mechanical cause of obstruction
        - Prepare clients for surgery and provide preoperative nursing care.
        - Withhold intake until peristalsis resumes.
- Therapeutic Procedures
    - Nasogastric tube to decompress the bowel
        - Nursing actions
            - Maintain intermittent suction as prescribed.
            - Check NG tube patency and irrigate every 4 hr, or as prescribed.
            - Measure gastric output.
            - Monitor nasal area for skin breakdown.
            - Monitor vital signs, skin integrity, weight, and I&O.
            - Clamp the NG tube while ambulating.
- Surgical Interventions
    - Exploratory laparotomy – Determine the cause of obstruction and rectify if possible.
        - Nursing actions
            - Provide pre and postoperative teaching and care.
            - Ensure clients understand the type of procedure (open or laparoscopic).
            - Monitor clients receiving IV fluid replacement and maintenance.
            - Monitor bowel sounds and document.
            - Maintain NG tube patency and measure output.
            - Clamp NG tube as prescribed to assess the client's tolerance prior to removing.
            - Advance diet as tolerated when prescribed beginning with clear liquids – clamp tube after eating for 1 to 2 hr.

- Client Outcomes
  - The client's bowel sounds will return.
  - The client will be able to eat and drink without nausea and vomiting.

Complications

- Dehydration (potential hypotension; small bowel obstruction)
  - Causes
    - Persistent vomiting
  - Nursing actions
    - Monitor the client's hydration through hematocrit, BUN, orthostatic vital signs, skin turgor/mucous membranes, urine output, and specific gravity. Notify the provider of a fluid imbalance.
    - Monitor clients receiving IV fluids.
- Electrolyte Imbalance (small bowel obstruction)
  - Causes
    - Persistent vomiting
  - Nursing actions
    - Monitor the client's electrolytes, especially potassium levels.
    - Notify the provider of an electrolyte imbalance.
    - Monitor clients receiving IV fluids.
- Metabolic Alkalosis
  - Causes
    - A higher-level obstruction due to a loss of hydrochloric acid and vomiting.
  - Nursing actions
    - Monitor clients for hypoventilation from compensatory action by the lungs (confusion, hypercarbia)
    - Obtain arterial blood gas.
    - Notify the provider of abnormal values.
- Metabolic Acidosis
  - Causes
    - A lower-level obstruction due to alkaline fluids not reabsorbed.
  - Nursing actions
    - Monitor clients for deep, rapid respirations (compensatory action by the lungs), confusion, hypotension, and flushed skin.
    - Obtain arterial blood gas.
    - Notify the provider of abnormal values.

Ⓐ **APPLICATION EXERCISES**

Scenario: A client who has a small bowel obstruction secondary to abdominal adhesions from a previous surgery is admitted to the hospital. The client has had several previous bowel obstructions but has been symptomatic with this exacerbation for the past 48 hr.

1. Which of the following findings should the nurse report to the provider? (Select all that apply.)

   _____ Urine specific gravity 1.040

   _____ Hematocrit 60%

   _____ Serum potassium 3.0 mEq/L

   _____ Oral temperature 38.5° C (99.5° F)

   _____ White blood cell count 9,800/mm³

2. A nasogastric tube (NG) is inserted as part of the treatment plan for the client. Which of the following actions is appropriate for the nurse to take? (Select all that apply.)

   _____ Subtract the NG drainage from the client's output.

   _____ Irrigate the NG with 20 mL 0.9% sodium chloride every 8 hr.

   _____ Check the client's abdomen for bowel sounds.

   _____ Provide the client with oral care as needed.

   _____ Clamp the NG while the client ambulates to the bathroom.

3. The nurse has been assigned another client who has a bowel obstruction. This client's obstruction is in the large intestine. Which of the following differences would the nurse expect between the client who has a small bowel obstruction and this client who has a large bowel obstruction? (Place an X in the box that correlates to the finding.)

FINDING	SMALL BOWEL OBSTRUCTION	LARGE BOWEL OBSTRUCTION
Pain is colicky in nature		
Peristaltic waves are visible		
Liquid diarrhea may be present		
Profuse vomiting is present		
Bowel sounds are high-pitched proximal to the obstruction		
Abdominal distension is present		
Vomitus has a fecal odor		
Pain is constant in nature		

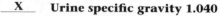

(A) APPLICATION EXERCISES ANSWER KEY

Scenario: A client who has a small bowel obstruction secondary to abdominal adhesions from a previous surgery is admitted to the hospital. The client has had several previous bowel obstructions but has been symptomatic with this exacerbation for the past 48 hr.

1. Which of the following findings should the nurse report to the provider? (Select all that apply.)

   X **Urine specific gravity 1.040**

   X **Hematocrit 60%**

   X **Serum potassium 3.0 mEq/L**

   _____ Oral temperature 38.5° C (99.5° F)

   _____ White blood cell count 9,800/mm³

   The urine specific gravity and hematocrit indicate significant dehydration and the potassium level is below the expected reference range. These findings should be reported to the provider. The temperature and white blood cell count are within the expected reference range.

   (N) NCLEX® Connection: Physiological Adaptation, Alterations in Body Systems

2. A nasogastric tube (NG) is inserted as part of the treatment plan for the client. Which of the following actions is appropriate for the nurse to take? (Select all that apply.)

   _____ Subtract the NG drainage from the client's output.

   _____ Irrigate the NG with 20 mL 0.9% sodium chloride every 8 hr.

   X **Check the client's abdomen for bowel sounds.**

   X **Provide the client with oral care as needed.**

   X **Clamp the NG while the client ambulates to the bathroom.**

   Nasogastric drainage, particularly in a small intestine obstruction, can be significant and is considered part of the output when planning fluid replacement. The NG is typically irrigated every 4 hr to maintain patency. Auscultating bowel sounds are part of the ongoing client data collection with an obstruction. An NG tube promotes mouth-breathing, and frequent oral care is needed. Clients can tolerate short-term clamping of the tube after the initial decompression; in fact, the client can be placed on a scheduled clamping routine before the tube is removed.

   (N) NCLEX® Connection: Physiological Adaptation, Alterations in Body Systems

3. The nurse has been assigned another client who has a bowel obstruction. This client's obstruction is in the large intestine. Which of the following differences would the nurse expect between the client who has a small bowel obstruction and this client who has a large bowel obstruction? (Place an X in the box that correlates to the finding.)

FINDING	SMALL BOWEL OBSTRUCTION	LARGE BOWEL OBSTRUCTION
Pain is colicky in nature	X	
Peristaltic waves are visible	X	
Liquid diarrhea may be present		X
Profuse vomiting is present	X	
Bowel sounds are high-pitched proximal to the obstruction	X	X
Abdominal distension is present	X	X
Vomitus has a fecal odor	X	
Pain is constant in nature		X

Ⓝ NCLEX® Connection: Physiological Adaptations, Basic Pathophysiology

UNIT 7	NURSING CARE OF CLIENTS WITH GASTROINTESTINAL DISORDERS
Section:	Lower Gastrointestinal Disorders
Chapter 47	Inflammatory Bowel Disease

Overview

- Inflammatory bowel disease (IBD) is an umbrella term that includes chronic inflammatory gastrointestinal (GI) diseases – ulcerative colitis, Crohn's disease, and diverticulitis. IBD is characterized by diarrhea (up to 20 stools during acute exacerbation), crampy abdominal pain, and exacerbations ("flare-ups")/remissions.

- Diverticulitis occurs when fecal matter becomes trapped in one or more diverticula resulting in inflammation and infection of the bowel mucosa. Diverticulosis is a condition that develops in the colon where small pouches form. Many clients with diverticulosis never develop diverticulitis.

DISORDER	DESCRIPTION OF DISEASE PROCESS	RELEVANT INFORMATION
Ulcerative colitis	• Edema and inflammation of the rectum may progress to the sigmoid colon and may expand the length of the colon. This usually begins in the rectum and the distal colon involving the mucosa and submucosa.	• Bowel obstruction may occur and intestinal mucosal cell changes may cause colon cancer.
Crohn's disease	• Crohn's disease is an inflammation and ulceration of the gastrointestinal tract, often at the distal ileum. • All bowel layers may become involved, and lesions are not continuous, but sporadic. • Fistulas are common with Crohn's disease.	• Crohn's disease can involve the entire GI tract from the mouth to the anus. • Malabsorption and malnutrition may develop when the jejunum and ileum become involved. Supplemental vitamins and minerals including vitamin B_{12} injections may be necessary.
Diverticulitis	• Diverticulitis is an inflammation of the diverticula (hernia in intestinal wall) that frequently occurs in the colon.	• Only about 10% of clients who have diverticula develop diverticulitis. Frequent episodes of inflammation from trapped feces or bacteria may lead to bleeding and infection. • Diverticula may bleed and the loss of blood may be minimal or severe. • Diverticula may perforate and cause peritonitis.

Data Collection

- Risk Factors

    o Genetics – Both ulcerative colitis and Crohn's disease are familial diseases.

    o Culture – Ulcerative colitis is higher in Caucasians and persons with a Jewish heritage.

    o Gender and age – The incidence of ulcerative colitis peaks at two points in life: adolescent to young adult (more often in females) and with older adults (more often in males).

        ▪ Crohn's disease may be diagnosed at any age.

        ▪ Diverticulitis occurs more often in older adults and affects men more frequently than women.

    o Diet – A diet low in fiber may predispose a client to ulcerative colitis and the development of diverticula.

    o Smoking – The incidence of ulcerative colitis is higher in nonsmokers.

    o Other factors – Stress, autoimmunity, and infection may be causative agents for both ulcerative colitis and Crohn's disease.

DISORDER	SUBJECTIVE DATA	OBJECTIVE DATA
Ulcerative colitis	• Abdominal pain/cramping – Often left lower quadrant pain • Anorexia and weight loss	• Fever • Diarrhea – May have up to 15 to 20 liquid stools/day • Mucus, blood, or pus may be present • Abdominal distension, tenderness and/or firmness upon palpitation • High-pitched bowel sounds • Rectal bleeding
Crohn's disease	• Abdominal pain/cramping – Often right-lower quadrant pain • Anorexia and weight loss	• Fever • Diarrhea – Five loose stools/day with mucous or pus • Abdominal distension, tenderness and/or firmness upon palpitation • High-pitched bowel sounds • Steatorrhea
Diverticulitis	• Abdominal pain in left-lower quadrant • Nausea and vomiting	• Fever • Chills • Tachycardia

LABORATORY FINDINGS			
LABORATORY TEST	**ULCERATIVE COLITIS**	**CROHN'S DISEASE**	**DIVERTICULITIS**
Hematocrit and hemoglobin	Decreased	Decreased	Decreased
Erythrocyte sedimentation rate (ESR)	Elevated	Elevated	–
WBC	Elevated	Elevated	Elevated
C-reactive protein	Elevated	Elevated	–
Platelet counts	Elevated	Elevated	–
Serum albumin	Decreased	Decreased	–
Folic acid and B_{12}	–	Decreased	–
pANCA (perinuclear anti-neutrophil cytoplasmic antibody	Elevated	–	–
Antiglycan antibody	–	Elevated	–
Stool for occult blood	May be positive	May be positive	Positive
Urinalysis	–	WBCs present	May have RBCs
K+, Mg, and Ca	Decreased	Decreased	–

- o Diagnostic procedures
  - ■ Abdominal x-ray and CT scan
  - ■ Barium enema – Barium is inserted into the rectum as a contrast medium for x-rays. This allows for the rectum and large intestine to be visualized, and is used to diagnose ulcerative colitis. A barium enema may show the presence of diverticulosis and is contraindicated in the presence of diverticulitis due to the risk of perforation.
  - ■ Colonoscopy (definitive for ulcerative colitis) and sigmoidoscopy – A lighted, flexible scope is inserted into the rectum to visualize the rectum and large intestine.
- o Findings
  - ■ Small intestine ulcerations and narrowing are consistent with Crohn's disease.
  - ■ Ulcerations and inflammation of the sigmoid colon and rectum are consistent with ulcerative colitis.
- o Nursing actions
  - ■ Monitor clients postprocedure for signs of bowel perforations (rectal bleeding, firm abdomen, tachycardia, hypotension).

○ Client education

■ Instruct clients to remain NPO after midnight and provide bowel preparation instructions.

■ Inform clients of possible abdominal discomfort and cramping during the barium enema.

Collaborative Care

- Nursing Care

  ○ Ulcerative colitis and Crohn's disease

  ■ Educate clients to eat foods that are high in protein and calories, and low in fiber. Clients may also take dietary supplements.

  ■ Instruct clients to avoid caffeine and alcohol, and take a multivitamin that contains iron.

  ■ Advise clients that small frequent meals may reduce the occurrence of symptoms.

  ■ Monitor clients for fluid and electrolyte imbalances, especially potassium due to frequent stools.

  ■ Educate clients regarding the use of vitamin supplements and B_{12} injections, if needed.

  ■ Assist clients in identifying foods that trigger symptoms.

  ■ Instruct clients to seek emergency care for signs of bowel obstruction or perforation (fever, severe abdominal pain, vomiting).

  ○ Diverticulitis

  ■ Clients with a mild case of diverticulitis may be treated at home. A health care provider may prescribe antibiotics, analgesics, antispasmodics, and rest.

  □ Instruct clients to limit oral intake to clear liquids initially, but may progress to a high-fiber, low-fat diet as tolerated.

  ■ Inpatient care includes:

  □ Maintaining NPO status

  □ Nasogastric suctioning

  □ Monitoring clients receiving IV fluids, IV antibiotics, total parenteral nutrition, and opioid analgesics for pain.

CLASSIFICATION/THERAPEUTIC INTENT	NURSING CONSIDERATIONS/CLIENT EDUCATION

5-aminosalicyllic acid (5-ASA)
• Sulfonamide
• Anti-inflammatory
   o Reduces inflammation of the intestinal mucosa
Medications:
• Sulfasalazine (Azulfidine)
• Olsalazine (Dipentum) for clients intolerant to sulfasalazine
Disorders:
• Ulcerative colitis
• Crohn's disease
	• Sulfasalazine is given orally.
	• These medications may be contraindicated if clients have a sulfa allergy.
	• Monitor CBC, renal, and hepatic function.
	• Advise clients of the following:
	   o Take with food.
	   o Avoid sun exposure.
	   o Increase fluid intake.
	   o Urine and skin may appear yellow or brown.
	   o Color may damage soft contact lenses. Notify the provider if sore throat, rash, bruising, and/or fever occur.

5-ASA • Anti-inflammatory Medication: • Mesalamine (Asacol, Pentasa, Rowasa) Disorder: • Ulcerative colitis	• Asacol and Pentasa may be given orally. • Rowasa is given by retention enema or rectal suppository. • These medications may be contraindicated if clients have a sulfa allergy. • Monitor CBC, renal, and hepatic function. • Clients should retain the suppository for at least 1 hr to promote effectiveness. • Clients should retain rectal suspension for at least 4 hr. • Inform clients to report headache or gastrointestinal problems (abdominal discomfort, diarrhea).

Corticosteroids
• Used to reduce inflammation and pain
Medications:
• Prednisone (Deltasone)
• Budesonide (Entocort)
• Hydrocortisone Enema (Cortenema)
• Rectal foam (Cortifoam)
• IV corticosteroids for fulminant disease (occurring suddenly)
Disorders:
• Ulcerative colitis
• Crohn's disease
	• Use corticosteroids in low doses to minimize adverse effects.
	• Monitor blood pressure.
	• Reduce systemic dose slowly.
	• Monitor electrolytes and blood glucose levels.
	• This medication may be slow-healing.
	• Advise clients to:
	   o Take oral dose with food.
	   o Avoid discontinuing dose suddenly.
	   o Report unexpected increase in weight or other signs of fluid retention.
	   o Avoid crowds and other exposures to infectious diseases.

CLASSIFICATION/THERAPEUTIC INTENT	NURSING CONSIDERATIONS/CLIENT EDUCATION
Immunosuppressants • The mechanism of action in treatment of IBD is unknown. Medication: • Cyclosporine (Sandimmune) and methotrexate (Rheumatrex) for severe refractory disease (resistant to treatment) Disorders: • Ulcerative colitis • Crohn's disease	• Reinforce to clients to avoid crowds and other chances of exposures to infectious diseases. • Advise clients to monitor for signs of bleeding, bruising, or infection. • Monitor kidney and hepatic function.
Immunomodulators • Acts by suppressing the immune response • An antibody used to reduce tumor necrosis factor Medications: • Infliximab (Remicade) • Certolizumab (Cimzia) Disorders: • Crohn's disease • Ulcerative colitis	• Many adverse effects are possible, including chills, fever, hypertension, dysrhythmias, and low levels of blood cells. • Monitor liver enzymes and hemoglobin and hematocrit. • Teach clients to avoid crowds and other environments that can increase exposure to infectious diseases. Clients are at risk for development or reactivation of tuberculosis. • Advise clients to monitor for signs of bleeding, bruising, or infection.
Antidiarrheals • Used to suppress the number of stools Medications: • Diphenoxylate hydrochloride and atropine (Lomotil) • Loperamide (Imodium) Disorders: • Crohn's disease • Ulcerative colitis	• These medications are used to decrease risk of fluid volume deficit and electrolyte imbalance. They also reduce discomfort. • Observe clients for signs of respiratory depression, especially in older adult clients. • Observe clients for signs of toxic megacolon (hypotension, abdominal distension, decrease or absence of bowel sounds). • Reinforce to clients to avoid hazardous activities until the response to the medication is established.
Antibiotics used to treat infections • Metronidazole (Flagyl) • Ciprofloxacin (Cipro)	

- Interdisciplinary Care

  ○ Refer clients for nutritional counseling.

  ○ Clients may benefit from complementary therapy (biofeedback, massage, yoga).

  ○ Clients may need a mental health referral for assistance with coping.

- Surgical Interventions
  - Surgical procedure for ulcerative colitis
    - Colectomy with or without ileostomy
  - Surgical procedures for Crohn's disease
    - Stricturoplasty may be performed laparoscopically in some cases
    - Surgical repair of fistulas or in response to other complications related to the disease (perforation)
  - Surgical procedures for diverticulitis
    - Colectomy, which may or may not include a colostomy that may be temporary
  - Preoperative care
    - Reinforce teaching on the type of surgery to be performed.
    - If the creation of stoma is planned, collaborate with an enterostomal therapy nurse regarding care related to the stoma.
    - Administer antibiotic bowel prep (neomycin sulfate), if prescribed.
    - Administer cleansing enema or laxative, if prescribed.
  - Postoperative care
    - Perform routine postoperative care.
    - Maintain clients on NPO status.
    - Monitor nasogastric tube with suction, unless the surgery was performed laparoscopically.
    - Monitor clients with an ileostomy for fluid volume deficit. An ileostomy may drain as much as 1,000 mL/day.
- Care after discharge
  - Client education
    - Request a referral for clients with an ostomy to an enterostomal therapist and to an ostomate support group.
- Client outcomes
  - The client's bowel elimination patterns will improve.
  - The client will be able to carry out ADLs.
  - The client's nutritional status will improve.
  - The client will identify family and community resources to aid in coping with a chronic illness.

Complications

- Bleeding

  - Bleeding occurs due to deterioration of the bowel.

    - Nursing actions

      - Observe clients for indications of rectal bleeding.

      - Monitor vital signs.

      - Check laboratory values, especially hematocrit, hemoglobin, and coagulation factors.

      - Administer oxygen as prescribed. Turn, cough, deep-breathe.

      - Maintain and monitor nasogastric suction.

      - Keep clients NPO.

      - Monitor fluid and electrolyte status (be alert for signs of hypovolemia).

      - Monitor clients receiving IV antibiotics.

      - If surgery is performed:

        - Monitor intake and output every hour immediately after surgery.

        - Use sterile technique to irrigate the peritoneal area via a catheter or drain (if ordered by the provider).

    - Client education

      - Instruct clients to report rectal bleeding.

      - Explain to clients the importance of bed rest.

- Toxic megacolon:

  - Toxic megacolon occurs due to inactivity of the colon. Massive dilation of the colon occurs and clients are at risk for perforation.

    - Nursing actions

      - Maintain nasogastric suction.

      - Monitor clients receiving IV fluids and electrolytes.

      - Administer prescribed medications (antibiotics, corticosteroids).

      - Prepare clients for surgery (usually an ileostomy) if clients do not begin to show signs of improvement within 72 hr or less.

IRRITABLE BOWEL SYNDROME

Overview

- IBS differs from IBD in that it does not cause structural damage to the GI tract and does not involve an inflammatory process.

- Additionally, it does not predispose clients to cancer.

Data Collection

- Risk Factors

  - Female

  - Stress

  - Eating large meals containing a large amount of fat

  - Caffeine

  - Alcohol

- Subjective and Objective Data

  - Physical assessment findings

    - Cramping pain in abdomen

    - Abdominal pain due to changes in bowel pattern and consistency

    - Nausea with meals or passing stool

    - Anorexia

    - Abdominal bloating

    - Belching

    - Diarrhea

    - Constipation

- Laboratory Tests

  - CBC, serum albumin, erythrocyte sedimentation rate (ESR), and occult stools are all laboratory findings that are obtained with clients with IBS.

- Diagnostic Tests

  - Difficult to diagnose with specific tests. A diagnosis is made by the presence of specific characteristics including: abdominal pain accompanied by changes in bowel patterns, abdominal distention, feeling that defecation is not complete, and the presence of mucus with stools.

Collaborative Care

- Nursing Care

  - Reinforce strategies to reduce stress.

  - Instruct clients to limit the intake of irritating agents (gas-forming foods, caffeine, alcohol).

  - Encourage a diet high in fiber.

Medications

- Alosetron (Lotronex) – An IBS-specific medication that selectively blocks 5-HT4 receptors, which innervate the viscera and result in increased firmness in stools, and decrease the urgency and frequency of defecation.

  o Indicated for irritable bowel syndrome with diarrhea (IBS-D) in women that has lasted more than 6 months and is resistant to conventional management.

  o Nursing considerations

    ▪ This medication is contraindicated for clients with chronic constipation, history of bowel obstruction, Crohn's disease, ulcerative colitis, impaired intestinal circulation, or thrombophlebitis.

    ▪ The dosage will start as once a day and may be increased to BID.

  o Client education

    ▪ Instruct clients that symptoms should resolve within 1 to 4 weeks, but will return 1 week after medication is discontinued.

- Lubiprostone (Amitiza) – An IBS-specific medication that increases fluid secretion in the intestine to promote intestinal motility. This is indicated for irritable bowel syndrome with constipation (IBS-C).

  o Nursing considerations

    ▪ These medications are contraindicated for clients with a history of bowel obstruction, Crohn's disease, ulcerative colitis, or diverticulitis.

  o Client education

    ▪ Instruct clients to take with food to decrease nausea.

- Care After Discharge

  o Encourage clients to avoid food that contains dairy, eggs, and wheat products.

  o Encourage clients to avoid alcoholic and caffeinated beverages. Beverages containing fructose and sorbitol should be avoided.

  o Encourage clients to drink 2 to 3 L/fluid per day from food and fluid sources.

  o Encourage clients to increase the amount of daily fiber intake (approximately 30 to 40 mg/day).

- Client Outcomes

  o The client's bowel elimination patterns will improve.

  o The client will be able to carry out ADLs.

  o The client's nutritional status will improve.

(A) APPLICATION EXERCISES

Scenario: A client who has Crohn's disease has been admitted for an acute exacerbation. A nurse is reviewing the laboratory findings for the client.

1. Which of the following laboratory results should the nurse expect to find elevated in the client? (Select all that apply.)

   _____ Hematocrit

   _____ Erythrocyte sedimentation rate (ESR)

   _____ WBC

   _____ Folic acid

   _____ Serum albumin

2. Sulfasalazine (Azulfidine) has been prescribed to treat the client's exacerbation of Crohn's disease. Which of the following statements should the nurse reinforce when explaining how to take the medication?

   A. "Take the medication 1 or 2 hr after eating."

   B. "Please let me know if you are allergic to penicillin."

   C. "Notify your provider if you experience a sore throat."

   D. "Your stools may turn black in color."

3. A client who has muscular dystrophy and resides in an extended care facility is experiencing an exacerbation of irritable bowel disease (IBD). The client has been placed on lubiprostone (Amitiza). The client's diet has been suspected as being a contributing factor in relation to the recurring episodes of irritable bowel disease (IBD). Which of the following foods should be eliminated from the client's diet? (Select all that apply.)

   _____ Nuts

   _____ Milk

   _____ Bread

   _____ Yogurt

   _____ Custard

   _____ Diet colas

   _____ Grapefruit juice

4. A nurse is reinforcing the type of diet a client who has chronic diverticulosis should eat. Which of the following should the nurse recommend?

    A. Low residue

    B. High fiber

    C. Low carbohydrate

    D. High protein

(A) APPLICATION EXERCISES ANSWER KEY

Scenario: A client who has Crohn's disease has been admitted for an acute exacerbation. A nurse is reviewing the laboratory findings for the client.

1. Which of the following laboratory results should the nurse expect to find elevated in the client? (Select all that apply.)

   _____ Hematocrit

   __X__ **Erythrocyte sedimentation rate (ESR)**

   __X__ **WBC**

   _____ Folic acid

   _____ Serum albumin

   In Crohn's disease, the ESR and WBC are elevated due to the inflammatory aspects of the disease. The hematocrit is low due to chronic blood loss. Malabsorption leads to a decrease in folic acid and serum albumin.

   (N) NCLEX® Connection: Physiological Adaptation, Pathophysiology

2. Sulfasalazine (Azulfidine) has been prescribed to treat the client's exacerbation of Crohn's disease. Which of the following statements should the nurse reinforce when explaining how to take the medication?

   A. "Take the medication 1 or 2 hr after eating."

   B. "Please let me know if you are allergic to penicillin."

   C. "Notify your provider if you experience a sore throat."

   D. "Your stools may turn black in color."

   The immune system of a client who is taking sulfasalazine (Azulfidine) can become depressed and subsequently more vulnerable to infection. Therefore, the client should notify the provider about signs of infection. The medication should be taken with food. The medication can be contraindicated if the client is allergic to sulfa. There is no contraindication with an allergy to penicillin. This medication does not cause a change in the color of the stool.

   (N) NCLEX® Connection: Pharmacological Therapies, Adverse Effects/Contraindications/Side Effects/Interactions

3. A client who has muscular dystrophy and resides in an extended care facility is experiencing an exacerbation of irritable bowel disease (IBD). The client has been placed on lubiprostone (Amitiza). The client's diet has been suspected as being a contributing factor in relation to the recurring episodes of irritable bowel disease (IBD). Which of the following foods should be eliminated from the client's diet? (Select all that apply.)

_____	Nuts	
X	**Milk**	
X	**Bread**	
X	**Yogurt**	
X	**Custard**	
X	**Diet colas**	
_____	Grapefruit juice	

Foods containing dairy, eggs, and wheat products as well as caffeine, fructose, and sorbitol should be avoided. Nuts and grapefruit juice are not dietary restrictions for a client who has IBD.

(N) NCLEX® Connection: Basic Care and Comfort, Nutrition and Oral Hydration

4. A nurse is reinforcing the type of diet a client who has chronic diverticulosis should eat. Which of the following should the nurse recommend?

A. Low residue

B. High fiber

C. Low carbohydrate

D. High protein

A client who has diverticulosis should eat a high-fiber diet to prevent constipation and promote soft stools. If the client develops an inflamed diverticulum, the client can be placed on NPO status initially and then progressed to a low-fiber diet as tolerated. A high-fiber diet should be resumed when the diverticulitis has resolved. A low-residue diet, low-carbohydrate, or high-protein diet are not appropriate for a client with diverticulosis.

(N) NCLEX® Connection: Basic Care and Comfort, Nutrition and Oral Hydration

UNIT 7	NURSING CARE OF CLIENTS WITH GASTROINTESTINAL DISORDERS
Section:	Lower Gastrointestinal Disorders
Chapter 48	Colorectal Cancer

Overview

- Colorectal cancer (CRC) is cancer of the rectum or colon. Most CRCs are adenocarcinoma, a tumor that arises from a gland in the epithelial layer of the colon.

- Adenocarcinoma grows slowly and begins as a polyp. If caught early when it is still benign, it can be removed during a colonoscopy. If left untreated, the polyp will grow and the risk of malignancy increases. Many times, the client is asymptomatic but occult blood is discovered in the stool during a rectal exam.

- CRC can metastasize (through blood or lymph) to the liver (most common), lungs, brain, or bones. Spreading can occur as a result of peritoneal seeding (during surgical resection of tumor).

- The most common location of CRC is the rectosigmoidal region.

Data Collection

- Risk Factors

    o Adenomatous colon polyps

    o Family history of CRC

    o Inflammatory Bowel Disease (ulcerative colitis, Crohn's disease)

    o High-fat, low-fiber diet

    o Older than 50 years of age

- Subjective and Objective Data

    o Blood in stool

    o Change in bowel habits (constipation, diarrhea)

    o Cramps and/or gas

        ▪ Palpable mass

        ▪ Weight loss and fatigue

        ▪ Vomiting

- Abdominal distention
- Abnormal bowel sounds indicative of obstruction (high-pitched tingling bowel sounds)
  - Laboratory tests
    - Fecal Occult Blood Test (FOBT) – Two stool samples within three consecutive days. False-positive results can occur with the ingestion of certain foods or drugs. In general, meat, NSAIDs, and vitamin C are avoided for the 48 hr prior to testing.
    - Carcinoembryonic Antigen (CEA) serum test – CEA levels are elevated in most individuals with CRC.
    - Hct and Hgb decreased due to intermittent bleeding
  - Diagnostic procedures
    - Sigmoidoscopy/Colonoscopy provides a definitive diagnosis of CRC.
      - This scope procedure permits visualization of tumors, removal of polyps, and tissue biopsy.
    - Barium enemas; computed tomography (CT) and magnetic resonance imaging (MRI) scans of the chest, abdomen, pelvis, lungs, and liver; chest x-rays may be done to further identify the specific location of cancer and to identify sites of metastases.

Collaborative Care

- Surgical Interventions
  - Colon resection, colectomy, colostomy, and abdominoperineal (AP) resection surgeries may be performed to remove all or portions of CRC.
  - CRC occurs in stages from 0 to IV according to the tissue depth of the lesion, and whether it has spread to local or distant sites.
  - Colectomy (surgical removal of part of the colon) with an end-to-end anastomosis or placement of external stoma is performed
  - An external stoma or colostomy may be temporary or permanent.
  - Nursing actions
    - Provide postoperative care to prevent complications.
    - Postoperatively, if clients have a stoma, observe the color and integrity of the stoma (an immediate postoperative stoma should be reddish pink, moist, and may have a small amount of visible blood; report any evidence of stoma ischemia or necrosis).

 View Media Supplement: Healthy Stoma (Image)

    - Maintain nasogastric suction (decompression).
    - Slowly progress the diet after nasogastric suctioning is discontinued, and monitor the client's response and bowel sounds.

- ○ Reinforce client education regarding activity limits (no lifting; use stool softeners to avoid straining).

- ○ Provide ostomy teaching (signs of ischemia to report, expected output, appliance management) if applicable.

 View Media Supplement: Ostomy Appliance (Image)

- ○ Support clients who are experiencing disturbed body image.

- Client Education

  - ○ Preoperatively

    - Instruct clients regarding preoperative diet (clear liquids several days prior to surgery).

    - Instruct clients to complete bowel prep with cathartics as prescribed.

    - Inform clients of the administration of antibiotics (neomycin, metronidazole [Flagyl]) to eradicate intestinal flora.

  - ○ Postoperatively

    - Instruct clients regarding the care of the incision, activity limits, and ostomy care, if applicable.

- Interdisciplinary Care

  - ○ Stoma nurse referral for instruction on care of colostomy

  - ○ Request referral to ostomy support group

- Therapeutic Procedures

  - ○ Chemotherapy

    - Classification and therapeutic intent

      - □ Adjuvant therapy may be given to decrease the chance of metastases for stage II, and distant metastases for type III cancers.

      - □ If stage IV cancer is found, chemotherapy is routinely given.

      - □ Targeted medication therapy – Monoclonal antibodies (MABs)

      - □ Angiogenesis inhibitors (inhibits growth of new blood vessels to tumors) – bevacizumab (Avastin)

      - □ Tyrosine kinase inhibitors (decreases cell proliferation and increases cell death of certain cancers) – Cetuximab (Erbitux) and panitumumab (Vectibix)

    - Radiation therapy

      - □ Radiation therapy is given in conjunction with chemotherapy to improve prognosis (usually used for rectal cancer to prevent lymph node involvement and recurrence).

- Care After Discharge
    - Client education
        - Recommend clients 50 yr of age or older to have regular colorectal screenings and fecal occult blood tests annually and more frequently if there is a family history of CRC.
        - Recommend clients to undergo a colonoscopy every 10 years after a baseline colonoscopy. If polyps are found, colonoscopies need to be done more frequently.
        - Suggest clients eat a diet high in fruits, vegetables, and whole grains.
        - Suggest clients decrease the intake of fats and meat proteins.
        - Recommend clients drink alcohol in moderation and stop smoking.
- Client Outcomes
    - The client will be cancer-free without recurrence for 5 years.
    - The client will adapt to bowel redirective surgery (colostomy).

Complications

- Recurrence
    - Causes
        - Recurrence of tumor at surgical or distant site (metastasis)
    - Nursing actions
        - Support clients with prognosis.
        - Ensure that clients understand treatment options.

Ⓐ APPLICATION EXERCISES

Scenario: A nurse is caring for an older adult client who has a preliminary diagnosis of colon cancer.

1. The nurse is collecting data from the client. Which of the following data are risks for colon cancer? (Select all that apply.)

    _____ Family history of colorectal cancer

    _____ Personal history of Crohn's disease

    _____ Consumption of a diet low in fat

    _____ Consumption of a diet high in fiber

    _____ Age

    _____ Gluten intolerance

2. Which of the following diagnostic tests will provide a definitive diagnosis for colorectal cancer (CRC)?

    A. Fecal occult blood test

    B. Colonoscopy

    C. Intravenous pyelogram

    D. Carcinoembryonic Antigen (CEA) serum test

3. The client is now postoperative following a colon resection with placement of a transverse colostomy with nasogastric tube placement. Postoperative care of the client by the nurse should include which of the following? (Select all that apply.)

    _____ Report serosanguineous discharge from the stoma.

    _____ Administer opioid analgesics for pain.

    _____ Start clear liquid diet.

    _____ Provide wound care using surgical aseptic technique.

    _____ Maintain patency of nasogastric tube.

(A) APPLICATION EXERCISES ANSWER KEY

Scenario: A nurse is caring for an older adult client who has a preliminary diagnosis of colon cancer.

1. The nurse is collecting data from the client. Which of the following data are risks for colon cancer? (Select all that apply.)

__X__	**Family history of colorectal cancer**
__X__	**Personal history of Crohn's disease**
_____	Consumption of a diet low in fat
_____	Consumption of a diet high in fiber
__X__	**Age**
_____	Gluten intolerance

    A family history of colorectal cancer, personal history of an inflammatory bowel disease such as Crohn's, and age over 50 are all risk factors for colorectal cancer. The consumption of a diet low in fat and high in fiber is protective against colorectal cancer. There is no relationship between gluten intolerance and colorectal cancer.

    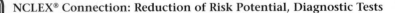 NCLEX® Connection: Physiological Adaptations, Basic Pathophysiology

2. Which of the following diagnostic tests will provide a definitive diagnosis for colorectal cancer (CRC)?

    A. Fecal occult blood test

    B. Colonoscopy

    C. Intravenous pyelogram

    D. Carcinoembryonic Antigen (CEA) serum test

    A colonoscopy is a procedure which permits visualization of tumors, removal of polyps, and tissue biopsy and can provide a definitive diagnosis for CRC. A fecal occult blood test will indicate if there is blood present in the stool, but blood is not always caused by CRC. CEA levels are elevated in most individuals with CRC but is not specific to CRC. An intravenous pyelogram is used to diagnose abnormalities of the urinary system.

    (N) NCLEX® Connection: Reduction of Risk Potential, Diagnostic Tests

3. The client is now postoperative following a colon resection with placement of a transverse colostomy with nasogastric tube placement. Postoperative care of the client by the nurse should include which of the following? (Select all that apply.)

    _____   Report serosanguineous discharge from the stoma.

    __X__   **Administer opioid analgesics for pain.**

    _____   Start clear liquid diet.

    __X__   **Provide wound care using surgical aseptic technique.**

    __X__   **Maintain patency of nasogastric tube.**

Pain should be routinely monitored, treated, and evaluated for treatment efficacy and can be managed with opioid analgesics. Use surgical aseptic technique for wound care to prevent infection. The nasogastric tube should remain patent to maintain decompression of the gastrointestinal tract. The client's stoma should be reddish pink in color, moist, and may have a small amount of serosanguineous drainage during the first few days after surgery. Oral intake should be delayed until the nasogastric tube is discontinued, but will usually start with ice chips, then progress to clear liquids, and will be advanced as tolerated.

Ⓝ NCLEX® Connection: Physiological Adaptation, Alterations in Body Systems

UNIT 7	NURSING CARE OF CLIENTS WITH GASTROINTESTINAL DISORDERS
Section:	Gallbladder and Pancreas Disorders
Chapter 49	Cholecystitis and Cholelithiasis

Overview

- Cholecystitis is an inflammation of the gallbladder wall.

- Cholecystitis is most often caused by gallstones (cholelithiasis) obstructing the cystic and/ or common bile ducts (bile flow from the gallbladder to the duodenum) causing bile to back up and the gallbladder to become inflamed.

- Cholelithiasis is the presence of stones in the gallbladder related to either the precipitation of bile or cholesterol into stones.

- Bile is used for the digestion of fats. It is produced in the liver and stored in the gallbladder.

- Cholecystitis can be acute or chronic, and can obstruct the pancreatic duct causing pancreatitis. It can also cause the gallbladder to rupture with secondary peritonitis.

Data Collection

- Risk Factors

  o   More common in females

  o   High-fat diet

  o   Obesity (impaired fat metabolism, high cholesterol levels)

  o   Genetic predisposition

  o   Older than 60 years of age (more likely to develop gallstones)

  o   Individuals who have type 1 diabetes mellitus (high triglycerides)

  o   Low-calorie, liquid protein diets

  o   Rapid weight loss (increases cholesterol)

- Subjective Data

  o   An episode of cholecystitis is characterized by:

  ▪   Sharp pain in the right upper quadrant of the abdomen, often radiating to the right shoulder

  ▪   Pain with deep inspiration during right subcostal palpation (Murphy's sign)

- Intense pain (increased heart rate, pallor, diaphoresis) caused by biliary colic with nausea and vomiting after ingestion of a large quantity of high-fat food
- Rebound tenderness
- Dyspepsia, eructation (belching), and flatulence
- Fever

- Objective Data

  - Physical assessment findings

    - Jaundice, clay-colored stools, steatorrhea (fatty stools), dark urine, and pruritus (accumulation of bile salts in the skin) may be seen in clients with chronic cholecystitis (due to biliary obstruction).
    - Older adult clients may have diabetes mellitus and have atypical presentations of cholecystitis (absence of pain or fever).

  - Laboratory tests

    - White blood cell count (elevations with left shift indicate inflammation)
    - Direct, indirect, and total serum bilirubin (elevated if bile duct obstruction)
    - Amylase and lipase (elevated if pancreatic involvement)
    - Aspartate aminotransferase (AST), lactate dehydrogenase (LDH), and alkaline phosphatase (elevated if liver dysfunction) may indicate the common bile duct is obstructed.
    - Serum cholesterol (elevated above 200 mg/dL)

  - Diagnostic procedures

    - A right-upper quadrant (RUQ) ultrasound visualizes gallstones and a dilated common bile duct.
    - An abdominal x-ray or CT scan can visualize calcified gallstones and an enlarged gall bladder.
    - A hepatobiliary scan (HIDA) assesses the patency of the biliary duct system after an IV injection of contrast.
    - An endoscopic retrograde cholangiopancreatography (ERCP) allows for direct visualization through the use of an endoscope that is inserted through the esophagus and into the common bile duct via the duodenum. A sphincterotomy with gallstone removal may be done during this procedure.
    - A percutaneous transhepatic cholangiography involves the direct injection of contrast into the biliary tract through the use of a flexible needle. The gallbladder and ducts can be visualized.

Collaborative Care

- Nursing Care

  - Administer analgesics as needed and prescribed.

- Medications

  - Meperidine (Demerol) or hydromorphone (Dilaudid) are analgesics that are preferred over morphine, as morphine sulfate may increase biliary spasms.

    - Analgesic and biliary antispasmodic

    - Nursing considerations

      - Monitor for seizures in older adults receiving meperidine.

  - Anticholinergics – dicyclomine (Bentyl)

    - Decrease ductal tone and biliary spasms

    - Nursing considerations

      - Monitor for constipation and urinary hesitancy/retention.

      - Monitor for confusion in older adults.

  - Bile acid – Chenodiol (Chenix), ursodiol (Ursodeoxycholic Acid)

    - Bile acid used to gradually dissolve cholesterol-based gallstones

    - Nursing considerations

      - Chenodiol – Monitor for excessive diarrhea and hepatotoxicity.

      - Ursodiol has few side effects.

    - Client education

      - Chenodiol – Inform clients that routine liver function tests must be done.

- Therapeutic Procedures

  - Extracorporeal shock wave lithotripsy (ESWL) – Shock waves are used to break up stones. This may be used more on nonsurgical candidates who have small, cholesterol-based stones and are not overweight.

    - Nursing actions

      - Prepare clients for immersion in water (fluid-filled bag may be used in place of immersion).

    - Client education

      - Inform clients that several procedures may be required to break up all stones.

      - Inform client that some hematuria may be present and to notify the provider if bleeding is excessive.

      - Instruct clients to avoid aspirin products.

- Surgical Interventions

  - Cholecystectomy – Removal of the gallbladder with a laparoscopic or an open approach

  - The client is usually discharged within 24 hr if a laparoscopic approach is used. An open approach requires the client to be hospitalized for 2 to 3 days.

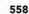

- Nursing actions
  - □ Laparoscopic approach
    - ▸ Provide immediate postoperative care.

  ⓜ View Media Supplement: Laparoscopic Cholecystectomy (Image)

  - □ Open approach
    - ▸ A T-tube may be placed in the common bile duct. This is only required when there is exploration of the common bile duct intraoperatively.
  - □ Provide postoperative care to prevent complications
  - □ Instruct clients to turn, cough and deep-breathe, splint incision
  - □ Instruct clients to use incentive spirometry every 1 to 2 hr
  - □ Promote early ambulation.
  - □ Care of the T-tube
    - ▸ Monitor and record drainage (initially bloody, then green-brown bile).
    - ▸ Initially, the T-tube may drain more than 400 mL/day and then gradually decrease in amount.
    - ▸ Instruct clients to report an absence of drainage with symptoms of nausea and pain (may indicate obstruction in the T-tube).
    - ▸ Instruct clients to report sudden increases in drainage or amounts exceeding 1,000 mL/day.
    - ▸ Inspect the surrounding skin for signs of infection or bile leakage.
    - ▸ Maintain flow by gravity and do not raise above level of gallbladder.
    - ▸ Empty the drainage bag every 8 hr.
    - ▸ Clamp the tube 1 to 2 hr before and after meals to assess the tolerance to food post-cholecystectomy, and prior to removal.
    - ▸ Observe stools for color (stools will be clay-colored until biliary flow is reestablished).
    - ▸ Monitor for bile peritonitis (pain, fever, jaundice).
    - ▸ Monitor and document the client's response to food.
- Client education
  - □ Laparoscopic approach
    - ▸ Reinforce to clients regarding pain from the carbon dioxide that is used to fill the abdomen during the procedure (under the right clavicle, shoulder, scapula), and that ambulation is helpful for this type of pain.
    - ▸ Instruct clients regarding pain control and incision care.
    - ▸ Instruct clients regarding complications (infection, bile leak [pain, vomiting, abdominal distension]).
    - ▸ Instruct clients that activities are often resumed in 1 week.

- □ Open approach
  - ▸ Inform clients regarding activity precautions for 4 to 6 weeks.
  - ▸ Tell clients that the T-tube is usually left in 1 to 2 weeks postoperatively.
  - ▸ Instruct clients to report sudden increase in drainage, foul odor, pain, fever, or jaundice.
  - ▸ Instruct clients to take showers instead of baths until T-tube is removed.
  - ▸ Tell clients to clamp T-tube 1 to 2 hr before and after meals as prescribed to prepare for removal.
  - ▸ Inform clients that the color of stools should return to brown in about a week, and diarrhea is common.
- ■ Dietary counseling
  - □ Encourage a low-fat diet (reduce dairy and avoid fried foods, chocolate, nuts, gravy).
  - □ Promote weight reduction.
  - □ Avoid gas-forming foods (beans, cabbage, cauliflower, broccoli).
  - □ Small, frequent meals may be tolerated.
- ● Care After Discharge
  - ○ Encourage clients to maintain ideal weight.
  - ○ Encourage clients to avoid heavy lifting.
- ● Client Outcomes
  - ○ The client will resume a regular diet without experiencing abdominal pain.
  - ○ The client's lipid profile will be within the expected reference range.

Complications

- ● Obstruction of the bile duct (pre-surgery)
  - ○ This can cause ischemia, gangrene, and a rupture of the gallbladder wall. A rupture of the gallbladder wall can cause a local abscess or peritonitis (rigid, board-like abdomen, guarding), which requires a surgical intervention and administration of broad spectrum antibiotics.
- ● Bile Peritonitis (post-surgery)
  - ○ This can occur if adequate amounts of bile are not drained from the surgical site. This is a rare complication, but it may be fatal.
  - ○ Nursing actions
    - ■ Monitor clients for pain, fever, and jaundice.
    - ■ Report to the provider immediately.

Ⓐ APPLICATION EXERCISES

Scenario: A client who has severe upper abdominal pain following a family dinner celebration is admitted. She reports vomiting once, frequent belching, and is febrile. Cholecystitis is suspected.

1. Which of the following foods might have triggered the cholecystitis attack? (Select all that apply.)

    _____ Ice cream

    _____ Brownie with nuts

    _____ Fruit salad

    _____ Turkey

    _____ Broccoli with cheese sauce

    _____ Potatoes and gravy

    _____ Deviled eggs and mayonnaise

2. Which of the following laboratory results should the nurse expect if the client is diagnosed with cholecystitis?

    _____ Clay-colored stools

    _____   Pale, yellow urine

    _____ Elevated WBC count

    _____ Decreased serum cholesterol level

    _____ Yellow sclera

3. The client undergoes an open cholecystectomy with T-tube placement. Which of the following instructions should the nurse reinforce when providing discharge teaching? (Select all that apply.)

    _____ Take baths rather than showers.

    _____ Clamp T-tube for 1 to 2 hr before and after meals.

    _____ Keep the drainage system at the level of the gallbladder.

    _____ Avoid heavy lifting and strenuous activities.

    _____ Empty drainage bag every 8 hr.

(A) **APPLICATION EXERCISES ANSWER KEY**

> **Scenario:** A client who has severe upper abdominal pain following a family dinner celebration is admitted. She reports vomiting once, frequent belching, and is febrile. Cholecystitis is suspected.

1. Which of the following foods might have triggered the cholecystitis attack? (Select all that apply.)

   __X__   **Ice cream**

   __X__   **Brownie with nuts**

   _____   Fruit salad

   _____   Turkey

   __X__   **Broccoli with cheese sauce**

   __X__   **Potatoes and gravy**

   __X__   **Deviled eggs and mayonnaise**

   Foods high in fat, such as ice cream, brownies, cheese sauce, gravy, and mayonnaise, could precipitate an attack of cholecystitis and should be avoided. Foods not high in fat, such as fruit and turkey, are usually better tolerated.

   (N) **NCLEX® Connection: Basic Care and Comfort Nutrition and Oral Hydration**

2. Which of the following laboratory results should the nurse expect if the client is diagnosed with cholecystitis?

   __X__   **Clay-colored stools**

   _____   Pale, yellow urine

   __X__   **Elevated WBC count**

   _____   Decreased serum cholesterol level

   __X__   **Yellow sclera**

   Clay-colored stools indicate bile is not being secreted into the small intestine due to biliary obstruction. An elevated WBC count indicates inflammation. Yellow sclera indicates jaundice secondary to an elevated bilirubin. Urine will likely be dark in color, and serum cholesterol levels will be elevated.

   (N) **NCLEX® Connection: Physiological Adaptation, Pathophysiology**

3. The client undergoes an open cholecystectomy with T-tube placement. Which of the following instructions should the nurse reinforce when providing discharge teaching? (Select all that apply.)

_____ Take baths rather than showers.

__X__ **Clamp T-tube for 1 to 2 hr before and after meals.**

_____ Keep the drainage system at the level of the gallbladder.

__X__ **Avoid heavy lifting and strenuous activities.**

__X__ **Empty drainage bag every 8 hr.**

Instruct the client to clamp the T-tube 1 to 2 hr before and after meals prior to removal to assess tolerance to food post-cholecystectomy. Also instruct the client to avoid heavy lifting to prevent evisceration, and to empty the drainage bag attached to the T-tube every 8 hr to prevent reflux back into the bile duct. The client should take showers rather than baths due to the increased risk for infection from entry of microorganisms into the wound. Instruct the client to maintain the flow of bile drainage by gravity. Do not place the drainage system at or above the level of the gallbladder, due to the risk of infection from reflux of drainage from the drainage tube into the wound bed.

 NCLEX® Connection: Reduction of Risk Potential, Potential for Complications from Surgical Procedures and Health Alterations

UNIT 7	NURSING CARE OF CLIENTS WITH GASTROINTESTINAL DISORDERS
Section:	Gallbladder and Pancreas Disorders
Chapter 50	Pancreatitis and Pancreatic Cancer

Overview

- The pancreas's islets of Langerhans secrete insulin and glucagon. The pancreatic tissues secrete digestive enzymes that break down carbohydrates, proteins, and fats.

PANCREATITIS

Overview

- Pancreatitis is an autodigestion of the pancreas from premature activation (before reaching the intestines) of pancreatic digestive enzymes (exact mechanism unknown). It can result in inflammation, necrosis, and hemorrhage.

- Classic signs and symptoms of an acute attack include severe, constant, and knife-like pain (left upper quadrant, midepigastric, and/or radiating to the back) that is unrelieved by nausea and vomiting.

- Acute pancreatitis is an inflammation of the pancreas from activated pancreatic enzymes autodigesting the pancreas. Severity varies, but overall mortality is 10% to 20%.

- Chronic pancreatitis is a progressive, destructive disease of the pancreas with the development of calcification and necrosis, possibly resulting in hemorrhagic pancreatitis. Mortality can be as high as 50%.

Data Collection

- Risk Factors

  - Two primary causes of pancreatitis are alcoholism and biliary tract disease (gallstones can cause a blockage where the common bile duct and pancreatic duct meet).

  - Triggering factors include an intake of large amounts of fat and/or alcohol.

  - The primary cause of chronic pancreatitis is alcoholism. This may occur more often in older adults as age-related changes reduce the ability to physiologically handle alcohol. Gallbladder disease can also cause pancreatitis.

- Subjective Data

  - Sudden onset of severe, boring pain

    - Epigastric, radiating to back, left flank, or left shoulder

    - Worse when lying down or while eating

    - Not relieved with vomiting

  - Pain relieved somewhat by fetal position

  - Nausea and vomiting

  - Anorexia and weight loss

- Objective Data

  - Physical assessment findings

    - Seepage of blood-stained exudates into tissue

      - Ecchymoses on the flanks (Turner's sign)

      - Bluish periumbilical discoloration (Cullen's sign)

> **(M) View Media Supplement:**
> - Turner's Sign (Image) • Cullen's Sign (Image) • Ascites (Image)

    - Generalized jaundice

    - Hypotension

    - Paralytic ileus

    - Hyperglycemia

    - Ascites

    - Tetany

      - Trousseau's sign (hand spasm when blood pressure cuff is inflated)

      - Chvostek's sign (facial twitching when facial nerve is tapped)

  - Laboratory tests

    - Serum amylase (rises within 12 hr, lasts 4 days) and serum lipase (rises slower but lasts up to 2 weeks).

      - Urine amylase remains elevated for up to 2 weeks.

      - Rises in enzymes indicate pancreatic cell injury.

      - Memory aid – During pancreatitis, the "ases" (aces) are high.

      - For amylase and lipase to be considered positive, the enzyme rise must be significant (2 to 3 times the normal value for amylase, and 3 to 5 times the normal value for lipase). The degree of enzyme elevation does not directly correlate with the severity of the disease.

- WBC – Elevated due to infection and inflammation
- Serum calcium and magnesium levels – Decreased due to fat necrosis with pancreatitis
- Serum liver enzymes and bilirubin levels – Elevated with associated biliary dysfunction
- Serum glucose level – Elevated due to a decrease in insulin production from the pancreas
  - o Diagnostic procedures
    - Computed tomography (CT) scan with contrast – Reliably diagnostic of acute pancreatitis

Collaborative Care

- Nursing Care
  - o Rest the pancreas.
    - NPO – No food until pain free
    - Administer antiemetic as needed
    - NG tube – Inserted for gastric decompression
    - Monitor clients receiving total parenteral nutrition (TPN) or jejunal feedings (less risk of hyperglycemia)
    - Resume diet – Bland, low-fat diet with no stimulants (caffeine); small, frequent meals
    - No alcohol consumption
    - No smoking
    - Limit stress
    - Manage pain
  - o Position clients for comfort (fetal, side-lying, the head of the bed elevated, sitting up or leaning forward).
  - o Administer analgesics and other medications as prescribed.
  - o Monitor blood glucose levels and provide insulin as needed (potential for hyperglycemia).
  - o Monitor hydration levels (orthostatic blood pressure, I&O, laboratory values).
  - o Assist with clients receiving IV fluids and electrolyte replacement as prescribed.
  - o Monitor bowel sounds related to potential for ileus development.

- Medications
  - Opioid analgesics – Morphine (Duramorph)
    - Acute pain management
    - Nursing considerations
      - Assist with clients who are receiving large doses of intravenous opioids for pain management.
  - Antibiotics – Imipenem (Primaxin)
    - Antibiotics may be used, but are generally indicated for clients with acute necrotizing pancreatitis.
    - Nursing considerations
      - Monitor for signs of infection.
  - Anticholinergics – Dicyclomine (Bentyl)
    - This is given to decrease intestinal motility and the flow of pancreatic enzymes.
  - Spasmolytics – Papaverine (Pavabid)
    - This medication relaxes smooth muscle.
  - Histamine$_2$ receptor antagonists – Ranitidine (Zantac) and proton pump inhibitors – Omeprazole (Prilosec)
    - These are given to decrease gastric acid secretion.
  - Pancreatic enzymes – Pancreatin (Donnazyme), pancrelipase (Viokase)
    - These aid with the digestion of fats and proteins when taken with meals and snacks.
- Interdisciplinary Care
  - Request dietary referral for post-pancreatitis diet and nutritional supplements when oral intake resumed.
- Therapeutic Procedures
  - ERCP to create an opening in the sphincter of Oddi if pancreatitis is caused by gallstones.
- Surgical Interventions
  - Cholecystectomy if pancreatitis is a result of cholecystitis and gallstones
  - Pancreaticojejunostomy (Roux-en-Y) reroutes drainage of pancreatic secretions into jejunum

- Care After Discharge

  o Recognize the need for home health services for clients needing assistance with nutritional needs, wound care, and ADLs.

  o Suggest participating in 12-step program for clients who have a history of alcohol abuse.

- Client Outcomes

  o The client will be able to tolerate an oral diet without the precipitation of pain or nausea.

  o The client's WBC count and pancreatic enzymes will return to values within their expected reference range.

Complications

- Hypovolemia

  o Causes

    ▪ Up to 6 L can be third-spaced; retroperitoneal loss of protein-rich fluid from proteolytic digestion

  o Nursing actions

    ▪ Monitor vital signs, electrolytes, and monitor IV fluid and electrolyte replacement.

- Chronic pancreatitis

  o Causes

    ▪ Alcohol abuse

  o Client education

    ▪ Encourage clients to avoid alcohol intake and caffeinated beverages, and to participate in alcoholic support groups.

- Pancreatic infection – Pseudocyst (outside pancreas); abscess (inside pancreas)

  o Causes

    ▪ Leakage of fluid out of damaged pancreatic duct

  o Nursing actions

    ▪ Monitor for rupture and hemorrhage.

    ▪ Maintain sump tube if placed for drainage of a cyst.

    ▪ Monitor the skin around the tube for breakdown secondary to corrosive enzymes.

- Type 1 diabetes mellitus

  o Causes

    ▪ Destruction of the beta cells of the Islets of Langerhans

- Nursing actions
  - Monitor blood glucose closely.
  - Administer insulin as needed.
- Client education
  - Inform clients about long-term diabetic management.

PANCREATIC CANCER

Overview

- Pancreatic carcinoma has vague symptoms and is usually diagnosed in late stages after liver or gallbladder involvement.
- It has a high mortality rate (less than 20% live longer than 1 year after diagnosis).

Data Collection

- Risk Factors
  - The cause is unknown, but there is a possible inherited risk.
  - Other risks may include:
    - Older age
    - Tobacco use
    - Chronic pancreatitis
    - Diabetes mellitus
- Subjective Data
  - Pain that radiates to the back and is unrelieved by change in position, and is more severe at night
  - Fatigue
  - Anorexia
  - Flatulence
  - Pruritus
- Objective Data
  - Physical assessment findings
    - Weight loss
    - Palpable abdominal mass
    - Hepatomegaly
    - Jaundice (late sign)

- Clay-colored stools
- Dark urine
- Ascites
  - Laboratory tests
    - Carcinoembryonic antigen (CEA) – Elevated
    - Serum amylase and lipase – Elevated
    - Serum alkaline phosphatase and bilirubin levels – Elevated
  - Diagnostic procedures
    - Ultrasound visualization of tumor
    - Computed tomography (CT) – Visualization of the tumor to determine size, location, and metastases
    - ERCP is the most definitive and allows for the placement of a drain or stent for biliary drainage.
    - Abdominal paracentesis can allow testing of abdominal fluid for malignant cells.

Collaborative Care

- Nursing Care
  - Implement palliative care measures.
    - Treat pain with opioid analgesics.
    - Employ other comfort measures as appropriate.
  - Monitor blood glucose levels and administer insulin as prescribed.
  - Monitor clients receiving nutritional support (enteral supplements, total parenteral nutrition).
- Medications
  - Opioid analgesics
    - Pain management is the priority intervention. Generally, large doses of opioids (morphine) are given.
    - Nursing considerations
      - Check the client's level of pain and administer an analgesic as prescribed.
      - Monitor the client's needs for analgesics frequently.
    - Client education
      - Advise clients to ask for analgesics before the pain becomes severe.

- Interdisciplinary Care

  ○ Palliative care

  ○ Cancer support group

- Therapeutic Procedures

  ○ Chemotherapy may be used to shrink the tumor size. Several medications are given to improve the results.

    ▪ Nursing actions

      □ Monitor for myelosuppression and pancytopenia.

  ○ Radiation may be used to shrink tumor size.

    ▪ Nursing actions

      □ Monitor clients for fatigue and diarrhea.

      □ A biliary stent is needed for clients who have a biliary obstruction.

- Surgical Interventions

  ○ Partial pancreatectomy – Done for small tumors. May be done laparoscopically.

  ○ Whipple procedure – Removal of the head of the pancreas, duodenum, parts of the jejunum and stomach, gallbladder, and possibly the spleen. The pancreatic duct is connected to the common bile duct, and the stomach is connected to the jejunum. This procedure may be done laparoscopically.

    ▪ Nursing actions

      □ Provide routine postoperative care

      □ Monitor NG tube output and ensure unimpeded drainage from NG tube and surgical drains. Observe for bloody or bile-tinged drainage which could indicate anastomotic disruption.

      □ Place clients in semi-Fowler's position to facilitate lung expansion and to prevent stress on the suture line.

      □ Monitor clients receiving IV fluids and blood.

      □ Monitor breath sounds and respirations and facilitate deep breathing. Encourage the use of incentive spirometer and administer oxygen as needed.

      □ Monitor blood glucose and administer insulin as needed.

    ▪ Client education (pre, post)

      □ Instruct clients to support measures for pain, anorexia, weight loss, and community resources.

- Client outcomes

  o The client will report pain level of 2-3 on a scale of 0-10.

  o The client will be able to maintain adequate oral or enteral nutrition.

  o The client and client's family will be able to verbalize a realistic prognosis and related care needs.

Complications

- Fistulas

  o Cause

    ▪ Breakdown of a site of anastomosis

  o Nursing actions

    ▪ Report drainage that is not serosanguineous from the drain, or drainage from the wound to the provider immediately.

- Peritonitis

  o Cause

    ▪ Internal leakage of corrosive pancreatic fluid

  o Nursing actions

    ▪ Monitor for signs and symptoms of peritonitis (elevated fever, WBC, abdominal pain, abdominal tenderness/rebound tenderness, alteration in bowel sounds, shoulder tip pain).

    ▪ Provide antibiotics as prescribed.

Ⓐ APPLICATION EXERCISES

Scenario: A nurse is caring for a client who has chronic pancreatitis. The client reports a history of alcohol abuse and gallstones. The client's prescriptions include keeping the client NPO, insertion of a nasogastric (NG) tube and applying suction, and administering dextrose 5% in normal saline at 125 mL/hr.

1. Which of the following laboratory results should the nurse expect? (Select all that apply.)

    _____ Increased serum lipase

    _____ Decreased WBC count

    _____ Increased serum calcium

    _____ Decreased bilirubin levels

    _____ Increased blood glucose levels

2. During the client's fourth hospital day he asks the nurse when he will be allowed to eat. Which of the following is an appropriate response by the nurse?

    A. "When your amylase value is within its expected reference range."

    B. "When you are no longer experiencing pain."

    C. "When your lipase value is within its expected reference range."

    D. "When you can ambulate without experiencing hypotension."

3. The nurse is preparing the client for discharge. Which of the following discharge instructions should the nurse reinforce? (Select all that apply.)

    _____ Avoid alcohol.

    _____ Avoid smoking.

    _____ Plan for rest periods during the day.

    _____ Sleep with the head of the bed elevated.

    _____ Use pursed-lip breathing during exercise.

4. A nurse is caring for a client with pancreatic cancer. Identify the findings the nurse should expect if the client develops peritonitis.

(A) **APPLICATION EXERCISES ANSWER KEY**

Scenario: A nurse is caring for a client who has chronic pancreatitis. The client reports a history of alcohol abuse and gallstones. The client's prescriptions include keeping the client NPO, insertion of a nasogastric (NG) tube and applying suction, and administering dextrose 5% in normal saline at 125 mL/hr.

1. Which of the following laboratory results should the nurse expect? (Select all that apply.)

   X   **Increased serum lipase**

   _____   Decreased WBC count

   _____   Increased serum calcium

   _____   Decreased bilirubin levels

   X   **Increased blood glucose levels**

   Serum lipase levels will be elevated due to pancreatic cell injury. Serum blood glucose levels will be elevated due to a decrease in insulin production from the pancreas. WBC count will more likely be increased due to the inflammatory response. Serum calcium levels will more likely be decreased due to fatty acid production. Serum bilirubin levels will likely be increased due to biliary obstruction and hepatobiliary inflammatory processes.

   (N) NCLEX® Connection: Reduction of Risk Potential, Laboratory Values

2. During the client's fourth hospital day he asks the nurse when he will be allowed to eat. Which of the following is an appropriate response by the nurse?

   A. "When your amylase value is within its expected reference range."

   B. "When you are no longer experiencing pain."

   C. "When your lipase value is within its expected reference range."

   D. "When you can ambulate without experiencing hypotension."

   The guideline used to determine when a client with pancreatitis can resume a diet is when the client is no longer experiencing pain. While the amylase and lipase levels can provide additional information about the stage of the disease, these levels are not used to determine when the client can resume a diet. Being able to ambulate without hypotension is not a factor in the client's ability to resume a diet.

   (N) NCLEX® Connection: Basic Care and Comfort and Oral Hydration

3. The nurse is preparing the client for discharge. Which of the following discharge instructions should the nurse reinforce? (Select all that apply.)

X	**Avoid alcohol.**
X	**Avoid smoking.**
X	**Plan for rest periods during the day.**
X	**Sleep with the head of the bed elevated.**
	Use pursed-lip breathing during exercise.

    The client's home care instructions for chronic pancreatitis should focus on preventing future exacerbations. Subsequently, instruct the client to avoid both alcohol and smoking and to plan rest periods during the day. Sleeping with the head of the bed elevated may promote comfort. It is not appropriate to recommend using pursed-lip breathing during exercise.

    (N) **NCLEX® Connection: Reduction of Risk Potential, Potential for Alterations in Body Systems**

4. A nurse is caring for a client with pancreatic cancer. Identify the findings the nurse should expect if the client develops peritonitis.

    Signs and symptoms of peritonitis include elevated fever, WBC, abdominal pain, abdominal tenderness/rebound tenderness, alteration in bowel sounds, and shoulder tip pain.

    (N) **NCLEX® Connection: Reduction of Risk Potential, Potential for Alterations in Body Systems**

UNIT 7	NURSING CARE OF CLIENTS WITH GASTROINTESTINAL DISORDERS
Section:	Liver Disorders
Chapter 51	**Hepatitis and Cirrhosis**

Overview

- Hepatitis is an inflammation of the liver.

- Hepatitis is caused by an infectious organism that enters the body through a chemical (alcohol, medications) or by a toxin (poisonous mushrooms).

- Cirrhosis occurs secondary to the inflammation of the liver, which replaces functional liver tissue with fibrotic, scar tissue.

- Cirrhosis is caused by infections (hepatitis, alcohol abuse, inflammatory disorders).

HEPATITIS

Overview

- Viral hepatitis can be acute or chronic.

- Noninfectious hepatitis may occur secondary to exposure to a chemical or medication.

- There are five major categories of viral hepatitis (hepatitis F and G have been identified but are uncommon).

  - Hepatitis A virus (HAV)

  - Hepatitis B virus (HBV)

  - Hepatitis C virus (HCV)

  - Hepatitis D virus (HDV)

  - Hepatitis E virus (HEV)

- All of the hepatitis viruses can cause an acute or short-term illness, and may become a chronic debilitating disease with increasing severity in symptoms over a long period of time. However, hepatitis A rarely results in long-term problems.

- Individuals with hepatitis are carriers and can spread the disease without showing any symptoms.

- People with hepatitis should never donate blood, body organs, or other body tissue.

- It is required to report all cases of hepatitis to the health department.

Data Collection

- Risk Factors

TYPE	ROUTE OF TRANSMISSION	RISK FACTORS
Hepatitis A (HAV)	Oral-fecal route	• Ingestion of contaminated food/water • Daycares and communal living facilities
Hepatitis B (HBV)	Blood	• Drug abuse • Sexual contact • Health care work
Hepatitis C (HCV)	Blood	• Drug abuse • Sexual contact
Hepatitis D (HDV)	Co-infection with HBV	• Drug abuse
Hepatitis E (HEV)	Oral-fecal route	• Ingestion of contaminated water

- High-risk behaviors
  - Percutaneous exposure (dirty needles, sharp instruments, body piercing, tattooing, use of another person's drug paraphernalia or personal hygiene tools)
  - Unprotected sexual intercourse with a hepatitis-infected person, sex with multiple partners, and/or anal sex
  - Unscreened blood transfusions (prior to 1992)
  - Hemodialysis
  - Ingestion of food prepared by a hepatitis-infected person who does not practice proper sanitation precautions
  - Travel/residence in underdeveloped country (using tap water to clean food products, drinking contaminated water)
  - Eating and/or living in crowded environments (correctional facilities, dormitories, universities, long-term care facilities, military base housing)

- Subjective Data
  - Influenza-like symptoms
    - Headache
    - Fatigue
    - Arthralgia and myalgia (joint and muscle pain, respectively)
    - Pruritus

- Objective Data
  - Physical findings
    - Low-grade fever
    - Right upper quadrant abdominal pain

- Nausea and vomiting
- Jaundice
- Dark urine
- Pruritus
- Weight loss
- Clay-colored stools

○ Laboratory tests

- Enzyme-linked immunosorbent assay (ELISA), or recombinant immunoblot assay (RIBA) may be done if hepatitis C is suspected. Assays confirm the presence of antibodies to hepatitis C.
- Serum liver enzymes – Elevated
  □ Alanine aminotransferase (ALT) – Elevated (expected reference range – 8 to 20units/L; 3 to 35 IU/L); most definitive for assessment of liver tissue damage.
  □ Aspartate aminotransferase (AST) – Elevated (expected reference range – 5 to 40 units/L)
  □ Alkaline phosphatase (ALP) – Elevated (expected reference range – 42 to 128 units/L; 30 to 85 IU/L)
- Serum bilirubin – Elevated
  □ Bilirubin – Direct (conjugated) – Elevated (expected reference range – 0.1 to 0.3 mg/dL)
  □ Bilirubin – Indirect (unconjugated) – Elevated (expected reference range – 0.1 to 1 mg/dL)
  □ Bilirubin – Total – Elevated (expected reference range – 0.1 to 1.0 mg/dL)
  □ Albumin – Decreased (expected reference range – 3.5 to 5 g/dL)
- Serologic markers – Identifies the presence of the virus (HAV, HBsAg and Anti HBc IgM, HCV, HDV, HEV). Serum presence of HBsAg for longer than 6 months indicates chronic hepatitis and/or hepatitis carrier status.
- Hepatitis antibody serum testing related to strain of hepatitis – anti-HAV, HBsAb, anti-HCV, anti-HDV, anti-HEV. Serum presence of HBsAb indicates immunity to HBV following the recovery from hepatitis B, or a successful vaccination.

○ Diagnostic procedures

- Abdominal films are used to visualize possible hepatomegaly, ascites, and spleen enlargement.
- Liver biopsy – This is the most definitive, and is used to identify the intensity of the infection, and the degree of tissue damage.
  □ Nursing actions
    ‣ Obtain the client's consent for liver biopsy.
    ‣ Review and explain to clients the biopsy procedure and what is expected following the procedure.

> ▸ Require clients to lie on the affected surgical side for a short period of time after the biopsy has been taken.

> ▸ Monitor the client's blood pressure and heart rate post procedure to detect bleeding.

Collaborative Care

- Nursing Care

  - Most clients will be cared for in the home unless they are acutely ill.

  - Enforce standard and contact precautions to include:

    - A private room or a room with other clients with the same infection.

    - Use of personal protective equipment appropriate to type of exposure (gown, gloves, goggles)

    - The use of disposable equipment or dedicated equipment and disposal of infectious dressing material into a single, nonporous bag without touching the outside of the bag.

    - Use of needleless system when delivering medications and parenteral solutions

  - Limit the client's activity (bed rest, rest periods) in order to promote hepatic healing.

  - Reinforce dietary instructions regarding a high-carbohydrate, high-calorie, low-to-moderate fat, and low-to-moderate protein diet, and small, frequent meals to promote nutrition and healing. Food aversion may make this difficult.

  - Administer interferon as prescribed for HBV and HCV. Monitor clients receiving interferon for side effects of flu-like symptoms, alopecia, and bone marrow suppression. Monitor CBC and administer an antiemetic as needed during interferon therapy.

  - Reinforce to clients and families regarding measures to prevent the transmission of the disease with others at home (avoid sexual intercourse until hepatitis antibody testing is negative).

  - Provide comfort measures.

  - Encourage all health care workers to have up-to-date Hepatitis B immunization.

  - Participate in community health educational programs on transmission and exposure.

  - Report hepatitis outbreaks to health authorities.

- Medications

  - Immunoglobulin – may be prescribed for household members and sexual partners of clients who have hepatitis A. Prophylactic injections may be given to individuals traveling to high-risk countries.

  - Biologic response modifiers (BMRs)

    - Peginterferon alfa-2a (Pegasys) Interferon alfa-2b (Intron-A) – Administered to clients who have chronic hepatitis B (Intron-A) or C (Pegasys, Intron-A) for several months to induce remission

- Nursing considerations
  - Note dose – Given in millions of units (10 MU [10 million units])
  - Monitor for bone marrow suppression and depression.
- Client education
  - Inform clients of possible flu-like symptoms after each injection
- Antivirals – Lamivudine (Epivir), adefovir (Hepsera) or ribavirin (Rebetol) – Can be given to clients who have chronic hepatitis B to decrease the incidence of cirrhosis, or clients waiting for a liver transplant. A combination of Peginterferon alfa-2a and ribavirin is used in clients who have hepatitis C to attain sustained virologic response (decreased viral load).
  - Nursing considerations
    - Monitor clients taking adefovir for nephrotoxicity.
  - Client education
    - Inform clients that an acute exacerbation of hepatitis B may occur if medication is abruptly discontinued.
    - Advise clients taking ribavirin and their sexual partners not to get pregnant while taking this medication.

- Interdisciplinary Care
  - Infection control services may be consulted.

- Care After Discharge
  - Client education
    - Instruct clients to avoid alcohol and all drugs not prescribed by a provider.
    - Instruct clients to avoid sexual intercourse until tests are negative for hepatitis.
    - Encourage frequent hand hygiene (before eating, after using the toilet).
    - Instruct clients who are traveling in underdeveloped countries to drink bottled water and limit sharing of bed linens and eating utensils.

- Client Outcomes
  - The client will recover from hepatitis A without liver damage.
  - The client's viral load of hepatitis B and C will be suppressed.
  - Clients who have hepatitis B and C will not experience liver failure.

Complications

- Chronic hepatitis
  - Results from hepatitis B, C, or D.
  - Increases the client's risk for liver cancer.

- Fulminating hepatitis

  o This is a fatal form of hepatitis due to the inability of the liver cells to regenerate with the progression of the necrotic process.

  o This disease results in hepatic encephalopathy and death.

  o Nursing actions

    ▪ Monitor clients for neurological changes, manage fluid and electrolytes, and provide comfort measures.

- Cirrhosis of the liver (See next section in this chapter)

  o Continued episodes of chronic hepatitis result in scarring and permanent injury to the liver, and are a risk factor for liver cancer.

- Liver cancer

- Liver failure

  o Chronic hepatitis, liver abscesses, and fatty liver infiltration all result in changes within the healthy liver and cause irreversible damage.

CIRRHOSIS

 Overview

- Cirrhosis refers to extensive scarring of the liver caused by necrotic injury or a chronic reaction to inflammation over a prolonged period of time. Normal liver tissue is replaced with fibrotic tissue that lacks function.

- Portal and periportal areas of the liver are primarily involved, affecting the liver's ability to handle the flow of bile. The development of new bile channels causes an overgrowth of tissue and liver scarring/enlargement. Jaundice is often the result.

Data Collection

- Risk Factors

  o Alcohol abuse

  o Chronic viral hepatitis (hepatitis B, C, or D)

  o Autoimmune hepatitis (destruction of the liver cells by the immune system)

  o Steatohepatitis (fatty liver disease causing chronic inflammation)

  o Damage to the liver caused by drugs, toxins, and other infections

  o Chronic biliary cirrhosis (bile duct obstruction, bile stasis, hepatic fibrosis)

  o Cardiac cirrhosis resulting from severe, right heart failure-inducing necrosis and fibrosis due to lack of blood flow

  o Obesity

- Subjective Data

  o Fatigue

  o Weight loss, abdominal pain, dyspepsia, and distention

  o Pruritus (severe itching of skin)

  o Confusion or difficulty thinking (due to the build-up of waste products in the blood and brain that the liver is unable to get rid of)

  o Personality and mentation changes, emotional lability, euphoria, sometimes depression

- Objective Data

  o Physical findings

    ▪ Gastrointestinal bleeding (enlarged veins [varices] develop and burst, causing vomiting and passing of blood in bowel movements)

    ▪ Ascites (bloating or swelling due to fluid build-up in abdomen and legs) and peripheral edema

    ▪ Jaundice (yellowing of skin) and icterus (yellowing of the eyes)

    ▪ Petechiae (round, pinpoint, red-purple lesions), ecchymosis (large yellow and purple blue bruises), nose bleeds, hematemesis, melena (decreased synthesis of prothrombin, deteriorating hepatic function)

    ▪ Palmar erythema (redness, warmth of the palms of the hands)

    ▪ Spider angiomas (red lesions vascular in nature with branches radiating on the nose, cheeks, upper thorax, shoulders)

    ▪ Dependent peripheral edema of extremities and sacrum

    ▪ Asterixis (liver flapping tremor) – Coarse tremor characterized by rapid, nonrhythmic extension, and flexion of the wrists and fingers

    ▪ Fetor hepaticus (liver breath) – Fruity or musty odor

  o Laboratory tests

    ▪ Serum liver enzymes – Elevated initially

      ☐ ALT

      ☐ AST

      ☐ ALP

      ☐ ALT and AST are elevated initially due to hepatic inflammation, and return to normal when liver cells are no longer able to create an inflammatory response. ALP increases in cirrhosis due to intrahepatic biliary obstruction.

    ▪ Serum bilirubin – Elevated

      ☐ Bilirubin – Direct (conjugated)

      ☐ Bilirubin – Indirect (unconjugated)

- □ Bilirubin – Total
- □ Bilirubin levels are elevated in cirrhosis due to the inability of the liver to excrete bilirubin.
- Serum proteins and serum albumin are lowered due to the lack of hepatic synthesis.
- Hematological tests – CBC, WBC, and platelets are decreased secondary to anemia.
- PT/INR is prolonged due to decreased synthesis of prothrombin.
- Ammonia levels (expected reference range 15 to 110 mg/dL) rise when hepatocellular injury (cirrhosis) prevents the conversion of ammonia to urea for excretion.
- Serum creatinine levels (expected reference range 0.6 to 1.2 mg/dL) may increase due to deteriorating kidney function which may occur as a result of advanced liver disease.
- ○ Diagnostic procedures
  - Abdominal x-rays and ultrasonography
    - □ This is used to visualize possible hepatomegaly, ascites, and spleen enlargement.
  - Liver biopsy (most definitive)
    - □ A liver biopsy identifies the progression and extent of the cirrhosis.
    - □ To minimize the risk of hemorrhage, a radiologist may perform the biopsy through the jugular vein, which is threaded to the hepatic vein to obtain tissue for a microscopic evaluation.
    - □ This is done under fluoroscopy for safety, as this procedure can be problematic for cirrhosis clients due to an increased risk for bleeding complications.
  - Esophagogastroduodenoscopy (EGD)
    - □ This is performed under moderate (conscious) sedation to detect the presence of esophageal varices.

Collaborative Care

- Nursing Care
  - ○ Monitor
    - Respiratory status – Monitor oxygen level. Provide comfort measures by positioning the client to ease respiratory effort (may be compromised by plasma volume excess and ascites). Have clients sit in a chair or elevate the head of the bed to 30°.
    - Skin integrity – Monitor clients closely for skin breakdown. Implement measures to prevent pressure ulcers. Pruritus will cause clients to scratch. Encourage washing with cold water and applying lotion to decrease the itching.

- Vital signs – Monitor clients for signs of fluid volume excess and keep strict I&O. Restrict fluids and sodium if prescribed and weigh daily.

- Neurological status – Monitor clients for deteriorating mental status and dementia consistent with hepatic encephalopathy. Lactulose may need to be given to aid in excretion of ammonia.

- Nutritional status – Encourage a high-caloric, high-protein (unless has hepatic encephalopathy), low fat and sodium diet and supplemental vitamins (B complex), folic acid, and iron.

- Gastrointestinal status – In the presence of ascites, measure abdominal girth daily. Mark the location of tape for consistency.

- Pain status – Monitor the client's pain level and administer analgesics and gastrointestinal antispasmodics as needed.

o Observe clients for potential bleeding complications. Assist with the care of clients receiving blood transfusions (packed RBCs, fresh frozen plasma). Monitor the trends in Hgb and Hct levels and note coagulation studies (aPTT, PT/INR).

o Provide medications as prescribed.

- Medications

o As the metabolism of most medications is dependent upon a functioning liver, general medications are administered sparingly, especially opioids, sedatives, and barbiturates.

o Diuretics are administered to decrease ascites.

o Proton pump inhibitors and H_2 receptor antagonists are administered to decrease gastric acid secretion and the risk of gastrointestinal bleeding.

o Lactulose is administered to promote ammonia excretion via the stool.

o Neomycin and metronidazole (Flagyl) are administered to remove intestinal bacteria, which produces ammonia.

- Interdisciplinary Care

o A dietary consult may be needed if hepatic encephalopathy requires a low-protein diet.

o Request appropriate referrals (social services, Alcoholics Anonymous, Al-Anon).

- Therapeutic Procedures

o Paracentesis

- Used to relieve ascites.

o Injection sclerotherapy/variceal band ligation

- The varices are either sclerosed or banded endoscopically.

- There is a decreased risk of hemorrhage with banding.

- Surgical Interventions
  - Transjugular intrahepatic portosystemic shunt (TIPS)
    - This is done to control ascites and variceal bleeding.
  - Surgical bypass shunting procedures
    - This is a last resort for clients with portal hypertension and esophageal varices. The ascites are shunted from the abdominal cavity to the superior vena cava.
  - Liver transplantation
    - Portions of healthy livers from trauma victims or living donors may be used for transplant.
    - The transplanted liver portion will regenerate and grow in size based on the needs of the body.
- Care After Discharge
  - Client education
    - Encourage clients to abstain from alcohol and engage in alcohol recovery program.
    - Instruct clients to follow dietary guidelines:
      - High-calorie, moderate-fat diet
      - Low-sodium diet (if the client has excessive fluid in the peritoneal cavity)
      - Low-protein diet (if encephalopathy, elevated ammonia)
      - Small, frequent, well-balanced nutritional meals
      - Supplemental vitamin-enriched liquids (Ensure, Boost)
      - Replacement and administration of vitamins due to the inability of the liver to store them
      - Fluid intake restrictions if serum sodium is low
- Client Outcomes
  - The client's Hct and electrolytes will return to their expected reference range.
  - The client will demonstrate orientation to person, place, and time.
  - The client's abdominal girth will demonstrate a decrease in circumference.

Complications

- Portal systemic encephalopathy (PSE)
  - Clients who have a poorly functioning liver are unable to convert ammonia and other waste products to a less toxic form. These products are carried to the brain and cause neurological symptoms. Clients are treated with medications such as lactulose to reduce the ammonia levels in the body via intestinal excretion. Reductions in dietary protein are indicated as ammonia is formed when protein is broken down by intestinal flora.

- o Nursing actions

  - Administer lactulose as prescribed, and monitor serum ammonia and potassium levels during treatment.

  - Monitor for changes in the level of consciousness and orientation.

  - Report asterixis (flapping of the hands) and fetor hepaticus (liver breath) immediately to the provider.

- o Client education

  - Instruct clients to follow a protein-restricted or vegetable protein diet.

- Esophageal varices

  - o Causes

    - Portal hypertension (elevated blood pressure in veins that carry blood from the intestines to the liver) is caused by impaired circulation of blood through the liver. Collateral circulation is subsequently developed creating varices in the upper stomach and esophagus. Varices are fragile and can bleed easily.

  - o Nursing actions

    - Assist with saline lavage (vasoconstriction), esophagogastric balloon tamponade, blood transfusions, ligation and sclerotherapy, and shunts to stop bleeding and reduce the risk for hypovolemic shock.

    - Monitor the client's hemoglobin level and vital signs.

Ⓐ APPLICATION EXERCISES

Scenario: A client who has a history of chronic biliary disease is admitted to the acute care facility with reports of anorexia, vomiting, chronic indigestion, and abdominal pain. The client's liver is enlarged and her abdomen is distended. The client's liver enzymes are elevated. Based on her history, physical examination, and laboratory values, the client is diagnosed with cirrhosis of the liver.

1. The nurse should recognize which of the following as the cause of the client's enlarged and distended abdomen?

    A. Asterixis

    B. Paralytic ileus

    C. Ascites

    D. Hyperglycemic-hyperosmolar state

2. The charge nurse has informed the nurse the client is at an increased risk for development of respiratory problems. Explain why the ascites can contribute to impaired oxygenation.

3. Which of the following client findings should the nurse recognize as consistent with an impending hepatic coma? (Select all that apply.)

    _____ Inability to state why she is in the hospital

    _____ Asterixis

    _____ Anorexia

    _____ Ascites

    _____ Fetor hepaticus

4. An older adult client presents to the clinic with an elevated temperature and reports a poor appetite and diarrhea for the past 2 weeks unrelieved by antidiarrheal medicine. He lives in a retirement community and eats at a restaurant every Sunday that serves a buffet. He denies any history of chemical abuse or recent sexual encounters. Which of the following types of hepatitis should the nurse anticipate is the most likely cause of these symptoms?

    A. Hepatitis A (HAV)

    B. Hepatitis B (HBV)

    C. Hepatitis C (HCV)

    D. Hepatitis E (HEV)

5. A nurse is reinforcing care instructions for a client who has Hepatitis B and the client's spouse and family. Which of the following information should the nurse include this client? (Select all that apply.)

_____ Limit physical activity.

_____ Avoid alcohol.

_____ Take acetaminophen (Tylenol) for comfort.

_____ Have family members wear masks.

_____ Take supplemental vitamins.

_____ Use condoms during sex.

(A) **APPLICATION EXERCISES ANSWER KEY**

> **Scenario:** A client who has a history of chronic biliary disease is admitted to the acute care facility with reports of anorexia, vomiting, chronic indigestion, and abdominal pain. The client's liver is enlarged and her abdomen is distended. The client's liver enzymes are elevated. Based on her history, physical examination, and laboratory values, the client is diagnosed with cirrhosis of the liver.

1. The nurse should recognize which of the following as the cause of the client's enlarged and distended abdomen?

    A. Asterixis

    B. Paralytic ileus

    C. Ascites

    D. Hyperglycemic-hyperosmolar state

    The client's large, protruding abdomen is consistent with ascites, which is commonly associated with cirrhosis. Ascites is due to portal hypertension, decreased synthesis of albumin, and obstruction of hepatic lymph flow. While asterixis is consistent with hepatitis, it does not manifest as abdominal ascites. Paralytic ileus and hyperglycemic-hyperosmolar state are unrelated to hepatitis.

(N) NCLEX® Connection: Reduction of Risk Potential, Potential for Alterations in Body Systems

2. The charge nurse has informed the nurse the client is at an increased risk for development of respiratory problems. Explain why the ascites can contribute to impaired oxygenation.

    The client's ascites, if not relieved by paracentesis, will place pressure on her diaphragm and subsequently the lungs. This will place her at risk for ineffective breathing patterns.

(N) NCLEX® Connection: Physiological Adaptation, Pathophysiology

3. Which of the following client findings should the nurse recognize as consistent with an impending hepatic coma? (Select all that apply.)

X	**Inability to state why she is in the hospital**
X	**Asterixis**
	Anorexia
	Ascites
X	**Fetor hepaticus**

    Impending signs of hepatic coma are deterioration in neurological status, abnormal flapping of the hands (asterixis), and foul breath (fetor hepaticus). Anorexia and ascites are findings of cirrhosis and may accompany hepatic coma, but they can also exist in the absence of hepatic coma.

(N) NCLEX® Connection: Physiological Adaptation, Medical Emergencies

4. An older adult client presents to the clinic with an elevated temperature and reports a poor appetite and diarrhea for the past 2 weeks unrelieved by antidiarrheal medicine. He lives in a retirement community and eats at a restaurant every Sunday that serves a buffet. He denies any history of chemical abuse or recent sexual encounters. Which of the following types of hepatitis should the nurse anticipate is the most likely cause of these symptoms?

   A. Hepatitis A (HAV)

   B. Hepatitis B (HBV)

   C. Hepatitis C (HCV)

   D. Hepatitis E (HEV)

   Because the client lives in a communal setting and eats at a restaurant on a regular basis it's most likely he has hepatitis A. HAV usually resolves on its own.

   Ⓝ NCLEX® Connection: Safety and Infection Control, Standard/Transmission-Based/Other Precautions/Surgical Asepsis

5. A nurse is reinforcing care instructions for a client who has Hepatitis B and the client's spouse and family. Which of the following information should the nurse include this client? (Select all that apply.)

   __X__ **Limit physical activity.**

   __X__ **Avoid alcohol.**

   _____ Take acetaminophen (Tylenol) for comfort.

   _____ Have family members wear masks.

   __X__ **Take supplemental vitamins.**

   __X__ **Use condoms during sex.**

   Instructions to the client should include limiting physical activity to promote healing, avoiding alcohol to prevent further damage to the liver, consuming a high-caloric, high-protein diet, and taking supplemental vitamins (B complex), folic acid, and iron. Clients should be advised to use a condom during sex to prevent exposing the spouse to the virus and to avoid acetaminophen due to potential for liver damage. It is not necessary for family members to wear a mask because Hepatitis B is a bloodborne pathogen.

   Ⓝ NCLEX® Connection: Physiological Adaptation, Illness Management

UNIT 7	NURSING CARE OF CLIENTS WITH GASTROINTESTINAL DISORDERS
Section:	Liver Disorders

Chapter 52   Liver Cancer

 Overview

- Liver cancer or hepatocellular carcinoma (HCC) is the most frequently occurring type of liver cancer. HCC is a primary liver cancer, not metastatic liver cancer.

Data Collection

- Risk Factors

  ○ Cirrhosis

     ■ Chronic hepatitis B and/or C infection

     ■ Alcoholic liver disease

     ■ Hemochromatosis (inability to break down iron)

  ○ Male

  ○ Tobacco use

  ○ Metastasis from another site

- Subjective Data

  ○ Abdominal pain

  ○ Nausea and vomiting

  ○ Loss of appetite

  ○ Weakness and fatigue

- Objective Data

  ○ Physical findings

     ■ Weight loss

     ■ Enlarged liver on palpation

     ■ Jaundice

     ■ Ascites and peripheral edema

     ■ Pruritus

     ■ Encephalopathy

- o Laboratory tests
  - Alpha-fetoprotein (AFP), a tumor marker, is elevated with primary liver cancer.
  - The alkaline phosphatase (ALP), serum aspartate aminotransferase (AST), and albumin and bilirubin are elevated in both primary and metastatic cancer.
  - Use an elevated CEA along with an elevated AFP to discriminate metastatic from primary liver cancer.
  - Prothrombin time predicts the severity of cirrhosis.
- o Diagnostic procedures
  - Use an ultrasound and a CT scan to visualize a tumor.
  - A liver biopsy is the most definitive diagnostic procedure and is done through the skin (percutaneously) with a biopsy needle.
- Nursing Care
  - o Observe clients for potential bleeding complications.
    - Assist with the care of clients receiving blood transfusions (packed red blood cells and fresh frozen plasma).
    - Monitor trends in hemoglobin and hematocrit levels.
    - Monitor coagulation studies (aPTT, PT/INR).
  - o Encourage clients to follow dietary guidelines.
    - High-calorie, moderate-fat diet
    - Low-sodium diet (if ascites is present)
    - Low-protein diet (if there is encephalopathy, elevated ammonia)
    - Small, frequent, well-balanced nutritional meals
    - Vitamin-enriched supplements (Ensure, Boost)
    - Replacement and administration of vitamins due to the inability of the liver to store them
    - Restriction of fluid intake (if serum sodium is low)
  - o Encourage clients to avoid drinking alcohol.
  - o Monitor for:
    - Abdominal discomfort and increase in ascites (measure abdominal girth daily)
    - Anorexia and weight loss
    - Signs of biliary obstruction (jaundice)
    - Pain
    - Fluid and electrolyte status

- - Hepatic function
  - Nutritional status
  - o Provide medications as prescribed.
    - As the metabolism of most drugs is dependent upon a functioning liver, medications generally are administered sparingly (especially opioids, sedatives, and barbiturates).
- Medications
  - o Systemically delivered chemotherapy has been found to be largely ineffective in treating tumors of the liver or prolonging life. Therefore, more direct delivery methods are used.
  - o Hepatic arterial infusion (HAI) is the direct infusion of chemotherapy via a catheter into the tumor. The client may go home with a catheter in place if continuous infusion is desired.
  - o Client education
    - Instruct clients and families to watch for signs of infection related to the pump site, hepatic toxicity (jaundice, liver functions tests), and immunosuppression (fatigue, decreased WBC).
    - Inform clients of the side effects of chemotherapy.
- Interdisciplinary Care
  - o Request referrals (social services, hospice, home health, Alcoholics Anonymous).
- Therapeutic Procedures
  - o Hepatic artery embolization/chemoembolization – Using a catheter threaded through the femoral artery and up to the liver, particles are injected into the arteries that supply blood to the tumor. If a chemotherapeutic drug is included, this procedure is called chemoembolization.
  - o Radiofrequency ablation involves the use of an electric current that is directly delivered to the tumor via thin needles.
  - o Percutaneous alcohol injections involve the direct injection of alcohol into the tumor mass, resulting in cell death.
  - o Cryotherapy uses liquid nitrogen injected directly into the tumor to destroy the tumor.
  - o External radiation is not generally used, as healthy liver tissue does not tolerate high doses of radiation.

- Surgical Interventions

    o Surgical resection – If liver cancer involves only one lobe of the liver, surgical removal may be indicated. A liver-lobe resection can result in a survival rate of up to 5 years.

        ▪ Nursing actions

            □ Support nutritional status.

            □ Inform clients about diagnostic tests that will be done to determine if the liver cancer has metastasized (chest x-ray, PET scan, MRI, laparoscopy).

            □ Provide preoperative teaching and postoperative care.

            □ Monitor clients for hypoglycemia after surgery and report findings.

            □ Monitor clients for bleeding. Assist with the care of clients receiving IV fluids and blood.

    o Liver transplantation – May be an option for clients who have small primary tumors

        ▪ Immunosuppressants that are given after the transplant can increase the risk for recurrence of cancer.

- Care After Discharge

    o Client education

        ▪ Encourage clients to avoid alcohol intake.

        ▪ Recommend clients eat a low-fat diet and maintain a BMI less than 30.

        ▪ Recommend clients receive a hepatitis B immunization.

        ▪ Recommend clients take precautions against hepatitis B and C (recognize that multiple sexual partners, IV drug use, and the sharing of needles all increase risk).

- Client Outcomes

    o The client's tumor will be surgically, chemically, or mechanically removed or demonstrate a decrease in size.

    o The client's appetite and nutritional status will improve.

Complications

- Acute graft rejection post-liver transplantation

Ⓐ APPLICATION EXERCISES

Scenario: A 65-year-old man is being evaluated for possible hepatocellular or liver carcinoma. The client is slightly jaundiced, and he has been experiencing nausea, anorexia, and abdominal pain. His provider has also discovered a small abdominal mass in the right upper quadrant. The client's serum sodium level is 140 mEq/L. His ammonia level is 40 mg/dL. There is no evidence of hepatic encephalopathy or ascites at this time.

1. Which of the following risk factors may have contributed to the development of the client's liver cancer? (Select all that apply.)

    _____ History of chronic hepatitis C

    _____ Biliary obstruction

    _____ History of smoking

    _____ History of alcoholism

    _____ Esophageal varices

    _____ Metastatic colon cancer

2. When the nurse reviews the client's chart, which of the following laboratory findings supports the diagnosis of primary liver cancer? (Select all that apply.)

    _____ Elevated alpha-fetoprotein (AFP)

    _____ Elevated alkaline phosphatase (ALP) 189 units/L

    _____ Hgb 14 g/dL

    _____ Serum total bilirubin 1.0 mg/dL

    _____ Elevated CEA

3. Which of the following dietary modifications should the nurse recommend for inclusion in the client's plan of care? (Select all that apply.)

    _____ High-calorie, moderate fat diet

    _____ Low-sodium diet

    _____ Low-protein diet

    _____ Small, frequent, well-balanced nutritional meals

    _____ Supplemental vitamin-enriched liquids

    _____ Replacement and administration of vitamins

    _____ Fluid restriction

(A) **APPLICATION EXERCISES ANSWER KEY**

Scenario: A 65-year-old man is being evaluated for possible hepatocellular or liver carcinoma. The client is slightly jaundiced, and he has been experiencing nausea, anorexia, and abdominal pain. His provider has also discovered a small abdominal mass in the right upper quadrant. The client's serum sodium level is 140 mEq/L. His ammonia level is 40 mg/dL. There is no evidence of hepatic encephalopathy or ascites at this time.

1. Which of the following risk factors may have contributed to the development of the client's liver cancer? (Select all that apply.)

   __X__ **History of chronic hepatitis C**

   _____ Biliary obstruction

   __X__ **History of smoking**

   __X__ **History of alcoholism**

   _____ Esophageal varices

   __X__ **Metastatic colon cancer**

   Chronic hepatitis C, smoking, alcoholism, and metastatic colon cancer could have been contributing factors in the development of the client's liver cancer. Biliary obstruction does not cause liver cancer. And while alcoholism can cause cirrhosis and secondarily esophageal varices, the esophageal varices themselves do not contribute to liver cancer.

   (N) NCLEX® Connection: Physiological Adaptations, Basic Pathophysiology

2. When the nurse reviews the client's chart, which of the following laboratory findings supports the diagnosis of primary liver cancer? (Select all that apply.)

   __X__ **Elevated alpha-fetoprotein (AFP)**

   __X__ **Elevated alkaline phosphatase (ALP) 189 units/L**

   _____ Hgb 14 g/dL

   _____ Serum total bilirubin 1.0 mg/dL

   __X__ **Elevated CEA**

   AFP, ALP, and CEA are elevated in a client who has liver cancer. The Hgb and serum total bilirubin levels are within the expected reference range.

   (N) NCLEX® Connection: Reduction of Risk Potential, Laboratory Values

3. Which of the following dietary modifications should the nurse recommend for inclusion in the client's plan of care? (Select all that apply.)

   __X__   **High-calorie, moderate fat diet**

   _____   Low-sodium diet

   _____   Low-protein diet

   __X__   **Small, frequent, well-balanced nutritional meals**

   __X__   **Supplemental vitamin-enriched liquids**

   __X__   **Replacement and administration of vitamins**

   _____   Fluid restriction

The client's diet should be developed around small, frequent, well-balanced meals that are high in calories, contain moderate amounts of fat, and are supplemented with vitamin-enriched liquids and vitamins. The client's sodium level is within the expected reference range, and there is no evidence of ascites at this time, so a low-sodium diet and fluid restriction are not necessary. The client's ammonia level is also within the expected reference range, and there is no evidence of hepatic encephalopathy, so a low-protein diet is not indicated.

(N) NCLEX® Connection: Basic Care and Comfort, Nutrition and Oral Hydration

UNIT 8: NURSING CARE OF CLIENTS WITH RENAL SYSTEM DISORDERS

- Diagnostic and Therapeutic Procedures
- Renal System Disorders

NCLEX® CONNECTIONS

When reviewing the chapters in this section, keep in mind the relevant sections of the NCLEX® outline, in particular:

CLIENT NEEDS: BASIC CARE AND COMFORT

Relevant topics/tasks include:
- Elimination
  - Use alternative methods to promote voiding.
- Nonpharmacological Comfort Interventions
  - Evaluate pain using rating scale.
- Nutrition and Oral Hydration
  - Monitor client intake/output.

CLIENT NEEDS: REDUCTION OF RISK POTENTIAL

Relevant topics/tasks include:
- Diagnostic Tests
  - Perform diagnostic testing.
- Laboratory Values
  - Monitor diagnostic or laboratory test results.
- Potential for Alterations in Body Systems
  - Compare current client clinical data to baseline information.

CLIENT NEEDS: PHYSIOLOGICAL ADAPTATION

Relevant topics/tasks include:
- Alterations in Body Systems
  - Provide care to client undergoing peritoneal dialysis.
- Basic Pathophysiology
  - Identify signs and symptoms related to acute or chronic illness.
- Fluid and Electrolyte Imbalances
  - Provide interventions to restore client fluid and/or electrolyte balance.

UNIT 8	NURSING CARE OF CLIENTS WITH RENAL SYSTEM DISORDERS

Section: Diagnostic and Therapeutic Procedures

Chapter 53   Renal Diagnostic Procedures

◎ Overview

- Laboratory tests and diagnostic procedures are performed to identify dysfunction of the renal system.

  ○ Responsibilities of the nurse include verifying information, reinforcing teaching, positioning clients, obtaining urine and blood samples using standard precautions or surgical asepsis, labeling containers with the client's identifying information, and transporting specimens to the laboratory.

- Laboratory tests

  ○ Urine specimens and blood samples

    ■ Indications

      □ Infection, renal dysfunction

PROCEDURE	NURSING INTERVENTIONS
Random nonsterile specimen – Usually for urinalysis and obtained with first void.	• Ask clients to urinate in clean container. • Pour urine into the specimen container.
Clean-catch midstream for culture and sensitivity (C&S)	• Instruct clients to: ○ Clean the urinary meatus with provided wipes. ○ Urinate a small amount, and while continuing to urinate, collect some urine in a sterile container. • Label the container with the client's identifying information. • Transport or send the specimen to the laboratory.
Catheter urine specimen for C&S	• Drain the catheter's tubing of urine. • Clamp the catheter's tubing below the port for 20 min. • Use surgical asepsis while withdrawing the required amount from the port with a syringe. • Unclamp the catheter. • Place the specimen in a sterile container.

PROCEDURE	NURSING INTERVENTIONS

Timed urine specimens	• Instruct clients to:
	  ○ Discard the first voiding.
	  ○ Collect all other voidings in a container placed on ice.
	  ○ Bring the container to the laboratory.

LABORATORY TEST	EXPECTED REFERENCE RANGE	SIGNIFICANCE OF FINDINGS
Serum BUN	• 10 to 20 mg/dL	• Increased with liver/kidney dysfunction, decreased renal perfusion, dehydration, high-protein diet, infection, GI bleeding, steroid use • Decreased with malnutrition, fluid volume excess, severe liver damage
Serum creatinine	• Males – 0.6 to 1.2 mg/dL • Females – 0.5 to 1.1mg/dL)	• Increased with kidney dysfunction • Decreased with decreased muscle mass
Creatinine clearance	• Males – 90 to 139 mL/min/m^2 • Females – 80 to 125 mL/min/m^2	• Best indication of overall kidney function
Urinalysis	• Clear, pale yellow, ammonia smell • Specific gravity 1.005-1.030 • pH 4.6-8 • Glucose – less than 0.5 g/day; protein 0.8 mg/dL; minimal RBCs, WBCs, casts • Bacteria – less than 1000 colonies/mL	• Infection, dehydration, fluid overload, hyperglycemia

Procedures

TEST	INDICATIONS/INTERPRETATION OF FINDINGS	NURSING INTERVENTIONS
Bedside sonogram/ Bladder scan	• Determines post-void residual volume of urine and if the client should have intermittent catheterization	• No preparation necessary • Choose male or female icon on scanner • Use conduction pad or gel and place the probe of the scanner at the midline about 4 cm (1.5 in) above the pubic bone, aiming towards the coccyx. • Take two readings by pressing and releasing the scan button.
Radiography	• An x-ray of the kidneys, ureters, and bladder (KUB) (can also be prescribed as a "flat plate") • Allows for visualization of these structures. Does not diagnose functional or structural problems.	• Ask female clients if they are pregnant. Inform clients that clothes over the area will need to be removed as well as all jewelry. X-ray will be taken with client in a supine position. • IV contrast dye (iodine-based) can be used to enhance images. ○ Determine if clients are allergic to iodine. Dye can cause renal failure. • Always check the client's creatinine levels. Parenteral fluid can be given to protect the function of the kidneys. • Steroids and/or antihistamines may be given. • Monitor for altered renal function following procedure. • Discontinue metformin (Glucophage) for at least 48 hr after the procedure.
CT scan	• Provides cross-sectional images to assess the size of the kidney and to assess for obstruction, cysts, or masses	• Same as KUB
MRI	• Useful in staging cancer, similar to a CT scan	• Clients will lie down and have to remain still for test. Determine if client is claustrophobic.

TEST	INDICATIONS/INTERPRETATION OF FINDINGS	NURSING INTERVENTIONS
Intravenous pyelography (IVP)	• Used to detect renal stones or injury and location, as well as assess renal function	• Not to be done during pregnancy • Relieving bowels produces better images. • IV bolus contrast dye (iodine based) can be used to enhance images. ○ Determine if clients are allergic to iodine. Dye can cause renal failure. • Always check the client's creatinine levels. Steroids and/or antihistamines may be given. • Monitor for altered renal function following procedure. • Metformin (glucophage) should be discontinued for at least 48 hr after the procedure.
Voiding cystourethrography (VCUG)	• Used to outline the bladder's shape and to detect urinary reflux	• This process can increase the risk of an infection due to urinary catheterization. Monitor clients for infection for the first 72 hr after the procedure.
Excretory urography	• Used to detect obstruction, assess for a parenchymal mass, and assess size of the kidney	• Same as KUB
Renal biopsy	• Removal of a sample of tissue by excision or needle aspiration for cytological (histological) examination to determine cause of renal problems	• Clients receive sedation and are monitored for this procedure. • Always check the client's coagulation studies. • Clients must lie on back postoperatively for 6 hr to prevent bleeding. Check for signs of bleeding and infection. • Hematuria may be present.
Cystoscopy	• Used to discover abnormalities of the bladder wall and/or occlusions of the ureter or urethra • May be used to remove tumors or enlarged prostate gland	• Clients are given anesthesia for the procedure. • Monitor vital signs. Check for signs of bleeding and infection. Monitor clients for infection for the first 72 hr after the procedure. Monitor urine output which may be pink tinged.

TEST	INDICATIONS/INTERPRETATION OF FINDINGS	NURSING INTERVENTIONS
Renal scan	• Used to assess renal blood flow and function	• Withhold ACE inhibitors 48 hr prior to the procedure. • No contrast dye is used for this procedure. • Medications can be given during the test. Watch for hypotension and make sure clients are well hydrated.
Renal ultrasound	• Used to assess the size of the kidney or for an obstruction in the lower urinary tract	• Minimal risk for clients. Good option if not able to do the excretory urography. • Requires full bladder.

- Complications
  - Bleeding
    - Bleeding can result from some of the above tests noted and should be monitored closely.
    - Nursing actions
      - If bleeding does occur, notify the provider immediately.
      - Notify provider immediately if client reports flank or abdominal pain.
  - Hematuria
    - Blood in the urine is one of the most common complications with a renal biopsy.
    - Nursing actions
      - Monitor the client's urinary output closely. Note the color and amount. If bright red blood or clots are observed, notify the provider immediately.
  - Renal failure
    - Using contrast dye can place the client at risk for renal failure.
    - Nursing actions
      - Always check the client's creatinine level prior to the procedure.
      - Monitor clients receiving IV fluids given for prevention of renal failure if needed.
  - Infection
    - Infection can be a result of some of the above tests noted and needs to be monitored for the first 48 to 72 hr after the procedure.
    - Nursing Actions
      - Notify the provider if clients have a temperature, are unable to void, or report pain.

Ⓐ **APPLICATION EXERCISES**

1. A nurse is caring for a client who is undergoing an x-ray of the kidneys, ureters, and bladder, or a KUB of the abdomen. Which of the following should the nurse reinforce when teaching the client about the test?

    A. "This test requires several position changes and will take most of the day."

    B. "You might experience some discomfort during the test."

    C. "You will be in the prone position for the test."

    D. "This test will help determine if you have a kidney stone."

2. A nurse is caring for a client who has just had a renal biopsy. Which of the following complications should the nurse monitor for during the immediate post-procedure period?

    A. Infection

    B. Bleeding

    C. Hematuria

    D. Decreased urine output

3. A nurse is caring for a client who has just had a cystoscopy to detect for bladder wall abnormalities and blockages in the ureters. The plan of care includes monitoring for infection. Which of the following data should be reported to the charge nurse?

    A. Temperature 36.8° C (98.2° F)

    B. Blood pressure 138/88 mm Hg

    C. Pain rating of 6 out of 10

    D. Urinary output 60 mL/2 hr

APPLICATION EXERCISES ANSWER KEY

1. A nurse is caring for a client who is undergoing an x-ray of the kidneys, ureters, and bladder, or a KUB of the abdomen. Which of the following should the nurse reinforce when teaching the client about the test?

    A. "This test requires several position changes and will take most of the day."

    B. "You might experience some discomfort during the test."

    C. "You will be in the prone position for the test."

    D. "This test will help determine if you have a kidney stone."

    A KUB is an x-ray that can identify kidney stones and other abnormalities of the kidneys, ureters, and bladder in regard to shape, strictures, or obstructions. This test is very brief unless a contrast dye is used, in which case the client will be monitored for side effects. There is no discomfort experienced during this test, and the client should be placed in the supine position.

     NCLEX® Connection: Reduction of Risk Potential, Therapeutic Procedures

2. A nurse is caring for a client who has just had a renal biopsy. Which of the following complications should the nurse monitor for during the immediate post-procedure period?

    A. Infection

    B. Bleeding

    C. Hematuria

    D. Decreased urine output

    The most immediate risk to the client is bleeding into the muscle or the kidney due to the invasiveness of the procedure. Infection, hematuria, and decreased urine output are potential complications but do not develop in the immediate post-operative period.

     NCLEX® Connection: Reduction of Risk Potential, Potential for Complications of Diagnostic Tests/Treatments/Procedures

3. A nurse is caring for a client who has just had a cystoscopy to detect for bladder wall abnormalities and blockages in the ureters. The plan of care includes monitoring for infection. Which of the following data should be reported to the charge nurse?

    A. Temperature 36.8° C (98.2° F)

    B. Blood pressure 138/88 mm Hg

    C. Pain rating of 6 out of 10

    D. Urinary output 60 mL/2 hr

    The nurse should report the pain rating to the charge nurse because pain can be a symptom of an infection. The other findings are within their expected reference range.

     NCLEX® Connection: Reduction of Risk Potential, Potential for Complications of Diagnostic Tests/Treatments/Procedures

UNIT 8	NURSING CARE OF CLIENTS WITH RENAL SYSTEM DISORDERS

Section: Diagnostic and Therapeutic Procedures

Chapter 54   Hemodialysis and Peritoneal Dialysis

Overview

- Functions of dialysis

    o   Rids the body of excess fluid and electrolytes.

    o   Achieves acid-base balance.

    o   Eliminates waste products.

    o   Restores internal homeostasis by osmosis, diffusion, and ultrafiltration.

- Dialysis can sustain life for clients who have both acute and chronic renal failure.

- Dialysis does not replace the hormonal functions of the kidneys.

- The two types of dialysis are hemodialysis and peritoneal dialysis.

Hemodialysis

- Hemodialysis shunts the client's blood from the body through a dialyzer and back into circulation. Vascular access is needed for hemodialysis.

- Indications

    o   Diagnoses

        ▪   Renal insufficiency

        ▪   Acute renal failure

        ▪   Chronic renal failure

        ▪   Drug overdose

        ▪   Persistent hyperkalemia

        ▪   Hypervolemia unresponsive to diuretics

    o   Client presentation

        ▪   Subjective data

            ▫   Fatigue, numbness and tingling of extremities, shortness of breath, anorexia, dry itchy skin, muscle pain

- Objective data
    - Lethargy, decreased attention span, seizures, tremors, hypertension, heart failure (edema of hands and feet, dyspnea, distended jugular veins, crackles), anemia, vomiting, pulmonary edema, cardiac dysrhythmias, pallor, bruising, halitosis, diminished or dark-colored urine

- Client Outcomes

    - The client will achieve and maintain a desired fluid and electrolyte balance, be free of infection, and perform self-care with minimum restrictions.

- Preprocedure

    - Nursing actions

        - Check patency of the access site (presence of bruit, palpable thrill, distal pulses, and circulation).

        - Avoid taking blood pressure, administering injections, performing venipunctures or inserting IV lines on an arm with an access site. Elevate the extremity following surgical development of AV fistula to reduce swelling.

        - Check vital signs, laboratory values (BUN, serum creatinine, electrolytes, Hct), and weight.

        - Discuss with the provider any medications that need to be withheld until after dialysis. Dialyzable medications and medications that lower blood pressure are usually withheld.

    - Client education

        - Instruct clients about the procedure. Tell clients that hemodialysis is usually done three times per week, for 3- to 5-hr sessions. Using sterile technique, two needles are inserted, one into an artery and the other into a vein.

        - Instruct clients to notify the nurse of muscle cramps, headache, nausea, or dizziness that occurs during the procedure.

- Intraprocedure

     View Media Supplement: Hemodialysis (Animation)

    - Nursing actions

        - Monitor vital signs and laboratory values during dialysis. Monitor for bleeding, such as oozing from insertion site. Monitor coagulation studies.

        - Administer anticoagulants as prescribed.

        - Have protamine sulfate ready to reverse heparin, if needed.

        - Provide emotional support. Offer activities, such as books, magazines, music, cards, or television, to occupy clients.

- Postprocedure
  - Nursing actions
    - Monitor vital signs, laboratory values (BUN, serum creatinine, electrolytes, Hct), and weight. Decreases in blood pressure, weight, and laboratory values are expected following dialysis.
    - Monitor for:
      - Complications (hypotension, clotting of vascular access, headache, muscle cramps, bleeding, disequilibrium syndrome)
      - Indications of bleeding, and/or infection at the access site
      - Nausea, vomiting, and change in level of consciousness
      - Signs of hypovolemia
    - Avoid invasive procedures for 4 to 6 hr after dialysis due to the risk of bleeding related to an intraprocedure anticoagulant.
  - Client education
    - Teach clients to:
      - Avoid lifting heavy objects with access-site arm.
      - Avoid carrying objects that compress the extremity.
      - Avoid sleeping on top of the extremity with the access device.
      - Perform hand exercises that promote fistula maturation.
      - Check the access site at intervals following dialysis. Apply light pressure if bleeding. Notify the provider if the site continues to bleed after 30 min following dialysis.
- Complications
  - Clotting/infection of access site
    - Anticoagulants are often given to prevent blood clots from forming. Infections of the access site are likely introduced during cannulation.
    - Advanced age is a risk factor for access site complications related to chronic illnesses and/or fragile veins.
    - Nursing actions
      - Avoid compression of access site and venipuncture or blood pressure on extremity with access site.
      - Administer anticoagulants as prescribed.
      - Observe graft site for palpable thrill or audible bruit indicating vascular flow.
      - Observe the access site for redness, swelling, or drainage. Monitor for fever.

- ■ Client education
  - □ Instruct clients to monitor the access site for signs of an infection such as fever, redness, drainage, or swelling.
  - □ Reinforce to clients to check the graft for patency by checking for thrill or bruit. Advise clients to contact the provider for absence of thrill/bruit and for signs of infection.
  - □ Advise clients to prevent any constriction of extremity with the vascular access.
- ○ Disequilibrium syndrome
  - ■ Disequilibrium syndrome is caused by too rapid a decrease of BUN and circulating fluid volume. It may result in cerebral edema and increased intracranial pressure (IICP).
    - □ Early recognition of disequilibrium syndrome is essential. Signs include nausea, vomiting, change in level of consciousness, seizures, and agitation.
    - □ Advanced age is a risk factor for dialysis disequilibrium and hypotension due to rapid changes in fluid and electrolyte status.
  - ■ Nursing actions
    - □ Use a slow dialysis exchange rate, especially for older adult clients and those being treated with hemodialysis for the first time.
    - □ Administer anticonvulsants/barbiturates if needed.
  - ■ Client education
    - □ Advise clients to alert the nurse of early signs of disequilibrium syndrome, such as nausea and headache.
- ○ Hypotension
  - ■ Rapid fluid depletion during dialysis may cause hypotension. Other causes include antihypertensives and splanchnic vasodilation due to food ingestion during dialysis.
  - ■ Nursing actions
    - □ Monitor clients receiving IV fluid or colloid replacement. Slow the dialysis exchange rate.
    - □ Lower the head of the client's bed.
    - □ For severe hypotension that is unresponsive to fluid replacement, discontinue the dialysis.
  - ■ Client education
    - □ Advise clients to notify the nurse of headache, nausea, or dizziness during dialysis. Advise clients not to eat during dialysis.

- ○ Anemia
  - ▪ Blood loss and removal of folate during dialysis may contribute to an existing anemia that often occurs with chronic renal failure (caused by decreased RBC production due to decreased erythropoietin secretion).
  - ▪ Nursing actions
    - ☐ Administer prescribed medication therapy (erythropoietin) to stimulate the production of RBCs.
    - ☐ Monitor Hgb and RBC level.
    - ☐ Monitor for hypotension and tachycardia.
  - ▪ Client education
    - ☐ Advise clients to take medications and supplements as prescribed.
    - ☐ Reinforce to clients about diet and nutrition, including foods high in folate (beans, green vegetables).

Peritoneal Dialysis

- • Peritoneal dialysis involves instillation of fluid into the peritoneal cavity. The peritoneum serves as the filtration membrane.
  - ○ Clients should have an intact peritoneal membrane, without adhesions from infection or multiple surgeries.

 View Media Supplement: Peritoneal Dialysis (Animation)

- • Indications
  - ○ Peritoneal dialysis is indicated for clients requiring dialysis who:
    - ▪ Are unable to tolerate anticoagulation.
    - ▪ Have difficulty with vascular access.
- • Client outcomes
  - ○ The client will achieve and maintain a desired fluid and electrolyte balance, be free of infection, and maintain an active lifestyle with minimum restrictions.
- • Preprocedure
  - ○ Nursing actions
    - ▪ Check dry weight (obtained when dialysate is drained), baseline vital signs, serum electrolytes, creatinine, BUN, and blood glucose.
    - ▪ Determine the client's ability to perform self-peritoneal dialysis.

- ○ Client education
  - Clients should be instructed about the procedure. Clients may feel fullness when the dialysate is dwelling. There may be discomfort initially with the dialysate infusion.
  - Continuous ambulatory peritoneal dialysis (CAPD) is usually done 7 days a week for 4 to 8 hr. Clients may continue normal activities during CAPD.

- Intraprocedure
  - ○ Nursing actions
    - Monitor the client's vital signs frequently during initial dialysis of clients in a hospital setting.
    - Monitor the client's serum glucose level.
    - Record the amount of inflow compared to outflow of dialysate.
    - Monitor the color (clear, light yellow is expected) and amount (expected to equal or exceed amount of dialysate inflow) of outflow. Outflow should be a continuous stream.
    - Monitor for signs of infection (fever; bloody, cloudy, or frothy dialysate return; drainage at access site) and for complications (respiratory distress, abdominal pain, insufficient outflow, discolored outflow).
    - Check the access site dressing for wetness (risk of dialysate leakage).
    - Warm the dialysate prior to instilling. Avoid the use of microwaves, which cause uneven heating.
    - Follow prescribed times for infusion, dwell, and outflow.
    - Maintain surgical asepsis of the catheter insertion site and when accessing the catheter.
    - Keep the outflow bag lower than the client's abdomen (drain by gravity, prevent reflux).
    - Reposition client if inflow or outflow is inadequate.
    - Carefully milk peritoneal dialysis catheter if fibrin clot has formed.
    - Provide emotional support to the client and family.

- Postprocedure
  - ○ Nursing actions
    - Monitor weight, serum electrolytes, creatinine, BUN, and blood glucose.

○ Client education

- Reinforce teaching to clients regarding home care of the access site.

  □ Instruct clients and their families how to perform peritoneal dialysis exchanges at home. Provide support for home peritoneal dialysis with home visits and support groups, such as the National Kidney Foundation. Instruct the client to follow directions carefully and to take all medications as prescribed.

  □ Older adult clients may be unable to care for a peritoneal access site due to cognitive or physical deficits.

- Complications

  ○ Peritonitis

  - Peritoneal dialysis can allow micro-organisms into the peritoneum and cause peritonitis.

  - Nursing actions

    □ Use sterile technique when connecting or disconnecting peritoneal catheter.

    □ Monitor for infection, such as fever, purulent drainage, redness or swelling, and cloudy or discolored drained dialysate.

    □ Obtain specimen for culture and sensitivity, along with Gram stain of dialysate outflow, if peritonitis is suspected.

  - Client education

    □ Educate clients to use strict sterile technique during exchanges.

    □ Instruct clients to notify the provider about any sign of infection.

  ○ Infection at the access site

  - Infection at the access site may be related to leakage of dialysate. Access site infections may cause peritonitis.

    □ Advanced age is a risk factor for access site complications related to chronic illnesses and/or fragile veins.

  - Nursing actions

    □ Maintain surgical asepsis of access site.

    □ Check site for wetness from a leaking catheter.

    □ Monitor for infection, such as fever, purulent drainage, redness, or swelling.

    □ Obtain specimen for culture and sensitivity along with Gram stain if purulent drainage is present at access site.

  - Client education

    □ Reinforce to clients the need to use strict sterile technique during exchanges.

    □ Instruct clients to notify the provider with any sign of infection.

    □ Advise clients to check the site for leaks and prevent tugging or twisting of tubing.

UNIT 8	NURSING CARE OF CLIENTS WITH RENAL SYSTEM DISORDERS
Section:	Renal System Disorders

Chapter 55   Acute and Chronic Glomerulonephritis

 Overview

- Glomerulonephritis is an inflammation of the glomerular capillaries, usually following a streptococcal infection. It is an immune complex disease, not an infection of the kidney.

- Glomerulonephritis exists as an acute, latent, and chronic disease.

- Acute glomerulonephritis (AGN)

  o Insoluble immune complexes develop and become trapped in the glomerular tissue, producing swelling and capillary cell death.

  o Prognosis varies depending upon the specific cause, but spontaneous recovery generally occurs after the acute illness.

- Chronic glomerulonephritis (CGN)

  o CGN can occur without a previous history or known onset.

  o This involves the progressive destruction of glomeruli and their eventual hardening (sclerosis).

  o CGN is the third-leading cause of end-stage renal disease (ESRD), with the prognosis varying depending on the specific cause.

(M) **View Media Supplement:** Glomerulonephritis (Image)

Data Collection

- Risk Factors

  o Immunological reactions

    ▪ Primary infection, particularly of the skin or upper respiratory tract, with group A beta-hemolytic streptococcal infection (most common)

    ▪ Systemic lupus erythematosus (SLE)

  o Vascular injury (hypertension)

  o Metabolic disease (diabetes mellitus)

    ○   Excessively high protein and high sodium diets

Ⓖ   ○   Older adult clients may report vague symptoms (nausea, fatigue, joint aches) which may mask glomerular disease.

    ○   Older adult clients tend to have a decreased number of working nephrons and are at increased risk for chronic renal failure.

- Subjective and Objective Data

  - Renal symptoms

    - Decreased urine output

    - Smoky or coffee-colored urine (hematuria)

    - Proteinuria

  - Fluid volume excess symptoms

    - Shortness of breath

    - Orthopnea

    - Bibasilar rales

    - Periorbital edema

    - Neck vein distention

    - S_3 heart sound

    - Mild to severe hypertension

  - Changes in the level of consciousness

  - Anorexia/nausea

  - Headache

  - Back pain

  - Fever (AGN)

  - Pruritus (CGN)

  - Laboratory tests

    - Throat culture to identify possible streptococcus infection

    - Serum BUN – Elevated: 100 to 200 mg/dL; expected reference range: 10 to 20 mg/dL

    - Creatinine – Elevated: greater than 6 mg/dL. Expected reference range: males, 0.6 to 1.2 mg/dL; females, 0.5 to 1.1mg/dL

    - Creatinine clearance – Decreased: 50 mL/min/m². Expected reference range: males: 90 to 139 mL/min/m², females: 80 to 125 mL/min/m²

    - Urinalysis – Proteinuria, hematuria, cell debris (red cells and casts), increased urine specific gravity

    - Electrolytes – Hyperkalemia and hyperphosphatemia

- Antistreptolysin-O (ASO) titer – Positive indicating the presence of strep antibodies
- Erythrocyte sedimentation rate (ESR) – Elevated indicating active inflammatory response
- WBC count – Elevated indicating inflammation and presence of active strep infection
- Glomerular filtration rate (GFR) – Decrease indicates loss of renal filtration function; best indicator of overall kidney function.
- Serum albumin levels are decreased due to protein loss in the urine and fluid retention.
- Diagnostic procedures
  - X-ray of kidney, ureter, bladder (KUB), and renal ultrasound (to detect structural abnormalities [atrophy])
  - Renal biopsy in early stages (to confirm or rule out diagnosis)
  - During acute glomerulonephritis, dialysis can be an intervention to treat severe uremia (large amounts of urea and other nitrogenous waste found in the blood)

Collaborative Care

- Nursing Care
  - Monitor the client's daily weight and note any recent weight gain.
  - Monitor I&O.
  - Observe clients for changes in urinary pattern.
  - Monitor serum electrolytes, BUN, and creatinine.
  - Maintain bed rest to decrease metabolic demands.
  - Maintain prescribed dietary restrictions.
    - Fluid restriction (24 hr output + 500 to 600 mL)
    - Sodium restriction
    - Protein restriction (if azotemia is present = increased BUN)
- Medications
  - Administer antibiotics on time to maintain blood levels for an effective elimination of the strep infection. Check for medication allergies clients may have.
  - Administer diuretics to reduce edema.
  - Use vasodilators to decrease blood pressure.
  - Administer corticosteroids to decrease the inflammatory response.
- Interdisciplinary Care
  - Request a referral for nutritional services for diet modifications and fluid restriction.
  - Request a referral for home care services if clients are homebound or living in a nursing facility.

- Therapeutic Procedures
  - Plasmapheresis (filters antibodies out of circulating blood volume)
    - Nursing actions
      - Monitor clients carefully during and following the procedure.
      - Take appropriate interventions to reduce the risk of coagulation.
    - Client education
      - Encourage clients to rest in order to conserve energy.
- Care after Discharge
  - Client education
    - Instruct clients to take medications as prescribed and to complete the entire course of any prescribed antibiotics.
    - Instruct clients to weigh themselves daily, at the same time, and to notify the provider for a weight gain of 2 lb in 24 hr or 5 lb in 1 week.
    - Instruct clients to take blood pressure reading daily at the same time, and notify the provider for any sudden increases.
    - Advise clients to maintain fluid and sodium restriction.
    - Inform clients of signs and symptoms of fluid retention and findings to report.
    - Reinforce to clients and families regarding the illness and encourage the expression of feelings.
- Client outcomes
  - The client will be free from pain.
  - The client will maintain fluid balance.
  - The client will improve tolerance to activity.
  - The client will follow a medication regimen.

Complications

- Uremia
  - Symptoms include muscle cramps, fatigue, pruritus, anorexia, and a metallic taste in mouth.
  - Nursing actions
    - Intervene to maintain skin integrity.
    - Assist with dialysis.
- Anemia
  - Nursing actions
    - Monitor hemoglobin.
    - Administer iron and erythropoietin as indicated.

- o Hyperlipidemia
- o Diseases of the vascular system
- o Renal function decreases with aging, which increases the risk for nephrotic syndrome.
- Subjective Data
  - o Edema (periorbital, dependent)
  - o Irritability
  - o Malaise, fatigue
  - o Anorexia, nausea
- Objective Data
  - o Proteinuria
  - o Hematuria
  - o Hypertension
  - o Anasarca (severe generalized edema)
  - o Foamy urine
  - o Oliguria
  - o Anemia (Hgb 12 g/dL or less)
  - o Azotemia (increased BUN)
  - o Uremia (symptoms of renal failure)
  - o Loss of skin integrity related to edema
  - o Laboratory Tests
    - ▪ Urinalysis/24 hr urine collection
      - □ Protein as high as +3 or +4 (> 3.5 g in 24 hr)
      - □ Casts
    - ▪ Serum lipid levels
      - □ Elevated serum cholesterol (> 200 mg/dL)
      - □ Elevated triglycerides
      - □ Elevated low-density and very low-density lipoproteins
    - ▪ Serum albumin
      - □ Less than 3 g/dL
    - ▪ Serum BUN, creatinine, and glomerular filtration rate (GFR) levels may indicate minimal to extensive loss of kidney function.
      - □ BUN and creatinine levels rise, while GFR levels decrease with the loss of kidney function.

- ○ Diagnostic Procedures
  - ■ Kidney biopsy
    - □ Minimal to extensive damage
    - □ Fatty deposits in tubules
    - □ Epithelium changes
    - □ Hypercellularity
    - □ Glomerular sclerosis
    - □ Immunoglobulins in capillary walls
    - □ Nursing Action
      - ▸ Explain the reason for the test.
      - ▸ Verify consent.
      - ▸ Prepare clients for the test.
      - ▸ Collect specimens accurately.

Collaborative Care

- • Nursing Care
  - ○ Monitor blood pressure and I&O.
  - ○ Report abnormal findings to the provider.
  - ○ Provide periods of rest with activities.
  - ○ Provide emotional support.
  - ○ Encourage adequate nutritional intake within restriction guidelines.
    - ■ Encourage lowering sodium intake.
    - ■ Adjust protein intake according to protein loss in urine over 24 hr.
    - ■ Provide high biologic value protein (lean meat, fish, poultry, dairy).
    - ■ Provide small, frequent feedings due to the client's loss of appetite.
  - ○ Administer medications as prescribed.
  - ○ Monitor skin and provide skin care.
- • Medications
  - ○ Loop diuretics – furosemide (Lasix), bumetanide (Bumex)
    - ■ Nursing Considerations
      - □ Monitor I&O.
      - □ Monitor for orthostatic hypotension.

- Client Education
    - Instruct clients to take the medication with food.
    - Inform clients that the medication may cause dizziness and lightheadedness and to change positions slowly.
- Angiotensin-converting enzyme (ACE) inhibitors – captopril (Capoten)
    - This is used to block the production of angiotensin II, resulting in the excretion of sodium and water.
    - Nursing Considerations
        - Monitor clients for increased potassium level.
        - Monitor clients for hypotension.
        - Use carefully for clients with renal impairment related to leukocyte depletion, and watch for infection.
    - Client Education
        - Inform clients that the medication may cause a dry cough that should be reported to the provider.
- Anticoagulants – Heparin
    - This can be used to decrease proteinuria and renal insufficiency.
    - Nursing Considerations
        - Monitor the client's aPTT level.
        - Monitor clients for signs of bleeding.
- Corticosteroid – Prednisone (Deltasone), cytotoxic or immunosuppressive agents – Cyclophosphamide (Cytoxan)
    - Use to improve immunologic processes.
    - Nursing Considerations
        - Monitor clients for infection.
    - Client Education
        - Instruct clients to avoid crowds and other situations that increase the risk for infection.
- Epoetin alfa (Epogen, Procrit)
    - This is used to stimulate the production of RBCs and is given for anemia.
    - Nursing Considerations
        - Monitor Hgb and Hct.
        - Monitor the client's blood pressure.
        - This is contraindicated for clients with uncontrolled hypertension.
    - Client Education
        - Instruct clients to have blood drawn twice a week to monitor Hgb and Hct.

- Interdisciplinary Care

  o Nephrology services may be consulted for renal impairment.

  o Nutritional services may be consulted for dietary modifications.

- Care after Discharge

  o Client Education

    ▪ Instruct clients to consume a diet low in sodium and restrict fluid intake.

    ▪ Encourage clients to provide periods of rest with activities.

    ▪ Encourage clients to take medications as prescribed.

    ▪ Instruct clients to notify the provider for a possible increased risk for bleeding.

    ▪ Instruct clients to take orthostatic hypotension precautions.

    ▪ Instruct clients to consult provider for decreasing urine output.

  o Client Outcomes

    ▪ The client will adhere to a prescribed medication regimen.

    ▪ The client will have a decrease in anxiety.

    ▪ The client will have an increase in activity level.

    ▪ The client will maintain an oral fluid restriction regimen.

    ▪ The client will have normal urine output.

Complications

- Respiratory Compromise

  o Nursing Actions

    ▪ Monitor breath sounds, respiratory rate, oxygen saturation.

- Peritonitis

  o Nursing Actions

    ▪ Monitor bowel sounds.

    ▪ Monitor for infection (rigid, tender abdomen, fever, elevated WBC count, tachycardia).

- Renal Failure

  o Nursing Actions

    ▪ Monitor renal status (BUN, serum creatinine, urinalysis).

    ▪ Monitor urine output.

    ▪ Prepare the client for dialysis, if indicated.

- Shock/Death

  o Nursing Actions

    ▪ Monitor for early indications of shock.

    ▪ Assist with emergency care.

ACUTE AND CHRONIC RENAL FAILURE

Overview

- The kidneys regulate fluid, acid-base, electrolyte balance, and hormone secretion, while also, eliminating wastes from the body.

- Renal failure may be diagnosed as acute or chronic. Acute renal failure can result in chronic renal failure without aggressive treatment, or when complicating pre-existing conditions exist.

- Acute renal failure (ARF) is the sudden cessation of renal function that occurs when blood flow to the kidneys is significantly compromised.

  o ARF is a leading cause of death among hospitalized clients and 50% is due to an iatrogenic cause.

  o ARF is comprised of four phases:

    ▪ Onset – begins with the onset of the event and lasts for hours to days. BUN and creatinine may begin to rise.

    ▪ Oliguria – begins with the renal insult and lasts for 1 to 3 weeks. Urine output –100 to 400/mL/day, which does not respond to treatment. Increasing BUN and creatinine and electrolyte imbalances begin.

    ▪ Diuresis – begins when the kidneys start to recover and can last for 2 to 6 weeks. In the high-output phase, output for dilute urine may be up to 10 L/day. BUN begins to fall.

    ▪ Recovery – continues until renal function is fully restored and can take up to 12 months. Clients are at higher risk for renal dysfunction during this phase.

  o Prerenal failure from volume depletion or prolonged reduction of blood pressure is the most common cause of acute renal deterioration and is usually reversible with prompt intervention.

- Clinical manifestations occur abruptly with ARF.

- Chronic renal failure (CRF) is a progressive, irreversible kidney disease.

  o End-stage renal failure exists when 90% of the functioning nephrons have been destroyed and are no longer able to maintain fluid, electrolyte, or acid-base homeostasis.

  o CRF is comprised of five stages:

    ▪ Stage 1 – Minimal kidney damage with normal GFR

    ▪ Stage 2 – Mild kidney damage with mildly decreased GFR

- - Stage 3 – Moderate kidney damage with a moderate decrease in GFR

    - Stage 4 – Severe kidney damage with a severe decrease in GFR

    - Stage 5 – Kidney failure and end-stage renal disease with little or no glomerular filtration; renal replacement therapy required

  - Dialysis or kidney transplantation can maintain life, but neither are cures for CRF.

- A client diagnosed with CRF may be asymptomatic except during periods of stress (infection, surgery, trauma). As renal failure progresses, clinical manifestations become apparent.

Data Collection

- Risk Factors of ARF

  - African Americans, Native Americans, and Asians have the highest incidence of end-stage renal disease.

  - Risk factors for acute renal failure include prerenal, intrarenal, and postrenal causes.

  - Prerenal – occurs before damage to the kidney occurs and includes hypovolemia (hemorrhage, dehydration), decreased cardiac output resulting in reduced renal perfusion (MI, cardiac dysrhythmias), decreased peripheral vascular resistance (anaphylaxis, septic shock), and renal vascular obstruction (embolism).

  - Intrarenal – occurs within the kidney and the damage is usually irreversible (acute tubular necrosis) and includes nephrotoxic injury (antibiotics, NSAIDs) and acute glomerulonephritis.

  - Postrenal – obstruction of structures leaving the kidney and includes renal calculi, urinary tract obstruction, and spinal cord disease.

  - Risk factors and causes of CRF

    - Acute renal failure

    - Diabetes mellitus

    - Chronic glomerulonephritis

    - Nephrotoxic medications (gentamicin, NSAIDs) or chemicals

    - Hypertension, especially if African American

    - Autoimmune disorders (systemic lupus erythematosus)

    - Polycystic kidney

    - Pyelonephrosis

    - Renal artery stenosis

    - Recurrent severe infections

  - Older adult clients are at an increased risk for renal failure related to the decreased number of functioning nephrons, decreased GFR, and water and sodium-conserving and compensating mechanisms.

    - An increased incidence of chronic renal failure may be related to the prevalence of diabetes mellitus, hypertension, and the use of NSAIDs in older adult clients.

- Subjective Data
    - Fatigue
    - Lethargy
    - Restless leg syndrome
    - Depression
    - Intractable hiccups
- Objective Data
    - In most cases, findings of renal failure are related to fluid volume overload and include:
        - Renal – polyuria, nocturia (early), oliguria, anuria (late), proteinuria, hematuria, and dilute urine color when present
        - Cardiovascular – hypertension, peripheral edema, pericardial effusion, heart failure, cardiomyopathy, and orthostatic hypotension
        - Respiratory – dyspnea, tachypnea, uremic pneumonitis, lung crackles, Kussmaul respirations, and pulmonary edema
        - Hematologic – anemia, bruising, and bleeding
        - Neurologic – lethargy, insomnia, confusion, encephalopathy, seizures, tremors, ataxia, paresthesias, and coma
        - Gastrointestinal – nausea, anorexia, vomiting, metallic taste, stomatitis, diarrhea, uremic halitosis, and gastritis
        - Skin – decreased skin turgor, yellow cast to skin, dry, pruritus, bruising, and uremic frost (late)
        - Musculoskeletal – osteomalacia (softening of bone), muscle weakness, pathologic fractures, and muscle cramps
        - Reproductive – erectile dysfunction
    - Laboratory Tests
        - Urinalysis
            - Hematuria, proteinuria, glucosuria, decreased osmolarity
            - Serum creatinine
                - Gradual increase of 1 to 2 mg/dL per every 24 to 48 hr for ARF
                - Gradual increase over months to years for CRF exceeding 4 mg/dL
        - BUN
            - 80 to 100 mg/dL within 1 week with ARF
            - Gradual increase with elevated serum creatinine over months to years for CRF
            - 180 to 200 mg/dL with CRF

- ■ Serum electrolytes
  - □ Normal, increased, or decreased sodium; decreased calcium; increased potassium, phosphorus, and magnesium
- ■ CBC
  - □ Decreased Hgb and Hct from anemia secondary to the loss of erythropoietin in CRF
- o Diagnostic Procedures
  - ■ Radiology
    - □ Demonstrates disease processes, obstruction, and arterial defects
    - □ Renal ultrasound
    - □ Kidneys, ureter, and bladder (KUB)
    - □ CT without contrast
    - □ Aortorenal angiography
    - □ Cystoscopy
    - □ Retrograde pyelography
    - □ Renal biopsy

Collaborative Care

- • Nursing Care
  - o Abnormal findings to be reported and monitored include:
    - ■ Urinary elimination patterns (amount, color, odor, and consistency; changes in stream or initiating urine).
    - ■ Vital signs (blood pressure may be increased or decreased).
    - ■ Weight – 1 kg (2.2 lb) daily weight increase is approximately 1 L of fluid retained.
  - o Provide clients a diet that is high in carbohydrates and moderate in fat. Monitor clients receiving total parenteral nutrition (TPN) or hyperalimentation.
  - o Restrict the client's intake of fluids (based on urinary output).
  - o Balance the client's activity and rest.
  - o Prepare clients for hemodialysis, peritoneal dialysis, and hemofiltration, if indicated.
  - o Provide skin care to clients to increase comfort and prevent breakdown.
  - o Protect clients from injury.
  - o Provide emotional support to clients and their families.
  - o Administer medications as prescribed.
  - o For clients with ARF, nurses should:

- Prepare for fluid challenge and diuretics during prerenal period of azotemia if the client is showing signs of fluid volume deficit.

- Restrict fluid intake during oliguric phase.

- Restrict dietary intake of protein, sodium, and potassium during oliguric phase (this restriction is for the client not requiring dialysis).

o For clients with CRF, nurses should:

- Obtain a detailed medication and herb history to determine the client's risk for continued renal insult.

- Control protein intake based on the client's stage of renal failure and type of dialysis.

- Restrict the client's dietary sodium, potassium, phosphorous, and magnesium.

- Encourage clients with diabetes mellitus to adhere to strict blood glucose control, as uncontrolled diabetes is a major risk factor for renal failure.

- Medications

  o Cardiac glycosides – digoxin (Lanoxin) increases myocardial contractility and promotes cardiac output.

    - Nursing Considerations

      □ Take apical pulse for 1 min prior to giving the medication. Notify the provider if the client's heart rate is less than 60/min.

    - Client Education

      □ Instruct clients to take apical pulse for 1 full min daily prior to self-administration of the medication.

      □ Instruct clients to notify the provider if apical pulse is less than 60/min.

      □ Instruct clients to notify the provider immediately if vision changes (blurred vision, seeing more yellow color), or if there is a sensitivity to light or behavior changes. These are signs of digoxin toxicity and need immediate attention.

  o Sodium polystyrene (Kayexalate) to increase elimination of potassium

    - Nursing Considerations

      □ Monitor levels of potassium.

      □ Monitor vital signs.

      □ Use cautiously with clients who have heart failure, hypertension, or edema.

  o Epoetin alfa (Epogen, Procrit) stimulates production of RBCs and is given for anemia

  o Iron supplement – ferrous sulfate (Feosol)

    - This increases the level of iron in the blood.

    - Nursing Considerations

      □ Administer medication after dialysis (if applicable).

      □ Administer stool softener to prevent constipation.

- ■ Client Education
  - □ Instruct clients to take the medication with food.
  - □ Instruct clients that blackish-green stools are expected when taking iron supplements.
  - o Aluminum hydroxide (Amphojel)
    - ■ A phosphate binder is used to increase the elimination of phosphate.
    - ■ Nursing Considerations
      - □ Administer a stool softener to prevent constipation.
      - □ Monitor phosphate levels.
    - ■ Client Education
      - □ Encourage clients to report signs of constipation.
  - o Diuretics (except in ESRD) – furosemide (Lasix)
- • Interdisciplinary Care
  - o Recognize the need for nutritional services to manage the nutritional needs of the client.
- • Therapeutic Procedures
  - o Hemodialysis
- • Care after Discharge
  - o Client Education
    - ■ Promote smoking cessation.
    - ■ Instruct clients to monitor the daily intake of carbohydrates, protein, sodium, and potassium, according to the provider.
    - ■ Instruct the client to monitor fluid intake according to fluid restriction prescribed by the provider.
    - ■ Instruct clients to avoid antacids containing magnesium.
    - ■ Instruct clients to take precautions with bleeding risks (avoid injury, use a soft toothbrush).
    - ■ Encourage clients to take rest periods from activity.
    - ■ Instruct clients how to measure blood pressure and weight at home.
    - ■ Encourage clients to ask questions and discuss fears.
    - ■ Encourage clients to diet, exercise, and take medication as prescribed.
    - ■ Advise the client to notify the provider if there are signs of skin breakdown.
    - ■ Advise clients to notify the provider if there are signs of infection.
    - ■ Instruct clients with vascular hemodialysis access to avoid blood pressure checks and venipunctures in that arm.

- Client Outcomes
    - The client will maintain fluid balance.
    - The client will improve tolerance to activity.
    - The client will report a decrease in anxiety.
    - The client will follow a medication regimen.
    - The client will have no signs of skin breakdown.
    - The client will have no episodes of bleeding.
    - The client will remain free from infection.
    - The client's hemodialysis access will maintain integrity.

Complications

- Potential complications of renal failure include electrolyte imbalance, dysrhythmias, fluid overload, metabolic acidosis, and secondary infection.

COMPLICATION	NURSING ACTIONS
Hyperkalemia	• Administer sodium polystyrene or insulin as prescribed.
Hypertension	• Administer antihypertensives and diuretics as prescribed.
Seizures	• Implement seizure precautions and administer antiepileptics as prescribed.
Cardiac dysrhythmias	• Assist with life-support interventions for life-threatening dysrhythmias. • Monitor the client for and report nonlethal dysrhythmias.
Pulmonary edema	• Prepare the client for hemodialysis.
Infection	• Maintain surgical asepsis of the client's invasive lines, monitor breath sounds, and turn the client every 2 hr. • Monitor clients for signs of localized and systemic infections and report.
Metabolic acidosis	• Prepare clients for hemodialysis.
Uremia	• Prepare the client for hemodialysis.

(A) APPLICATION EXERCISES

1. A nurse is caring for a client who has nephrotic syndrome. The client asks the nurse about his swollen legs, feet, and eyes. Which of the following statements by the nurse reinforces teaching about the client's concern?

   A. "The kidneys are not able to rid the body of excess fluids, so they collect in the tissues."

   B. "It is common to have swelling while on bedrest."

   C. "I'll notify the provider. Maybe the amount of prescribed diuretic needs to be reduced."

   D. "The dietician will be coming to talk to you about restricting calcium in your diet."

2. Which of the following findings should the nurse monitor for in a client who has nephrotic syndrome? (Select all that apply.)

   _____ Proteinuria

   _____ Hematuria

   _____ Hypotension

   _____ Polyuria

   _____ Decreased BUN

3. Match the medications that are administered for nephrotic syndrome with their potential side effects.

   _____ Captopril (Capoten)   A. Infection

   _____ Heparin   B. Elevated blood pressure

   _____ Prednisone (Deltasone)   C. Bleeding

   _____ Epoetin alfa (Epogen)   D. Orthostatic hypotension)

4. A nurse is caring for a client who has acute renal failure (ARF). Which of the following laboratory values should the nurse expect to be increased? (Select all that apply.)

   _____ BUN

   _____ Serum calcium

   _____ Serum potassium

   _____ Serum creatinine

   _____ Serum phosphorous

5. A nurse is caring for a client who has ARF.

   To increase myocardial contractility and promote cardiac output, the nurse should administer _____.

   To stimulate production of RBCs, the nurse should administer _____.

   To increase elimination of potassium, the nurse should administer sodium _____.

   To increase the elimination of phosphate, the nurse should administer _____.

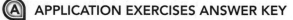 **APPLICATION EXERCISES ANSWER KEY**

1. A nurse is caring for a client who has nephrotic syndrome. The client asks the nurse about his swollen legs, feet, and eyes. Which of the following statements by the nurse reinforces teaching about the client's concern?

   A. "The kidneys are not able to rid the body of excess fluids, so they collect in the tissues."

   B. "It is common to have swelling while on bedrest."

   C. "I'll notify the provider. Maybe the amount of prescribed diuretic needs to be reduced."

   D. "The dietician will be coming to talk to you about restricting calcium in your diet."

   The nurse should reinforce teaching about the function of the kidneys. The kidneys are not able to rid the body of excess fluids, so the fluids collect in the tissues. The remaining statements are direct contradictions of appropriate care practices.

   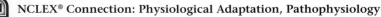 NCLEX® Connection: Physiological Adaptation, Pathophysiology

2. Which of the following findings should the nurse monitor for in a client who has nephrotic syndrome? (Select all that apply.)

X	**Proteinuria**
X	**Hematuria**
_____	Hypotension
_____	Polyuria
X	**Decreased BUN**

   Proteinuria, hematuria, and decreased BUN are all expected findings in a client who has nephrotic syndrome. Hypertension and oliguria, rather than hypotension and polyuria, are findings associated with nephrotic syndrome.

    NCLEX® Connection: Physiological Adaptation, Pathophysiology

3. Match the medications that are administered for nephrotic syndrome with their potential side effects.

D	Captopril (Capoten)	A. Infection
C	Heparin	B. Elevated blood pressure
A	Prednisone (Deltasone)	C. Bleeding
B	Epoetin alfa (Epogen)	D. Orthostatic hypotension)

    NCLEX® Connection: Pharmacological Therapies, Adverse Effects/ Contraindications/Side Effects/Interactions

4. A nurse is caring for a client who has acute renal failure (ARF). Which of the following laboratory values should the nurse expect to be increased? (Select all that apply.)

　__X__　**BUN**

　_____　Serum calcium

　__X__　**Serum potassium**

　__X__　**Serum creatinine**

　__X__　**Serum phosphorous**

BUN, serum potassium, creatinine, and phosphorous will increase with ARF. Serum calcium will be decreased.

(N) NCLEX® Connection: Reduction of Risk Potential, Laboratory Values

5. A nurse is caring for a client who has ARF.

To increase myocardial contractility and promote cardiac output, the nurse should administer **digoxin (Lanoxin)**.

To stimulate production of RBCs, the nurse should administer **epoetin alfa (Epogen)**.

To increase elimination of potassium, the nurse should administer sodium **polystyrene (Kayexalate)**.

To increase the elimination of phosphate, the nurse should administer **aluminum hydroxide**.

(N) NCLEX® Connection: Pharmacological Therapies, Expected Actions/Outcomes

UNIT 8	NURSING CARE OF CLIENTS WITH RENAL SYSTEM DISORDERS
Section:	Renal System Disorders
Chapter 57	Infections of the Renal System

 Overview

- There are three components to the urinary system: the ureter, bladder, and urethra. The goal of the urinary system is to promote optimal kidney function. Infections that affect the urinary system may be of the lower urinary tract (urethritis, cystitis and prostatitis) or the upper urinary tract (pyelonephritis).

LOWER URINARY TRACT INFECTIONS

 Overview

- Lower urinary tract infections (UTIs) are caused by Enterobacteriaceae micro-organisms (Klebsiella, Proteus), Pseudomonas, Serratia, and most commonly, *Escherichia coli*.

- Untreated UTIs may lead to urosepsis, which can cause septic shock and death.

- The use of urinary catheters is the most common cause of hospital-acquired UTIs.

Data Collection

- Risk Factors

  - Female gender

    - Short urethra, close proximity of the urethra to the rectum, sexual intercourse

    - Frequent use of feminine hygiene sprays, tampons, sanitary napkins, and spermicidal jellies

    - Pregnancy

    - Hormonal influences within the vaginal flora

    - Synthetic underwear and pantyhose, wet bathing suits

    - Frequent submersion into baths or hot tubs

  - Indwelling urinary catheters (hospital-acquired UTIs)

  - Urinary conditions (anomalies, stasis, calculi, residual urine)

  - Disease (diabetes mellitus)

- o Decreased estrogen in aging women promotes atrophy of the urethral opening toward the rectum (increases the risk of urosepsis in women)

Ⓖ
- o Older adult clients have an increased risk of bacteremia, sepsis, and shock.

- Subjective Data

  - o Lower back or lower abdominal discomfort and tenderness over the bladder area
  - o Nausea
  - o Urinary frequency and urgency
  - o Dysuria, bladder cramping, or spasms
  - o Perineal itching
  - o Hematuria (red-tinged, smoky, coffee-colored urine)
  - o Pyuria

- Objective Data

  - o Fever
  - o Vomiting
  - o Voiding in small amounts
  - o Nocturia
  - o Urethral discharge
  - o Cloudy or foul smelling urine
  - o Laboratory Tests
    - ▪ Urinalysis and urine culture and sensitivity
      - □ Nursing Actions
        - ▸ Instruct clients regarding proper technique for the collection of a clean catch urine specimen.
        - ▸ Collect catheterized urine specimens using sterile technique.
      - □ Expected findings include:
        - ▸ Bacteria, sediment, WBCs, and RBCs.
        - ▸ Positive leukocyte esterase (85% to 90% specific).
        - ▸ Positive nitrate (95% specific).
    - ▪ WBC count and differential if urosepsis is suspected
      - □ WBC count at or above 10,000/mm^3 with a shift to the left (indicating an increased number of immature cells in response to infection).
    - ▪ Rule out sexually transmitted diseases.

       ○   Diagnostic Procedures

          ■   Cystoscopy is used for complicated UTIs.

Collaborative Care

- Nursing Care

  ○ Promote fluid intake up to 2 to 3 L daily from food and beverage sources.

  ○ Consult with the provider regarding prescribed fluid restrictions if needed.

  ○ Administer medications as prescribed.

  ○ Provide frequent perineal hygiene to clients with indwelling catheters.

- Medications

  ○ Fluoroquinolones (Ciprofloxacin), nitrofurantoin (Macrobid), or sulfonamides (Bactrim or Septra) are antibiotics used to treat urinary infections.

    ■ Nursing Considerations

      □ If sulfonamide is prescribed, ask clients if they are allergic to sulfa.

    ■ Client Education

      □ Reinforce to clients regarding the need to take all of the prescribed antibiotics even if symptoms subside.

      □ Encourage clients to take the medication with food.

  ○ Phenazopyridine (Pyridium) is a bladder analgesic used to treat UTIs.

    ■ Nursing Considerations

      □ Inform clients that the medication will not treat the infection, but will help relieve bladder discomfort.

      □ Inform clients that the medication will turn urine orange.

    ■ Client Education

      □ Encourage clients to take the medication with food.

- Interdisciplinary Care

  ○ Initiate urology services for the occurrence of chronic UTIs.

- Client Education

  ○ Instruct clients to consume 2 to 3 L of fluid daily from food and beverage sources.

  ○ Instruct clients to bathe daily to promote good body hygiene.

  ○ Instruct clients to get proper rest and nutrition.

  ○ Instruct clients to notify the provider if symptoms reoccur.

  ○ Advise clients to empty the bladder every 3 to 4 hr instead of waiting until the bladder is completely full.

- o Advise clients to urinate before and after intercourse.

- o Advise clients to drink cranberry juice as an alternative to water to decrease the risk of infection.

- o Advise clients to empty the bladder as soon as there is an urgency to void.

- o Instruct female clients to:

    - Wipe the perineal area from front to back.

    - Avoid using bubble baths, or feminine products or toilet paper containing perfumes.

    - Avoid sitting in wet bathing suits.

    - Avoid wearing synthetic underwear and pantyhose with slacks or tight clothing.

- Client Outcomes

  - o The client will be free from pain.

  - o The client will be free of infection.

  - o The client will take the medication as prescribed.

  - o The client will drink at least 2 to 3 L of fluids daily to decrease the risk of infection.

Complications

- Urethral obstruction, pyelonephritis, chronic renal failure, urosepsis, septic shock, and death

  - o Nursing Actions

    - Monitor vital signs for worsening infection and report abnormal data promptly.

    - Maintain medication schedules to assure adequate medication blood levels to eradicate infection.

PYELONEPHRITIS

Overview

- Pyelonephritis is an infection and inflammation of the renal pelvis, calyces, and medulla. The infection usually begins in the lower urinary tract with organisms ascending into the renal pelvis.

- *Escherichia coli* organisms are the cause of most acute cases of pyelonephritis.

- Repeated infections create scarring that changes the blood flow to the kidney, glomerulus, and tubular structure.

- Filtration, reabsorption, and secretion are impaired, which results in a decrease in renal function.

- Acute pyelonephritis is an active bacterial infection that can cause:

  ○ Interstitial inflammation.

  ○ Tubular cell necrosis.

  ○ Abscess formation in the capsule, cortex, or medulla.

  ○ Temporarily altered renal function (this rarely progresses to renal failure).

- Chronic pyelonephritis is the result of repeated infections that cause progressive inflammation and scarring.

  ○ This can result in the thickening of the calyces and postinflammatory fibrosis with permanent renal tissue scarring.

  ○ It is more common with obstructions, urinary anomaly, and vesicoureteral urine reflux.

  ○ Reflux of urine occurs at the junction where the ureter connects to the bladder.

Data Collection

- Risk Factors

  ○ Chronic urinary stone disorders

  ○ Spinal cord injury

  ○ Pregnancy

  ○ Congenital malformations

  ○ Bladder tumors

  ○ Chronic illness (diabetes mellitus, hypertension, chronic cystitis)

  ○ Older age

    ▪ Women over 65 years of age

    ▪ Men with enlarged prostate

    ▪ A decrease in vascular flow may decrease blood flow to the kidneys.

    ▪ Increased urine pH promotes bacterial growth.

    ▪ Incomplete bladder emptying

    ▪ Older adult clients may exhibit gastrointestinal or pulmonary symptoms instead of febrile responses.

- Subjective Data

  ○ Chills

  ○ Colicky-type abdominal pain

  ○ Nausea

  ○ Malaise, fatigue

- o   Burning, urgency, and frequency with urination

- o   Costovertebral tenderness indicating inflammation and/or infection

- Objective Data

  - o   Fever, tachycardia, tachypnea, hypertension

  - o   Flank and back pain

  - o   Costovertebral edema or erythema indicating inflammation and/or infection

  - o   Vomiting

  - o   Nocturia

  - o   Inability to concentrate urine or conserve sodium (chronic pyelonephritis)

  - o   Asymptomatic bacteremia

- Laboratory Tests

  - o   Urinalysis and urine culture and sensitivity

    - ■   Monitor for:

      - □   Dark color, cloudy appearance, and foul odor.

      - □   Bacteria, sediment, WBCs, and RBCs.

      - □   Positive leukocyte esterase (85% to 90% specific).

      - □   Positive nitrate (95% specific).

  - o   WBC count and differential – A WBC count at or above 10,000/mm³ with a shift to the left indicates an increased number of immature cells in response to an infection.

  - o   Blood cultures will be positive for the presence of bacteria if a systemic infection is present.

  - o   Serum creatinine and BUN are elevated during acute episodes and consistently elevated with chronic infection.

  - o   C-reactive protein is elevated during exacerbating inflammatory processes.

    - ■   Erythrocyte sedimentation rate (ESR) is elevated during acute or chronic inflammation.

- Diagnostic Procedures

  - o   An x-ray of the kidneys, ureters, and bladder (KUB) may demonstrate calculi or structural abnormalities.

  - o   A gallium scan should be used to identify active pyelonephritis or an abscess related to specific enzymes present.

  - o   Intravenous pyelogram (IVP) may demonstrate calculi, structural, or vascular abnormalities.

- Nursing Actions
  - Check for allergy to contrast dye prior to the procedure.
  - Verify consent as indicated.
- Client Education
  - Inform clients that bowel preparation may be prescribed prior to the procedure for image clarity.
  - Inform clients of hydration prior to the procedure and that diuretic administration following the procedure may be prescribed to reduce the risk of nephrotoxicity.

Collaborative Care

- Nursing Care
  - Increase fluid intake to 2 to 3 L per day unless contraindicated.
  - Administer antipyretic as needed.
  - Administer antibiotics as prescribed.
  - Provide emotional support.
  - Assist with personal hygiene.
- Medications
  - Opioid analgesics (opioid agonists), morphine sulfate, and morphine
    - Opioid agents are used to treat moderate to severe pain. These medications act on the mu and kappa receptors that help alleviate pain. Activation of these receptors produces analgesia (pain relief), respiratory depression, euphoria, sedation, and a decrease in gastrointestinal (GI) motility.
    - Use cautiously with clients who have asthma or emphysema due to the risk of respiratory depression.
    - Nursing Considerations
      - Monitor the client's pain level every 4 hr.
      - Watch clients for signs of respiratory depression, especially in older adults. If respirations are 12/min or less, stop the medication and notify the provider immediately.
      - Monitor the client's vital signs closely for sign of hypotension and decreased respirations.
      - Observe the client's level of sedation (drowsiness, LOC [level of consciousness]).

- Client Education
  - Encourage clients to suck on hard candies to help with dry mouth.
  - Encourage clients to drink plenty of fluids to help prevent constipation.
  - Reinforce to clients to request pain medication before pain becomes severe.
- Nonsteroidal anti-inflammatory agents (NSAIDs – ibuprofen [Advil])
  - Use to treat mild to moderate pain, fever, and inflammation.
  - Nursing Considerations
    - Encourage clients to take with food to decrease GI distress.
    - Observe for signs of bleeding.
  - Client Education
    - Instruct clients to watch for signs of bleeding.
    - Instruct clients to notify the provider if signs of gastric discomfort of ulceration occur.
- Antibiotics: nitrofurantoin (Macrodantin)
  - Use this medication to eradicate infection.
  - Nursing Considerations
    - Encourage clients to notify the provider immediately if persistent cough begins after starting the medication.
    - Inform clients that the medication may turn urine the color brown.
  - Client Education
    - Encourage clients to take with food.
    - Instruct the client to take full regimen of antibiotics as prescribed.

- Interdisciplinary Care
  - Initiate referral for urology services to manage pyelonephritis.
  - Recognize the need for nutritional services to promote adequate calories for clients.
- Surgical Interventions
  - Pyelolithotomy
    - This is the removal of a stone from the kidney.
  - Nephrectomy
    - This is the removal of the kidney.
  - Ureteroplasty
    - This is done to repair or revise the ureter.

- ▪ Nursing Actions
  - ▫ Inform clients of the purpose of the surgery and expected outcomes.
  - ▫ Monitor clients receiving IV antibiotics and analgesics.
- Care after Discharge
  - Client Education
  - o Educate clients regarding adequate nutritional status.
  - o Encourage clients to consume 2 to 3 L of fluids daily from food and beverage sources unless otherwise indicated by the provider.
  - o Instruct clients to take medications as prescribed.
  - o Instruct clients to notify the provider if acute onset of pain occurs or a fever is present.
  - o Encourage clients and family to express their fears and anxiety related to the disease.
  - o Encourage clients to take rest periods as needed from activity.
- Client Outcomes
  - o The client will be free from pain.
  - o The client will have a decrease in anxiety.
  - o The client will be compliant with a medication regimen.
  - o The client will have an increase in activity level.

Complications

- Septic Shock
  - o Nursing Actions
    - ▪ Identify signs (hypotension, tachycardia, fever).
    - ▪ Assist with emergency care interventions as needed.
- Renal Failure
  - o Nursing Actions
    - ▪ Monitor I&O.
    - ▪ Monitor renal function studies for elevations in BUN and creatinine.
    - ▪ Encourage increased fluid intake.
- Hypertension
  - o Nursing Actions
    - ▪ Monitor blood pressure for trends.
    - ▪ Report changes from baseline.

(A) APPLICATION EXERCISES

1. A nurse is caring for a client who has just been diagnosed with a UTI. The client reports pain and a burning sensation upon urination, and also reports that the urine is cloudy and has an odor. Which of the following is the priority action by the nurse?

   A. Offer a warm sitz bath.

   B. Obtain a set of vital signs.

   C. Encourage increased fluids.

   D. Administer a prescribed antibiotic.

2. A client reports repeated UTIs over the past year. To prevent reoccurrence of a UTI, a nurse should reinforce teaching regarding (Select all that apply.)

   _____ not wearing tight pants.

   _____ urinating every 3 to 4 hr.

   _____ wiping the perineal area back to front.

   _____ increasing fluid intake up to 3 L a day.

   _____ wearing nylon underwear.

3. A nurse is reinforcing teaching to a client who is prescribed phenazopyridine (Pyridium) for a UTI. Which of the following should the nurse include in the teaching?

   A. Take the medication on an empty stomach.

   B. Continue the medication even if the symptoms subside.

   C. The drug of choice for documented sulfa allergies.

   D. Expect urine to turn orange.

4. Which of the following should a nurse identify as expected laboratory results of a client who has pyelonephritis? (Select all that apply.)

   _____ Presence of bacteria in urine

   _____ Decreased serum protein

   _____ Decreased C-reactive protein

   _____ Positive leukocyte esterase

   _____ Decreased erythrocyte sedimentation rate (ESR)

   _____ Elevated BUN

APPLICATION EXERCISES ANSWER KEY

1. A nurse is caring for a client who has just been diagnosed with a UTI. The client reports pain and a burning sensation upon urination, and also reports that the urine is cloudy and has an odor. Which of the following is the priority action by the nurse?

    A. Offer a warm sitz bath.

    B. Obtain a set of vital signs.

    C. Encourage increased fluids.

    D. Administer a prescribed antibiotic.

    The greatest risk to the client is injury of the urinary tract infection. Therefore, the first action the nurse should take is to administer the prescribed antibiotic. Offering a warm sitz bath, obtaining a set of vital signs, and encouraging increased fluid intake are all important actions, but are not the priority action by the nurse.

     NCLEX® Connection: Pharmacological Therapies, Expected Actions/Outcomes

2. A client reports repeated UTIs over the past year. To prevent reoccurrence of a UTI, a nurse should reinforce teaching regarding (Select all that apply.)

    __X__ **not wearing tight pants.**

    __X__ **urinating every 3 to 4 hr.**

    _____ wiping the perineal area back to front.

    __X__ **increasing fluid intake up to 3 L a day.**

    _____ wearing nylon underwear.

    The nurse should reinforce to the client to avoid wearing tight pants, urinating every 3 to 4 hr, and increasing fluid intake up to 3 L a day. The client should wipe the perineal area from front to back and should wear cotton, not nylon, underwear.

     NCLEX® Connection: Basic Care and Comfort, Elimination

3. A nurse is reinforcing teaching to a client who is prescribed phenazopyridine (Pyridium) for a UTI. Which of the following should the nurse include in the teaching?

    A. Take the medication on an empty stomach.

    B. Continue the medication even if the symptoms subside.

    C. The drug of choice for documented sulfa allergies.

    D. Expect urine to turn orange.

    Inform the client that urine will turn orange and can stain clothing. Phenazopyridine can upset the stomach, so it might be better tolerated with food. Take only if experiencing discomfort. Phenazopyridine is not an antibiotic, so it is not a replacement medication for sulfa.

     NCLEX® Connection: Pharmacological Therapies, Adverse Effects/Contraindications/Side Effects/Interactions

4. Which of the following should a nurse identify as expected laboratory results of a client who has pyelonephritis? (Select all that apply.)

    X   **Presence of bacteria in urine**

    _____   Decreased serum protein

    _____   Decreased C-reactive protein

    X   **Positive leukocyte esterase**

    _____   Decreased erythrocyte sedimentation rate (ESR)

    X   **Elevated BUN**

The presence of bacteria in urine, positive leukocyte esterase, and an elevated BUN are all expected findings for a client who has pyelonephritis. A decreased serum protein, decreased C-reactive protein, and decreased ESR are not be expected findings for the client.

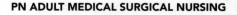 NCLEX® Connection: Reduction of Risk Potential, Laboratory Values

UNIT 8	NURSING CARE OF CLIENTS WITH RENAL SYSTEM DISORDERS
Section:	Renal System Disorders
Chapter 58	Renal Calculi

Overview

- Urolithiasis is the presence of calculi (stones) in the urinary tract.

- The majority of stones (75%) are composed of calcium phosphate or calcium oxalate, but may contain other substances (uric acid, struvite, cystine).

- A diet high in calcium is not believed to increase the risk of stone formation unless there is a pre-existing metabolic disorder or renal tubular defect.

- Reoccurrence is increased (35% to 50%) in individuals with calcium stones who have a family history, or whose first occurrence of urinary calculi is prior to the age of 25.

- Most clients can expel stones without invasive procedures. Factors that influence whether a stone will pass spontaneously or not include the composition, size, and location of the stone.

(M) View Media Supplement: Renal Calculus (Image)

Data Collection

- Risk Factors

  o The cause of urolithiasis is unknown.

  o There is an increased incidence of urolithiasis in males.

  o Urolithiasis formation is associated with damaged urinary tract lining, concentrated urine, increased oxalate production (genetic) or ingestion from foods, and increased production or decreased clearance of purines (contributing to increased uric-acid levels).

  o Stone formation can be attributed to high alkalinity or acidity in the urine.

  o Urinary stasis, urinary retention, immobilization, and dehydration contribute to an environment favorable for stone formation.

  o Decreased fluid intake or increased incidence of dehydration among older adult clients can increase the risk of stone formation.

- Subjective Data
  - Severe pain (renal colic)
    - Pain intensifies as the stone moves through the ureter.
    - Flank pain suggests stones are located in the kidney or upper ureter.
    - Flank pain that radiates to the abdomen, scrotum, testes, or vulva is suggestive of stones in the ureter or bladder.
  - Urinary frequency or dysuria (occurs with stones in the bladder)
- Objective Data
  - Fever with infection
  - Diaphoresis
  - Pallor
  - Nausea/vomiting
  - Vital signs – Tachycardia, tachypnea, increased or decreased blood pressure with pain
  - Oliguria/anuria (occurs with stones that obstruct urinary flow)
  - Hematuria (smoky-looking urine)
  - Laboratory Tests
    - Urinalysis is used to detect:
      - The odor of the urine and increased urine turbidity if infection is present.
      - Increased RBCs, WBCs, and bacteria.
      - Crystals noted on a microscopic exam.
      - Elevated WBC if infection is present.
      - Abnormal serum calcium, phosphate, and uric-acid levels in the presence of metabolic disorders/defects.
  - Diagnostic Procedures
    - Radiology examination
      - KUB (x-ray of kidney, ureters, bladder), noncontrast helical CT scan, or IVP (IV pyelogram) is used to confirm the presence and location of stones. IVP is contraindicated if there is a urinary obstruction.
    - CT or MRI
      - A CT or MRI is used to identify cystine or uric-acid stones, which cannot be seen on standard x-rays.
    - A renal ultrasound or cystoscopy may confirm the diagnosis.

Collaborative Care

- Nursing Care

  o Report abnormal findings to the provider.

  o Provide preoperative and postoperative care as indicated.

  o Monitor:

    ▪ Pain status.

    ▪ Vital signs.

    ▪ I&O.

    ▪ Urinary pH.

  o Administer prescribed medications.

  o Strain all urine to check for passage of the stone and save the stone for laboratory analysis.

  o Encourage increased oral intake to 3 L/day unless contraindicated.

  o Administer IV fluids as prescribed.

  o Encourage ambulation to promote passage of the stone.

- Medications

  o Analgesics

    ▪ Opioids – Morphine

      □ Use for moderate to severe pain for the acute onset of stones within the first 24 hr.

      □ Nursing Considerations

        ▸ Monitor the client's pain level every 4 hr.

        ▸ Watch clients for signs of respiratory depression, especially in older adult clients. If respirations are 12/min or less, stop the medication and notify the provider immediately.

        ▸ Monitor the client's vital signs closely for signs of hypotension and decreased respirations.

        ▸ Observe the client's level of sedation (drowsiness, LOC [level of consciousness]).

        ▸ Check for response of therapy.

      □ Client Education

        ▸ Encourage clients to suck on hard candies to help with dry mouth.

        ▸ Encourage clients to drink plenty of fluids to help prevent constipation.

- NSAIDs – ketorolac (Toradol)
  - □ NSAIDs are used to treat mild to moderate pain, fever, and inflammation.
  - □ Nursing Considerations
    - ▸ Observe for signs of bleeding.
    - ▸ Check for response to therapy.
  - □ Client Education
    - ▸ Instruct clients to watch for signs of bleeding.
    - ▸ Instruct clients to notify the provider if signs of gastric discomfort or ulceration occur.
- Spasmolytic medications
  - ■ Oxybutynin chloride (Ditropan)
    - □ Use to help alleviate pain with a neurogenic or overactive bladder.
  - ■ Nursing Considerations
    - □ Ask clients if there is a history of glaucoma, as this medication increases intraocular pressure.
    - □ Monitor for dizziness and tachycardia.
    - □ Monitor for urinary retention.
    - □ Check for response to therapy.
  - ■ Client Education
    - □ Instruct clients to report problems with voiding or constipation.
    - □ Inform clients to report palpitations.
    - □ Inform clients that dizziness and dry mouth are common with the medication.
- Antibiotics – Gentamicin (Garamycin); cephalexin (Keflex)
  - ■ Use to treat infection.
  - ■ Nursing Considerations
    - □ Administer medication with food to decrease gastrointestinal distress.
    - □ Monitor blood levels of antibiotics as indicated.
  - ■ Client Education
    - □ Inform clients that urine may have a foul odor related to the antibiotic.
    - □ Instruct clients to report loose stools related to the medication.
- Interdisciplinary Care
  - Recognize the need for nutritional services for dietary modifications concerning foods related to stone formation.

- Therapeutic Procedures

  - Extracorporeal shock wave lithotripsy (ESWL)

    - ESWL uses sound, laser, or shock-wave energies to break the stone into fragments.

    - Requires moderate (conscious) sedation and ECG monitoring during the procedure.

    - Nursing Actions

      □ Reinforce teaching to clients regarding ESWL.

      □ Observe for gross hematuria following the procedure.

      □ Strain urine following the procedure.

      □ Provide pain relief following procedure.

    - Client Education

      □ Inform clients that bruising is normal at the site where waves are applied.

      □ Explain to clients that there will be hematuria postprocedure.

- Surgical Interventions

  - Stenting

    - Stenting is the placement of a small tube in the ureter during a ureteroscopy to dilate the ureter, enlarging the passageway for the stone to be passed.

  - Retrograde ureteroscopy

    - Retrograde ureteroscopy uses a basket, forceps, or loop on the end of the ureteroscope to grasp and remove the stone.

  - Percutaneous ureterolithotomy/nephrolithotomy

    - Percutaneous ureterolithotomy/nephrolithotomy is the insertion of an ultrasonic or laser lithotripter into the ureter or kidney to grasp and extract the stone through the skin.

  - Open surgery

    - Open surgery uses a surgical incision to remove the stone. This surgery is used for large or impacted stones (staghorn calculi), or for stones not removed by other approaches.

    - Ureterolithotomy (into the ureter)

    - Pyelolithotomy (into the kidney pelvis)

    - Nephrolithotomy (into the kidney)

- Care after Discharge

  - Client Education

    - Reinforce to clients regarding the role of diet and medications in the treatment and prevention of urinary stones.

- Calcium phosphate
  - ☐ Limit intake of foods high in animal protein (reduction of protein intake decreases calcium precipitation).
  - ☐ Limit sodium intake.
  - ☐ Reduced calcium intake (dairy products) is individualized.
  - ☐ Medications
    - ▸ Use thiazide diuretics to increase calcium reabsorption.
    - ▸ Use orthophosphates to decrease urine saturation of calcium oxalate.
    - ▸ Use sodium cellulose phosphate to reduce the intestinal absorption of calcium.
- Calcium oxalate
  - ☐ Avoid oxalate sources – Spinach, black tea, rhubarb, cocoa, beets, pecans, peanuts, okra, chocolate, wheat germ, lime peel, and Swiss chard.
  - ☐ Limit sodium intake.
- Struvite (magnesium ammonium phosphate)
  - ☐ Avoid high-phosphate foods (dairy products, red and organ meats, whole grains).
- Uric acid (urate)
  - ☐ Decrease intake of purine sources (organ meats, poultry, fish, gravies, red wine, sardines).
  - ☐ Medications
    - ▸ Allopurinol (Zyloprim) is used to prevent the formation of uric acid.
    - ▸ Potassium or sodium citrate or sodium bicarbonate is used to alkalinize the urine.
- Cystine
  - ☐ Limit animal protein intake.
  - ☐ Encourage fluid intake if not contraindicated.
  - ☐ Medications
    - ▸ Alpha mercapto propionylglycine (AMPG) is used to lower urine cystine.
    - ▸ Captopril (Capoten) is used to lower urine cystine.

- Client Outcomes

  o The client will have a decrease in anxiety.

  o The client will be free from pain.

  o The client will be free of infection.

  o The client will take the medication as prescribed and follow dietary restrictions.

Complications

- Obstruction

  o A stone may block the passage of urine into the kidney, ureter, or bladder. The client's urinary output may be greatly diminished or absent.

  o Nursing Actions

    ▪ Notify the provider immediately.

    ▪ Prepare clients for removal of the stone.

- Hydronephrosis

  o This occurs when a stone has blocked a portion of the urinary tract. The urine becomes backed up and causes distension of the kidney.

  o Nursing Actions

    ▪ Notify the provider immediately.

    ▪ Prepare clients for removal of the stone.

Ⓐ APPLICATION EXERCISES

1. A nurse is caring for a client who is admitted to the nursing unit with a diagnosis of left renal calculus, has an indwelling urinary catheter, and is receiving 0.9% sodium chloride IV infusing at 150 mL/hr. Which of the following data is the priority?

    A. Flank pain that radiates to the lower abdomen

    B. Nausea that requires management with an antiemetic

    C. No urine output for 2 hr

    D. Client reports feeling sweaty

2. A middle-aged adult client is scheduled for extracorporeal shock wave lithotripsy (ESWL). Which of the following statements by the client demonstrates a correct understanding of the procedure?

    A. "I will be fully awake during the procedure."

    B. "I should report blood in my urine after the test."

    C. "Lithotripsy will reduce my chances of stone reoccurrence."

    D. "Straining my urine following the procedure is important."

3. A client is being discharged after spontaneously passing a calcium phosphate stone. The nurse encourages the client to take action to prevent reoccurrences. Which of the following should the nurse encourage? (Select all that apply.)

    _____ Strain all urine.

    _____ Reduce sodium intake in diet.

    _____ Avoid drinking fluids at bedtime.

    _____ Increase fluid intake to 3 L/day if not contraindicated.

    _____ Limit physical activity throughout the day.

    _____ Report burning or dysuria to the provider.

    _____ Limit intake of foods high in animal protein.

APPLICATION EXERCISES ANSWER KEY

1. A nurse is caring for a client who is admitted to the nursing unit with a diagnosis of left renal calculus, has an indwelling urinary catheter, and is receiving 0.9% sodium chloride IV infusing at 150 mL/hr. Which of the following data is the priority?

   A. Flank pain that radiates to the lower abdomen

   B. Nausea that requires management with an antiemetic

   C. No urine output for 2 hr

   D. Client reports feeling sweaty

   The greatest risk to the client is kidney damage that may occur from an obstruction. Therefore, the priority finding is no urine output for the past 2 hr. Flank pain that radiates to the abdomen, nausea, and sweating are all important findings, but are not the priority.

 NCLEX® Connection: Physiological Adaptations, Alterations in Body Systems

2. A middle-aged adult client is scheduled for extracorporeal shock wave lithotripsy (ESWL). Which of the following statements by the client demonstrates a correct understanding of the procedure?

   A. "I will be fully awake during the procedure."

   B. "I should report blood in my urine after the test."

   C. "Lithotripsy will reduce my chances of stone reoccurrence."

   D. "Straining my urine following the procedure is important."

   Straining the urine and capture of the stone will allow for analysis of the stone. The client will receive moderate sedation during the procedure, hematuria is an expected finding, and lithotripsy does not reduce the risk of stone reoccurrence.

 NCLEX® Connection: Reduction of Risk Potential, Potential for Complications from Surgical Procedures and Health Alterations

3. A client is being discharged after spontaneously passing a calcium phosphate stone. The nurse encourages the client to take action to prevent reoccurrences. Which of the following should the nurse encourage? (Select all that apply.)

     _____ Strain all urine.

     __X__ **Reduce sodium intake in diet.**

     _____ Avoid drinking fluids at bedtime.

     __X__ **Increase fluid intake to 3 L/day if not contraindicated.**

     _____ Limit physical activity throughout the day.

     __X__ **Report burning or dysuria to the provider.**

     __X__ **Limit intake of foods high in animal protein.**

Reducing sodium intake, increasing fluid intake to 3 L/day, reporting burning or dysuria to the provider, and limiting intake of foods high in animal protein should be encouraged by the nurse. Straining the urine and restriction of fluids at bedtime and activity will not prevent a reoccurrence of a calcium phosphate stone.

NCLEX® Connection: Physiological Adaptations, Basic Pathophysiology

UNIT 8	NURSING CARE OF CLIENTS WITH RENAL SYSTEM DISORDERS
Section:	Renal System Disorders
Chapter 59	Voiding Disorders

 Overview

- There are six major types of urinary incontinence:

  - Stress – The loss of small amounts of urine when laughing, sneezing, or lifting. Stress incontinence is related primarily to weak pelvic muscles, urethra, or surrounding tissues.

  - Urge – The inability to stop urine flow long enough to reach the bathroom. Urge incontinence is related to an overactive detrusor muscle with increased bladder pressure.

  - Overflow – Urinary retention associated with bladder overdistention and frequent loss of small amounts of urine. Overflow incontinence is related to obstruction of the urinary outlet or an impaired detrusor muscle.

  - Reflex – The involuntary loss of a moderate amount of urine usually with warning. Reflex incontinence is related to hyperreflexia of the detrusor muscle, usually from altered spinal cord activity.

  - Functional – The inability to make it to the bathroom to urinate. Functional incontinence is related to physical, cognitive, or social impairment.

  - Total incontinence – The unpredictable, involuntary loss of urine that does not generally respond to treatment.

- Urinary incontinence is a significant contributing factor to altered skin integrity and falls, especially in older adults.

Data Collection

- Risk Factors

  - Female

  - History of multiple pregnancies and vaginal births, aging, chronic urinary retention, urinary bladder spasm, renal disease, chronic bladder infection (cystitis), lower pelvic procedures, or surgery

  - Neurological disorders – Parkinson's disease, cerebrovascular accident, spinal cord injury, multiple sclerosis

- ○ Medication therapy – Diuretics, narcotics, anticholinergics, calcium channel blockers, sedative/hypnotics, and adrenergic antagonists

- ○ Obesity

- ○ Confusion, dementia, immobility, and depression

- ○ Older adult client (due to physiological changes secondary to aging)

- ○ Decreased estrogen levels and decreased pelvic-muscle tone

- ○ Risks may be attributed to immobility, chronic degenerative diseases, dementia, diabetes mellitus, stroke, and medications

- ○ Urinary incontinence is associated with a risk for falls, fractures, pressure ulcers, and depression.

- • Subjective Data

  - ○ Loss of urine when laughing, coughing, or sneezing

  - ○ Enuresis (bed-wetting)

  - ○ Bladder spasms

  - ○ Urinary retention

  - ○ Frequency, urgency, nocturia

- • Objective Data

  - ○ Laboratory Tests

    - ■ Urinalysis and urine culture/sensitivity – To rule out urinary tract infection (presence of RBCs, WBCs, microorganisms).

    - ■ Serum creatinine and BUN – To assess renal function (elevated with renal dysfunction).

  - ○ Diagnostic Procedures

    - ■ Postvoid residual urine using a pelvis ultrasonographic scanner or postvoid catheterization– To rule out urinary retention (greater than 100 mL retained urine post voiding)

    - ■ Voiding cystourethrography (VCUG)

      - □ Used to assess the size, shape, support, and function of the urinary bladder, identify obstruction (prostate), and postvoid residual urine

    - ■ Urodynamic Testing

      - □ Cystourethroscopy

        - ▸ Visualization of the inside of the bladder and urethra

      - □ Cystometrogram (CMG)

        - ▸ Measures pressure inside the bladder while urine is filling

- □ Uroflowmetry
  - ‣ Measures rate and degree of bladder emptying
- □ Urethral pressure profilometry (UPP)
  - ‣ Compares urethral pressure to bladder pressure during certain activities (coughing, lifting)
- Electromyography (EMG)
  - □ Measures strength of pelvic muscle contractions
- Ultrasound
  - □ Used to detect bladder abnormalities and/or residual urine

Collaborative Care

- Nursing Care
  - ○ Establish a toileting schedule.
  - ○ Monitor fluid intake during the daytime, and decrease fluid intake prior to bedtime.
  - ○ Remove or control barriers to toileting.
  - ○ Apply and monitor electrical stimulation of the pelvic floor muscles if ordered.
  - ○ Provide incontinence garments.
  - ○ Apply an external or condom catheter to males.
  - ○ Avoid the use of indwelling urinary catheters.
  - ○ Provide incontinence care.
  - ○ Reinforce to clients:
    - To keep an incontinence diary.
    - How to perform Kegel exercises. Tighten pelvic muscles for a count of 10, relax slowly for a count of 10, and repeat in sequences of 15 in the lying-down, sitting, and standing positions.
    - Bladder compression techniques (Credé, Valsalva, double-voiding, splinting).
    - To avoid caffeine and alcohol consumption, as these produce diuresis and the urge to urinate.
    - Space consumption of fluids at regular intervals throughout the day. Limit fluid intake in the evening hours.
    - Weight reduction may decrease stress incontinence in obese clients.
    - The side effects of prescribed medications that may stimulate voiding.
    - Vaginal cone therapy to strengthen pelvic muscles (stress incontinence).

- Medications
  - Antibiotics
    - Gentamicin (Garamycin) and cephalexin (Keflex) are given if an infection is present to treat bacteria.
    - Nursing Considerations
      - Administer medication with food to decrease gastrointestinal distress.
    - Client Education
      - Inform clients that urine may have a foul odor related to the antibiotic.
      - Instruct clients to report loose stools related to the medication.
      - Encourage clients to complete the full course of therapy even if symptoms resolve.
  - Tricyclic antidepressants
    - Nortriptyline (Pamelor) contains anticholinergic effects that can relieve urinary incontinence.
    - Nursing Considerations
      - This medication can cause dizziness.
      - Monitor blood pressure and for signs of orthostatic hypotension.
    - Client Education
      - Encourage clients to get up slowly.
  - Urinary antispasmodics or anticholinergic agents
    - Oxybutynin (Ditropan) and dicyclomine (Bentyl) are used to decrease urgency and help alleviate pain with a neurogenic or overactive bladder.
    - Nursing Considerations
      - Ask clients if there is a history of glaucoma.
      - The medication increases intraocular pressure.
      - Monitor for dizziness and tachycardia.
      - Inform clients that dry mouth and constipation are common with this medication.
      - Monitor for urinary retention.
    - Client Education
      - Instruct clients to report voiding problems or constipation.
      - Instruct clients to report palpitations.
      - Inform clients that dizziness and dry mouth are common with this medication.

- o Phenazopyridine (Pyridium)
  - This is a bladder analgesic used to treat urinary tract infections.
  - Nursing Considerations
    - □ The medication will not treat infection, but will help with bladder discomfort.
    - □ Remind clients that the medication will turn urine orange.
    - □ Monitor for a decrease in Hgb and Hct.
    - □ This is contraindicated in clients with hepatic disorders or renal insufficiency.
  - Client Education
    - □ Encourage clients to take with food.
    - □ Inform clients that the medication turns urine orange in color.
    - □ Instruct clients to notify the provider immediately if skin becomes yellow-tinged.
- o Hormone replacement therapy
  - This is controversial, but it increases blood supply to the pelvis.

- Interdisciplinary Care
  - o Urology services may be consulted for urinary incontinence.
  - o To alleviate stress incontinence, nutritional services may be consulted for dietary modifications if the client is obese.
  - o Home care services may be consulted to provide intermittent catheter, portable commode, or stool riser. Handrails can be installed to assist clients with bathroom needs.

- Therapeutic Procedures
  - o Bladder training program
    - Urinary bladder training increases the bladder's ability to hold urine and the client's ability to suppress urination.
    - Nursing Actions
      - □ Instruct clients to void at scheduled intervals.
      - □ Gradually increase the client's voiding intervals if clients have no incontinence episodes for 3 days until the optimal 4 hr interval is achieved.
    - Client Education
      - □ Remind clients to consciously hold urine until the scheduled toileting time.
      - □ Encourage clients to keep track of voiding times.

- o Urinary habit training

  - Urinary habit training helps clients with limited cognitive ability to establish a predictable pattern of bladder emptying.

  - Nursing Actions

    - □ Instruct clients to void at scheduled intervals.

  - Client Education

    - □ Inform clients that the toileting schedules are based on voiding patterns.

    - □ Encourage clients to maintain a voiding schedule according to the pattern in which no incontinence occurs (every 2 hr).

- o Intermittent urinary catheterization

  - Intermittent urinary catheterization is periodic catheterization to empty the bladder. Intermittent catheterization is recommended over an indwelling urinary catheter due to the risk of infection. Indwelling urinary catheters should be used only when clients are at risk for skin breakdown, or when other options have failed. Their use should be temporary.

  - Nursing Actions

    - □ Adjust the frequency of catheterization to maintain an output of 300 mL or less.

    - □ Explain the procedure to clients.

  - Client Education

    - □ Encourage clients to maintain a voiding schedule according to the pattern in which no incontinence occurs (every 2 hr).

- Surgical Interventions

  - o Anterior vaginal repair, retropubic suspension, pubovaginal sling, and/or insertion of an artificial sphincter

    - Catheters (suprapubic and/or urinary) are typically inserted and maintained until clients have a postvoid residual of less than 50 mL. Traction (with tape) is applied to the catheter to prevent movement of the bladder.

    - Suprapubic catheters are surgically inserted into the abdomen above the pubic bone and in the bladder. This can be performed under a local anesthetic and the catheter is sutured in place. The care for the catheter tubing and drainage bag is the same as for an indwelling catheter.

    - Nursing Actions

      - □ Monitor the client's output closely and for any signs of infection (color of urine, sediment, level of output).

      - □ Keep the catheter patent at all times.

      - □ Determine the client's ability to detect the urge to void.

UNIT 9: NURSING CARE OF CLIENTS WITH REPRODUCTIVE DISORDERS

- Female Reproductive Disorders
- Male Reproductive Disorders

NCLEX® CONNECTIONS

When reviewing the chapters in this section, keep in mind the relevant sections of the NCLEX® outline, in particular:

CLIENT NEEDS: HEALTH PROMOTION AND MAINTENANCE	CLIENT NEEDS: REDUCTION OF RISK POTENTIAL	CLIENT NEEDS: PHYSIOLOGICAL ADAPTATION

Relevant topics/tasks include:
- Data Collection Techniques
  ○ Prepare client for physical examination.
- Health Promotion/Disease Prevention
  ○ Identify client health-seeking behaviors.
- High Risk Behaviors
  ○ Reinforce client teaching related to client high-risk behavior.
	Relevant topics/tasks include:
	- Diagnostic Tests
	  ○ Reinforce client teaching about diagnostic test.
	- Laboratory Values
	  ○ Compare client laboratory values to normal laboratory values.
	- Potential for Complications of Diagnostic Tests/Treatments/Procedures
	  ○ Perform risk monitoring and provide follow up.
		Relevant topics/tasks include:
		- Alterations in Body Systems
		  ○ Provide care to correct client alteration in body system.
		- Basic Pathophysiology
		  ○ Identify signs and symptoms related to acute or chronic illness.
		- Radiation Therapy
		  ○ Monitor client for signs and symptoms of adverse effects of radiation therapy.

UNIT 9	NURSING CARE OF CLIENTS WITH REPRODUCTIVE DISORDERS
Section:	Female Reproductive Disorders

Chapter 60 Diagnostic and Therapeutic Procedures for Female Reproductive Disorders

Overview

- Diagnostic and therapeutic procedures used to evaluate the structure, condition, and function of a female client's reproductive tissues and organs

  o Pelvic exam with Papanicolaou (Pap) test

  o Colposcopy and cervical biopsy, cone biopsy, and endometrial biopsy

  o Serologic studies

  o Mammography

  o Hysterectomy

- Biopsies can also serve as therapeutic purposes in removing abnormal tissue. Another therapeutic procedure that nurses should be knowledgeable about is a hysterectomy.

Pelvic Exam with Pap Test

- Bimanual examination of the cervix, uterus, fallopian tubes, and ovaries is performed by the provider. The provider inserts two gloved fingers into the vagina and traps the reproductive structures between the fingers of the one hand and the fingers of the opposite hand that is on the abdomen. Palpation of the structures is done during this time.

- A Pap test is a screening test to detect precancerous or cancerous process. The cervix is scraped with a wooden spatula, cytology brush, cotton-tipped applicator, or a combination of these tools, and specimens are placed on glass slides with a fixative immediately applied. The slide is sent to a laboratory for analysis.

  o All women should undergo a Pap test for cervical cancer on a regular basis. The frequency of this test is related to several factors.

  o A Pap test can also detect the presence of fungal, viral, and parasitic disorders.

- Indications

  o Begin testing at age 21 or within 3 years of becoming sexually active.

  o Have a yearly Pap test until age 30. If all tests have been negative, a longer period of time such as every 2 to 3 years may be recommended by the provider.

- ○ Pap tests may be discontinued after cervical removal during a hysterectomy or at age 65 if they have been normal for the past several years.
- ○ Interpretation of Findings
  - Analysis of the Pap test will yield either a "negative" result or description of cell abnormalities as outlined by either the Bethesda or cervical intraepithelial neoplasia (CIN) systems. False positives may be obtained in the presence of infection.
  - Atypical squamous cells (ASC)
    - □ ASC-US – atypical squamous cells of undetermined significance (considered mildly abnormal)
    - □ ASC-H – atypical squamous cells of which high-grade squamous intraepithelial lesions cannot be excluded (indicates high risk of being precancerous)
  - Squamous cell carcinoma
    - □ LSIL – low-grade squamous intraepithelial lesion (indicates mild abnormality that demonstrates early changes in shape and size of squamous cells)
    - □ HSIL – high-grade squamous intraepithelial lesion (indicates a more severe abnormality in size and shape of cells that can progress to invasive cancer)
  - Atypical glandular cells (AGC)
    - □ AGC – indicates a change in the glandular cells of the cervix rather than the squamous cells
  - Adenocarcinoma in situ (AIS)
    - □ AIS – indicates the presence of precancerous cells in the glandular tissue
- Preprocedure
  - ○ Nursing Actions
    - Ask clients if they have refrained from douching in the past 24 hr. Douching may wash away abnormal cells.
    - Inform client that use of vaginal medications or sexual intercourse within the last 24 hr may alter test results.
    - Have client empty the bladder.
    - Place clients in the lithotomy position and drape appropriately.
    - Explain to clients how the procedure will be carried out.
    - Have all necessary equipment available (light source, cervical scraping tools, glass slides, fixative, perineal pad, gloves, and speculum).

- Intraprocedure
  - Nursing Actions
    - Have necessary equipment ready for the provider during the procedure.
    - Transfer specimens to slides and apply fixative to slides.
- Postprocedure
  - Nursing Actions
    - Provide clients with a perineal pad and tissues.
  - Client Education
    - Inform clients that minimal bleeding may occur from the cervix.
    - Inform clients of the time frame for results to be available.

Colposcopy and Cervical Biopsy, Cone Biopsy, and Endometrial Biopsy

PROCEDURE	INDICATIONS
Colposcopy and Cervical Biopsy • A colposcope is used to inspect the cervix and take a cervical biopsy. All suspicious areas are biopsied and sent to a laboratory for microscopic examination.	Atypical or abnormal cells found on Pap tests
Cone Biopsy • This is an extensive cervical biopsy that excises a cone-shaped sample of tissue.	To remove potentially harmful cells, and done if a cervical lesion is clearly visible
Endometrial Biopsy • A thin, hollow tube is inserted through the cervix, and a curette or suction equipment is used to obtain the endometrial tissue sample.	To assess for uterine cancer as well as evaluate for menstrual irregularities and potential causes of infertility

- Preprocedure
  - Nursing Actions
    - Preprocedure care is the same as that for a Pap test, except a sterile biopsy cup will be needed instead of the other equipment.
    - Confirm that clients have withheld medications (anticoagulants, aspirin) if ordered by the provider.
    - Give clients pain reliever 30 min prior to the procedure. Inform clients that some discomfort will be experienced.
    - Verify informed consent has been given.
  - Client Education
    - Educate clients about the procedure.
    - Instruct clients to empty their bladder.

- Postprocedure
  - Nursing Actions
    - Postprocedure care is the same as that for a Pap test.
  - Client Education
    - Instruct clients to abstain from sexual intercourse and avoid using a douche, vaginal creams, or tampons until all discharge has stopped (usually about 2 weeks).
    - Have clients notify the provider of heavy vaginal bleeding, fever, severe pain, and/or foul discharge.
- Complications
  - Bleeding
    - Heavy bleeding can result from the excision of tissue.
    - Nursing Actions
      - Monitor clients for heavy bleeding.
    - Client Education
      - Instruct clients to notify the provider of abnormal vaginal bleeding.
  - Infection
    - Infection can result from this invasive procedure.
    - Nursing Actions
      - Monitor clients for fever, chills, severe pain, foul odor, or purulent vaginal discharge.
    - Client Education
      - Instruct clients to notify the provider regarding these symptoms.

Serologic (Blood) Studies

- Venereal disease research laboratory (VDRL) – the oldest test for syphilis that is still performed
- Rapid plasma regain (RPR) – a newer test for syphilis and has replaced the VDRL test in many institutions
- Indications
  - Client Presentation
    - Primary chancre – a firm, painless skin ulceration localized at point of initial exposure, and heals without treatment (clients still positive for syphilis)
    - Local lymph node swelling
    - Secondary symptoms – headache, anorexia, rash on trunk and extremities, fever, sore throat, malaise, and weight loss

- Interpretation of Findings
  - ○ Both tests are done using a sample of blood and reported as nonreactive (negative for syphilis) or reactive (positive for syphilis).
  - ○ False positives may occur secondary to infection, pregnancy, malignancies, and autoimmune disorders.
  - ○ If either test comes back as reactive, diagnosis should be done by confirming the results using one of the following tests:
    - ▪ Fluorescent treponemal antibody absorbed (FTA-ABS)
    - ▪ Treponema pallidum particle agglutination assay (TPPA)

Mammography

- A mammogram is an x-ray of the breast that is used as a screening tool for breast cancer. Tumors that are too small to be palpated can be visualized on a mammogram.
  - ○ During a mammogram, a woman's breast is mechanically compressed both vertically and horizontally by the x-ray machine while radiologic pictures are taken of each breast.
- Indications
  - ○ Mammograms should be done every 1 to 2 years beginning at age 40 during a wellness screening. If there is a family history of breast cancer, mammograms should begin at an earlier age.
  - ○ Diagnostic mammograms are also performed to evaluate a lesion or lump.
- Interpretation of Findings
  - ○ If a suspicious lesion is identified, a fine needle aspiration or open biopsy is usually performed.
- Preprocedure
  - ○ Nursing Actions
    - ▪ Instruct clients to avoid the use of deodorant, perfume, lotions, or powders in the axillary region or on the breasts prior to the exam.
    - ▪ Instruct clients that caffeine may increase discomfort and should be avoided.
    - ▪ Inform clients to tell the provider if pregnant.
- Intraprocedure
  - ○ Nursing Actions
    - ▪ Radiologic technicians are often the members of the health care team that perform mammograms.
- Postprocedure
  - ○ Client Education
    - ▪ Instruct clients to return every 1 to 2 years for a follow-up mammogram.
    - ▪ If follow-up is needed, the client will be contacted.

Hysterectomy

- A hysterectomy is the removal of the uterus and, in some cases, removal of the ovaries and fallopian tubes.
  - There are three methods of performing a hysterectomy
    - Abdominal approach, also known as a total abdominal hysterectomy
    - Vaginal approach
    - Laparoscopy hysterectomy
      - LAVH (Laparoscopy-assisted vaginal hysterectomy)
      - Uterine vessel ligation laparoscopic hysterectomy
      - Total laparoscopic
- Indications
  - Diagnoses
    - Uterine cancer
    - Noncancerous conditions – fibroids, endometriosis (inflammation of the endometrium), and genital prolapse – that cause pain, bleeding, or emotional stress
  - Client Presentation
    - Painful intercourse
    - Menorrhagia
    - Pelvic pressure
    - Urinary urgency or frequency
    - Constipation
- Preprocedure
  - Nursing Actions
    - Confirm that clients have withheld medications (anticoagulants, aspirin) if ordered by the provider.
    - Maintain NPO status.
    - Verify that informed consent has been obtained.
  - Client Education
    - Teach clients how to turn, cough, and deep breathe.
    - Instruct clients how to use an incentive spirometer.

- Postprocedure
  - Nursing Actions
    - Provide routine postoperative care to prevent complications.
    - Monitor clients for vaginal bleeding. Excess bleeding is more than one saturated pad in 4 hr.
    - Monitor urine output via indwelling urinary catheter. Notify the provider if output is less than 30 mL/hr.
    - Monitor the client's incision (infection, integrity, risk of dehiscence).
  - Client Education
    - Instruct clients about a well-balanced diet that is high in protein and vitamin C for wound healing, and high in iron if the client is anemic.
    - Instruct clients to avoid tampons, douches, and feminine deodorant spray.
    - Instruct clients to restrict activity (heavy lifting, strenuous activity, driving, stairs, sexual activity) for 4 to 6 weeks.
- Complications
  - Hypovolemic shock
    - Hypovolemic shock due to blood loss is a potential complication following a hysterectomy.
    - Nursing Actions
      - Monitor vital signs.
      - Monitor the client's Hgb and Hct.
      - Assist with care of clients receiving IV fluid replacement and/or blood transfusions.
  - Psychological reactions
    - Psychological reactions can occur months to years after surgery.
    - Nursing Actions
      - Encourage clients to discuss the positive aspects of life.
      - Monitor clients for persistent sadness or depression. Request a referral for counseling if indicated.
    - Client Education
      - Encourage clients to attend a support group.

Ⓐ APPLICATION EXERCISES

1. A nurse is preparing a sexually-active adolescent for her first Papanicolaou (Pap) test. Which of the following information should the nurse reinforce to the client?

    A. You will not feel any discomfort.

    B. You will need to hold your breath during the procedure.

    C. You may experience some bleeding after the procedure.

    D. You should urinate immediately after the procedure.

2. The Pap test analysis is classified as AIS. AIS is interpreted as

    A. atypical squamous cells of undetermined significance.

    B. evidence of precancerous cells.

    C. low-grade squamous intraepithelial lesion.

    D. a change in the glandular cells of the cervix rather than the squamous cells.

3. A nurse is reviewing the plan of care for a client who is postoperative a total abdominal hysterectomy. Postoperatively, the RN documented vital signs as: temperature 38.6° C (101.4° F), heart rate 88/min, respiratory rate 18/min, and blood pressure 124/82 mm Hg. Breath sounds are clear bilaterally. Bowel sounds are absent. An indwelling urinary catheter is patent and urinary output is 30 mL/hr. Four hours after surgery, the nurse's data now reveals vital signs as: temperature 38.7° C (101.6° F), heart rate 110/min, respiratory rate 32/min, blood pressure 102/68 mm Hg, and urinary output 20 mL/hour. Which of the following are appropriate nursing actions at this time? (Select all that apply.)

    _____ Change the dressing.

    _____ Call for assistance.

    _____ Calculate urine output.

    _____ Check for vaginal bleeding.

    _____ Continue IV fluid and electrolyte replacement.

4. A nurse is reinforcing premammogram instructions to a client. Which of the following should the nurse advise the client to avoid prior to the procedure?

    A. Exercise

    B. Deodorant

    C. Facial makeup

    D. Citrus fruit drinks

(A) APPLICATION EXERCISES ANSWER KEY

1. A nurse is preparing a sexually-active adolescent for her first Papanicolaou (Pap) test. Which of the following information should the nurse reinforce to the client?

   A. You will not feel any discomfort.

   B. You will need to hold your breath during the procedure.

   C. You may experience some bleeding after the procedure.

   D. You should urinate immediately after the procedure.

   It is normal and expected for a small amount of bleeding to occur after the procedure secondary to the scraping of the cervix. It is unnecessary for the client to urinate immediately after the procedure. Some discomfort can be felt when the speculum is introduced and the cervical scraping is done. The client should breath normally or take a few deep breaths during the procedure.

   (N) **NCLEX® Connection: Reduction of Risk Potential, Diagnostic Tests**

2. The Pap test analysis is classified as AIS. AIS is interpreted as

   A. atypical squamous cells of undetermined significance.

   B. evidence of precancerous cells.

   C. low-grade squamous intraepithelial lesion.

   D. a change in the glandular cells of the cervix rather than the squamous cells.

   Adenocarcinoma in situ, which indicates presence of precancerous cells in the glandular tissue is classified as AIS. Women with atypical cells are urged to have follow-up testing. Atypical squamous cells of undetermined significance is classified as ASC-US; low-grade squamous intraepithelial lesion is classified as LSIL; a change in the glandular cells of the cervix rather than the squamous cells is classified as AGC.

   (N) **NCLEX® Connection: Physiological Adaptations, Basic Pathophysiology**

3. A nurse is reviewing the plan of care for a client who is postoperative a total abdominal hysterectomy. Postoperatively, the RN documented vital signs as: temperature 38.6° C (101.4° F), heart rate 88/min, respiratory rate 18/min, and blood pressure 124/82 mm Hg. Breath sounds are clear bilaterally. Bowel sounds are absent. An indwelling urinary catheter is patent and urinary output is 30 mL/hr. Four hours after surgery, the nurse's data now reveals vital signs as: temperature 38.7° C (101.6° F), heart rate 110/min, respiratory rate 32/min, blood pressure 102/68 mm Hg, and urinary output 20 mL/hour. Which of the following are appropriate nursing actions at this time? (Select all that apply.)

_____	Change the dressing.
__X__	**Call for assistance.**
__X__	**Calculate urine output.**
__X__	**Check for vaginal bleeding.**
__X__	**Continue IV fluid and electrolyte replacement.**

    The client is showing signs of hypovolemic shock, possibly due to excessive bleeding. Because the client is becoming unstable, the nurse should call for assistance from the charge nurse. Calculating the urinary output as another parameter that provides data regarding possible shock, checking for vaginal bleeding, and continuing the IV fluid are appropriate actions at this time. Changing the dressing is not an appropriate action.

    Ⓝ NCLEX® Connection: Physiological Adaptations, Medical Emergencies

4. A nurse is reinforcing premammogram instructions to a client. Which of the following should the nurse advise the client to avoid prior to the procedure?

    A. Exercise

    B. Deodorant

    C. Facial makeup

    D. Citrus fruit drinks

    A client should not apply deodorant prior to a mammogram because it can appear on the film as a shadow that could be mistaken for a lesion. Exercising, using facial makeup, or consuming citrus drinks are not contraindicated prior to having a mammogram.

    Ⓝ NCLEX® Connection: Reduction of Risk Potential, Diagnostic Tests

UNIT 9	NURSING CARE OF CLIENTS WITH REPRODUCTIVE DISORDERS
Section:	Female Reproductive Disorders
Chapter 61	Menstrual Disorders and Menopause

Overview

- The average age of menarche (first menses) in the United States is 13 years of age. If an adolescent has not begun having periods by 15 years of age, possible causes should be investigated.

- Menstrual cycles are typically 28 days long, with a range from 21 to 35 days. The first day of menstruation is day 1 of a menstrual cycle. Ovulation typically occurs around day 14. Bleeding begins 14 days after ovulation and typically lasts 4 to 5 days, but it can continue for up to 7 days.

- Menstrual cycles continue until menopause or surgical removal of the uterus. Menopause is the time when ovulation ceases and menstrual cycles become irregular and eventually stop. The median age of onset of menopause is 51 years of age.

MENSTRUAL DISORDERS

Overview

- Painful menstruation, or dysmenorrhea, is common in adolescents and young women.

- Dysfunctional uterine bleeding (DUB) is believed to be due to a hormonal imbalance and may include menorrhagia and metrorrhagia. Menorrhagia is excessive bleeding (in amount and duration), possibly with clots and for longer than 7 days. Metrorrhagia is bleeding between menstrual periods more frequently than every 21 days.

- Amenorrhea is the absence of menses. In a woman who has had menstrual cycles, this can be a sign of a medical disorder. A common cause is low percentage of body fat in women who are involved in sports or women who over exercise.

- Premenstrual syndrome (PMS) involves a number of symptoms immediately prior to menstruation. The monthly fluctuation of hormones as well as a change in the level of serotonin has been considered a possible cause for these symptoms.

- Premenstrual dysphoric disorder (PMDD) is similar to premenstrual syndrome, but the symptoms occur for at least two consecutive cycles and are so severe they interfere with a women's ability to function. The symptoms include depression, irritability, changes in appetite, abdominal bloating, fatigue, emotional lability, and fluid retention. Treatment includes decreasing intake of sugar, salt, and alcohol, as well as increasing exercise. Antidepressants have been helpful for some women who experience severe PMDD.

- Endometriosis is characterized by an over growth of endometrial tissue that extends outside the uterus into the fallopian tubes, onto the ovaries, and into the pelvis. Blockage of the fallopian tubes by endometrial tissue is a common cause of infertility.

Data Collection

- Subjective data

  o Menstrual history (age of first menses, monthly cycle)

  o Report of premenstrual depression, irritability, changes in appetite, abdominal bloating, fatigue, emotional lability, or fluid retention

  o Characteristics of menstrual flow

  o Characteristics and location of pain during menstrual cycle

  o Painful intercourse

  o Objective data

    ■ Pelvic tenderness during palpation of the lower abdomen and the pelvic examination

    ■ Metabolic disorders (hypothyroidism)

  o Laboratory tests

    ■ Hgb and Hct

      □ May be below reference range due to excessive blood loss

  o Diagnostic procedures

    ■ Endometrial biopsy

      □ Determines the relationship between menstrual flow and the hormone cycle, as well as possible pathologic reasons for bleeding, such as uterine cancer

    ■ Transvaginal ultrasound

      □ Can identify the presence of uterine fibroids or leiomyomas

Collaborative Care

- Medications

  o Hormonal contraceptives

    ■ Use to decrease symptoms of PMS and PMDD.

- Use for DUB such as metrorrhagia, menorrhagia, or dysmenorrhea.
- These may be the initial treatment for endometriosis.
  - Leuprolide (Lupron) – Synthetic luteinizing hormone
    - This suppresses estrogen and testosterone production in the body, making it an effective treatment for endometriosis (promotes atrophy of ectopic tissue).
    - It can cause birth defects, so a reliable form of contraception should be used.
    - May cause decreased libido and increased risk of osteoporosis
  - NSAIDs – Ibuprofen (Motrin)
    - Use for endometriosis to inhibit production of prostaglandins.
    - These aid in the treatment of pain and discomfort related to PMS and PMDD.
  - SSRIs
    - Use for PMDD if other treatments are unsuccessful.
- Surgical Interventions
  - DUB
    - Endometrial ablation
      - Use to remove endometrial tissue in the uterus.
      - The tissue may be removed by laser, heat, electricity, or cryotherapy.
  - Endometriosis
    - Laparoscopic removal of ectopic tissue and adhesions
      - A laser may be used to remove tissue.
- Client Outcomes
  - DUB
    - The client will re-establish a menstrual cycle of approximately 28 days, with menstruation lasting no more than 7 days.
  - PMDD
    - The client will resume regular ADLs.
  - Endometriosis
    - The client will experience less pain and discomfort and be able to become pregnant if desired.

Complications

- Ectopic pregnancy
  - Due to the presence of endometrial tissue outside of the uterus, the ovum may implant in the fallopian tubes or abdominal cavity.
  - As the ovum increases in size, the fallopian tube may rupture and the client may bleed to death.

- ○ The fallopian tube may need to be surgically removed if bleeding is severe or the tube is irreparably damaged.

- ○ If ectopic pregnancy is identified prior to rupture of the fallopian tube, a salpingostomy may be performed to remove the fetus, or a medication (methotrexate [Rheumatrex]) may be given to terminate the pregnancy and promote reabsorption of the fetal products.

MENOPAUSE

Overview

- Menopause is the cessation of menses. Menses will appear on an infrequent cycle for a period of time that does not exceed 2 years. Menopause is considered complete when no menses have occurred for 12 months.

- Menopause may be natural or surgically induced.

Data Collection

- Subjective and Objective Data

  - ○ Vasomotor symptoms – Hot flashes and irregular menses

  - ○ Genitourinary – Atrophic vaginitis, vaginal dryness, and incontinence

  - ○ Psychologic – Mood swings, changes in sleep patterns, and decreased REM sleep

  - ○ Skeletal – Decreased bone density

  - ○ Cardiovascular – Decreased HDL and increased LDL

  - ○ Dermatologic – Decreased skin elasticity and loss of hair on head and in the pubic area

  - ○ Reproductive – Breast tissue changes

  - ○ Laboratory Tests

    - ▪ Follicle stimulating hormone (FSH) – Increased during menopause

    - ▪ Blood, urine, and saliva hormone levels (estrogens, progesterone, dehydroepiandrosterone sulfate [DHEA-S], testosterone)

  - ○ Diagnostic Procedures

    - ▪ Pelvic examination with Papanicolaou smear to rule out cancer in cases of abnormal bleeding

    - ▪ Breast examination with mammogram to rule out cancer in cases of a palpable change from predominantly glandular tissue to fatty tissue

- Biopsy of uterine lining in cases of undiagnosed abnormal uterine bleeding in a woman over 40 years of age or in a woman whose menses has stopped for a year and bleeding has begun again

- Bone mass measurements to determine a baseline measurement of density and strength and subsequently confirm the development of osteopenia/osteoporosis

Collaborative Care

- Medications

  - Hormone replacement therapy (HRT)

    - HRT may be prescribed to help control symptoms associated with the estrogen deficiency that occurs during and after menopause. Estrogen deficiency symptoms (hot flashes, atrophy of vaginal tissues, osteoporosis) occur naturally as part of the aging process during menopause. For a woman who has a uterus, HRT will include estrogen and progesterone. For a woman who no longer has a uterus (following a hysterectomy), HRT will only include estrogen.

    - Many different preparations of HRT are available (oral, transdermal, intravaginal, intramuscular). HRT may be prescribed as a continuous, combined estrogen-progesterone therapy or a variety of cyclic patterns.

    - If a woman and her health care provider believe that the use of HRT is required for management of menopausal symptoms, the best recommendation is to use HRT on a short-term basis, generally less than 5 years.

    - HRT is not indicated for prophylaxis of heart disease and generally is not prescribed for women at high risk for heart disease.

    - Risk factors that increase the incidence of adverse effects from HRT

      - Pregnancy – HRT should not be taken during pregnancy due to the risk of teratogenic effects.

      - Smoking

      - Cancer

        - Cancer of the breast or family history of breast cancer

        - Cancer of the uterus

        - Undiagnosed abnormal vaginal bleeding

      - Embolism

        - Active thrombophlebitis

        - Thromboembolic disorder or history of thrombus

        - Stroke

        - Heart disease or high risk for heart disease (hypertension)

- Nursing Actions
  - Monitor
    - Increased blood pressure
    - Breast tenderness, lumps, or abnormalities
    - Vaginal bleeding
    - Venous thrombosis
- Client Education
  - Reinforce to clients the advantages and disadvantages of HRT.
  - Instruct clients in self-administration of HRT.
  - Advise clients to immediately quit smoking if applicable.
  - Reinforce to clients how to prevent and check for the development of venous thrombosis.
    - Avoid wearing knee-high stockings and clothing or socks that are restrictive.
    - Note and report symptoms of unilateral leg pain, edema, warmth, and redness.
    - Avoid sitting for long periods of time.
    - Take short walks throughout the day to promote circulation.
    - Perform frequent ankle pumps, and move and stretch legs.
  - Recommend that clients schedule annual physicals, pelvic examinations, mammograms, and bone density tests.
  - Instruct clients about atypical presentation of MI signs and symptoms in women (abdominal pain, vague chest symptoms, arm pain, pain between the shoulders) and instruct the client to seek assistance immediately.
  - Instruct clients to take oral doses with food to alleviate nausea.
  - Advise clients to refrain from inserting vaginal creams or suppositories prior to intercourse to prevent the client's partner from absorbing the product.
- Alternative therapies
  - Dong quai and black cohosh have reportedly been effective in some women. Research regarding their usefulness has been inconsistent.
  - Phytoestrogens interact with estrogen receptors in the body. Vegetables such as dandelion greens, alfalfa sprouts, black beans, and soy beans contain phytoestrogens.
  - Vitamin E has been reported to decrease hot flashes in some women.

- ○ Client Education
  - ■ HRT is beneficial in the prevention of age-related problems.
    - □ Osteoporosis
      - ‣ Older adult clients may also decrease the risk of osteoporosis by performing regular weight-bearing exercises; increasing intake of high-protein and high-calcium foods; avoiding alcohol, caffeine, and tobacco; and taking calcium with vitamin D supplements.
    - □ Atrophic vaginitis, which is characterized by vaginal burning and bleeding, pruritus, and painful intercourse may improve with HRT. Vaginal instillations of estrogen may be an option and may result in less systemic absorption.
  - ■ Client Outcomes
    - □ The client will report a decrease in estrogen deficiency symptoms.
    - □ The client's bone scans will not demonstrate demineralization.

Complications

- Embolic complications (risk increased by concurrent smoking)
  - ○ MI, especially during the first year of therapy
  - ○ Stroke
  - ○ Venous thrombosis – Thrombophlebitis, especially during the first year of therapy
- Cancer
  - ○ In some studies, long-term use of HRT has been found to increase the risk for breast cancer.
  - ○ Long-term use of estrogen-only HRT increases the risk for ovarian and endometrial cancer, but this risk is decreased with 12 or more days of progesterone per month.

Ⓐ APPLICATION EXERCISES

1. Identify the signs and symptoms associated with premenstrual syndrome (PMS) and premenstrual dysphoric disorder (PMDD). What is one difference between these two disorders?

Scenario: A 51-year-old woman who is nulliparous presents to the women's health clinic with reports of hot flashes and irregular menses. She states she cannot sleep at night because the hot flashes awaken her. She is requesting hormone replacement therapy (HRT) for relief of menopausal symptoms. She stopped using oral contraceptive pills several years ago when her husband passed away. She has not been sexually active since his death. This is her first visit to a healthcare provider in 3 years.

2. Which of the following assumptions can a nurse make about the client's irregular menses? (Select all that apply.)

   _____ The client is probably menopausal.

   _____ The hot flashes are vasomotor symptoms.

   _____ Sleep disturbance can be associated with the irregular menses.

   _____ Cessation of oral contraceptives precipitated menopause.

   _____ The client is too young for menopausal symptoms.

3. While the nurse is collecting data from the client, the history reveals information that is contraindicated for HRT. Which of the following should the nurse consider as possible contraindications for HRT with this client? (Select all that apply.)

   _____ Type 2 diabetes mellitus

   _____ Family history of osteoporosis

   _____ Smokes one pack of cigarettes per day

   _____ History of a blood clot in the leg

   _____ Family history of breast cancer

4. A nurse is advising a client who was recently diagnosed with endometriosis. Which of the following should the nurse reinforce when teaching about the implications of endometriosis?

   A. Infertility

   B. Risk for multiple births

   C. Contraindication for use of contraceptives

   D. Increased susceptibility for pelvic inflammatory disease (PID)

Ⓐ APPLICATION EXERCISES ANSWER KEY

1. Identify the signs and symptoms associated with premenstrual syndrome (PMS) and premenstrual dysphoric disorder (PMDD). What is one difference between these two disorders?

   Signs and symptoms include depression, irritability, changes in appetite, abdominal bloating, fatigue, emotional lability, and fluid retention. Even though the findings are similar, the severity of the symptoms of PMDD are such that they interfere with a women's ability to function.

   NCLEX® Connection: Physiological Adaptations, Basic Pathophysiology

Scenario: A 51-year-old woman who is nulliparous presents to the women's health clinic with reports of hot flashes and irregular menses. She states she cannot sleep at night because the hot flashes awaken her. She is requesting hormone replacement therapy (HRT) for relief of menopausal symptoms. She stopped using oral contraceptive pills several years ago when her husband passed away. She has not been sexually active since his death. This is her first visit to a healthcare provider in 3 years.

2. Which of the following assumptions can a nurse make about the client's irregular menses? (Select all that apply.)

   __X__ **The client is probably menopausal.**

   __X__ **The hot flashes are vasomotor symptoms.**

   __X__ **Sleep disturbance can be associated with the irregular menses.**

   _____ Cessation of oral contraceptives precipitated menopause.

   _____ The client is too young for menopausal symptoms.

   The client is probably menopausal. Hot flashes and sleep disturbances are commonly associated with menopause. Cessation of oral contraceptives does not cause menopause, and 51 years is the average age for women to experience menopause.

Ⓝ NCLEX® Connection: Physiological Adaptations, Basic Pathophysiology

3. While the nurse is collecting data from the client, the history reveals information that is contraindicated for HRT. Which of the following should the nurse consider as possible contraindications for HRT with this client? (Select all that apply.)

_____	Type 2 diabetes mellitus
_____	Family history of osteoporosis
X	**Smokes one pack of cigarettes per day**
X	**History of a blood clot in the leg**
X	**Family history of breast cancer**

Smoking can increase the risk for thrombus development and should be discouraged prior to beginning therapy. HRT is contraindicated for clients who have experienced a blood clot before, since venous thrombi can develop as a side effect of HRT. Clients who have a family history of breast cancer should consider other options until research can determine if there is a relationship between HRT and increased risk for breast cancer. Type 2 diabetes mellitus and a family history of osteoporosis are not contraindications for HRT.

NCLEX® Connection: Pharmacological Therapies, Adverse Effects/Contraindications/Side Effects/Interactions

4. A nurse is advising a client who was recently diagnosed with endometriosis. Which of the following should the nurse reinforce when teaching about the implications of endometriosis?

A. Infertility

B. Risk for multiple births

C. Contraindication for use of contraceptives

D. Increased susceptibility for pelvic inflammatory disease (PID)

Endometriosis is an overgrowth of endometrial tissue that can block the fallopian tubes, causing infertility. The risk for multiple births or PID does not increase. Contraceptives are sometimes prescribed to treat endometriosis due to the suppression of endometrial growth.

NCLEX® Connection: Reduction of Risk Potential, Potential for Alterations in Body Systems

UNIT 9	NURSING CARE OF CLIENTS WITH REPRODUCTIVE DISORDERS
Section:	Female Reproductive Disorders

Chapter 62 Disorders and Cancers of the Female Reproductive System

Overview

- A cystocele is a protrusion of the posterior bladder through the posterior vaginal wall. It is caused by weakened pelvic muscles and/or structures.

  ○ Treatment for a cystocele includes estrogen therapy, Kegel exercises, vaginal pessary, or surgery (anterior colporrhaphy).

- A rectocele is a protrusion of the anterior rectal wall through the posterior vaginal wall. It is caused by a defect of the pelvic structures, a difficult delivery, or a forceps delivery.

  ○ Treatment for a rectocele includes a posterior colporrhaphy or anterior-posterior repair.

Data Collection

- Risk Factors

  ○ Cystocele

    ▪ Obesity

    ▪ Advanced age (loss of estrogen)

    ▪ Chronic constipation

    ▪ Family history

    ▪ Childbearing

    ▪ Hysterectomy

  ○ Rectocele

    ▪ Pelvic structure defects

    ▪ Obesity

    ▪ Aging

    ▪ Family history

    ▪ Difficult childbirth necessitating repair of a tear

    ▪ Forceps delivery

    ▪ Previous hysterectomy

- o Cystocele and rectocele may develop in older adult females, usually following menopause.

- o Older adult clients are more susceptible to constipation and chronic bearing down during elimination, which can displace weakened structures.

- Subjective Data

  - o Cystocele

    - Urinary frequency and/or urgency

    - Stress incontinence

    - Report of frequent UTIs

    - Sense of vaginal fullness

  - o Rectocele

    - Constipation and/or the need to place fingers in the vagina to elevate the rectocele to complete evacuation of feces

    - Sensation of a mass in the vagina

    - Pelvic pressure or pain

    - Pain with intercourse

    - Pain in the back or pelvis

- Objective Data

  - o Diagnostic Procedures

    - Cystocele

      - □ A pelvic examination reveals a bulging of the anterior wall when the client is instructed to bear down.

      - □ A voiding cystourethrography is performed to identify the degree of bladder protrusion and the amount of urine residual.

    - Rectocele

      - □ A pelvic examination reveals a bulging of the posterior wall when the client is instructed to bear down.

      - □ A rectal examination and/or barium enema reveals the presence of a rectocele.

Collaborative Care

- Therapeutic Procedures
  - Vaginal pessary
    - A removable rubber, plastic, or silicone device inserted into the vagina to provide support and block protrusion of other organs into the vagina

     View Media Supplement: Pessary (Image)

    - Nursing Actions
      - Teach clients how to insert, remove, and clean the device.
      - Monitor for possible bleeding or fistula formation.
  - Kegel exercises
    - Exercises done to strengthen the pelvic floor
    - Client Education
      - Instruct clients how to perform the exercises.
        - Tighten pelvic muscles for 10 counts.
        - Relax slowly for 10 counts, pause for 10 to 15 seconds, and repeat in sequences of 15.
        - Perform while lying, sitting, and standing.
        - Perform at least 4 times daily.
        - Keep abdominal muscles relaxed during contractions.
- Surgical Interventions
  - Cystocele
    - Anterior colporrhaphy
      - Using a vaginal approach, the pelvic muscles are shortened and tightened.
  - Rectocele
    - Posterior colporrhaphy
      - Using a vaginal/perineal approach, the pelvic muscles are shortened and tightened.
      - A biological mesh graft may be used to provide extra support to weakened tissue.

- ○ Anterior-Posterior repair

  - In some cases, surgery for both a cystocele and a rectocele is needed; this is called an anterior-posterior repair.

  - A hysterectomy may be performed at the same time as any of the procedures listed above.

  - Nursing Actions

    - □ Postoperative

      - ‣ Provide routine postoperative care to prevent complications.

      - ‣ Administer analgesics, antimicrobials, and stool softeners/laxatives as prescribed.

      - ‣ Provide perineal care at least twice daily following surgery and after every urination or bowel movement.

      - ‣ Apply an ice pack to the perineal area to relieve pain and swelling.

      - ‣ Suggest that clients take frequent sitz baths to soothe the perineal area.

      - ‣ Provide a liquid diet immediately following surgery followed by a low-residue diet until normal bowel function returns.

      - ‣ Recommend that clients drink 2 to 3 L of fluid daily from food and beverage sources, unless contraindicated.

      - ‣ Following removal of the indwelling urinary catheter, instruct the client to void every 2 to 3 hr to prevent a full bladder and stress on stitches.

- • Care After Discharge

  - ○ Client Education

    - Administer estrogen therapy to prevent uterine atrophy and atrophic vaginitis if the client is not at risk for complications from hormone therapy (cardiovascular or embolic history).

    - Instruct clients on how to care for an indwelling urinary catheter at home. Remind the client to thoroughly wash her hands before and after handling the catheter and to remove any crust or debris collected around the catheter.

    - Instruct clients to tighten and support pelvic muscles when coughing or sneezing.

    - Advise clients of postoperative restrictions, including avoidance of strenuous activity, lifting anything weighing greater than 5 lb, and sexual intercourse.

    - Inform clients that if the provider did not schedule her for removal of stitches, they will be absorbed by the body, negating the need for removal.

    - Advise clients who are at risk to lose weight if obese.

    - Instruct clients to eat high-fiber diets and drink adequate fluids to prevent constipation.

- - Caution clients to avoid straining at defecation.
  - Caution clients to avoid sitting, walking, or standing for prolonged periods following surgery.
- Client Outcomes
  - The client will not experience urine leakage when coughing, laughing, or bearing down.
  - The client will be able to have bowel movement without trapping of feces in the rectal pouch.

Complications

- Dyspareunia (painful sexual intercourse) is a possible surgical complication due to surgical alteration of the vaginal orifice.

CANCER

Overview

- Cancer may affect the various parts of the female reproductive system
  - Breasts
  - Cervix
  - Uterus
  - Ovaries
- Cervical cancer is a slow-growing cancer. With proper screening, it may be detected early and treated with good results.
- The exact etiology of ovarian cancer is unknown; however, the more times a woman ovulates in her lifetime seems to be a risk factor since ovarian cancer is more prevalent in women with early menarche, late-onset menopause, nulliparity, and those who use infertility agents. Birth control pills may offer protection against ovarian cancer.

BREAST CANCER

Overview

- A combination of breast self-examination (BSE), a clinical breast exam, and mammography is effective in detecting early breast cancer and reducing mortality rates.

Health Promotion and Disease Prevention

- Client Education
  - Recommend that women over age 20 to conduct a monthly BSE and schedule an annual clinical breast examination.
  - Recommend women over age 40 to receive mammograms every 1 to 2 years.

- Instruct clients to eat five servings of fruits and vegetables daily.

- Instruct clients to maintain a healthy weight and exercise regularly.

- Instruct clients to limit alcohol intake and avoid smoking.

Data Collection

- Risk Factors

  - High genetic risk

    - First-degree relative with breast cancer (parent, sibling, or child)

    - Early age at diagnosis

  - Female sex (less than 1% of males develop breast cancer)

  - Age over 40

  - Early menarche, late menopause

  - First pregnancy after age 30

  - Early or prolonged use of oral contraceptives

  - High-fat diet (possible risk)

  - Low-fiber diet (possible risk)

  - Excessive alcohol intake (possibly related to folic acid depletion)

  - Cigarette smoking

  - Exposure to low-level radiation

  - Hormone replacement therapy

  - Obesity

  - History of endometrial or ovarian cancer

- Subjective Data

  - Breast pain or soreness

  - Report of change in physical appearance of the breast

- Objective Data

  - Physical Findings

    - Skin changes (peau d'orange)

(M) View Media Supplement: Breast Changes: Peau d' Orange (Image)

- Dimpling
- Palpable lump (usually small, irregularly shaped, firm, nontender, and nonmobile)
- Increased vascularity
- Nipple retraction or ulceration
- Enlarged lymph nodes

○ Laboratory Tests

- BRCA1 and BRCA2 gene test
  □ Recommend this for women who have two first-degree relatives who were diagnosed with breast cancer before age 50 or women who have a family history of both breast and ovarian cancer.
  □ This cannot be done within 3 months of a blood transfusion.
  □ Test results are either positive or negative for presence of the gene.
- HER2 gene cell
  □ A pathology report from a biopsy may determine if cancer cells contain the HER2 gene.
  □ If the result is positive, this gene may be responsible for the rapidly cancerous growing cells.
  □ Additional chemotherapy may be needed postoperatively.

○ Diagnostic Procedures

- Mammogram, ultrasound, MRI
- Biopsy-definitive diagnosis
  □ An open biopsy is done by excising a small portion of the mass for histologic exam.
  □ Fine needle aspiration is the removal of tissue or fluid from the breast mass through a large-bore needle.

Collaborative Care

- Interdisciplinary Care

  ○ Arrange for a visitor from Reach for Recovery to speak with clients.

  ○ Request a referral to a community support group as appropriate.

  ○ Request a referral for home health care services for care of drains and dressings and for help with ADLs.

- Therapeutic Procedures

  ○ The choice of treatment depends on the stage and size of the tumor, nodal involvement, client's age, hormone status related to menopause, and genetic predisposition.

  ○ Adjuvant therapy (radiation therapy, chemotherapy, or hormonal therapy) follows surgery to decrease the risk of recurrence.

- Hormone therapy
  - Gonadotropin-releasing hormone (GnRH) – leuprolide (Lupron)
    - Inhibits estrogen synthesis.
    - May be used in premenopausal women to stop or prevent the growth of breast tumors.
  - Selective estrogen receptor modulators (SERMs) – tamoxifen (Nolvadex) and raloxifene (Evista)
    - SERMs are used in women who are at high risk for breast cancer or who have advanced breast cancer.
    - SERMs suppress the growth of remaining cancer cells postmastectomy or lumpectomy.
    - Tamoxifen has been found to increase the risk of endometrial cancer, DVT, and pulmonary embolism; raloxifene does not share these side effects.
- Chemotherapy/radiation therapy
  - Clients who undergo chemotherapy are usually given a combination of several medications (Cytoxan, Adriamycin, and fluorouracil).
  - Clients who have the HER2/neu gene may receive trastuzumab (Herceptin).
  - Clients who have metastatic cancer may receive a vascular endothelial growth factor inhibitor, such as bevacizumab (Avastin).
  - Stem-cell transplants are being researched in regard to treating clients who are at high risk of recurrence.
  - Radiation therapy is usually reserved for clients who had a lumpectomy or breast-conserving procedure.
    - Whole or partial breast radiation may be prescribed. Skin care will be a high priority due to radiation damage as well as generalized fatigue.
    - Brachytherapy with radioactive seeds may also be an option.
    - Intraoperative radiation therapy allows an intense dose of radiation to be delivered directly to the surgical site.

- Surgical Interventions
  - Surgical procedures include lumpectomy (breast-conserving), wide excision or partial mastectomy, total mastectomy, modified radical mastectomy, radical mastectomy, and reconstructive surgery.

 View Media Supplement: Total Mastectomy with Lymph Node Dissection (Image)

- Nursing Actions
  - Provide routine postoperative care to prevent postoperative complications.
  - Position clients with the head of the bed elevated 30° when awake and with arm supported on a pillow.
  - Assist clients in supporting the arm on the operative side with a sling while ambulating, and encourage good posture.
  - Encourage clients to lie on the unaffected side postoperatively to relieve pain.
  - Avoid administering injections, taking blood pressure, or drawing blood from the client's affected arm. Place a sign above the client's bed regarding these precautions.
  - Emphasize the importance of a well-fitting breast prosthesis for clients who have had a mastectomy.
  - Provide emotional support to clients and their families.
- Client Education
  - Reinforce to clients how to care for the incision and drainage tubes. Drains are usually left in for 1 to 3 weeks.
  - Advise clients to avoid placing the affected arm in a dependent arm position. This position will interfere with wound healing.
  - Encourage early arm and hand exercises (squeezing a rubber ball, elbow flexion and extension, and hand-wall climbing) to prevent lymphedema and to regain full range of motion.
  - Instruct clients not to wear constrictive clothing, to avoid cuts and injuries, and to not allow blood pressure to be taken in the affected arm.
  - Reinforce techniques for breast self-examination.
  - Instruct clients to report numbness, pain, heaviness, or impaired motor function of the affected arm to the surgeon.
  - Encourage clients to discuss breast reconstruction alternatives with the surgeon.
    - Reconstruction may begin during the original breast removal procedure or after some healing has occurred.
    - A tissue expander (a saline-filled implant that has a port through which additional saline can be injected, gradually expanding the tissue prior to permanent implant) is often placed during the original procedure.
    - Saline or silicone implants are used for permanent placement.
    - Autologous flaps may also be used for reconstruction.
    - Nipple reconstruction may be done using tissue from the labia, abdomen, or inner thigh.

- Client Outcomes

  o The client will regain full use of the arm on the side where the mastectomy occurred.

  o The client will integrate the mastectomy scar or reconstructive appearance of the breast into her new body image.

Complications

- Tumor invasion

  o A tumor invasion can occur in the lymphatic channels and seed cancer cells into the blood and lymphatic systems. The most common areas of metastases are the nearby bone, lungs, brain, and liver.

  o Client Education

    ▪ Reinforce the importance of continuing adjuvant therapy if prescribed.

    ▪ Instruct clients about signs and symptoms of metastatic breast cancer and common locations.

CERVICAL CANCER

Overview

- Early cervical cancer is generally asymptomatic. Symptoms do not develop until the cancer has become invasive.

- Papanicolaou (Pap) tests are an effective screening tool for detecting the earliest changes associated with cervical cancer. Findings of a Pap smear are usually classified according to the Bethesda system.

Data Collection

- Risk Factors

  o Early sexual activity (before 18 years of age)

  o Client and/or male partner has had multiple sexual partners

  o Male partner who had a female partner with cervical cancer

  o Low economic status

  o Family history of cervical cancer

  o African American

  o Chronic cervical inflammation/infections

  o Infection with human papilloma virus (HPV), which is associated in 90% of cases

  o History of sexually transmitted diseases

  o Infection with HIV or other immunosuppressive disorder

- o Cigarette smoking
- o Intrauterine exposure to diethylstilbestrol during pregnancy
- Subjective Data
  - o Painless vaginal bleeding between periods
  - o Watery, blood-tinged vaginal discharge
  - o Unexplained weight loss
  - o Pelvic pain
  - o Pain during and after intercourse
- Objective Data
  - o Diagnostic Procedures
    - Pap test – microscopic examination of cervical cells
    - Cervical biopsy (definitive) is performed for cytologic studies when a cervical lesion is identified. Biopsy is usually performed during colposcopy as a follow up to an abnormal Pap smear.

Collaborative Care

- Nursing Care
  - o Treat anemia as indicated.
  - o Administer antibiotics for pelvic, vaginal, or UTIs.
  - o Administer pain medications as prescribed.
  - o Provide emotional support to clients and their families.
- Interdisciplinary Care
  - o Request referral to a community support group as appropriate.
  - o Request referral for clients to counseling if depressed or expressing concerns over sexuality.
  - o Request referral for home care needs (ostomy nurse, home health nurse, home health aide, and emotional support).
- Therapeutic Procedures
  - o Removal of the lesion by conization, cryotherapy, laser ablation, hysterectomy, or a loop electrosurgical excision procedure.
    - Nursing Actions
      - □ Prepare clients for the procedure indicated.

- Client Education
  - □ Reinforce to clients signs and symptoms of infection.
  - □ Inform clients that vaginal discharge, consistent with the type of procedure, is normal after the procedure.
  - □ Reinforce home care instructions following special procedures (vaginal discharge, pain, avoiding douches, avoiding tampons, avoiding sexual intercourse, safety precautions, and postradiation treatments).
  - ○ Radiation
    - Brachytherapy and external radiation therapy may be options for cancer that is no longer limited to local invasion.
- Surgical Interventions
  - ○ Clients who have early stage cervical cancer may require a simple hysterectomy (removal of the uterus and cervix) or a radical hysterectomy (removal of the uterus, upper third of the vagina, uterosacral uterovesical ligaments, and pelvic nodes).

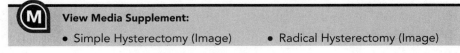

View Media Supplement:
- Simple Hysterectomy (Image)   • Radical Hysterectomy (Image)

  - ○ Clients with more extensive cancer may require a more extensive pelvic surgery called exenteration.
    - Anterior exenteration involves removal of the uterus, cervix, fallopian tubes, vagina, ovaries, bladder, urethra, and pelvic lymph nodes. An ileal conduit will need to be established for urinary diversion.
    - Posterior exenteration involves removal of the uterus, cervix, fallopian tubes, vagina, ovaries, anal canal, rectum, and descending colon. A colostomy will need to be established for bowel diversion.
    - A total exenteration involves removal of all of the above organs and establishment of both urinary and bowel diversions.
    - Nursing Actions
      - □ Provide routine postoperative care to prevent complications.
      - □ Manage drains as well as urinary and bowel diversions.
      - □ Monitor clients for body image disturbance and encourage speaking openly about it.
      - □ Discuss the client's understanding and expectations of treatment.
    - Client Education
      - □ Teach clients signs and symptoms of wound infection and how to care for drains that may remain after discharge.

□ Instruct clients about how to care for urinary and bowel diversion.

□ Instruct clients about how to care for perineal wounds and expectations regarding discharge.

- Care After Discharge

  o Client Education

    ■ Encourage all women to have Pap tests on a regular basis as recommended by the provider.

    ■ Recommend that clients limit the number of sexual partners.

    ■ Recommend clients use condoms during sex.

    ■ Promote smoking cessation.

  o Client Outcomes

    ■ The client will reestablish urinary and bowel function via a diversional method.

    ■ The client will reestablish positive self-image, integrating alterations caused by the surgical procedure.

Complications

  o Fistula development can occur after pelvic exenteration.

  o Kidney infections are also common secondary to the urinary diversion.

UTERINE (ENDOMETRIAL) CANCER

Overview

- Endometrial cancer is more common in older adult women and is related to prolonged exposure to estrogen.

- Estrogen therapy in postmenopausal women who have a uterus should include progesterone to decrease the risk of endometrial cancer.

Data Collection

- Risk Factors

  o Over 55 years of age

  o Obesity

  o Unopposed estrogen hormone replacement therapy

  o Nulliparity

  o Use of tamoxifen to prevent breast cancer

  o Late menopause

- Subjective Data
  - Irregular and/or postmenopausal bleeding
- Objective Data
  - Diagnostic Procedures
    - Endometrial biopsy

Collaborative Care

- Therapeutic Procedures
  - Radiation
    - Radiation therapy is given as adjuvant therapy, usually after a hysterectomy.
    - Brachytherapy and external radiation therapy may be options for cancer that is no longer limited to the uterus.
- Surgical Interventions
  - Treatment of endometrial cancer usually involves a total hysterectomy (uterus and cervix).
  - Removal of the fallopian tubes (salpingectomy), ovaries (oophorectomy) or both (bilateral salpingo-oophorectomy [BSO]) may also be done in the presence of a malignancy. The vagina remains for sexual intercourse to continue.
    - Either an open, laparoscopic, or vaginal approach may be used for either of the above procedures.
  - Nursing Actions
    - Provide routine postoperative care to prevent postoperative complications.
    - Observe for urinary retention and difficulty voiding due to the proximity of the urethra (more common after vaginal hysterectomies).
    - Monitor for a paralytic ileus due to manipulation of the bowel during surgery.
    - Discuss sexuality, surgically induced menopause, and other self-image issues with clients.
  - Client Education
    - Instruct clients to avoid straining, driving, lifting more than 5 lb, douching, and participating in sexual intercourse until the provider gives release.
- Care After Discharge
  - Client Education
    - Instruct clients to immediately report signs and symptoms of infection, as well as vaginal discharge that is excessive or has a foul odor.
    - Discuss hormone replacement therapy options with the client if she is premenopausal.

- Client Outcomes

  o The client will reestablish positive self-image in regard to removal of the reproductive organs.

  o The client will not develop an infection of the incision or bladder.

OVARIAN CANCER

Overview

- Metastases frequently occurs before the primary ovarian malignancy is diagnosed.

- The most reliable indicator of prognosis is related to the stage of the cancer at the time of diagnosis.

Data Collection

- Risk Factors

  o Over 40 years of age

  o Nulliparity or first pregnancy after 30 years of age

  o Family history of ovarian, breast, or colon cancer

  o History of dysmenorrhea or heavy bleeding

  o Endometriosis

  o High-fat diet (possible risk)

  o Hormone replacement therapy

  o Use of infertility medications

  o Older adult clients following surgery for cancer.

- Subjective Data

  o Abdominal pain or swelling

  o Abdominal discomfort (dyspepsia, indigestion, gas, distention)

  o Abdominal mass

  o Urinary frequency

- Objective Data

  o Laboratory Tests

    - Cancer antigen test (CA-125 antigen)

      □ Elevates in the presence of damaged endometrial tissue, in response to endometriosis, pregnancy, and fibroids

      □ Elevated value is greater than 35 units/mL

- ○ Diagnostic Procedures

  - ▪ Bimanual examination may reveal an enlarged ovary. The finding may not be apparent until the ovarian tumor is 4 to 6 inches in size.

  - ▪ A vaginal ultrasound may also be helpful in determining the presurgical size and location of tumors as well as a 1 year follow up that evaluates success of treatment and recurrence or metastases of tumors.

  - ▪ Staging of ovarian cancer is determined at the time of the hysterectomy or exploratory laparotomy when the tumor is removed and examined by the pathologist.

Collaborative Care

- • Interdisciplinary Care

  - ○ Arrange for clients to visit with a cancer survivor if possible.

  - ○ Provide clients with information about cancer support groups (Gilda's Club and National Ovarian Cancer Coalition).

  - ○ Provide information about hospice care when appropriate.

- • Therapeutic Procedures

  - ○ Chemotherapy (traditional or intraperitoneal)

    - ▪ Chemotherapy is always given for ovarian cancer, even if surgery was performed. Cisplatin and carboplatin are the most common chemotherapeutic mediations used for ovarian cancer.

    - ▪ Intracavitary chemotherapy involves the placement of an intraperitoneal catheter through which the chemotherapy is administered.

      - □ With the client in a semi-Fowler's position, the chemotherapeutic agent is infused into the abdomen. Discomfort will be felt related to the pressure from the infusion, but may also indicate dislocation of the catheter.

      - □ "Dwell time" is the amount of time the agent remains in the abdominal cavity.

      - □ Agent is drained via the catheter after the prescribed amount of dwell time.

      - □ Clients should be instructed to report signs and symptoms of infection, including peritonitis.

  - ○ Pelvic or abdominal irradiation

    - ▪ Radiation is only used if the disease is localized to a small area or if palliative treatment of tumors is the goal.

- • Surgical Interventions

  - ○ A total abdominal hysterectomy with bilateral salpingectomy and oophorectomy (TAH with BSO) is the usual treatment for ovarian cancer.

- A TAH with BSO also helps determine the extent of the disease as well as local and distant metastases. Staging of the cancer is done at this time.
- Nursing Actions
  - Provide postoperative care and prevent postoperative complications.
  - Observe clients for urinary retention and difficulty voiding.
  - Observe clients for paralytic ileus common due to manipulation of the bowel during surgery.
  - Discuss sexuality, surgically induced menopause, and other self-image issues with clients.
  - Encourage clients to express feelings about the cancer and fears of death.
  - Help clients and their families to develop coping strategies.
  - Monitor the client's progress through the stages of grief.
- Client Education
  - Instruct clients to avoid straining, driving, lifting more than 5 lb, douching, and participating in sexual intercourse until the provider gives release.
  - Instruct clients to immediately report signs and symptoms of infection, as well as vaginal discharge that is excessive or has a foul odor.

- Client Outcomes
  - The client will experience minimal side effects from chemotherapy.
  - The client will set realistic personal goals in view of the stage of the disease and prognosis.

(A) APPLICATION EXERCISES

1. Which of the following instructions should a nurse reinforce to a client concerning Kegel exercises for conservative management of a cystocele or rectocele? (Select all that apply.)

    _____ Perform exercises at least 4 times a day.

    _____ Hold the contraction for 6 to 10 seconds.

    _____ Pause for 1 min between each exercise.

    _____ Perform exercises in, lying, sitting and standing positions.

    _____ Tighten abdominal muscles during contractions.

    _____ Tighten pelvic muscles for a count of 10.

2. A nurse is collecting data from a client admitted to the gynecology unit for an anterior colporrhaphy to repair a cystocele. Which of the following client statements should the nurse expect?

    A. "I have to push the feces out of a pouch in my vagina with my fingers."

    B. "I have pain and bleeding when I have a bowel movement."

    C. "I have had frequent urinary tract infections."

    D. "I have pain during intercourse."

3. A nurse is preparing to discharge a client who has had an anterior and posterior colporrhaphy. Which of the following instructions should the nurse reinforce in the teaching?

    A. Do not bend over for at least 6 weeks.

    B. Take showers, not tub baths for at least 2 weeks.

    C. Do not engage in intercourse for at least 6 weeks.

    D. Expect to have a urinary catheter in place for at least 2 weeks.

Scenario: A 47-year-old woman presents to the health screening clinic for the first time in 8 years. She is in a new relationship and is planning to resume sexual activity for the first time since the death of her husband 8 years ago. Her medical history is significant for hypercholesteremia, which resolved with dietary changes and exercise. She lost 25 lb last year, but has hypertension. Her body mass index is 25. She smokes three to four cigarettes daily. She engages in vigorous exercise four to five times a week. Family history is significant for the death of her mother at age 25 due to ovarian cancer. She has no siblings. She was married for 17 years prior to the death of her husband and was unable to conceive during that time. The couple did not seek infertility treatment. The client has had one sexual partner in her lifetime. Her menstrual history is: menarche at age 13, regular 31 day cycles, gravida 0.

4. Which of the following findings place the client at risk for cancers of the reproductive system? (Select all that apply.)

    _____ Nullipara

    _____ Hypertensive

    _____ Female gender

    _____ Menarche at age 13

    _____ Cigarette smoking

    _____ Over 40 years of age

    _____ Previous history of obesity

    _____ Ovarian cancer in a first-degree relative

5. Which of the following diagnostic procedures should the nurse anticipate will need to be performed on the client to assess for ovarian cancer?

    A. Pap smear

    B. Mammogram

    C. Stool for occult blood

    D. Bimanual pelvic examination

6. A nurse is caring for a client who has breast cancer and is to undergo hormone therapy. Identify two agents used for this type of treatment and their intended effect.

(A) **APPLICATION EXERCISES ANSWER KEY**

1. Which of the following instructions should a nurse reinforce to a client concerning Kegel exercises for conservative management of a cystocele or rectocele? (Select all that apply.)

    ___X___ **Perform exercises at least 4 times a day.**

    ___X___ **Hold the contraction for 6 to 10 seconds.**

    _____ Pause for 1 min between each exercise.

    ___X___ **Perform exercises in, lying, sitting and standing positions.**

    _____ Tighten abdominal muscles during contractions.

    ___X___ **Tighten pelvic muscles for a count of 10.**

    Kegel exercises should be done at least 4 times a day. Contractions should be held for 6 to 10 seconds followed by a 10- to 15-min relaxation period. Perform exercises lying, sitting, and standing. Exercises are done by tightening pelvic muscles. Keep abdominal muscles relaxed during the contractions.

(N) NCLEX® Connection: Reduction of Risk Potential, Therapeutic Procedures

2. A nurse is collecting data from a client admitted to the gynecology unit for an anterior colporrhaphy to repair a cystocele. Which of the following client statements should the nurse expect?

    A. "I have to push the feces out of a pouch in my vagina with my fingers."

    B. "I have pain and bleeding when I have a bowel movement."

    C. "I have had frequent urinary tract infections."

    D. "I have pain during intercourse."

    Clients with a cystocele experience frequent urinary tract infections due to the trapping of urine in the urovaginal pouch. Pushing feces out of a pouch in the vagina, pain and bleeding during urination, and pain during intercourse are consistent with a rectocele, not a cystocele.

(N) NCLEX® Connection: Physiological Adaptation, Pathophysiology

3. A nurse is preparing to discharge a client who has had an anterior and posterior colporrhaphy. Which of the following instructions should the nurse reinforce in the teaching?

   A. Do not bend over for at least 6 weeks.

   B. Take showers, not tub baths for at least 2 weeks.

   C. Do not engage in intercourse for at least 6 weeks.

   D. Expect to have a urinary catheter in place for at least 2 weeks.

   The nurse should tell the client to not engage in intercourse for at least 6 weeks. There are no restrictions in regard to bending over. Tub baths are encouraged for comfort and hygiene. The client's indwelling urinary catheter will be removed when swelling permits unimpeded urination, which is usually less than 2 weeks.

NCLEX® Connection: Reduction of Risk Potential, Potential for Complications from Surgical Procedures and Health Alterations

Scenario: A 47-year-old woman presents to the health screening clinic for the first time in 8 years. She is in a new relationship and is planning to resume sexual activity for the first time since the death of her husband 8 years ago. Her medical history is significant for hypercholesteremia, which resolved with dietary changes and exercise. She lost 25 lb last year, but has hypertension. Her body mass index is 25. She smokes three to four cigarettes daily. She engages in vigorous exercise four to five times a week. Family history is significant for the death of her mother at age 25 due to ovarian cancer. She has no siblings. She was married for 17 years prior to the death of her husband and was unable to conceive during that time. The couple did not seek infertility treatment. The client has had one sexual partner in her lifetime. Her menstrual history is: menarche at age 13, regular 31 day cycles, gravida 0.

4. Which of the following findings place the client at risk for cancers of the reproductive system? (Select all that apply.)

__X__	**Nullipara**
_____	Hypertensive
__X__	**Female gender**
_____	Menarche at age 13
__X__	**Cigarette smoking**
__X__	**Over 40 years of age**
__X__	**Previous history of obesity**
__X__	**Ovarian cancer in a first-degree relative**

   Nulliparity, female gender, cigarette smoking, age over 40, previous history of obesity, and ovarian cancer in a first-degree relative are all risk factors for cancer of a reproductive organ. Hypertension is not a risk factor for reproductive cancer and menarche at age 13 is within the expected reference range (it is not considered early menarche).

NCLEX® Connection: Physiological Adaptation, Alterations in Body Systems

5. Which of the following diagnostic procedures should the nurse anticipate will need to be performed on the client to assess for ovarian cancer?

    A. Pap smear

    B. Mammogram

    C. Stool for occult blood

    D. Bimanual pelvic examination

    Due to the location of ovarian cancer, a bimanual pelvic examination should be performed to assess for an ovarian mass or enlarged ovary. A Pap test is done to screen for cervical cancer, a mammogram is done to screen for breast cancer, and a stool for occult blood is done to screen for colon cancer.

    NCLEX® Connection: Reduction of Risk Potential, Diagnostic Tests

6. A nurse is caring for a client who has breast cancer and is to undergo hormone therapy. Identify two agents used for this type of treatment and their intended effect.

    Leuprolide (Lupron) is a gonadotropin-releasing hormone (GnRH) that inhibits estrogen synthesis. Tamoxifen (Nolvadex) and raloxifene (Evista) are selective estrogen receptor modulators (SERMs) that suppress the growth of remaining cancer cells postmastectomy or lumpectomy.

    NCLEX® Connection: Pharmacological Therapies, Expected Actions/Outcomes

UNIT 9	NURSING CARE OF CLIENTS WITH REPRODUCTIVE DISORDERS
Section:	Male Reproductive Disorders
Chapter 63	Diagnostic Procedures for Male Reproductive Disorders

Overview

- Changes to the prostate gland are common as men age, and routine diagnostic procedures should be performed to evaluate it.

  o Enlargement of the prostate gland is usually benign and is called benign prostatic hypertrophy.

  o Prostate cancer is the most common type of cancer in men.

- Diagnostic procedures for male reproductive disorders that nurses should be knowledgeable about

  o Prostatic specific antigen

  o Digital rectal exam

  o Transrectal ultrasound

Prostatic Specific Antigen (PSA) and Digital Rectal Exam (DRE)

- The PSA measures the amount of a protein produced by the prostate gland in the bloodstream.

  o The PSA is done on a sample of blood, and its value is reported.

  o Clients who have an elevated PSA should undergo a DRE by a provider to validate the findings.

- The DRE is done by a provider in an office or clinic.

  o With the client leaning over the examination table, the provider places a gloved finger in the client's anus and palpates the posterior portion of the prostate gland through the rectal wall.

  o If the DRE reveals an abnormality, the location of the potentially cancerous prostate lesion is determined by ultrasonography and confirmed by a biopsy.

- Indications

  o Many providers recommend an annual PSA and DRE on men over 50 to better ensure early detection of prostate cancer. African-American men and men who have a family history of prostate cancer should begin screening at an earlier age.

- o Client Presentation
    - As men age, their prostate glands enlarge. As the prostate gland enlarges, it puts pressure on the urethra and causes diminished flow and retention of urine. Blood may also be found in the urine. These symptoms could be indicative of BPH or prostate cancer.
- Interpretation of Findings
    - o PSA
        - An increase in PSA may indicate that a client has prostatic cancer.
            - □ The expected reference range for the PSA is from 2 to 4 ng/mL.
            - □ A PSA is considered elevated if its value is above 4 to 10 ng/mL.
    - o DRE
        - Abnormal findings during the DRE include an abnormally large and hard prostate with an irregular shape or lumps.

Transrectal Ultrasound (TRUS)

- With the client in a left, side-lying position, a probe is inserted into the client's rectum, and sound waves are bounced off the surface of the prostate gland.
    - o The sound waves provide an image of the gland.
- Indications
    - o A TRUS is done if a client's PSA and/or DRE reveal a possible abnormality.
- Interpretation of Findings
    - o If an irregularity is found, the image from the TRUS will be used to guide a needle biopsy.

(A) APPLICATION EXERCISES

1. An older adult client is having an annual physical exam at a provider's office. Which of the following client findings indicates additional follow-up is needed in regard to the prostate gland? (Select all that apply.)

   _____ Report of weak urine stream

   _____ Report of urinating once during the night

   _____ Smegma present below the glans of the penis

   _____ Prostatic specific antigen (PSA) is 4.2 ng/mL

   _____ Digital rectal exam (DRE) reveals an enlarged prostate that is hard with an irregular shape

2. A nurse is reinforcing teaching to a client who is to undergo a transrectal ultrasound (TRUS). Which of the following information should the nurse include in the teaching?

   A. "This procedure will determine if you have prostate cancer."

   B. "The provider will insert a finger into your anus during the procedure."

   C. "Sound waves will be used to create a picture of your prostate."

   D. "An anesthetic will be used prior to insertion of the biopsy needle."

Ⓐ APPLICATION EXERCISES ANSWER KEY

1. An older adult client is having an annual physical exam at a provider's office. Which of the following client findings indicates additional follow-up is needed in regard to the prostate gland? (Select all that apply.)

    X   **Report of weak urine stream**

    _____ Report of urinating once during the night

    _____ Smegma present below the glans of the penis

    X   **Prostatic specific antigen (PSA) is 4.2 ng/mL**

    X   **Digital rectal exam (DRE) reveals an enlarged prostate that is hard with an irregular shape**

    Follow up is indicated for the client because he reports a weak urine stream; his PSA is above 4.0 ng/mL; and his prostate is enlarged, hard, and has an irregular shape. Urinating once during the night is common in older adults due to redistribution of blood trapped in lower extremities during the day. Smegma is a common secretion that can accumulate beneath the glans of the penis if not removed during hygiene. An enlarged prostate that is smooth and firm is expected for an older adult because the prostate gland enlarges with age.

    Ⓝ NCLEX® Connection: Reduction of Risk Potential, Diagnostic Tests

2. A nurse is reinforcing teaching to a client who is to undergo a transrectal ultrasound (TRUS). Which of the following information should the nurse include in the teaching?

    A. "This procedure will determine if you have prostate cancer."

    B. "The provider will insert a finger into your anus during the procedure."

    C. "Sound waves will be used to create a picture of your prostate."

    D. "An anesthetic will be used prior to insertion of the biopsy needle."

    A TRUS is done using sound waves to create a picture of the prostate gland. It is done by introducing a transducer into the client's rectum and bouncing sound waves off the prostate to determine the presence of lumps or irregularities. This procedure cannot determine if a client has prostate cancer. Only a biopsy of the tissue can make this determination.

    Ⓝ NCLEX® Connection: Reduction of Risk Potential, Diagnostic Tests

Overview

- There are several disorders that are associated with the male reproductive system.

  o Testicular cancer

  o Benign prostatic hypertrophy

  o Prostate cancer

- Testicular cancer is the most common malignancy in men 15 to 35 years old.

- As an adult male ages, the prostate gland enlarges. When the enlargement of the gland begins to cause urinary dysfunction, it is called benign prostatic hypertrophy (BPH).

- Prostate cancer is a slow-growing cancer. Conservative treatment may be the treatment of choice for a client, based on age and life expectancy and if the cancer if growing and/or spreading.

TESTICULAR CANCER

Overview

- The cause of testicular cancer is unknown.

Health Promotion and Disease Prevention

- Reinforce to clients how to perform testicular self-examination (TSE). Tell clients to look and feel for any lumps or change in the size, shape, or consistency of the testes by gently rolling them between the thumbs and fingers.

- Recommend clients perform TSE, starting at puberty, monthly after a shower and in front of a mirror.

Data Collection

- Risk Factors

  o Undescended testis (cryptorchidism)

  o Genetic disposition

  o Metastases

  o Age 15 to 35 (but can occur at any age)

- Subjective Data

  - Lumps and/or swelling of testes

  - Feeling of heaviness in the testicles

  - Reports of back pain (evidence of metastasis)

- Objective Data

  - Enlarged testes without pain

  - Palpable lump

  - Swelling of lymph nodes in the groin

  - Abdominal mass, gynecomastia (evidence of metastasis)

  - Laboratory Tests

    - Bio-markers for testicular tumors – Alpha-fetoprotein and human chorionic gonadotropin (hCG)

      - Elevated values in testicular cancer

      - May use for diagnostic purposes as well as for treatment efficacy

  - Diagnostic Procedures

    - Ultrasonography

      - Determines if palpable mass is solid or fluid-filled

    - Computed tomography (CT) imaging scan, chest x-rays, and bone scans

      - Evaluates the extent of the cancer

      - Localized or metastasized to other organs in the body (brain, spinal cord and bones)

    - Lymphangiography

      - Evaluates spread to lymph nodes

Collaborative Care

- Surgical Interventions

  - Orchiectomy – Removal of the testis (unilateral orchiectomy) is the treatment of choice for testicular cancer.

    - This procedure is performed using an inguinal incision.

    - Gel-filled prostheses are implanted in the scrotum after removal of diseased testes.

    - If the lymph nodes are involved or the risk of spread is high, retroperitoneal lymph node dissection may also be performed.

    - Depending on the type of tumor and stage of cancer, chemotherapy or radiation may be prescribed postoperatively.

- Nursing Actions
  - Preoperative
    - Discuss with clients any concerns about sexual functioning.
      - ▷ Erectile and climactic functions are usually not affected.
      - ▷ Fertility may be affected. Arrange for sperm banking prior to surgery, if desired.
    - Discuss with clients what to expect in relation to incisions and pain.
    - Lymph node dissection will require larger and more extensive incision unless it is done laparoscopically.
  - Postoperative
    - Provide routine postoperative care to prevent complications.
    - Manage pain with analgesics and ice packs.
    - Observe the client's incisions for signs and symptoms of infection.
- Client Education
  - Instruct clients to report symptoms of infection.
  - Instruct clients to avoid heavy lifting and strenuous activity for the prescribed period of time.
  - Reinforce the importance of performing TSE, follow-up testing, and reporting any signs or symptoms that may indicate reoccurrence.
- Client Outcomes
  - The client will not have any recurrence of cancer.
  - The client will re-establish a positive body image.

BENIGN PROSTATIC HYPERTROPHY (BPH)

Overview

- BPH can significantly impair the outflow of urine from the bladder, making a client susceptible to infection and retention. Excessive amounts of retained urine can cause reflux of urine into the kidney, dilating the ureter and causing kidney infections.

Data Collection

- Risk Factors
  - Age
  - Family history
- Subjective Data
  - Urinary hesitancy, frequency and nocturia
  - Recurrent bladder infections

- ○ Feeling of incomplete emptying of bladder
- ○ Painless hematuria
- • Objective Data
  - ○ Small amounts of urine voided at one time with significant, residual weak stream, and posturination dribble
  - ○ Hematuria and/or bacteruria
  - ○ Elevated BUN and creatinine (indicates kidney damage)
  - ○ Diagnostic Procedures
    - ▪ A digital rectal exam (DRE) will reveal an enlarged, smooth prostate.
    - ▪ Use uroflowmetry to measure rate and degree of bladder emptying.

Collaborative Care

- • Nursing Care
  - ▪ Client Teaching
    - □ Tell clients that frequent ejaculation has been found to release prostatic fluids, therefore, decreasing the size of the prostate.
    - □ Tell clients to avoid drinking large amounts of fluids at one time and urinate when the urge is initially felt.
    - □ Tell clients to avoid bladder stimulants, such as alcohol and caffeine.
    - □ Tell clients to avoid medications that cause decreased bladder tone, such as anticholinergics, decongestants, and antihistamines.
    - □ BPH may initially be treated conservatively with medication.
- • Medications
  - ○ The goal of medication for BPH is to re-establish an uninhibited urine flow out of the bladder.
    - ▪ 5-alpha reductase inhibitors – Finasteride (Proscar), dutasteride (Avodart)
      - □ Used to inhibit the enzyme – 5-alpha reductase from converting testosterone to dihydrotestosterone (DHT) and thus decrease the production of testosterone in the prostate gland.
      - □ Decreasing a male client's DHT will often cause a decrease in the size of the prostate.
      - □ Client Education
        - ‣ Reinforce to clients that medication must be taken daily on a long-term basis.
        - ‣ Inform clients that impotence and a decrease in libido are possible side effects.

- ▸ Inform clients taking dutasteride that it can be absorbed through the skin. Clients taking dutasteride should not donate blood for 6 months after discontinuing the medication. Women who are pregnant or may become pregnant should use caution when handling the medication, and avoid exposure to semen of a partner taking these medications due to risk to male fetus.

- ■ Alpha-blocking agents – Tamsulosin (Flomax)

  - ☐ Alpha-adrenergic receptor antagonists cause relaxation of the bladder outlet and prostate gland.

  - ☐ These agents cause less pressure to be placed on the urethra, therefore, re-establishing a stronger urine flow.

  - ☐ Client Education

    - ▸ Warn clients that postural hypotension may occur and that changes in position must be made slowly.

    - ▸ Warn clients that concurrent use with cimetidine (Tagamet) can potentiate the hypotensive effect.

- ● Surgical Interventions

  - ○ Clients who do not receive adequate relief from conservative measures may need to have a transurethral resection of the prostate (TURP) performed.

    - ■ A TURP is performed using a resectoscope (similar to a cystoscope) that is inserted through the urethra and trims away excess prostatic tissue, enlarging the passageway of the urethra through the prostate gland.

    - ■ Nursing Actions

      - ☐ Preoperatively

        - ▸ Perform routine preoperative care.

      - ☐ Postoperatively

        - ▸ Provide routine postoperative care to prevent complications.

        - ▸ Manage continuous bladder irrigation through a large balloon (30 to 45 mL), indwelling urinary three-way catheter. The catheter tubing is taped tightly to the leg, creating traction so that the balloon will apply firm pressure to the prostatic fossa to prevent bleeding.

          - ▷ The catheter drains urine and allows for instillation of a continuous bladder irrigation (CBI) of 0.9% sodium chloride (isotonic) or another prescribed irrigating solution to keep the catheter free of obstruction.

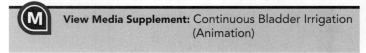

View Media Supplement: Continuous Bladder Irrigation (Animation)

- ▷ Adjust the rate of the CBI to keep the irrigation return pink or lighter. For example, if bright-red or ketchup-appearing (arterial) bleeding with clots is observed, increase the CBI rate.

▷ If the catheter becomes obstructed (bladder spasms, reduced irrigation outflow), turn off the CBI and irrigate with 50 mL of irrigation solution using a large piston syringe. Contact the provider if unable to dislodge the clot.

▷ Record the amount of irrigating solution instilled (generally very large volumes) and the amount of return. The difference equals urine output.

▷ Provide reassurance to clients who feel a continuous need to urinate. Instruct clients to not void around the catheter as this causes bladder spasms.

▷ Avoid kinks in the tubing.

▸ Monitor the client's vital signs and urinary output.

▸ Monitor clients for bleeding (persistent bright-red bleeding unresponsive to increase in CBI and traction on the catheter or reduced Hgb levels) and report it to the provider.

▸ If blood is present, monitor the incision and change the dressing as appropriate.

▸ Administer medications to clients as prescribed.

▷ Analgesics

▷ Antispasmodics (bladder spasms)

▷ Antibiotics (prophylaxis)

▷ Stool softeners (avoid straining)

▸ Discontinue CBI and catheter as prescribed. Monitor the client's urinary output. The initial voiding following removal may be uncomfortable, red in color and contain clots. The color of the urine should progress toward amber in 2 to 3 days. Instruct clients that expected output is 150 to 200 mL every 3 to 4 hr.

■ Client Education

□ Instruct clients to contact provider for difficulty or inability to void and/or persistent bleeding.

□ Tell clients to avoid heavy lifting, strenuous exercise, straining, and sexual intercourse for the prescribed length of time (usually 2 to 6 weeks).

□ Tell clients to consume 2 to 3 L/day of fluids from food and beverage sources.

□ Tell clients to avoid bladder stimulants, such as caffeine and alcohol.

□ Tell clients that if urine becomes bloody, stop activity, rest, and increase fluid intake.

● Client Outcomes

○ The client's urine will be pink without clots postoperatively.

○ The client's flow of urine will allow the bladder to empty completely.

Complications

- TURP Complications

    ○ Urethral trauma, urinary retention, bleeding, and infection are complications associated with TURP.

    ○ Nursing Actions

    ▪ Monitor clients and intervene for bleeding.

    ▪ Provide antibiotic prophylaxis to clients.

PROSTATE CANCER

Overview

- The incidence of prostate cancer increases with age.

- Symptoms are often similar to those of BPH.

Health Promotion and Disease Prevention

- Instruct clients to have a prostate-specific antigen (PSA) and DRE done annually after age 50. African-American men and men who have a close relative who had prostate cancer may begin screenings earlier.

Data Collection

- Risk Factors

    ○ Age greater than 65 years

    ○ Family history

    ○ African-American heritage

    ○ High-fat diet

    ○ BRCA2 mutation may be associated with an increased risk

- Subjective Data

    ○ Urinary hesitancy and weak stream

    ○ Recurrent bladder infections

    ○ Urinary retention

    ○ Blood in urine and semen

    ○ Painful ejaculation

- Objective Data

    ○ Small amounts of urine voided at one time with significant residual

    ○ Hematuria and/or bacteruria

- ○ Elevated BUN and creatinine (indicates kidney damage)
- ○ Laboratory Tests
  - PSA serum levels are elevated with prostate cancer (abnormal levels are greater than 4 ng/mL).
- ○ Diagnostic Procedures
  - DRE – Reveals a hard prostate with palpable irregularities
  - A transrectal ultrasound (TRUS) may be performed to definitively diagnose or rule out prostate cancer in the presence of an enlarged prostate. Can indicate the location of the lesion or lesions.
  - Needle or aspiration biopsy of the lesion – Definitively diagnose or rule out prostate cancer
  - Magnetic resonance imaging (MRI), computed tomography (CT) scans, and bone scans – Assess for metastases

Collaborative Care

- Medications
  - ○ Hormone therapy
    - Leuprolide acetate (Lupron), Triptorelin (Trelstar Depot) – Gonadotropin-releasing hormone (GnRH)
      - □ Used in advanced prostate cancer to produce a chemical castration
      - □ Nursing Actions
        - ▸ Monitor clients for osteoporosis, which can occur due to testosterone suppression.
        - ▸ Administer by subcutaneous or IM injection.
      - □ Client Education
        - ▸ Warn clients that hot flashes are an adverse effect.
        - ▸ Tell clients that impotence and decreased libido may also be side effects.
    - Flutamide (Eulexin), bicalutamide (Casodex) – Androgen receptor blocker
      - □ Used in conjunction with a GnRH
      - □ Client Education
        - ▸ Inform clients that gynecomastia is a side effect.
        - ▸ Instruct clients to adhere to follow up for periodic liver function tests.
  - ○ Chemotherapy – Used for clients whose cancer has spread or who have had little improvement with other therapies
    - Docetaxel (Taxotere) – Usually used to treat breast cancer

□ Client Education

▸ Instruct clients to adhere to follow-up for periodic routine blood tests for neutropenia, leukopenia, thrombocytopenia, and anemia.

- Therapeutic Procedures

  ○ Radiation therapy – External beam radiation therapy or implanted radioactive seeds (brachytherapy)

- Surgical Interventions

  ○ Radical prostatectomy

    ■ Involves the removal of the entire prostate gland, along with the seminal vesicles, the cuff at the bladder neck, and the regional lymph nodes

    ■ Procedure of choice for treatment of prostate cancer

    ■ May be done using a suprapubic, perineal, or retropubic approach.

    ■ A laparoscopic approach may be an option for treatment of localized prostate cancer.

    ■ Nursing Actions

      □ Preoperatively

        ▸ Ensure that clients fully understand the procedure and what to expect postoperatively.

      □ Postoperatively

        ▸ Provide routine postoperative care to prevent complications.

        ▸ Provide catheter care and administer bladder antispasmodics to clients as prescribed.

        ▸ If clients have a suprapubic prostatectomy, a suprapubic catheter, in addition to the urethral catheter, will be placed. Usually, it will be removed when residual urine measurements are less than 75 mL.

    ■ Client Education

      □ Instruct clients to report signs and symptoms of infection.

      □ Reinforce to clients catheter care if they will be going home with one in place.

      □ Tell clients to avoid heavy lifting and strenuous activity for the prescribed period of time.

      □ Instruct clients to avoid tub baths for at least 2 to 3 weeks.

- Client Outcomes

  ○ The client's incisions will heal without infection.

  ○ The client will redefine sexuality.

Complications

- A radical prostatectomy puts clients at risk for the following complications:
  - Irreversible erectile dysfunction
    - This is due to pudendal nerve damage during the operation. In certain circumstances, the surgeon may be able to perform a nerve-sparing prostatectomy.
    - Client Education
      - Recommend to clients that they attend a community support group.
  - Refractory postoperative urinary incontinence
    - This requires implantation of an artificial urinary sphincter (AUS). An AUS is a device that prevents incontinence and allows clients some control over bladder elimination pattern.
    - Reinforce to clients to perform perineal exercises to reduce urinary incontinence.

(A) APPLICATION EXERCISES

1. When instructing a client in testicular self-examination (TSE), a nurse should reinforce which of the following instructions? (Select all that apply.)

   _____ Perform every 6 months.

   _____ Examine testicles while lying down.

   _____ Examine testicles following a shower.

   _____ Roll testes between thumb and fingers.

   _____ Report changes in the size, shape, or consistency of the testes.

2. Label each of the following findings as a characteristic of prostate (P) or testicular cancer (T).

   _____ Testicular lump

   _____ Urinary hesitancy

   _____ Urinary retention

   _____ Painless hematuria

   _____ Recurrent bladder infections

   _____ Elevated alpha fetoprotein (AFP)

   _____ Elevated prostate-specific antigen (PSA)

3. A nurse is caring for a client who has undergone a transurethral resection of the prostate (TURP) and is receiving continuous bladder irrigation (CBI). The nurse observes that the urine is bright red and contains many clots. Which of the following actions should the nurse take at this time? (Select all that apply.)

   _____ Encourage oral fluid intake.

   _____ Change monitoring of vital signs to every hour.

   _____ Contact the provider if the problem persists.

   _____ Continue monitoring the color of the urine.

   _____ Check the drainage tube for occlusions.

   _____ Decrease CBI flow rate.

4. A nurse is caring for a client who is preparing to undergo a radical prostatectomy. Which of the following complications should the client be informed of prior to the surgery?

   A. Impotence

   B. Constipation

   C. Urethral strictures

   D. Bowel incontinence

APPLICATION EXERCISES ANSWER KEY

1. When instructing a client in testicular self-examination (TSE), a nurse should reinforce which of the following instructions? (Select all that apply.)

   _____ Perform every 6 months.

   _____ Examine testicles while lying down.

   __X__ **Examine testicles following a shower.**

   __X__ **Roll testes between thumb and fingers.**

   __X__ **Report changes in the size, shape, or consistency of the testes.**

   TSE should be performed monthly following a shower by rolling the testes between the thumb and fingers while standing. Any lumps, changes in the size, shape, or consistency of the testes should be reported to the provider.

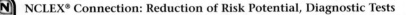

 NCLEX® Connection: Reduction of Risk Potential, Diagnostic Tests

2. Label each of the following findings as a characteristic of prostate (P) or testicular cancer (T).

   __T__ Testicular lump

   __P__ Urinary hesitancy

   __P__ Urinary retention

   __P__ Painless hematuria

   __P__ Recurrent bladder infections

   __T__ Elevated alpha fetoprotein (AFP)

   __P__ Elevated prostate-specific antigen (PSA)

   Urinary hesitancy, urinary retention, painless hematuria, recurrent bladder infections, and elevated PSA are findings of prostate cancer. Testicular lumps and an elevated AFP are findings of testicular cancer.

 NCLEX® Connection: Physiological Adaptations, Basic Pathophysiology

3. A nurse is caring for a client who has undergone a transurethral resection of the prostate (TURP) and is receiving continuous bladder irrigation (CBI). The nurse observes that the urine is bright red and contains many clots. Which of the following actions should the nurse take at this time? (Select all that apply.)

   __X__ Encourage oral fluid intake.

   __X__ Change monitoring of vital signs to every hour.

   __X__ Contact the provider if the problem persists.

   __X__ Continue monitoring the color of the urine.

   __X__ Check the drainage tube for occlusions.

   _____ Decrease CBI flow rate.

   Encouraging oral fluid intake, checking vital signs more frequently, contacting the provider if the problem persists, continuing to monitor color of urine, checking the drainage tube for occlusions, and increasing, rather than decreasing, CBI flow rate are appropriate interventions at this time.

   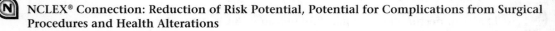 NCLEX® Connection: Reduction of Risk Potential, Potential for Complications from Surgical Procedures and Health Alterations

4. A nurse is caring for a client who is preparing to undergo a radical prostatectomy. Which of the following complications should the client be informed of prior to the surgery?

   A. Impotence

   B. Constipation

   C. Urethral strictures

   D. Bowel incontinence

   Due to the possibility of damaging the pudendal nerve during the operation, impotence is a potential complication. Constipation, urethral strictures, and bowel incontinence are not complications related to a radical prostatectomy.

   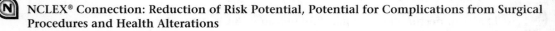 NCLEX® Connection: Reduction of Risk Potential, Potential for Complications from Surgical Procedures and Health Alterations

UNIT 10: NURSING CARE OF CLIENTS WITH MUSCULOSKELETAL DISORDERS

- Diagnostic and Therapeutic Procedures
- Musculoskeletal Disorders

NCLEX® CONNECTIONS

When reviewing the chapters in this section, keep in mind the relevant sections of the NCLEX® outline, in particular:

CLIENT NEEDS: BASIC CARE AND COMFORT

Relevant topics/tasks include:
- Assistive Devices
  - Reinforce teaching for client using assistive device.
- Mobility/Immobility
  - Check client for mobility, gait, strength, motor skills.
- Non-Pharmacological Comfort Interventions
  - Apply therapies for comfort and treatment of inflammation/swelling.

CLIENT NEEDS: REDUCTION OF RISK POTENTIAL

Relevant topics/tasks include:
- Diagnostic Tests
  - Reinforce client teaching about diagnostic test.
- Potential for Alterations in Body Systems
  - Administer and check proper use of compression stockings/sequential compression devices (SCD).
- Potential for Complications from Surgical Procedures and Health Alterations
  - Reinforce teaching to prevent complications due to surgery or health alterations.

CLIENT NEEDS: PHYSIOLOGICAL ADAPTATION

Relevant topics/tasks include:
- Alterations in Body Systems
  - Provide care for client drainage device.
- Medical Emergencies
  - Notify primary health care provider about client unexpected response/emergency situation.
- Unexpected Response to Therapies
  - Promote recovery from client unexpected negative response to therapy.

Chapter 65   Musculoskeletal Diagnostic Procedures

Overview

- Imaging studies are the primary diagnostic procedures used for musculoskeletal disorders.

- Evaluation of the conduction of electrical impulses in muscles may also be assessed in the presence of muscle weakness.

- Endoscopic studies (arthroscopy) are done to assess the condition of a joint and may simultaneously repair tears and other joint defects that are identified.

- Musculoskeletal diagnostic procedures that nurses should be knowledgeable about:

  o   Arthroscopy

  o   Bone scans

  o   Dual-energy x-ray absorptiometry (DEXA) scans

  o   Electromyography and nerve conduction studies

Arthroscopy

- Arthroscopy is an endoscopic procedure done to visualize the internal structures of a joint, usually of the knee and shoulder.

- Small incisions are made near the joints through which the scope is passed.

- Number and placement of incisions depend on the area of the joint to be visualized and the extent of the needed repair.

- Arthroscopy cannot be done if infection is present in the joint.

- Indications

  o   Potential Diagnoses

    ▪   Clients who have sustained injuries to the joints, ligaments or meniscus may undergo arthroscopy to ascertain the extent of damage, during which time repair may also be done using the endoscope.

- ○ Client Presentation
    - Joint swelling, pain, and crepitus
    - Joint instability
- Interpretation of Findings
    - ○ Knee joint and articular surfaces are visualized for injury or damage.
    - ○ Surgery may be done at the time of the arthroscopy if damage is visualized.
- Preprocedure
    - ○ Nursing Actions
        - Instruct clients in postprocedure exercises (straight leg raising, quadriceps setting isometrics) or request a referral to a physical therapist.
        - Verify that clients have signed the informed consent form.
    - ○ Client Education
        - Postoperative joint exercises
- Postprocedure
    - ○ Nursing Actions
        - Teach clients postprocedure care as arthroscopy is done on an outpatient basis.
        - Check the neurovascular status of the client's limb prior to discharge.
    - ○ Client Education
        - Instruct clients to:
            - □ Apply ice for 15-20 min and then allow area to warm for at least 45 min to 1 hr, or before applying ice again. Continue this routine for 24 hr.
            - □ Elevate the client's extremity for 24 hr.
            - □ Take a prescribed analgesic for pain.
            - □ Maintain a splint or sling if prescribed.
            - □ Use crutches if limited weight bearing is prescribed.
- Complications
    - ○ Infection
        - Complications are uncommon after this procedure, but infection may occur as with any procedure that disrupts the integrity of the skin.
        - Client Education
            - □ Instruct clients to notify the provider immediately of any signs of infection, such as swelling, redness, or fever.

Bone Scan

- Bone scans are done when a client's entire skeletal system is to be evaluated.

- It is done using a radionuclide such as gallium or thallium.

- Radionuclide is injected 4 to 6 hr before scanning.

- The scan takes 30 to 60 min during which time clients must lay still.

- Indications

  o Potential Diagnoses

    ▪ Osteoporosis

    ▪ Primary or metastatic bone cancer

    ▪ Bone pain of unknown origin

  o Client Presentation

    ▪ Bone pain

- Interpretation of Findings

  o Provides size and location of tumors in the bones which are often metastases from a primary cancer.

- Preprocedure

  o Nursing Actions

    ▪ Inform clients about how the procedure will be done.

  o Client Education

    ▪ Tell clients to lie still during the length of the procedure.

- Postprocedure

  o Client Education

    ▪ Encourage clients to drink fluids to increase excretion of radionuclide. Inform clients that radioactive precautions are not necessary.

Dual-Energy X-ray Absorptiometry (DEXA) Scans

- DEXA scans are done to estimate the density of a client's bone mass and presence/extent of osteoporosis.

- These scans are usually done on the wrist, hip, or spine.

- Contrast material is not used.

- A DEXA scan uses two beams of radiation and findings are analyzed by a computer and interpreted by a radiologist. Clients receive a score (T-score) that relates their amount of bone density to other people in their age group and gender.

- Clients will lie on an x-ray table while a scan of a selected area is done.

- Indications

  o Potential Diagnoses

    ■ Osteoporosis

    ■ Postmenopausal state (baseline may be done at age 40)

  o Client Presentation

    ■ Loss of height

    ■ Bone pain

    ■ Fractures

- Interpretation of Findings

  o Lower than expected density of bone for age of client is diagnostic for osteoporosis.

- Preprocedure

  o Nursing Actions

    ■ Inform clients about how the procedure will be done.

  o Client Education

    ■ Instruct clients to avoid taking a calcium supplement 24 hr prior to the procedure.

- Postprocedure

  o Client Education

    ■ Remind clients to follow up with the provider regarding supplements and medications that may be needed if bone loss is present.

Electromyography and Nerve Conduction Studies

- Electromyography (EMG) and nerve conduction studies are done to determine the presence and cause of muscle weakness.

- EMG

  o Thin needles are placed in the muscle under study and attached to an electrode.

  o An electrode is attached to an oscilloscope and electrical activity is recorded during a muscle contraction.

- Nerve conduction study

  o Flat electrodes are taped on the skin.

  o Low, electrical currents are sent through the electrodes and muscle response to the stimulus is recorded.

- Indications

  - Potential Diagnoses

    - Lower motor neuron disease (amyotrophic lateral sclerosis, myasthenia gravis)

    - Peripheral nerve disorders (carpal tunnel, Guillain Barré)

- Interpretation of findings

  - Low or absent electrical potentials elicited by the muscle in response to an electrical stimulus indicate lower motor neuron and peripheral nerve disorders.

- Preprocedure

  - Nursing Actions

    - Inform clients about what to expect.

    - Inform clients to avoid caffeine products before the exam, due to stimulatory effect on the CNS.

    - Ask if clients are taking an anticoagulant or muscle relaxants (contraindicated for this procedure).

  - Client Education

    - Inform clients that discomfort may be felt during needle insertion and when electrical current is sent through electrodes.

    - Tell clients they may be asked to flex muscles while the needle is inserted.

- Postprocedure

  - Client Education

    - Inform clients that some bruising may occur at needle insertion sites.

    - Have clients report swelling or tenderness at any of the sites to provider.

    - Instruct clients to apply ice to the insertion sites to reduce swelling and pain.

(A) APPLICATION EXERCISES

1. A 55 year-old woman is scheduled for a dual-energy x-ray absorptiometry (DEXA) scan. A nurse recognizes this has been prescribed in relation to which of the following client factors?

    A. Age is 55
    B. Rheumatoid arthritis
    C. Mother had osteoarthritis
    D. Body mass index (BMI) is 30

2. Which of the following statements should a nurse reinforce for a client who is preparing to undergo a bone scan?

    A. "The entire procedure will take about 1 hr."
    B. "A radioactive substance will be injected into a vein."
    C. "You will be placed in a tube-like structure during the exam."
    D. "You will need to take precautions with your urine for 24 hr."

3. A nurse is preparing a client for an arthroscopy during which time a repair of the meniscus is planned. Which of the following should the nurse reinforce from the preoperative teaching? (Select all that apply.)

    _____ Apply ice for 15 to 20 min alternating with 1 hr rest for the first 24 hr.
    _____ Keep the joint in a dependent position.
    _____ Perform isometric exercises on the affected extremity.
    _____ Expect the affected extremity to be placed in a cast after the procedure.
    _____ Monitor the incisions for infection.

(A) **APPLICATION EXERCISES ANSWER KEY**

1. A 55 year-old woman is scheduled for a dual-energy x-ray absorptiometry (DEXA) scan. A nurse recognizes this has been prescribed in relation to which of the following client factors?

    A. Age is 55

    B. Rheumatoid arthritis

    C. Mother had osteoarthritis

    D. Body mass index (BMI) is 30

    At age 55, the client is probably postmenopausal. Postmenopausal women often have their bone mass monitored to identify osteoporosis prior to significant loss of bone mass. There is no relationship between rheumatoid arthritis or osteoarthritis and osteoporosis. A BMI of 30 has no relationship to bone mass.

(N) **NCLEX® Connection: Reduction of Risk Potential, Diagnostic Tests**

2. Which of the following statements should a nurse reinforce for a client who is preparing to undergo a bone scan?

    A. "The entire procedure will take about 1 hr."

    B. "A radioactive substance will be injected into a vein."

    C. "You will be placed in a tube-like structure during the exam."

    D. "You will need to take precautions with your urine for 24 hr."

    A radioactive substance is injected into a vein and takes 4 to 6 hr to be absorbed by the bone before the scan can begin. The scan itself takes approximately 30 to 60 min. The client will be instructed to lie still on the table. The client does not need to take precautions with the urine after the procedure.

(N) **NCLEX® Connection: Reduction of Risk Potential, Diagnostic Tests**

3. A nurse is preparing a client for an arthroscopy during which time a repair of the meniscus is planned. Which of the following should the nurse reinforce from the preoperative teaching? (Select all that apply.)

   X   **Apply ice for 15 to 20 min alternating with 1 hr rest for the first 24 hr.**

          Keep the joint in a dependent position.

   X   **Perform isometric exercises on the affected extremity.**

          Expect the affected extremity to be placed in a cast after the procedure.

   X   **Monitor the incisions for infection.**

During the arthroscopy, small incisions will be made through which the arthroscope will be inserted. Apply ice for 15-20 min and then allow the area to warm for at least 45 min to an hr or before applying ice again. Continue this routine for 24 hr. Begin isometric exercises of the muscles in the affected extremity as soon as possible. Monitor the incisions for infection. Keep the extremity elevated, not placed in a dependent position, to reduce swelling. Splints, not casts, are placed postprocedure.

NCLEX® Connection: Reduction of Risk Potential, Potential for Complications of Diagnostic Tests/Treatments/Procedures

UNIT 10	NURSING CARE OF CLIENTS WITH MUSCULOSKELETAL DISORDERS
Section:	Diagnostic and Therapeutic Procedures
Chapter 66	**Musculoskeletal Surgical Procedures**

 Overview

- Most musculoskeletal surgical procedures are performed to repair damaged joints, in particular the knees and the hips.

- Arthroplasty refers to the surgical removal of a diseased joint and replacement with prosthetics or artificial components made of metal and/or plastic.

- Total joint arthroplasty, which can also be called total joint replacement, involves replacement of all components of an articulating joint.

- Musculoskeletal surgical procedures that nurses should be knowledgeable about:

  ○ Knee arthroplasty

  ○ Hip arthroplasty

Knee and Hip Arthroplasty

- Total knee arthroplasty involves the replacement of the distal femoral component, the tibial plate, and the patellar button. Total knee arthroplasty is a surgical option when conservative measures fail.

 View Media Supplement: Artificial Knee Joint (Image)

- Unicondylar knee replacements are done when the client's joint may be diseased in one compartment of the joint.

- Total hip arthroplasty involves the replacement of the acetabular cup, the femoral head, and the femoral stem.

View Media Supplement: Artificial Hip Joint (Image)

- Hemiarthroplasty refers to half of a joint replacement. Fractures of the femoral neck can be treated with the replacement of the femoral component only.

- Indications

  - Diagnoses

    - Knee and hip arthroplasty is used to treat degenerative disease (osteoarthritis, rheumatoid arthritis).

      - Clients who generally require total-joint arthroplasty are older than 65 years.

  - Client Presentation

    - Pain when bearing weight on the joint (walking, running)

    - Joint crepitus and stiffness

    - Joint swelling (primarily occurs in the knees)

- Client Outcomes

  - The client will be free from pain.

  - The client will regain joint mobility.

- Preprocedure

  - Nursing Actions

    - Review diagnostic test results.

      - CBC, urinalysis, electrolytes, BUN, creatinine – Epoetin alfa may be prescribed preoperatively to increase Hgb.

      - Chest x-ray

      - ECG

      - Administer prophylactic broad-spectrum antibiotic if prescribed.

  - Client Education

    - Inform clients regarding autologous blood donation (client donates blood prior to procedure to be used postoperatively).

    - Inform clients regarding postoperative care (incentive spirometry, transfusion, surgical drains, dressing, pain control, transfer, postoperative exercises, activity limits).

- Intraprocedure

  - General or spinal anesthesia may be used.

  - Joint components are removed and replaced with artificial components.

  - Components may or may not be cemented in place. Components that do not use cement allow the bone to grow into the prosthesis to stabilize it. Weight bearing is delayed several weeks until femoral shaft has grown into prosthesis.

  - Artificial joints have a limited life span ranging from 10 to 20 years.

- Postprocedure
  - Nursing Actions
    - Frequently monitor older adult clients who are at a higher risk for medical complications related to chronic conditions, including hypertension, diabetes mellitus, coronary artery disease, and obstructive pulmonary disease.
    - Knee arthroplasty
      - □ Provide postoperative care to prevent postoperative complications.
      - □ Maintain continuous passive motion machine, which is used to promote motion in the knee and prevent scar tissue formation. It is usually placed and initiated immediately after surgery. It provides passive range of motion from full extension to the prescribed amount of flexion. May be turned off during meals.
      - □ Positions of flexion of the knee are limited to avoid flexion contractures. Avoid knee gatch and pillows placed behind the knee.
      - □ Provide medications as prescribed.
        - ‣ Analgesics – Opioids (epidural, PCA, IV, oral), NSAIDs
        - ‣ Antibiotics
        - ‣ Anticoagulant – Aspirin; low-molecular weight heparin, such as enoxaparin (Lovenox); warfarin (Coumadin)
      - □ Apply ice or cold therapy to reduce postoperative swelling.
      - □ Monitor the client's neurovascular status of surgical extremity every 2 to 4 hr for circulation, movement, and sensation (CMS).
      - □ Observe clients frequently for overt bleeding and signs of hypovolemia, such as hypotension and tachycardia.
    - Hip arthroplasty
      - □ Provide postoperative care to prevent postoperative complications.
      - □ Monitor clients for bleeding.
        - ‣ Check the dressing site frequently, noting any evidence of bleeding. Monitor and record drainage from surgical drains.
        - ‣ Monitor daily laboratory values, including Hgb and Hct levels. The client's Hgb and Hct may continue to drop 24 to 48 hr after surgery. Autologous blood from presurgery donation or blood salvaged intraoperatively or postoperatively using special collection devices may be used for postoperative blood replacement. Blood transfusions are relatively common for Hgb levels less than 9 g/dL.
      - □ Perform CMS checks every 2 to 4 hr.

- Provide medications as prescribed.
  - ▸ Analgesics – Opioids (epidural, PCA, IV, oral), NSAIDs
  - ▸ Antibiotics
  - ▸ Anticoagulant – Aspirin; low-molecular weight heparin, such as enoxaparin (Lovenox); warfarin (Coumadin)
- Early Ambulation
  - ▸ Transfer clients out of bed from the unaffected side into a reclining wheelchair.
  - ▸ The client's weight-bearing status is determined by the orthopedic surgeon and by choice of cemented (usually partial/full weight-bearing as tolerated) versus noncemented prostheses (usually only partial weight-bearing until after a few weeks of bone growth).
  - ▸ Use assistive devices (walker) and adaptive devices (raised toilet seat) when caring for client.
- Client position – Place clients supine with the head slightly elevated and the affected leg in neutral position. A pillow or abduction device may be placed between legs when turning client to the unaffected side or if client is nonadherent with restrictions. Clients should not be turned to the operative side, which could cause hip dislocation.
- Use total hip precautions to prevent dislocation of new joint.

DO	DON'T
Use elevated seating/raised toilet set.	Avoid flexion of hip greater than 90°.
Use straight chairs with arms.	Avoid low chairs.
Use an abduction pillow between the client's legs while in bed (and with turning).	Do not cross the client's legs.
Externally rotate the client's toes.	Do not internally rotate the client's toes.

- ○ Client Education
  - ■ Knee and hip arthroplasty
    - Inform clients of the need for extensive physical therapy to regain mobility. Clients may be discharged to home or an extended care facility for rehabilitation. If discharged to home, outpatient or in-home therapy must be provided. Home care should be available for 4 to 6 weeks.
    - Instruct clients to monitor signs and symptoms of incisional infection (fever, increased redness, swelling, purulent drainage) and care for the incision (clean daily with soap and water).
    - Instruct clients to monitor for signs and symptoms of deep vein thrombosis (swelling, redness, pain in calf), pulmonary embolism (shortness of breath, chest pain), and bleeding if clients are taking an anticoagulant.

- Knee arthroplasty – Inform clients that dislocation is not common following total knee arthroplasty but that kneeling and deep-knee bends are limited indefinitely.

- Hip arthroplasty – Instruct clients to follow position restrictions to avoid dislocation (See table above). Arrange for and instruct clients about the use of raised toilet seats, and care items (long-handled shoehorn, dressing sticks).

- Complications

  - Deep vein thrombosis

    - Deep vein thrombosis is a complication and can result in a pulmonary embolism.

    - Nursing Actions

      - Monitor clients for symptoms of pulmonary embolism, including acute onset of dyspnea, tachycardia, and pleuritic chest pain.

      - Deep vein thrombosis prophylaxis includes pharmacological management, the use of anti-embolic stockings and sequential compression devices, ankle exercises while in bed, and early mobilization with physical and occupational therapy.

    - Hip dislocation and subluxation

      - Since the muscle surrounding the hip joint has been cut to expose and replace the diseased joint, clients are at risk for hip dislocation.

    - Nursing Actions

      - Monitor clients for symptoms, including acute onset of pain, the client's report of hearing "a pop," internal rotation of the affected extremity, and shortened affected extremity.

      - An abductor pillow or splint is used to prevent adduction, which can cause dislocation of the surgical hip.

- o Chronic disease processes

  - ▪ Peripheral vascular disease resulting in ischemia/gangrene

  - ▪ Diabetes mellitus resulting in peripheral neuropathy and peripheral vascular disease

  - ▪ Infection (osteomyelitis)

- o Older adult clients have a higher risk of peripheral vascular disease and diabetes mellitus, resulting in decreased tissue perfusion and peripheral neuropathy. Both conditions place older adult clients at risk for lower extremity amputation.

- • Subjective Data

  - o Clients may or may not report pain.

  - o History of injury or disease process precipitating amputation

- • Objective Data

  - o Impaired neurovascular status as evidenced by absent or weak pulses, cool extremities, pallor, cyanosis, decreased sensation and movement.

 View Media Supplement: Doppler Assessment of Pulses (Video)

  - o Presence of infection and wounds

- • Diagnostic Procedures

  - o Several studies are done to determine blood flow at various levels of an extremity.

    - ▪ Angiography – Allows visualization of peripheral vasculature and areas of impaired circulation

    - ▪ Doppler laser and ultrasonography studies – Measures speed of blood flow in an extremity

    - ▪ Transcutaneous oxygen pressure ($TcPO_2$) – Measures oxygen pressures in an extremity

    - ▪ Ankle-brachial index – Measures difference between ankle and brachial systolic pressures

    - ▪ Level of amputation will be determined by level at which adequate blood flow is available for healing.

 View Media Supplement: AK and BK Amputation (Images)

Collaborative Care

- Surgical Interventions – Surgical amputation techniques

  - Closed amputation

    - This is the most common technique used. Skin flap is sutured over end of residual limb, closing site.

  - Open amputation

    - This technique is used when an active infection is present. Skin flap is not sutured over end of residual limb allowing for drainage of infection. Skin flap is closed at a later date.

- Nursing Actions

  - Provide routine postoperative care to prevent complications.

  - Check surgical site for bleeding, infection and/or non-healing of incision. Monitor tissue perfusion at end of residual limb.

    - Palpate residual limb for warmth. Heat may indicate infection.

    - Compare pulse most proximal to incision with pulse in other extremity.

  - Monitor and treat pain.

    - Differentiate between phantom limb and incisional and residual limb pain.

    - Treat incisional and residual limb pain with opioid analgesics.

    - Treat phantom limb pain

      □ Administer beta blockers such as propranolol (Inderal) for constant, dull, burning pain.

      □ Administer antiepileptics such as gabapentin (Neurontin) for sharp, knife-like pain.

      □ Monitor clients receiving calcitonin (Miacalcin) IV.

      □ Administer antispasmodics such as baclofen (Lioresal) to treat muscle spasms.

    - Encourage use of complementary and alternative therapies as appropriate, such as massage and distraction.

  - Position the affected extremity in dependent position to promote blood flow/oxygenation.

  - Provide firm mattress.

  - Facilitate mobility by providing overhead frame with trapeze.

  - Administer antibiotics and change dressings as prescribed if open amputation was performed.

- ○ Record characteristics of drainage, such as color, odor, consistency, and amount (COCA).

  - ▪ Facilitate supportive environment for both clients and their families so grief can be processed.

    - ☐ Monitor for anger, withdrawal, and sadness.

    - ☐ Allow time for grieving for the loss of the body part and change in body image.

    - ☐ Assist with residual limb preparation and prosthesis fitting.

  - ▪ Residual limb must be shaped and shrunk in preparation for prosthetic training.

  - ▪ Shrinkage interventions include:

    - ☐ Wrapping the stump using elastic bandages (figure-eight wrap) to prevent restriction of blood flow.

    - ☐ Using a stump shrinker sock (easier for clients to apply).

    - ☐ Using an air splint (plastic inflatable device) inflated to 20 to 22 mm Hg for 22 of 24 hr/day.

 View Media Supplement: Amputation Stump Wrapping (Video)

- ○ Client Education

  - ▪ Explain to clients how to care for and wrap the residual limb and perform limb-strengthening exercises.

  - ▪ Demonstrate proper application and care of the prosthesis to clients.

  - ▪ Explain to clients how to safely transfer and use mobility devices and adaptive aids.

  - ▪ Explain to clients how to manage phantom limb pain.

- • Interdisciplinary Care

  - ○ Request a referral for a certified prosthetic orthotist who will fit client with prosthesis after wound is healed and stump has shrunk.

  - ○ Request a referral for physical therapy that may be able to provide pain management with ultrasound, massage, exercises, TENS, and assistance with care of prosthesis and mobility aids.

  - ○ Request a referral for counseling if indicated to assist clients with adjustment to loss of extremity.

- Care After Discharge

  o Client Education

    ▪ Recommend that clients who have diabetes monitor blood glucose levels and maintain levels within the expected reference range.

    ▪ Encourage smoking cessation.

    ▪ Instruct clients to practice good foot care and seek early medical attention for nonhealing wounds.

- Client Outcomes

  o Client will adapt physically and emotionally to prosthesis.

  o Client will integrate residual limb and prosthesis into body image.

Complications

- Phantom Limb Pain

  o Phantom limb pain is the sensation of pain in the location of the extremity following the amputation. Clients may experience phantom limb pain because the nerve endings at the site of the amputation continue to send pain signals to the brain. It also tends to lessen with time, but some clients experience phantom limb pain or sensation indefinitely. It may be described as deep and burning, cramping, shooting, or aching.

  o Nursing Actions

    ▪ Acknowledge the client's pain.

    ▪ Administer appropriate medications.

- Flexion Contractures

  o Flexion contractures can occur in the hip or knee joint following amputation due to improper positioning.

  o Nursing Actions

    ▪ Provide firm mattress.

    ▪ Avoid elevating the stump on a pillow after the first 24 hr.

    ▪ Assist clients to lie prone several times a day for 20 to 30 min at a time to prevent hip flexion contractions.

    ▪ Encourage range-of-motion exercises.

    ▪ Discourage prolonged sitting.

  o Client Education

    ▪ Instruct clients to perform range-of-motion exercises to prevent contractures.

    ▪ Remind clients to stand using good posture with residual limb in extension. This will also aid in balance.

Ⓐ APPLICATION EXERCISES

Scenario: A nurse is caring for a young adult client who is 32 hr postoperative above-the-knee amputation of his left leg as treatment for osteogenic sarcoma. The gauze and elastic dressings are dry and intact. His vital signs are stable and he is controlling his pain by self-administration of morphine through a patient-controlled analgesic pump.

1. Which of the following postoperative measures should the nurse provide to the client to avoid hip flexion contractures?

    A. Elevate the residual limb on a pillow.

    B. Encourage the use of the over-bed trapeze.

    C. Have the client lie in a prone position.

    D. Wrap the stump using a figure-eight pattern.

2. The client reports that he is experiencing pain in the foot that is no longer there. Which of the following statements by the nurse reinforces teaching about this phenomenon?

    A. "This pain is referred pain from the bone that was cut."

    B. "This pain is incisional pain coming from the amputated limb."

    C. "This pain is imaginary pain because the limb is no longer there."

    D. "This pain is phantom limb pain, because pain signals are still being sent to your brain."

3. The client tells the nurse that he is feeling sharp, knife-like pain. Which of the following medications should the nurse administer?

    A. Propranolol (Inderal)

    B. Gabapentin (Neurontin)

    C. Baclofen (Lioresal)

    D. Morphine (MS Contin)

(A) **APPLICATION EXERCISES ANSWER KEY**

Scenario: A nurse is caring for a young adult client who is 32 hr postoperative above-the-knee amputation of his left leg as treatment for osteogenic sarcoma. The gauze and elastic dressings are dry and intact. His vital signs are stable and he is controlling his pain by self-administration of morphine through a patient-controlled analgesic pump.

1. Which of the following postoperative measures should the nurse provide to the client to avoid hip flexion contractures?

    A. Elevate the residual limb on a pillow.

    B. Encourage the use of the over-bed trapeze.

    C. Have the client lie in a prone position.

    D. Wrap the stump using a figure-eight pattern.

    The client should be placed in the prone position several times a day to prevent hip flexion contractions. Elevating the residual limb on a pillow can increase the risk for hip flexion contractures. Use of the over-bed trapeze by the client will promote independence and mobility, but it will not prevent contractures. Wrapping the stump will decrease swelling, but this will not prevent contractures.

     NCLEX® Connection: Potential for Complications from Surgical Procedures and Health Alterations

2. The client reports that he is experiencing pain in the foot that is no longer there. Which of the following statements by the nurse reinforces teaching about this phenomenon?

    A. "This pain is referred pain from the bone that was cut."

    B. "This pain is incisional pain coming from the amputated limb."

    C. "This pain is imaginary pain because the limb is no longer there."

    D. "This pain is phantom limb pain, because pain signals are still being sent to your brain."

    Phantom limb pain is real pain that is experienced by clients who have undergone amputations. This may be experienced as pain because the nerve endings at the site of the amputation continue to send pain signals to the brain. Incisional pain would be experienced at the incisional site, not in the amputated foot. Referred pain is not a complication after amputation of a limb. If the client feels pain then it is not imaginary.

    (N) NCLEX® Connection: Potential for Complications from Surgical Procedures and Health Alterations

3. The client tells the nurse that he is feeling sharp, knife-like pain. Which of the following medications should the nurse administer?

    A. Propranolol (Inderal)

    B. Gabapentin (Neurontin)

    C. Baclofen (Lioresal)

    D. Morphine (MS Contin)

Gabapentin, an antiepileptic, can be administered for sharp, knife-like pain. Propranolol, an adrenergic blocking agent, can be administered for constant, dull, burning pain. Baclofen, an antispasmodic, can be administered to treat muscle spasms. Morphine is not specific for phantom limb pain.

Ⓝ NCLEX® Connection: Pharmacological Therapies, Pharmacological Pain Management

UNIT 10	NURSING CARE OF CLIENTS WITH MUSCULOSKELETAL DISORDERS
Section:	Musculoskeletal Disorders
Chapter 68	Osteoporosis and Osteoarthritis

Overview

- Osteoporosis is the most common metabolic bone disorder resulting in low bone density. Osteoporosis occurs when the rate of bone resorption (osteoclast cells) exceeds the rate of bone formation (osteoblast cells) resulting in fragile bone tissue and subsequent fractures.

- Osteopenia, the precursor to osteoporosis, refers to low bone mineral density for what is expected for the client's age and sex.

- Peak bone mineral density occurs between the ages of 30 and 35. After peak years, bone density decreases, with a significant increase in the rate of loss in postmenopausal women due to estrogen loss.

- Fragile, thin bone tissue is susceptible to fracture.

Data Collection

- Risk Factors

  o Female

  o Age over 60 (over 75, if male)

  o Postmenopausal estrogen deficiency

  o Family history

  o Thin, lean body build

  o History of low calcium intake with suboptimal levels of vitamin D

  o History of smoking

  o History of high alcohol intake

  o Lack of physical activity/prolonged immobility

  o Secondary osteoporosis results from medical conditions including:

    ▪ Hyperparathyroidism

    ▪ Long-term corticosteroid use (asthma, systemic lupus erythematosus)

    ▪ Long-term lack of weight-bearing (spinal cord injury)

o   Primary osteoporosis most frequently occurs in postmenopausal women

o   Older adult clients have an increased risk of falls related to impaired balance, generalized weakness, gait changes, and impaired vision and hearing. Medication side effects can cause orthostatic hypotension, urinary frequency, or confusion, which can also raise the client's risk for falls.

- Subjective Data

  o   Reduced height (postmenopausal)

  o   Acute back pain after lifting or bending (worse with activity, relieved by rest)

  o   Restriction in movement

  o   History of fractures

- Objective Data

  o   Reduced height (postmenopausal)

  o   Thoracic (kyphosis)

View Media Supplement: Kyphosis (Image)

  o   Pain upon palpation over affected area

  o   Laboratory Tests

  ■   Serum calcium, vitamin D, phosphorus, and alkaline phosphatase levels are drawn to rule out other metabolic bone diseases (Paget's disease or osteomalacia).

  o   Diagnostic Procedures

  ■   Radiographs

  □   Radiographs of the spine and long bones reveal low bone density and fractures.

  ■   Dual energy x-ray absorptiometry (DEXA)

  □   DEXA is used to screen for early changes in bone density. This painless test measures bone mineral density in the wrist, hip, and vertebral column.

  ■   Quantitative ultrasound (QUS)

  □   An ultrasound, usually of the heel. QUS is an inexpensive, portable, and low-risk method to determine osteoporosis and assessing for risk of fracture.

Collaborative Care

- Nursing Care

  o   Administer medications as prescribed.

  o   Instruct clients regarding dietary calcium food sources (broccoli, calcium-fortified orange juice, milk, yogurt, cheese).

- Recommend clients consume appropriate amount of daily calcium and vitamin D for age
  - For adults under 50 yr of age – A minimum of 1,000 mg of calcium and 5 ug of vitamin D
  - For adults age 50 or older – A minimum of 1,200 mg of calcium and 10 ug of vitamin D
- Encourage clients to take a calcium supplement with vitamin D if dietary intake is inadequate (lactose intolerant).
- Provide information regarding calcium supplementation (take with food).
- Instruct clients of the need for adequate amounts of calcium, vitamin D, protein, magnesium, vitamin K, and other trace minerals needed for bone formation.
- Reinforce the need for exposure to vitamin D (sunlight, fortified milk). Encourage clients to expose areas of skin to sun 5 to 30 min twice a week.
- Recommend that clients minimize alcohol, soft drinks, and caffeine.
- Recommend smoking cessation for clients who smoke.
- Encourage weight-bearing exercises to improve strength and reduce bone loss. Tell clients that the best way to prevent osteoporosis is to walk 30 min 3 to 5 times/week.

- Medications
  - Several medications can be taken to slow the development of osteoporosis. Clients may be prescribed a combination of several of these medications.

CLASSIFICATION/MEDICATION	THERAPEUTIC INTENT	NURSING CONSIDERATIONS/ CLIENT EDUCATION
Estrogen Hormone Supplement • Estrogen (Premarin) • Estrogen and medroxyprogesterone (Prempro)	• Replaces estrogen lost due to menopause or surgical removal of ovaries	• Instruct clients on potential complications, including breast and endometrial cancers and deep vein thrombosis (DVT). • Reinforce monthly breast self-examinations.
Selective Estrogen Receptor Modulators • Raloxifene hydrochloride (Evista)	• Decreases osteoclast activity, subsequently decreasing bone resorption • Treats postmenopausal osteoporosis	• Avoid for clients with a history of DVT. • Monitor liver function tests.
Calcium Supplement • Calcium-carbonate (Os-Cal, Caltrate-600) • Calcium-citrate (Citracal)	• Supplements calcium that is consumed in food products	• Instruct clients to take with food in divided doses with 6 to 8 oz of water to prevent gastrointestinal upset. • Monitor for kidney stones.

CLASSIFICATION/MEDICATION	THERAPEUTIC INTENT	NURSING CONSIDERATIONS/ CLIENT EDUCATION
Vitamin D Supplement	• Increases absorption of calcium from the intestinal tract and availability of calcium in the serum needed for remineralization of bone • Needed by individuals who are not exposed to adequate amounts of sunlight or who do not meet daily requirements	• Vitamin D is a fat-soluble vitamin, so toxicity can occur. Instruct clients to watch for signs and symptoms of toxicity, including nausea, constipation, and kidney stones.
Bisphosphonates (inhibit bone resorption) • PO • Alendronate (Fosamax) • Risedronate (Actonel) • PO, IV • Ibandronate (Boniva) Etidronate (Didronel) ○ IV • Zoledronate (Reclast)	• Decreases number and actions of osteoclasts, subsequently inhibiting bone resorption	• Instruct clients to oral medications take with 8 oz of water in the early morning before eating and to remain upright for 30 min. • Instruct clients to report indigestion, chest pain, difficulty swallowing, or bloody emesis to provider immediately.
Thyroid Hormone • Calcitonin (Miacalcin)	• Decreases bone resorption by inhibiting osteoclast activity	• Can be taken IM/SC or nasally; instruct clients to alternate nostrils.

- Interdisciplinary Care

  - Request a referral for physical therapy to establish an exercise regimen.

  - Recognize the need for rehabilitation if fractures cause immobilization or disability.

- Therapeutic Procedures

  - Orthotic devices are available for immobilization of the spine immediately after a compression fracture of the spine.

    - Provides support and decreases pain

    - A physical therapist fits the device for clients and teaches how to apply it.

    - Nursing Actions

      - Instruct clients how to check for skin breakdown under the orthotic device.

- Surgical Interventions

    o Joint repair or joint arthroplasty may be necessary to repair or replace a joint weakened by osteoporosis. This is most often the hip joint.

    o Vertebroplasty and kyphoplasty may be performed for vertebral body compression and fractures to reduce pain and improve function.

Care After Discharge

- Client Education

    o Encourage clients to adhere to the therapeutic regimen.

    o Have clients check the home environment for safety (remove throw rugs, provide adequate lighting, clear walkways). Have clients clearly mark thresholds, doorways, and steps.

    o Reinforce the use of safety equipment and assistive devices.

        ▪ Encourage clients to discuss the pros and cons of hormone replacement therapy with the provider.

- Client Outcomes

    o The client will participate in weight-bearing exercises on a regular basis.

    o The client with consume a diet with adequate calcium and vitamin D.

    o The client will be free from injury.

OSTEOARTHRITIS

Overview

- Osteoarthritis (OA) is a disorder characterized by progressive deterioration of the articular cartilage. It is a noninflammatory (unless localized), nonsystemic disease. Changes within joints lead to pain, immobility, muscle spasms, and potential inflammation.

- Early in the disease process of OA, it may be difficult to distinguish from rheumatoid arthritis (RA).

CHARACTERISTIC	OSTEOARTHRITIS	RHEUMATOID ARTHRITIS
Disease process	Cartilage destruction with bone spur growth at joint ends; degenerative	Synovial membrane inflammation resulting in cartilage destruction and bone erosion; inflammatory
Signs and symptoms	Pain with activity that improves at rest	Swelling, redness, warmth, pain at rest or after immobility (morning stiffness)
Effusions	Localized inflammatory response	All joints
Body Size	Usually overweight	Usually underweight

CHARACTERISTIC	OSTEOARTHRITIS	RHEUMATOID ARTHRITIS
Nodes	Heberden's and Bouchard's nodes	Swan neck and boutonnière deformities of hands
Systemic involvement	No; articular	Yes; lungs, heart, skin, and extra-articular
Symmetrical	No	Yes
Diagnostic tests	X-rays	X-rays, and positive rheumatoid factor

Data Collection

- Risk Factors

    o Age (a majority of adults over the age of 55 have joint changes on x-ray).

    o Female sex

    o Obesity

    o Possible genetic link

    o History of repetitive stress on joints (manual laborers, professional athletes, marathon runners)

- Subjective Data

    o Joint pain and stiffness that resolves with rest or inactivity

    o History of injury or repetitive stress

    o History of obesity

- Objective Data

    o Pain with joint palpation or range of motion (observe for muscle atrophy, loss of function, limp when walking, and restricted activity due to pain)

    o Crepitus in one or more of the affected joints

    o Enlarged joint related to bone hypertrophy

    o Heberden's nodes enlarged at the distal interphalangeal (DIP) joints

    o Bouchard's nodes located at the proximal interphalangeal (PIP) joints (OA is not a symmetrical disease, but these nodes can occur bilaterally).

    o Inflammation resulting from secondary synovitis, indicating advanced disease

    o Laboratory Tests

        ▪ Erythrocyte sedimentation rate (ESR) and high-sensitivity C-reactive protein may be increased slightly related to secondary synovitis. Osteoarthritis without synovitis is not an inflammatory disorder.

○ Diagnostic Procedures

▪ Radiographs and CT scans can determine structural changes within the joint.

☐ Decreased joint space

☐ Bone spurs

Collaborative Care

● Nursing Care

○ Monitor

▪ Pain – Level (0 to 10), location, characteristics, quality, and severity

▪ Degree of functional limitation

▪ Levels of fatigue and pain after activity

▪ Range of motion

▪ Proper functional/joint alignment

▪ Home barriers

▪ Ability to perform ADLs

○ Instruct clients about the use of analgesics and NSAIDs prior to activity and around the clock as needed.

○ Instruct clients on proper body mechanics.

○ Encourage the use of thermal applications — heat to alleviate pain and ice for acute inflammation.

○ Encourage the use of complementary and alternative therapies, including acupuncture, tai chi, hypnosis, magnets, and music therapy.

○ Encourage the use of splinting for joint protection and the use of larger joints.

● Medications

○ Analgesic therapy

▪ Acetaminophen

☐ Does not provide anti-inflammatory benefits, which may not be needed if synovitis is not present

☐ Nursing Actions

▸ Monitor liver function tests.

▪ NSAIDs

☐ Analgesics and anti-inflammatories that are used to relieve pain and synovitis if present

☐ May replace acetaminophen with an NSAID if adequate relief is not obtained

- Topical analgesics

  □ Trolamine salicylate (Aspercreme) – It may provide varying amounts of temporary pain relief, depending on the client's response. Apply topically over the area of involvement. It contains salicylate.

  □ Capsaicin (Axsain, Capsin) – It may provide varying amounts of temporary pain relief depending on the client's response. Apply topically over an area of involvement. It is made from alkaloid that is derived from hot peppers. It is thought to prevent transmission of pain sensations from peripheral neural transmitters.

  □ Client Education

    ‣ Instruct clients to wear gloves during application (capsaicin).

    ‣ Explain to clients that a burning sensation of the skin after application is normal and should subside.

    ‣ Instruct clients to apply frequently (up to 4 times a day) for maximum benefit.

- Glucosamine (rebuilds cartilage)

  □ Glucosamine is a naturally occurring chemical involved in the makeup of cartilage. Glucosamine sulfate is believed to aid glycosaminoglycan synthesis and subsequently rebuilds cartilage. Glucosamine is often taken in combination with chondroitin, a glycosaminoglycan also involved in the makeup of articular cartilage.

  □ Client Education

    ‣ Instruct clients to consult the provider regarding dosage.

  ‣ Intra-articular injections

  ‣ Glucocorticoids – Used to treat localized inflammation

  ‣ Hyaluronic acid (Hyalgan, Synvisc) – It is used to replace the body's natural hyaluronic acid, which is destroyed by joint inflammation. It is currently only approved for treatment of knee joints.

    □ Client Education

      ‣ Hyaluronic acid – Instruct clients to notify the provider if allergic to birds, feathers, or eggs because this medication is made from combs of chickens.

- Interdisciplinary Care

  ○ Request a referral for physical therapy for the application of heat, diathermy (treatment with electrical currents), ultrasonography (treatment with sound waves), a transcutaneous electrical nerve stimulation (TENS) unit, or stretching and strengthening exercises.

  ○ Request a referral to a nutritionist to assist clients in diet for weight loss or control in relation to reduced activity level.

- Therapeutic Procedures

  - Conservative therapy

    - Conservative therapy includes balancing rest with activity, using bracing or splints, and applying thermal therapies (heat or cold).

- Surgical Interventions

  - Total joint arthroplasty

    - When all other conservative measures fail, clients may choose to undergo total joint arthroplasty to relieve the pain and improve mobility and quality of life.

- Care After Discharge

  - Encourage clients to balance rest with activity.

  - Encourage the use of assistive devices to promote safety and independence, including an elevated toilet seat, shower bench, and long-handled reacher and shoe horn.

  - Encourage the use of a daily schedule of activities that will promote independence (high-energy activities in the morning).

  - Encourage a well-balanced diet and ideal body weight. Consult a dietitian to provide meal planning for balanced nutrition.

- Client Outcomes

  - The client will schedule activities and use conservative therapies that allow completion of ADLs.

  - The client will make lifestyle alterations that will slow or stop progression of the disease.

(A) APPLICATION EXERCISES

1. Identify risk factors for developing osteoporosis.

2. When reinforcing dietary instructions to a client to minimize the risk of osteoporosis, the nurse should recommend which of the following foods?

    A. Bread

    B. Yogurt

    C. Chicken

    D. Carrots

3. Match the medication classification in column A with the therapeutic intent in column B.

    _____ Estrogen Hormone Supplement

    _____ Selective Estrogen Receptor Modulators

    _____ Calcium Supplement

    _____ Vitamin D Supplement

    _____ Bisphosphonates

    A. Decreases osteoclast activity, subsequently decreasing bone resorption

    B. Decreases number and actions of osteoclasts, subsequently inhibiting bone resorption

    C. Replaces estrogen lost due to menopause

    D. Supplements calcium that is consumed in food products

    E. Increases absorption of calcium from the intestinal tract and availability of calcium in the serum needed for remineralization of bone

4. Identify which of the following characteristics may indicate osteoarthritis (OA). (Select all that apply.)

    _____ Heberden's nodes

    _____ Systemic involvement

    _____ Small body frame

    _____ Pain that occurs with activity

    _____ Need for total joint arthroplasty

5. A nurse is reinforcing teaching to a client about a newly prescribed medication, capsaicin (Axsain, Capsin). Which of the following information should the nurse include?

    A. Apply the medication while wearing gloves.

    B. Avoid drinking alcohol after applying the medication.

    C. Take the medication in combination with chondroitin.

    D. Apply the medication once daily.

APPLICATION EXERCISES ANSWER KEY

1. Identify risk factors for developing osteoporosis.

    Risk factors include: female; age over 60 (over 75, if male); postmenopausal estrogen deficiency; family history; thin, lean body build; history of low calcium intake with suboptimal levels of vitamin D; history of smoking; history of high alcohol intake; and lack of physical activity/prolonged immobility.

    NCLEX® Connection: Physiological Adaptation, Pathophysiology

2. When reinforcing dietary instructions to a client to minimize the risk of osteoporosis, the nurse should recommend which of the following foods?

    A. Bread

    B. Yogurt

    C. Chicken

    D. Carrots

    Dairy products are high in calcium, and yogurt is a dairy product. Bread, chicken, and carrots do not provide high sources of calcium.

    NCLEX® Connection: Basic Care and Comfort, Nutrition and Oral Hydration

3. Match the medication classification in column A with the therapeutic intent in column B.

C	Estrogen Hormone Supplement	A. Decreases osteoclast activity, subsequently decreasing bone resorption
A	Selective Estrogen Receptor Modulators	B. Decreases number and actions of osteoclasts, subsequently inhibiting bone resorption
D	Calcium Supplement	C. Replaces estrogen lost due to menopause
E	Vitamin D Supplement	D. Supplements calcium that is consumed in food products
B	Bisphosphonates	E. Increases absorption of calcium from the intestinal tract and availability of calcium in the serum needed for remineralization of bone

    NCLEX® Connection: Pharmacological Therapies, Expected Actions/Outcomes

4. Identify which of the following characteristics may indicate osteoarthritis (OA). (Select all that apply.)

     __X__ **Heberden's nodes**

     _____ Systemic involvement

     _____ Small body frame

     __X__ **Pain that occurs with activity**

     __X__ **Need for total joint arthroplasty**

     OA is a localized disease that can produce Heberden's nodes on the interphalangeal joints, pain that worsens with activity, and degeneration of the joint's cartilage and articular surfaces that can necessitate joint arthroplasty. It is more frequent in individuals who are overweight. Individuals with a small body frame are at risk for osteoporosis.

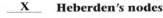 NCLEX® Connection: Physiological Adaptation, Pathophysiology

5. A nurse is reinforcing teaching to a client about a newly prescribed medication, capsaicin (Axsain, Capsin). Which of the following information should the nurse include?

     A. Apply the medication while wearing gloves.

     B. Avoid drinking alcohol after applying the medication.

     C. Take the medication in combination with chondroitin.

     D. Apply the medication once daily.

     Capsaicin is made from hot peppers so gloves should be worn during application. It is not necessary to avoid alcohol when using this medication. Glucosamine can be taken with chondroitin for osteoarthritis, but its use with capsaicin will yield no additional therapeutic effects. Instruct the client to apply the medication frequently (up to 4 times a day) for maximum benefit.

 NCLEX® Connection: Pharmacological Therapies, Medication Administration

UNIT 10   NURSING CARE OF CLIENTS WITH MUSCULOSKELETAL DISORDERS

Section: Musculoskeletal Disorders

Chapter 69   Fractures

Overview

- A fracture is a break in a bone secondary to trauma or a pathological condition.

- Fractures caused by trauma are the most common type of fracture.

- Pathological fractures may be caused by metastatic cancer, osteoporosis, or Paget's disease.

- A closed fracture does not break through the skin surface. An open, or compound, fracture disrupts the skin integrity, causing an open wound with a risk of infection.

- Open fractures are graded based upon the extent of tissue injury.

  ○ Grade I – minimal skin damage

  ○ Grade II – damage includes skin and muscle contusions

  ○ Grade III – damage to skin, muscles, nerves, and blood vessels

- A complete fracture goes through the entire bone, dividing it into two parts. An incomplete fracture goes through part of the bone.

- A simple fracture has one fracture line, while a comminuted fracture has multiple fracture lines splitting the bone into multiple pieces.

- A displaced fracture has bone fragments that are not in alignment, and a non-displaced fracture has bone fragments that remain in alignment.

- Common Types of Fractures

  ○ Comminuted – Bone is fragmented

  ○ Oblique – Fracture occurs at oblique angle

  ○ Spiral – Fracture occurs from twisting motion (common with physical abuse)

  ○ Impacted – Fractured bone is wedged inside opposite fractured fragment

  ○ Greenstick – Fracture that occurs on one side (cortex), but does not extend completely through the bone. Occurs most often in children.

- Hip fractures are the most common injury in older adults.

> (M) **View Media Supplement:** X-Ray of Leg Fracture (Image)

- Treatments for fractures include surgery and immobilizing interventions such as splints, casts and traction. Immobilization secures the injured extremity in order to:

  o Prevent further injury.

  o Promote healing/circulation.

  o Reduce pain.

  o Correct a deformity.

- Types of immobilization devices include:

  o Splints/immobilizers.

  o Casts.

  o Traction.

  o External fixation.

  o Internal fixation.

- Closed reduction is when a pulling force (traction) is applied manually to realign the displaced fractured bone fragments. Once the fracture is reduced, immobilization is used to allow the bone to heal.

- Open reduction is when a surgical incision is made and the bone is manually aligned and kept in place with plates and screws. This is known as an open reduction and internal fixation (ORIF) procedure.

Data Collection

- Risk Factors

  o Osteoporosis

    ▪ Women who do not use estrogen replacement therapy after menopause lose estrogen and are unable to form strong new bone.

  o Long-term corticosteroid therapy

  o Falls

  o Motor vehicle crashes

  o Substance abuse

  o Diseases (bone cancer, Paget's disease)

  o Contact sports and hazardous recreational activities (football, skiing)

  o Physical abuse

(G)

- o Lactose intolerance
- o Age, as bone becomes less dense with advancing age
- Subjective Data
  - o Collect data regarding trauma, metabolic bone disorders, chronic conditions, and possible use of corticosteroid therapy.
  - o Pain and/or reduced movement at the area of fracture or the area distal to the fracture.
- Objective Data
  - o Physical Findings
    - Crepitus – A grating sound created by the rubbing of bone fragments
    - Deformity – May observe internal rotation of extremity, shortened extremity, visible bone with open fracture
    - Muscle spasms – Occur from the pulling forces of the bone when not aligned
    - Edema – Swelling from trauma
    - Ecchymosis – Bleeding into underlying soft tissues from trauma
  - o Diagnostic Procedures
    - Standard radiographs, CT scan, and/or magnetic resonance imagery.
    - Identify the type of fracture and location.
    - Indicate pathological fracture resulting from tumor or mass.
    - Determine soft tissue damage.
    - A bone scan is used to determine fracture complications/delayed healing.

Collaborative Care

- Nursing Care
  - o Provide emergency care at time of injury.
    - Maintain ABCs.
    - Monitor the client's vital signs and neurological status.
    - Check neurovascular status of injured extremity.
    - Place clients in supine position.
    - Stabilize the injured area including the joints above and below the fracture, avoiding unnecessary movement.
    - Elevate the limb and apply ice.
    - Observe for bleeding and apply pressure, if needed.
    - Cover open wounds with a sterile dressing.

- Remove clothing and jewelry near injury.
- Keep clients warm.
  - In an urgent care clinic:
    - Frequently check pain and follow pain management protocols, both pharmacologic and nonpharmacologic.
    - Initiate and continue neurovascular checks on a regular schedule. Immediately report any change in status.
    - Maintain proper alignment.
    - Prepare clients for immobilization procedure appropriate for fracture.
  - Perform neurovascular data collection
    - Pain. Check the client's pain level, location, and frequency. Assess pain using a 0-to-10 pain rating scale and have clients describe the pain.
    - Sensation. Check for presence of sensation in affected extremity. Loss of sensation may indicate nerve damage. Check for numbness and tingling (paresthesia)
    - Skin color and temperature. Skin should be pink, not pale or cyanotic. Check the temperature of the affected extremity. The extremity should be warm, not cool, to touch.
    - Capillary refill. Press nail beds of affected extremity until blanching occurs. Blood return should be within 3 seconds.
    - Pulses. Pulses should be palpable and strong. Pulses should also be equal to the pulses of the unaffected extremity with passive or active motion.
    - Movement. Clients should be able to move affected extremity.

- Splints and Immobilizers
  - Splints are removable and allow for monitoring of skin swelling or integrity.
  - Splints can be used to support fractured/injured areas until casting can be done or used for post-paralysis injuries to avoid joint contracture.
  - Immobilizers are prefabricated and typically fasten with Velcro straps.
  - Client Education
    - Ensure clients are aware of application protocol regarding full-time or part-time use.
    - Instruct clients to observe for skin breakdown at pressure points.
  - Casts
    - Types of casts include:
      - Short- and long-arm and leg casts.
      - Spica casts, which refer to a portion of the trunk and one or two extremities. Typically used on children with congenital hip dysplasia
      - Body casts, which encircle the trunk of the body.

- Casting materials
  - Plaster of Paris casts are heavy, not water-resistant, and can take 24 to 48 hr to dry.
  - Synthetic fiberglass casts are light, water-resistant, and dry very quickly (in 30 min).
- Casts, as circumferential immobilizers, are applied once the swelling has subsided (to avoid compartment syndrome). If the swelling continues after cast application and causes unrelieved pain, the cast can be split on one side (univalved) or on both sides (bivalved).
- A window can be placed in an area of the cast to allow for skin inspection (clients have a wound under the cast).
- Moleskin is used over any rough area of the cast that may rub against the client's skin.
- Nursing Actions
  - Prior to casting, the area is cleaned and dried. Tubular cotton web roll is placed over the affected area to maintain skin integrity. The casting material is then applied.
  - After cast application, position clients so that warm, dry air circulates around and under the cast (support the casted area without pressure under or directly on the cast) for faster drying and to prevent pressure from changing the shape of the cast. Use gloves to touch the cast until the cast is completely dry.
  - Elevate cast above the level of the heart during the first 24 to 48 hr to prevent swelling.
  - If any drainage is seen on the cast, it should be outlined, dated, and timed, so it can be monitored for any additional drainage.
  - Older adult clients have an increased risk for impaired skin integrity due to the loss of elasticity of the skin and decreased sensation (comorbidities).
- Client Education
  - Instruct clients not to place any foreign objects under the cast to avoid trauma to the skin.
  - Tell clients that itching under the cast can be relieved by blowing cool air from a hair dryer under the cast.
  - Use plastic coverings over the cast to avoid soiling from urine or feces and to keep casts dry during baths and showers.

- ○ Traction
  - ■ Traction uses a pulling force to promote and maintain alignment to the injured area.
  - ■ Goals of traction include:
    - □ Realignment of bone fragments.
    - □ Decreasing muscle spasms and pain.
    - □ Correcting or preventing further deformities.
  - ■ Traction prescriptions should include the type of traction, amount of weight, and whether traction can be removed for nursing care.
  - ■ Types of Traction
    - □ In straight or running traction, the countertraction is provided by the client's body. Movement of the client's body can alter the traction provided. In balanced suspension traction, the countertraction is produced by devices such as slings or splints. The client's body can be moved vertically without altering the traction.
    - □ Manual – A pulling force is applied by the hands of the provider for temporary immobilization, usually with sedation or anesthesia, in conjunction with the application of an immobilizing device.
    - □ Skin – Used intermittently. The pulling force is applied by weights that are attached by rope to clients with tape, straps, boots, or cuffs. Examples include chin halter straps, Bryant's traction (used for congenital hip dislocation in children), and Buck's traction (used for hip fractures preoperatively for immobilization in adult clients).

 View Media Supplement: Buck's Traction (Image)

    - □ Skeletal – Used continuously. The pulling force is applied directly to the bone by weights attached by rope directly to a rod/screw placed through the bone. Examples include skeletal tongs (Gardner-Wells) and femoral or tibial pins (Steinmann pin). Weights up to 25 pounds can be applied as needed.

View Media Supplement: Skeletal Traction (Image)

    - □ Halo – Screws are placed through a halo-type bar that encircles the head into the outer table of the bone of the skull. This halo is attached to either bed traction or rods that are secured to a vest worn by clients. Assure that the wrench to release the rods is attached to the vest when using halo traction in the event CPR is necessary.
  - ■ Nursing Actions
    - □ Maintain body alignment and realign if clients seem uncomfortable or report pain.
    - □ Avoid lifting or removing weights.

- □ Assure that weights hang freely.

- □ If the weights are accidentally displaced, replace the weights. If the problem is not corrected, notify the provider.

- □ Assure that pulley ropes are free of knots.

- □ Notify the provider if clients experience severe pain from muscle spasms unrelieved with medications and/or repositioning. Move clients in halo traction as a unit, without applying pressure to the rods. This will prevent loosening of the pins and pain.

- □ Routinely monitor skin integrity and document.

- ○ Pin Site Care

  - ■ Pin care is done frequently throughout immobilization (skeletal traction and external fixation methods) to prevent and to monitor for signs of infection including:

    - □ Drainage (COCA – color, odor, consistency, amount).

    - □ Loosening of pins.

    - □ Tenting of skin at pin site (skin rising up pin).

  - ■ Pin care protocols (chlorhexidine) are based on provider preference and institution policy. A primary concept of pin care is that one cotton-tip swab is designated for each pin to avoid cross-contamination.

  - ■ Pin care is provided three times a day or per facility protocol.

  - ■ Crusting at the pin site should not be removed as this provides a natural barrier from bacteria.

- • Medications

  - ○ Prophylactic antibiotics

    - ■ Prophylactic antibiotics are used to prevent infection when fracture immobilization is achieved, using pins, metal screws, or wires. Typically, a broad-spectrum IV antibiotic such as cefazolin (Ancef) is administered for 24 to 48 hr post-injury.

  - ○ Analgesics

    - ■ Opioid and nonopioid analgesics may be used as needed to control pain.

  - ○ Muscle relaxants

    - ■ Muscle relaxants may be given to relieve muscle spasms.

- Surgical Interventions
  - External Fixation
    - External fixation involves fracture immobilization using percutaneous pins and wires that are attached to a rigid external frame.
    - Used to treat:
      - Comminuted fracture with extensive soft tissue damage.
      - Leg length discrepancies from congenital defects.
      - Bone loss related to tumors or osteomyelitis.
    - Advantages include:
      - Immediate fracture stabilization.
      - Allowing three-plane correction of the injury.
      - Minimal blood loss occurring in comparison with internal fixation.
      - Allowing for early mobilization and ambulation.
      - Maintaining alignment of closed fractures that could not be maintained in cast or splint.
      - Permitting wound care with open fractures.
    - Disadvantages include:
      - Risk of pin tract infection.
      - Potential overwhelming appearance to client.
      - Noncompliance issues.
    - Nursing Actions
      - Provide pin care.
      - Observe for signs of fat and pulmonary embolism.
      - Provide anti-embolism stockings and sequential compression device to prevent DVT.
    - Client Education
      - Reinforce to clients how to perform pin care.
      - Discuss clothing and other materials that can be used to cover the device.
      - If activity is restricted, advise client to perform deep breathing and leg exercises and other techniques to prevent complications of immobilization, such as pneumonia or thrombus formation.

- ○ ORIF
    - Open reduction refers to visualization of a fracture through an incision in the skin, with repair made with plates, screws, pins, rods, and prosthetics as needed.
    - After the bone heals, the hardware may be removed, depending on the location and type of hardware.
    - Nursing Actions
        - □ Collect data regarding neurovascular status.
        - □ Observe the cast or dressing for postoperative drainage. The cast may have a window cut in it through which the incision can be viewed.
        - □ Observe for signs of fat and pulmonary embolism.
        - □ Provide antiembolism stockings and sequential compression device to prevent DVT.
        - □ Monitor the client's pain level.
        - □ Monitor for signs of infection.
            - ▸ Monitor the client's vital signs, watching for fever and tachycardia.
            - ▸ Monitor laboratory values (WBC, ESR).
            - ▸ Provide surgical aseptic wound care.
        - □ Increase physical mobility as appropriate.
            - ▸ Consult physical and occupational therapy for ambulation and activities of daily living (ADLs).
            - ▸ Monitor orthostatic blood pressure when clients get out of bed for the first time.
            - ▸ Turn and reposition clients every 2 hr.
            - ▸ Have clients get out of bed from the unaffected side.
            - ▸ Position clients for comfort (within restrictions).
        - □ Support nutrition.
            - ▸ Encourage increased calorie intake.
            - ▸ Ensure use of calcium supplements.
            - ▸ Encourage small, frequent meals with snacks.
            - ▸ Monitor for constipation.
- Client Outcomes
    - ○ Client will not develop complications related to a bone fracture or its treatment (compartment syndrome, fat embolism, osteomyelitis).
    - ○ Client will demonstrate proper use of mobility devices such as crutches or walker.

Complications

- Compartment syndrome

    o Compartment syndrome occurs when pressure within one or more of the muscle compartments of the extremity compromises circulation, resulting in an ischemia–edema cycle. Capillaries dilate in an attempt to pull oxygen into the tissue. Increased capillary permeability from the release of histamine leads to edema from plasma proteins leaking into the interstitial fluid space. Increased edema causes pressure on the nerve endings, resulting in pain. Blood flow is further reduced and ischemia persists resulting in compromised neurovascular status.

    o Pressure can result from external sources, such as a tight cast or a constrictive bulky dressing.

    o Internal sources, such as an accumulation of blood or fluid within the muscle compartment, can cause pressure as well.

    o Compartment pressure is monitored with a handheld device or with a catheter connected to a transducer. Normal compartmental pressure is 0 to 8 mm Hg. Clinical manifestations (evolving neurovascular compromise) and compartmental pressure readings greater than 8 mm Hg are used to indicate an emergent need for treatment.

    o Findings include:

        ▪ Weak pulses, rarely disappearing

        ▪ Increased pain unrelieved with elevation or analgesia.

        ▪ Intense pain with passive motion.

        ▪ Paresthesia or numbness.

        ▪ Color of tissue is pale (pallor), becoming cyanotic.

        ▪ Edema

    o If untreated, tissue necrosis can result. Neuromuscular damage occurs within 4 to 6 hr.

    o Surgical treatment is a fasciotomy.

        ▪ A surgical incision is made through the subcutaneous tissue and fascia of the affected compartment to relieve the pressure and restore circulation.

        ▪ After the fasciotomy, the open wounds require sterile packings and dressings until secondary closure occurs. Skin grafts may be necessary.

    o Nursing Actions

        ▪ Prevention includes:

            □ Cutting the cast on one side (univalve) or both sides (bivalve).

            □ Loosening the constrictive dressing or cutting the bandage or tape.

            □ Elevating the extremity and applying ice. If compartment syndrome is suspected, the extremity should not be elevated above the level of the heart to ensure adequate perfusion.

- ○ Client Education
  - Instruct clients to report pain not relieved by analgesics or pain that continues to increase in intensity.
  - Instruct clients to report numbness, tingling, or a change in color of the extremity.

- Fat embolism
  - ○ Fat embolism can occur, usually within 48 hr following long bone fractures. Fat globules from the bone marrow are released into the vasculature and travel to the small blood vessels, including those in the lungs, resulting in acute respiratory insufficiency. Careful diagnosis should differentiate between fat embolism and pulmonary embolism.
  - ○ Clinical manifestations include:
    - Decreased mental acuity related to low arterial oxygen level (earliest sign).
    - Respiratory distress.
    - Tachycardia.
    - Tachypnea.
    - Fever.
    - Cutaneous petechiae – pinpoint-sized subdermal hemorrhages that occur on the neck, chest, upper arms, and abdomen (from the blockage of the capillaries by the fat globules). This is a discriminating finding from a pulmonary embolism.
  - ○ Nursing Actions
    - Prevention includes immobilization of fractures of the long bones and minimal manipulation during turning if immobilization procedure has not yet been performed.
    - Treatment includes oxygen for respiratory compromise, corticosteroids for cerebral edema, vasopressors, and fluid replacement for shock, as well as pain and antianxiety medications as needed.

- Deep vein thrombosis
  - ○ Deep vein thrombosis is the most common complication following trauma, surgery, or disability related to immobility.
  - ○ Nursing Actions
    - Administer anticoagulants as prescribed.
    - Encourage intake of fluids to prevent hemoconcentration.
    - Instruct clients to rotate feet at the ankles and perform other lower extremity exercises as permitted by immobilization device employed.

- Osteomyelitis

  o Osteomyelitis is an inflammation within the bone secondary to penetration by infectious organisms (trauma, surgery).

  o Signs and symptoms

    - Bone pain that is worse with movement

    - Erythema and edema at the site of the infection

    - Fever

    - Leukocytosis and possible elevated sedimentation rate

    - Many of these signs will disappear if the infection becomes chronic.

  o Diagnostic procedures

    - Definitive diagnosis is with a bone biopsy.

    - Cultures are performed for detection of possible aerobic and anaerobic organisms.

    - If septicemia develops, blood cultures will be positive for offending microbes.

  o Treatment

    - Long course (3 months) of IV and oral antibiotic therapy.

    - Surgical debridement may also be indicated. If a significant amount of the bone requires removal, a bone graft may be necessary.

    - Hyperbaric oxygen treatments may be needed to promote healing in chronic cases of osteomyelitis.

    - Unsuccessful treatment can result in amputation.

  o Nursing Actions

    - Administer antibiotics as prescribed to maintain a constant blood level.

    - Administer analgesics as needed.

    - Conduct neurovascular assessments if debridement is done.

    - If wound is left open to heal, standard precautions are adequate and clean technique can be used during dressing changes.

- Avascular necrosis

  o Avascular necrosis results from the circulatory compromise that occurs after a fracture. Blood flow is disrupted to the fracture site and the resulting ischemia leads to tissue (bone) necrosis.

  o Replacement of damaged bone with a bone graft or prosthetic replacement may be necessary.

- Failure of Fracture to Heal

  o A fracture that has not healed within 6 months of injury is considered to be experiencing delayed union.

  o Malunion – Fracture heals incorrectly

  o Nonunion – Fracture that never heals

    ■ Electrical bone stimulation and bone grafting can be used to treat nonunion.

    ■ May occur more frequently in older adults due to impaired healing process.

  o Malunion or nonunion may cause immobilizing deformity of bone involved.

Overview

- A wound is a result of injury to the skin. Although there are many different types and degrees of injury, the basic phases of healing are essentially the same for most wounds.

- A pressure ulcer is a specific type of tissue injury caused by unrelieved pressure that results in ischemia and damage to the underlying tissue.

PRESSURE ULCERS

Overview

- Pressure ulcers range from nonblanchable tissue redness to full thickness skin loss with damage to underlying muscle and bone.

- The primary focus of prevention and treatment is to relieve the pressure and provide optimal nutrition and hydration.

- All clients must be checked regularly for skin integrity status and evaluated regularly for risk factors that contribute to impaired skin integrity.

Data Collection

- Risk Factors
  - Skin changes related to aging
  - Immobility
  - Incontinence or excessive moisture
  - Skin friction and shearing
  - Vascular disorders
  - Obesity
  - Inadequate nutrition and/or hydration
  - Anemia
  - Fever
  - Impaired circulation
  - Edema
  - Sensory deficits

- ○ Impaired cognitive functioning, neurological disorders

- ○ Chronic diseases (diabetes mellitus, chronic renal failure, congestive heart disease, chronic lung disease)

- ○ Sedation that impairs spontaneous repositioning

- Pressure ulcers are classified according to a staging system developed by the National Pressure Ulcer Advisory Panel. The stages are:

  - ○ Suspected deep tissue injury – Discolored but intact skin caused by damage to underlying tissue

  - ○ Stage I – Intact skin with an area of persistent, nonblanchable redness, typically over a bony prominence, which may feel warm or cool to touch. The tissue is swollen and congested, with possible discomfort at the site. With darker skin tones, the ulcer may appear blue or purple.

  - ○ Stage II – Partial-thickness skin loss involving the epidermis and the dermis. The ulcer is visible and superficial and may appear as an abrasion, blister, or shallow cavity. Edema persists, and the ulcer may become infected, possibly with pain and scant drainage.

  - ○ Stage III – Full-thickness tissue loss with damage to or necrosis of subcutaneous tissue. The ulcer may reach, but not extend thorough the fascia below. The ulcer appears as a deep crater with or without undermining of adjacent tissue and without exposed muscle or bone. Drainage and infection are common.

  - ○ Stage IV – Full-thickness tissue loss with destruction, tissue necrosis, or damage to muscle, bone, or supporting structures. There may be sinus tracts, deep pockets of infection, tunneling, undermining, eschar (black scab-like material), or slough (tan, yellow, or green scab-like material).

  - ○ Unstageable – Ulcers whose stages cannot be determined because eschar or slough obscures the wound.

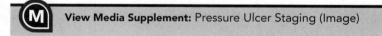

View Media Supplement: Pressure Ulcer Staging (Image)

Collaborative Care

- Nursing Care

  - ○ Reposition clients in bed at least every 2 hr and every 1 hr in a chair. Document position changes.

    - ▪ Place pillows strategically between bony surfaces.

    - ▪ Maintain the head of the bed at or below a 30° angle, unless contraindicated, to relieve pressure on the sacrum, buttocks, and heels.

    - ▪ Keep clients from sliding down in bed, as this increases shearing forces that pull tissue layers apart and cause damage.

    - ▪ Lift, rather than pull, clients up in bed or in a chair, because pulling creates friction that can damage the outer layer of the skin (epidermis).

    - ▪ Raise the client's heels off of the bed to prevent pressure on the heels.

    - ▪ Ambulate clients as soon as possible and as often as possible.

- Client Outcomes

  ○ The client will have improved skin integrity.

  ○ The client will be free of infection.

  ○ The client will be free of pain.

Complications

- Deterioration to a higher stage ulceration and/or infection

  ○ Nursing Actions

    ▪ Monitor the ulcer frequently and report increases in the size or depth of the lesion, changes in granulation tissue (color, texture), and changes in exudate (color, quantity, odor).

    ▪ Follow the facility's protocol for ulcer treatment.

- Systemic infection

  ○ Nursing Actions

    ▪ Monitor clients for signs of sepsis (changes in level of consciousness, persistent recurrent fever, tachycardia, tachypnea, hypotension, oliguria, increased WBC).

    ▪ Prevent infection by using appropriate asepsis when performing ulcer treatment and dressing changes.

    ▪ Provide optimal nutrition to promote the immune response.

    ▪ Provide for adequate rest to promote healing.

    ▪ Administer antibiotic therapy as prescribed.

WOUND HEALING AND MANAGEMENT

Overview

- General Principles of Wound Management

  ○ Wounds impair skin integrity.

  ○ Inflammation is a localized protective response triggered by injury or destruction of tissue.

  ○ Wounds heal by various processes and in stages.

  ○ Wounds may become infected by the invasion of pathogenic microorganisms.

  ○ Principles of wound care include data collection, cleansing, and protection.

- Stages of Wound Healing

  o The inflammatory stage occurs in the first 3 days after the initial trauma. Attempts are made at the site to:

    - Control bleeding with clot formation.

    - Deliver oxygen, WBCs, and nutrients to the area via the blood supply.

  o The proliferative stage lasts the next 3 to 24 days. Effects to the wound include:

    - Replacing lost tissue with connective or granulated tissue.

    - Contraction of the wound's edges.

    - Resurfacing of new epithelial cells.

  o The maturation or remodeling stage involves the strengthening of the collagen scar and the restoration of a more normal appearance. It can take more than 1 year to complete, depending on the extent of the original wound.

- Healing Process

TYPE OF HEALING	CHARACTERISTICS	WOUND TYPE
Primary intention	• Little or no tissue loss • Edges are approximated, as with a surgical incision	• Heals rapidly • Low risk of infection • Minimal or no scarring
Secondary intention	• Loss of tissue • Wound edges widely separated, as with pressure ulcers and stab wounds	• Increased risk of infection • Scarring
Tertiary intention	• Widely separated • Deep • Spontaneous opening of a previously closed wound • Risk of infection	• Extensive drainage and tissue debris • Closes later • Long healing time

Data Collection

- Risk Factors

  o Increased age delays healing because of:

    - Loss of skin turgor

    - Skin fragility

    - Decreased peripheral circulation and oxygenation

    - Slower tissue regeneration

    - Decreased absorption of nutrients

    - Decreased collagen

- Impaired function of the immune system
- Impaired immune function
- Medications (glucocorticoids) may interfere with the body's ability to respond to and/or prevent infection.
- Poor nutritional status
- Obesity – Fatty tissue lacks blood supply.
- Chronic diseases, such as diabetes mellitus, place additional stress on the body's healing mechanisms.
- Chronic stress further impedes healing.
- Smoking impairs oxygenation and clotting.

- Subjective and Objective Data

  - Note the color of open wounds.
    - Red – Healthy regeneration of tissue
    - Yellow – Presence of purulent drainage and slough
    - Black – Presence of eschar that hinders healing and must be removed
  - Note skin edges for closed wounds – Skin edges should be well-approximated.
  - Note the amount of drainage from a drain or on a dressing.
  - Note the character of drainage (COCA – color, odor, consistency, amount)
    - Serous drainage is the portion of the blood (serum) that is watery and clear or slightly yellow in appearance.
    - Sanguineous drainage contains serum and red blood cells. It is thick and appears reddish.
    - Serosanguineous drainage contains both serum and blood. It is watery and appears blood streaked or blood tinged.
    - Purulent drainage is the result of infection. It is thick and contains white blood cells, tissue debris, and bacteria. It may have a foul odor, and its color reflects the type of organism present (green may indicate a pseudomonas infection).
  - Note wound closure (staples, sutures, wound closure strips [Steri-strips])

Collaborative Care

- Nursing Care

  - Provide adequate hydration and meet protein and calorie needs.
    - Encourage an intake of 2,000 to 3,000 mL of water/day if not contraindicated (due to heart failure or renal failure).
    - Provide education about good sources of protein (meat, fish, poultry, eggs, dairy products, beans, nuts, whole grains).

- Note if serum albumin levels are low (below 3.5 g/dL), because a lack of protein puts the client at greater risk for delayed wound healing and infection.

- Provide nutritional support as indicated (vitamin and mineral supplements, nutritional supplements, enteral nutrition, parenteral nutrition).

o Perform wound cleansing.

- Cleanse in a direction from the least contaminated toward the most contaminated.

- Use gentle friction when cleansing or applying solutions to the skin to avoid bleeding or further injury to the wound.

- While other mild cleansing agents may be prescribed, isotonic solutions remain the preferred cleansing agents.

- Never use the same gauze to cleanse across an incision or wound more than once.

- Irrigate with a solution-filled syringe held 2.5 cm (1 in) above the wound.

- With each cleansing, observe the skin around a drain for irritation and breakdown.

o For wound dressings, use:

- Woven gauze (sponges) – Absorb exudate from the wound

- Nonadherent material – Does not adhere to the wound bed

- Self-adhesive, transparent film – A temporary "second skin" ideal for small, superficial wounds

- Hydrocolloid – An occlusive dressing that swells in the presence of exudate

  □ Used to maintain a granulating wound bed

  □ May be left in place up to 5 days

- Hydrogel (Aquasorb)

  □ May be used on infected, deep wounds

  □ Provides a moist wound bed

o Use the negative pressure of a wound vacuum-assisted closure if prescribed.

o Remove sutures/staples as prescribed.

o Administer analgesics as prescribed.

o Administer antimicrobials (topical and/or systemic) as prescribed.

o Document the location and type of wound/incision, the status of the wound and the type of drainage, the type of dressing and materials used, the client teaching reinforced, and how the client tolerated the procedure.

o Use pressure-reducing surfaces and pressure-relieving devices.

o Inspect the skin frequently and document the client's risk using a tool such as the Braden scale.

- o Clean and dry the skin immediately following urine or stool incontinence.

- o Keep linens dry and wrinkle free.

- o Apply moisture barrier creams to the skin of clients who are incontinent.

- o Use tepid water (not hot), use minimal scrubbing, and pat the skin dry.

- Medications

  - o Antimicrobial Therapy

    - Antimicrobial therapy kills or inhibits the growth of microorganisms such as bacteria, fungi, viruses, and protozoans. Antimicrobial medications either kill pathogens or prevent their growth.

    - Nursing Considerations

      - □ Administer antimicrobial therapy as prescribed.

      - □ Monitor for medication effectiveness (reduced fever, increased level of comfort, decreasing white blood cell count).

      - □ Maintain medication schedule to assure consistent blood levels of antibiotic.

  - o Antipyretics (acetaminophen, aspirin) are used for fever and discomfort as prescribed.

    - Nursing Considerations

      - □ Monitor fever to determine effectiveness.

      - □ Monitor client's temperature fluctuations.

  - o Analgesics (hydrocodone [Vicodin] and morphine).

    - Nursing Considerations

      - □ Administer analgesics therapy as prescribed.

      - □ Monitor effectiveness of medication related to pain.

      - □ Monitor level of consciousness, especially respiratory distress with morphine.

- Interdisciplinary Care

  - o Request referral services, such as home health, nutritional services, pharmacy services, or wound care consultants, to provide items such as wound dressing materials.

  - o Contact community outreach programs, such as Meals on Wheels, or a nutritionist to provide meals high in protein and vitamin C to promote wound healing.

- Care After Discharge

  - o Client Education

    - Instruct clients on how to perform wound care.

    - Vitamin C to promote wound healing. to promote wound healing

    - Encourage clients to take vitamins and supplements to promote wound healing.

- Remind clients to keep skin clean and dry.
- Remind clients to report any signs of infection or further skin breakdown.
- Client Outcomes
  - The client will have improved skin integrity.
  - The client will be free of infection.
  - The client will be free of pain.

Complications

- Dehiscence is a partial or total rupture (separation) of a sutured wound, usually with separation of underlying skin layers. Evisceration is a dehiscence that involves the protrusion of visceral organs through a wound opening. It is usually caused by the increased flow of serosanguineous fluid about 3 to 11 days postoperatively.
  - Signs/symptoms of dehiscence include:
    - A significant increase in the flow of serosanguineous fluid on the wound dressings
    - Immediate history of sudden straining (coughing, sneezing, vomiting)
    - Clients reporting a change or "popping" or "giving way" in the wound area
    - Visualization of viscera
  - Evisceration/dehiscence requires emergency treatment.
  - Nursing Actions
    - Call for help.
    - Stay with the client.
    - Cover the wound and any protruding organs with sterile towels or dressings that have been soaked in a sterile 0.9% sodium chloride solution. Do not attempt to reinsert the organs.
    - Position the client supine with the hips and knees bent.
    - Observe the client for signs of shock.
    - Maintain a calm environment.

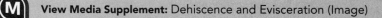

View Media Supplement: Dehiscence and Evisceration (Image)

- Infection
  - Risk factors
    - Extremes in age (immature immune system, decreased immune function)
    - Impaired circulation and oxygenation (COPD, peripheral vascular disease)
    - Wound condition/nature (gunshot wound vs. surgical incision)
    - Impaired/suppressed immune system

UNIT 11	NURSING CARE OF CLIENTS WITH INTEGUMENTARY DISORDERS

Chapter 71   Chronic Skin Conditions

 Overview

- Psoriasis is a skin disorder that is characterized by scaly, dermal patches and is caused by an overproduction of keratin. This overproduction can occur at a rate up to nine times the rate of normal cells. It is thought to be an autoimmune disorder and has periods of exacerbations and remissions.

- In some clients, psoriasis can also affect the joints, causing arthritis-type changes and pain.

> **View Media Supplement:** Psoriasis (Image)

- Seborrheic dermatitis is a skin disorder caused by inflammation of areas of the skin that contain a high number of sebaceous glands. It is characterized by papulopustules (oily form) or flaky plaques (dry form) that form on the surface of the skin. Dandruff is a type of seborrheic dermatitis.

- Seborrheic dermatitis also occurs for periods of time interspersed with symptom-free periods.

PSORIASIS

Data Collection

- Risk Factors

  o   Genetics

  o   Stress

  o   Seasons

  o   Hormones

- Subjective Data

  o   Exacerbation and remission of pruritic lesions

- Objective Data
  - Physical Findings
    - Scaly patches
    - Bleeding stimulated by removal of scales
    - Skin lesions primarily on the scalp, elbows and knees, and genitals
    - Pitting, crumbling nails

Collaborative Care

- Medications
  - Topical Corticosteroids – Triamcinolone acetonide (Kenalog)
    - Reduces secondary inflammatory response of lesions
    - Nursing Actions
      - Observe skin for thinning, striae with high-potency corticosteroids.
    - Client Education
      - Instruct clients to apply high-potency corticosteroids as prescribed to prevent side effects (avoid use on face or in skin folds, and take periodic medication vacations).
      - Instruct clients to use occlusive dressings on smaller areas, gloves on the hands, and socks on the feet after applying medication to increase absorption if prescribed.
  - Tar Preparations – Coal Tar (Balnetar)
    - Suppresses cell division and decreases inflammation and itching
    - May stain skin and hair
    - May stimulate growth of skin cancers
    - Nursing Actions
      - Instruct clients on proper application.
      - Instruct clients on how to check for cancerous lesions.
    - Client Education
      - Due to odor and staining, clients should apply this product at night and cover areas of body with old pajamas, gloves, and socks.
  - Topical epidermopoiesis suppressive medications – Calcipotriene (Dovonex), tazarotene (Tazorac)
    - Reduces accelerated development of epidermal cells
    - Not recommended for older adults
    - Tazarotene (Tazorac) may cause birth defects. Women should be advised to use birth control during use.

- Nursing Actions
    - Calcipotriene (Dovonex) – Monitor for symptoms of hypercalcemia (elevated serum calcium, muscle weakness, fatigue, anorexia).
- Client Education
    - Instruct clients to avoid using the product on the face or in skin folds.
    - Instruct clients that burning and stinging can occur upon application.
    - Instruct clients to not use the product concurrently with corticosteroids.
    - Tazarotene (Tazorac) – Advise clients to use sunscreen and avoid sun exposure.
  - Cytotoxic medications (severe, intractable cases) – Methotrexate (Mexate), azathioprine (Imuran), cyclosporine (Neoral)
    - Reduces turnover of epidermal cells
    - Contraindicated in pregnant women
- Nursing Actions
    - Monitor laboratory tests for organ toxicity and bone marrow suppression.
- Client Education
    - Instruct clients to avoid alcohol while taking this medication.
    - Advise clients to monitor for fever, sore throat, increased bleeding or bruising, and fatigue.

- Therapeutic Procedures
  - PUVA - Psoralen (photosensitizing medication) and ultraviolet light A
    - Psoralen is given 2 hr before light treatments.
    - Treatments are given 2 to 3 times per week, avoiding consecutive days.
- Nursing Actions
    - Monitor the skin's response to light.
    - Ensure that clients wear eye protection during treatment.
- Client Education
    - Instruct clients to notify the provider of extreme redness, swelling, and discomfort.
  - Oil or coal tar baths
    - Removal of scales can be done using oil or coal tar bath.
    - Treatments are done on a regular basis.
- Client Education
    - Reinforce to clients how to add oil/tar to water and remove scales using a soft brush after soaking followed by acid based emollient.

- Client Outcomes

  - The client will experience a decrease in the number and size of the lesions.

  - The client will verbalize increased coping with chronic condition.

  - The client will experience extended periods of remission from disease.

SEBORRHEIC DERMATITIS

Data Collection

- Risk Factors

  - Genetics

  - Stress

  - Hormones

  - Older adults can develop seborrheic keratoses, which are more plaque-like in appearance.

  View Media Supplement: Seborrheic Keratoses (Image)

- Subjective Data

  - Report of periods of exacerbations and remissions

  - Pruritic lesions

- Objective Data

  - Physical Findings

    - Waxy- or flaky-appearing plaques and/or scales

    - Skin lesions primarily on the oily areas of the body (scalp, forehead, nose, axilla, groin)

    - Seborrheic keratoses lesions may be pigmented tan, brown, or black.

Collaborative Care

- Medications

  - Topical corticosteroids

    - Reduces secondary inflammatory response of lesions

    - Client Education

      - Instruct clients to avoid getting medication in the eyes or skin folds.

- o Antiseborrheic shampoos
  - ▪ Contain selenium sulfide, sulfur, or salicylic acid
  - ▪ Client education
    - □ Clients should use at least three times per week.
    - □ Clients should leave shampoo on for 3 to 5 min.
- Care After Discharge
  - o Client Education
    - ▪ Encourage clients to keep skin dry.
    - ▪ Recommend that clients avoid overheating and perspiring.
    - ▪ Instruct clients not to scratch pruritic lesions.
- Client Outcomes
  - o The client will report decreased pruritus of affected areas.
  - o The client will report increased periods of remissions.

Ⓐ **APPLICATION EXERCISES**

1. A nurse is caring for a client who has a long history of psoriasis and has consented to phototherapy with ultraviolet light A (PUVA). Which of the following information should the nurse reinforce about this type of therapy?

    A. PUVA will need to be done every night.

    B. Avoid NSAIDs during treatment.

    C. A medication will be given to enhance photosensitivity.

    D. Gently remove scales on lesions after each treatment.

2. A nurse is caring for a client who has been prescribed topical corticosteroids. Which of the following should the nurse reinforce the client to do to enhance the efficacy of the medication? (Select all that apply.)

    _____   Apply 3 to 4 times per day.

    _____   Apply an occlusive dressing after application.

    _____   Wear gloves after application for lesions on the hands.

    _____   Avoid using the medication in the skin folds.

    _____   Avoid applying close to the eyes.

3. A nurse is caring for a client who has been using a shampoo to treat seborrhea of the scalp. Which of the following instructions should the nurse reinforce to the client to enhance the efficacy of the medication?

    A. Scrub your scalp vigorously after application.

    B. Follow the shampoo with a conditioner.

    C. Use shampoo once a week

    D. Leave the shampoo in for at least 3 to 5 min.

(A) APPLICATION EXERCISES ANSWER KEY

1. A nurse is caring for a client who has a long history of psoriasis and has consented to phototherapy with ultraviolet light A (PUVA). Which of the following information should the nurse reinforce about this type of therapy?

   A. PUVA will need to be done every night.

   B. Avoid NSAIDs during treatment.

   C. A medication will be given to enhance photosensitivity.

   D. Gently remove scales on lesions after each treatment.

   PUVA treatments involve taking a medication, such as a psoralen, to enhance photosensitivity. It is given 2 hr prior to the PUVA treatment. This type of light treatment decreases cellular proliferation. Treatments are given 2 to 3 times per week, avoiding consecutive days. There are no contraindications to taking NSAIDs during treatment. Do not remove scales on the lesions after each treatment.

   (N) NCLEX® Connection: Pharmacological Therapies, Expected Actions/Outcomes

2. A nurse is caring for a client who has been prescribed topical corticosteroids. Which of the following should the nurse reinforce the client to do to enhance the efficacy of the medication? (Select all that apply.)

	Apply 3 to 4 times per day.
X	**Apply an occlusive dressing after application.**
X	**Wear gloves after application for lesions on the hands.**
X	**Avoid using the medication in the skin folds.**
X	**Avoid applying close to the eyes.**

   Topical corticosteroids can be used over a period of several months for chronic skin disorders. The efficacy of topical corticosteroids can be enhanced by using occlusive dressings that enhance the exposure of the lesions to the medication. If the lesions are on the hands, gloves should be worn after application. Do not apply corticosteroids close to the eyes due to risk of cataracts or skin folds due to risk of yeast infections. Only apply topical corticosteroids 2 times per day and periodically stop to prevent development of local and systemic side effects.

   (N) NCLEX® Connection: Pharmacological Therapies, Medication Administration

3. A nurse is caring for a client who has been using a shampoo to treat seborrhea of the scalp. Which of the following instructions should the nurse reinforce to the client to enhance the efficacy of the medication?

    A. Scrub your scalp vigorously after application.

    B. Follow the shampoo with a conditioner.

    C. Use shampoo once a week

    D. Leave the shampoo in for at least 3 to 5 min.

To enhance the efficacy of the shampoo it must be used at least 3 times a week leaving it in for 3 to 5 min. Scrubbing the scalp vigorously and using a conditioner does not enhance the efficacy.

Ⓝ NCLEX® Connection: Pharmacological Therapies, Medication Administration

UNIT 11	NURSING CARE OF CLIENTS WITH INTEGUMENTARY DISORDERS
Chapter 72	Skin Cancer

Overview

- Sunlight exposure is the leading cause of skin cancer. The most effective strategy for prevention of skin cancer is avoidance or reduction of skin exposure to sunlight.

- Precancerous skin lesions, called actinic keratoses, are common in people with chronically sun-damaged skin, such as older adults.

- There are three types of skin cancer:

  o Squamous cell carcinoma is a cancer of the top layer of the epidermis that can be localized, but it may metastasize to other tissue and organs.

  o Basal cell carcinoma is a cancer of the basal cell layer (under the squamous layer) of the epidermis, that can damage surrounding tissue and can advance to include underlying structures. This type of cancer is not usually metastatic, but the rate of recurrence is very high.

  o Malignant melanoma is an aggressive, metastatic cancer that originates in the melanin-producing cells of the epidermis.

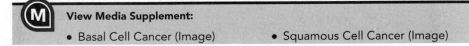

View Media Supplement:
- Basal Cell Cancer (Image)   • Squamous Cell Cancer (Image)

Health Promotion and Disease Prevention

- Advise clients to:

  o Limit exposure to sunlight, especially between 1000 and 1500 hr.

  o Use sunblock that has an SPF of at least 15, with both UVA and UVB protection. Sunblock should be reapplied at least every 2 hr.

  o Wear protective clothing, hats, sunglasses, and lip balm that has an SPF of at least 15.

  o Avoid tanning beds/equipment.

  o Examine body monthly for suspicious lesions and develop a body map (diagram of skin scars or lesions) to monitor for changes.

Data Collection

- Risk Factors

  - Exposure to ultraviolet light (such as natural light or tanning beds/equipment) over long periods of time

  - Chronic skin irritation and burn scars

  - Fair complexion (blonde or red hair, fair skin, freckles, blue eyes) with a tendency to burn easily

  - Presence of several large or many small moles

  - Family or personal history of melanoma

  - Residing in locations in upper elevations or close proximity to equator (thinner layer of ozone and rays of sun are strongest)

- Subjective Data

  - Report of change in appearance of mole or lesion

- Objective Data

  - Physical Findings

    - Basal and squamous cell carcinomas

      □ Small, waxy nodule with small, superficial blood vessels (basal cell)

      □ Rough, scaly lesion that may bleed and has a central area of ulceration or crusting (squamous cell)

      □ Size varies in relation to duration of lesion

    - Melanoma

      □ Check for suspicious lesions on the: face and scalp, the shoulders and back, legs, feet, and between the toes. Lesions may occur on the palms and soles of individuals who have dark skin. Satellite lesions (secondary lesions in close proximity to the primary lesion) may also be present.

      □ The ABCDs of suspicious lesions

        ▸ Asymmetry – One side does not match the other

        ▸ Borders – Ragged, notched, irregular, or blurred edges

        ▸ Color – Lack of uniformity in pigmentation (shades of tan, brown, or black)

        ▸ Diameter – Width greater than 6 mm, or about the size of a pencil eraser or a pea

 View Media Supplement: Melanomas (Images)

□ Palpate regional lymph nodes for enlargement.

□ Because of the cumulative effects of sun damage over the lifespan, screening for suspicious lesions is an essential part of the routine physical assessment of older adult clients.

○ Laboratory Tests

- No test is available to help diagnose skin cancer. If melanoma is diagnosed, blood tests will be ordered (CBC, liver) to check for organ involvement.

○ Diagnostic Procedures

- Biopsy

□ A biopsy is the extraction of a very small amount of skin tissue by excision or needle aspiration, to definitively diagnose cell type and to confirm or rule out malignancy. Biopsies can also be performed on bone marrow, cervical, endometrial, brain, liver, lung, pleural, renal, skin, and lymph node tissue. Biopsies can be performed with local anesthesia or moderate sedation in an ambulatory setting, intraoperatively, and/or during scope procedures.

□ Indications

▸ Evidence of skin lesion, which may include an area of discoloration that is thickened, thinned, raised, flat, rough, painful, open, dry and/or itchy.

□ Interpretation of Findings

▸ After a biopsy is completed, the tissue sample is sent to pathology for interpretation.

□ Preprocedure

▸ Nursing Actions

▷ Verify clients have signed the informed consent form.

▷ Explain the procedure.

▷ Establish a sterile field and assemble supplies and instruments, including local anesthetic, specimen containers, and dressings.

□ Client Education

▸ Reinforce to clients about what to expect about the test/procedure.

▸ Inform clients about what to expect in regard to the formation of a scar.

▸ Instruct clients how to perform dressing changes and care for wound.

□ Intraprocedure

▸ Nursing Actions

▷ Assist the provider with the test/procedure as needed.

▷ As appropriate, apply pressure to the biopsy site to control bleeding.

▷ As appropriate, place a sterile dressing over the biopsy site.

▫ Types of biopsies

INSTRUMENT		PROCEDURE
Punch	A circular instrument (punch) that is 2 to 6 mm in diameter	• The punch is placed over the lesion and slowly rotated to remove a small circle of tissue to the depth of subcutaneous fat. • The area may be sutured.
Shave	Scalpel or razor blade	• The skin elevated above the surrounding tissue by an injection of a local anesthetic is shaved off. • Use for superficial or raised lesions
Excision	Scalpel	• A deep incision is made and then sutured after the entire lesion is removed. • Use for large or deep lesions.

▫ Postprocedure

▸ Nursing Actions

▹ Monitor clients for pain and bleeding at the biopsy site.

▹ Provide analgesia for pain management.

▸ Client Education

▹ Reinforce to clients to check the incision daily. The incision should be clean, dry, and intact.

▹ Reinforce to clients to report excessive bleeding and/or signs of infection (fever, increased redness, swelling, presence of purulent drainage) to the provider.

▹ If sutures are in place, remind clients to return in 7 to 10 days to have them removed.

▹ Ensure that clients are knowledgeable about how to assess for suspicious lesions on a regular basis.

▫ Complications

▸ Infection

▹ Infection may occur after a biopsy.

◆ Nursing Actions

◇ Monitor the biopsy site for signs of infection. Monitor for fever and increase in WBC count.

◇ Apply an antibacterial ointment.

◇ Keep the incisional site clean and dry.

▸ Bleeding

▹ Bleeding can occur from the site and needs to be reported to the provider immediately.

Collaborative Care

- Therapeutic Procedures

    o Cryosurgery

        ■ Freeze tissue by applying liquid nitrogen (-200° C).

        ■ Client Education

            □ Reinforce to clients to cleanse with hydrogen peroxide and apply a topical antimicrobial until healed.

    o Topical chemotherapy

        ■ Topical chemotherapy with 5-fluorouracil cream for treatment of actinic keratoses

        ■ Client Education

            □ Prepare clients for extended treatment that will cause the lesion to weep, crust, and erode.

            □ Reassure clients that the appearance will improve after treatment.

    o Interferon

        ■ Used for postoperative treatment of stage III or greater melanomas

        ■ Nursing Actions

            □ Report and provide relief for side effects or toxic effects of chemotherapy.

            □ Encourage adequate nutrition and fluid intake.

- Surgical Interventions

    o Excision

        ■ The extent of excision is based on the size and depth of the invasion.

        ■ Sentinel lymph node may also be biopsied to assess for metastasis.

        ■ The incision will be closed with sutures if possible. A skin graft may be necessary for large areas.

        ■ Client Education

            □ Advise clients about postoperative wound care and care of the skin graft if used.

- Client Outcomes

    o The client will identify suspicious lesions during the early stage and notify the provider.

    o The client will take precautions to prevent unnecessary exposure to ultraviolet light and direct sunlight.

(A) APPLICATION EXERCISES

Scenario: A nurse is caring for a client who comes to the clinic to undergo a procedure to remove a large mole from his right shoulder. He reports the mole has bothered him for a couple of weeks, ever since he scraped it while painting the outside of a house. He also reports working on a daily basis without wearing a shirt. Because of the injury, the mole has been oozing and crusting.

1. When conducting an initial interview, which of the following data should a nurse collect in order to determine the client's risk factors for malignant melanoma? (Select all that apply.)

    _____ Recent changes in size, color, or shape of the lesion

    _____ Geographic location where client previously and currently resides

    _____ Family history of colon cancer

    _____ Recreational activities

    _____ Use of oral corticosteroids

    _____ Occupational exposure to chemicals

2. Which of the following are characteristics of the client's mole that might suggest it is malignant? (Select all that apply.)

    _____ Mole is 4 mm in diameter

    _____ Mole is located in an area that receives daily exposure to the sun

    _____ Border of mole is irregular

    _____ Recurrent oozing and crusting of the mole

    _____ Color is consistent throughout mole

3. A nurse working in a dermatology clinic knows that which of the following has the highest risk for metastases?

    A. Melanoma

    B. Basal cell carcinoma

    C. Squamous cell carcinoma

    D. Actinic keratosis

(A) APPLICATION EXERCISES ANSWER KEY

Scenario: A nurse is caring for a client who comes to the clinic to undergo a procedure to remove a large mole from his right shoulder. He reports the mole has bothered him for a couple of weeks, ever since he scraped it while painting the outside of a house. He also reports working on a daily basis without wearing a shirt. Because of the injury, the mole has been oozing and crusting.

1. When conducting an initial interview, which of the following data should a nurse collect in order to determine the client's risk factors for malignant melanoma? (Select all that apply.)

   __X__   **Recent changes in size, color, or shape of the lesion**

   __X__   **Geographic location where client previously and currently resides**

   _____   Family history of colon cancer

   __X__   **Recreational activities**

   _____   Use of oral corticosteroids

   __X__   **Occupational exposure to chemicals**

   Recent changes in size, color, or shape of the lesion, geographic location where the client previously and currently resides, recreational activities, and occupational exposure to chemicals are important questions to ask because they are risk factors for malignant melanoma. A family history of colon cancer and use of oral corticosteroids are not risk factors for developing malignant melanoma.

   (N) NCLEX® Connection: Health Promotion and Maintenance, Health Promotion/Disease Prevention

2. Which of the following are characteristics of the client's mole that might suggest it is malignant? (Select all that apply.)

   _____   Mole is 4 mm in diameter

   __X__   **Mole is located in an area that receives daily exposure to the sun**

   __X__   **Border of mole is irregular**

   __X__   **Recurrent oozing and crusting of the mole**

   _____   Color is consistent throughout mole

   Injury to a lesion located on a part of the body prone to chronic sun exposure, border irregularity, and oozing and crusting suggest a malignancy. A mole 5 mm or less in diameter that is consistent in color does not suggest malignancy.

   (N) NCLEX® Connection: Physiological Adaptation, Pathophysiology

3. A nurse working in a dermatology clinic knows that which of the following has the highest risk for metastases?

   A. Melanoma

   B. Basal cell carcinoma

   C. Squamous cell carcinoma

   D. Actinic keratosis

   A melanoma has the highest risk of metastasis. Basal cell carcinoma rarely metastasizes. Squamous cell carcinomas can metastasize but do so much less quickly than a melanoma. Actinic keratosis is a precancerous lesion and poses no risk for metastases until it changes into a malignant lesion.

   Ⓝ NCLEX® Connection: Physiological Adaptation, Pathophysiology

UNIT 11	NURSING CARE OF CLIENTS WITH INTEGUMENTARY DISORDERS
Chapter 73	Burns

Overview

- Thermal, chemical, electrical, and radioactive agents can cause burns, which result in cellular destruction of the skin layers and underlying tissue. The type of burn and the severity of the burn impact the treatment plan.

    o Thermal burns occur when there is exposure to flames, steam, or hot liquids. This type of burn occurs most frequently, especially in older adults and children.

    o Chemical burns occur when there is exposure to a caustic agent. Cleaning agents used in the home (drain cleaner, bleach) and agents used in the industrial setting (caustic soda, sulfuric acid) cause chemical burns.

    o Electrical burns occur when an electrical current passes through the body and can result in severe damage, including loss of organ function, tissue destruction with subsequent need for amputation of a limb, and cardiac and/or respiratory arrest.

    o Radiation burns most frequently occur as a result of therapeutic treatment for cancer or from sunburn.

- In addition to destruction of body tissue, a burn injury results in the loss of:

    o Temperature regulation

    o Sweat and sebaceous gland function

    o Sensory function

    o Body heat, which increases metabolic rate

- The severity of the burn is based on the:

    o Percentage of total body surface area (TBSA) – Standardized charts for age groups are used to identify the extent of the injury.

    o Depth of the burn

    o Body location of the burn

    o Age of clients

    o Causative agent

    o Presence of other injuries

    o Involvement of the respiratory system

    o Overall health of clients

- Three Phases of Burn Care
    - Emergent (Resuscitative phase)
        - First 24 to 48 hr after the burn occurs
    - Acute
        - Begins when fluid resuscitation is finished
        - Ends when the wound is covered by tissue
    - Rehabilitative
        - Begins when most of the burn area is healed
        - Ends when reconstructive and corrective procedures are complete (may last for years)

Data Collection

- Risk Factors

    (G)
    - Age greater than 60 years
    - Burn involves greater than 40% total body surface area
    - Inhalation injury
    - Age

    (G)
        - Older adults are at higher risk for damage to subcutaneous tissue, muscle, connective tissue, and bone because their skin is thinner.
        - Older adults have a higher risk for complications from burns because of chronic illnesses (e.g., diabetes mellitus, cardiovascular disease).
- Subjective Data
    - To evaluate the extent of damage when observing burns, it is important to know:
        - The type of burning agent (dry heat, moist heat, chemical, electrical, ionizing radiation)
        - The duration of contact
        - The area of the body in which the burn occurred

- Objective Data

  o Physical Findings

DEPTH	AREA INVOLVED/ APPEARANCE	SENSATION/HEALING	EXAMPLE
Superficial – damage to epidermis	• Pink to red, tender, no blisters, mild edema, and no eschar	• Painful • Heals within 5 to 10 days • No scarring	• Sunburn
Superficial partial thickness – damage to the entire epidermis and some parts of the dermis	• Pink to red, blisters, mild to moderate edema, and no eschar	• Painful • Heals within 14 days • No scarring	• Flame or burn scalds
Deep partial thickness – damage to entire epidermis and deep into the dermis	• Red to white, with moderate edema, free of blisters, and soft and dry eschar	• Painful and sensitive to touch • Heals within 14 to 36 days • Scarring likely • Possible grafting involved	• Flame and burn scalds • Grease, tar, or chemical burns • Exposure to hot objects for prolonged time
Full thickness – damage to the entire epidermis and dermis, and may extend into the subcutaneous tissue. Nerve damage also occurs.	• Red to tan, black, brown, or white • Free from blisters, severe edema, and hard and inelastic eschar	• Pain may or may not be present. • As burn heals, painful sensations return and severity of pain increases. • Heals within weeks to months • Scarring • Grafting required	• Burn scalds • Grease, tar, chemical, or electrical burns • Exposure to hot objects for prolonged time
Deep full thickness – damage to all layers of skin and extends to muscle, tendons and bones.	• Black, no edema	• Heals within weeks to months • Scarring • Grafting required	• Chemical burns

Ⓜ **View Media Supplement:** Burn Staging (Images)

- Inhalation damage findings may include singed nasal hair, eye brows, and eye lashes; a sooty appearance to sputum; hoarseness; and wheezing. Clinical manifestations may not be evident for 24 to 48 hr and are seen as wheezing, hoarseness, and increased respiratory secretions.

- Carbon monoxide inhalation (suspected if the injury took place in an enclosed area) findings include erythema (pink or cherry red color of skin) and upper airway edema, followed by sloughing of the respiratory tract mucosa.

  □ Hypotension, tachycardia, and decreased cardiac output may occur indicating hypovolemia or shock.

  o Laboratory Tests

  - White blood cell (WBC) count – identifies infection

  - Hgb and Hct – may be decreased due to blood loss

  - Serum electrolytes – imbalances such as hyperkalemia or hyponatremia

  - Blood glucose – elevated due to stress response

  - ABGs – slight hypoxemia and metabolic acidosis

  - Total protein and albumin – low due to fluid loss

  - BUN – elevated due to enhanced metabolism of proteins

Collaborative Care

- Nursing Care

  o Minor Burns

  - Stop the burning process.

    □ Remove clothing or jewelry that might conduct heat.

    □ Apply cool water soaks or run cool water over injury; do not use ice.

    □ Flush chemical burns with large amounts of water.

    □ Cover the burn with clean cloth to prevent contamination and hypothermia.

    □ Provide warmth.

    □ If necessary, have client go to a health care facility for medical care.

  - Provide analgesia.

  - Cleanse with mild soap and tepid water (avoid excess friction).

  - Use antimicrobial ointment.

  - Apply dressing (nonadherent, hydrocolloid) if the burn area is irritated by clothing.

  - Educate families to avoid using greasy lotions or butter on burn.

- Educate families to monitor for signs of infection.
- Check immunization status for tetanus and determine need for immunization.

○ Moderate and Major Burns

- Maintain airway and ventilation.
- Provide humidified supplemental oxygen as ordered.
- Monitor vital signs.
- Maintain cardiac output.
  □ Monitor fluid replacement.
    ‣ Rapid fluid replacement is needed during the emergent phase to maintain tissue perfusion and prevent hypovolemic (burn) shock.
    ‣ Fluid resuscitation is based on individual client needs (evaluation of urine output, cardiac output, blood pressure, status of electrolytes).
    ‣ Isotonic crystalloid solutions, such as 0.9% sodium chloride, or lactated Ringer's solution, are used during the early stage of burn recovery.
    ‣ Colloid solutions, such as albumin, or synthetic plasma expanders (Hespan, Plasma-Lyte), may be used after the first 24 hr of burn recovery.
    ‣ Maintain urine output of 30 mL/hr (0.5 to 1.0 mL/kg/hr).
    ‣ Monitor clients receiving blood products.
  □ Monitor for manifestations of shock.
    ‣ Alterations in sensorium (confusion)
    ‣ Increased capillary refill time
    ‣ Urine output less than 30 mL/hr
    ‣ Spiking fever
    ‣ Decreased bowel sounds
    ‣ Blood pressure may remain normotensive, even in hypovolemia.
    ‣ Notify the provider of findings.

○ Pain Management

- Establish ongoing monitoring of pain and effectiveness of pain treatment.
- Monitor clients receiving IV bolus pain medications or IV patient-controlled analgesia.
- Avoid IM or subcutaneous injections.
- Monitor for respiratory depression when using opioid analgesics.

- Administer pain medication prior to dressing changes or procedures.
- Use nonpharmacologic methods for pain control, such as guided imagery, music therapy, and therapeutic touch, to enhance the effects of analgesic medications and lead to more effective pain management.

○ Prevent Infection

- Follow standard precautions when performing wound care.
- Restrict plants and flowers due to the risk of contact with pseudomonas.
- Restrict consumption of fresh fruits and vegetables.
- Limit visitors.
- Use reverse isolation if prescribed.
- Monitor for signs and symptoms of infection and report to provider.
- Use client-designated equipment such as BP cuffs, thermometers.
- Administer tetanus toxoid if indicated.
- Administer antibiotics if infection present.

○ Nutritional Support

- Encourage increased caloric intake to meet increased metabolic demands and prevent hypoglycemia.
- Encourage increased protein intake to prevent tissue breakdown and to promote healing.
- Encourage vitamin C intake for wound healing.
- Provide enteral therapy if necessary due to decreased gastrointestinal motility and increased caloric needs.
- Monitor clients receiving TPN.

○ Restoration of Mobility

- Maintain correct body alignment, splint extremities, and facilitate position changes to prevent contractures.
- Maintain active and passive range of motion.
- Assist with ambulation as soon as clients are stable.
- Apply pressure dressings to prevent contractures and scarring.
- Closely monitor areas at high risk for pressure sores (heels, sacrum, back of head).

○ Psychological Support

- Provide emotional support.
- Assist with coping.

- Medications
  - Topical Agents

ANTIMICROBIAL CREAM	USES AND ADVANTAGES	DISADVANTAGES
Silver nitrate 0.5%	• Use on wounds exposed to air, or with modified or occlusive dressing. • May affect joint movement • Reduces fluid evaporation • Bacteriostatic against pseudomonas and staphylococcus • Inexpensive	• Does not penetrate eschar • Stains clothing and linen • Discolors wound, making observation difficult • Painful on application
Silver sulfadiazine 1% (Silvadene)	• Use with occlusive dressings. • Maintains joint mobility • Effective against gram-negative bacteria, gram-positive bacteria, and yeast	• May cause transient neutropenia • Contraindicated with allergies to sulfa • Does not penetrate eschar • Painful to remove from wound • Decreases granulocyte formation
Mafenide acetate (Sulfamylon)	• Use on wounds exposed to air. • Use as a solution for occlusive dressings to keep the dressing moist. • Penetrates eschar and goes into underlying tissues • Effective with electrical and infected wounds • Biostatic against gram-negative and gram-positive bacteria	• Painful to apply and remove • May cause metabolic acidosis or hyperpnea • Inhibits wound healing • Hypersensitivity may develop
Bacitracin	• Use on wounds exposed to air or with modified dressings. • Maintains joint mobility • Bacteriostatic against gram-positive organisms • Painless and easy to apply	• Limited effectiveness on gram-negative organisms

- Morphine
  - Analgesia
  - Nursing Considerations
    - Monitor for respiratory depression.
    - Monitor pain relief.
  - Client Education
    - Educate clients on the safety precautions needed with opioid administration.
- Midazolam (Versed), fentanyl (Sublimaze), propofol (Diprivan), and nitrous oxide
  - Sedation and analgesia
  - Nursing Considerations
    - Identify the need for sedation.
    - Monitor pain relief.
  - Client Education
    - Educate clients about the safety precautions needed with opioid administration.
- Interdisciplinary Care
  - Request referrals to a registered dietitian, social worker, home health nursing care, psychological counselor, or occupational/physical therapist if indicated.
  - Coordinate care with respiratory therapy to improve pulmonary function.
  - Initiate referral for home health nursing care.
  - Initiate referral to occupational therapy for evaluation of the home environment and assistance to relearn how to perform ADLs.
  - Initiate referral to social services for community support services
- Therapeutic Procedures
  - Wound Care
    - Nonsurgical management
    - Nursing Actions
      - Monitor pain and discomfort level.
      - Ensure clients are premedicated with analgesic and antipruritic agents as prescribed prior to all wound care.
      - Remove all previous dressings.
      - Observe for odors, drainage, and discharge.
      - Cleanse the wound as prescribed, removing all previous ointments (it is important to cleanse the wound thoroughly).

□ Assist with debridement.

▸ Mechanical – Use of scissors and forceps to cut away the dead tissue during the hydrotherapy treatment

▸ Hydrotherapy (clients placed in a warm tub of water or use of warm running water, as if to shower) to cleanse the wound.

▷ Assist with hydrotherapy by using mild soap or detergent to gently wash burns and then rinsing with room-temperature water. Usually performed once or twice a day for up to 20 min.

▷ Encourage clients to exercise joints during the hydrotherapy treatment.

▷ Ensure that clients do not become hypothermic during the treatment.

▸ Enzymatic – Apply a topical enzyme to break down and remove dead tissue.

□ Apply a thin layer of topical antibiotic ointment as prescribed and cover with dressing, using surgical aseptic technique.

○ Skin Coverings

■ Biologic skin coverings are temporarily used to promote healing of large burns.

□ Allograft (homograft) – Skin is obtained from human cadavers that is used for partial- and full-thickness burn wounds.

□ Xenograft (heterograft) – Obtained from animals, such as pigs, for partial-thickness burn wounds.

□ Amnion – Obtained from human placenta; requires frequent changes.

□ Synthetic skin coverings – Used for partial-thickness burn wounds.

■ Permanent skin coverings may be the treatment of choice for burns covering large areas of the body.

□ Autografts

▸ Sheet graft – Sheet of skin used to cover wound

▸ Mesh graft – Sheet of skin placed in mesher so skin graft has small slits in it; allows graft to cover larger areas of the burn wound

□ Artificial skin – Synthetic product that is used for partial- and full-thickness burn wounds (healing is faster)

□ Cultured epithelium – Epithelial cells cultured for use when grafting sites are limited

■ Nursing Actions

□ Maintain immobilization of graft site.

□ Elevate extremity.

□ Provide wound care to the donor site.

□ Administer pain medication.

□ Monitor for signs of infection before and after skin coverings or grafts are applied.

▸ Discoloration of unburned skin surrounding burn wound

▸ Green color to subcutaneous fat

▸ Degeneration of granulation tissue

▸ Development of subeschar hemorrhage

▸ Hyperventilation indicating systemic involvement of infection

▸ Unstable body temperature

■ Client Education

□ Instruct clients to keep extremity elevated.

□ Instruct clients to report signs and symptoms of infection.

- Care After Discharge

  ○ Client Education

    ■ Instruct clients to continue to perform range-of-motion exercises and to work with a physical therapist to prevent contractures.

    ■ Provide instructions about how to observe the wound for infection and how to perform wound care.

    ■ Instruct clients to have adequate number and placement of fire extinguishers and smoke alarms in the home and that they are operable.

    ■ Instruct clients to keep emergency numbers near the phone.

    ■ Have clients develop an exit and meeting plan for fires.

    ■ Review with clients of all ages that in the event that clothing or skin is on fire, they should "Stop, drop, and roll" to extinguish the fire.

    ■ Instruct clients to store matches and lighters out of reach and out of sight of adults who lack the ability to protect themselves.

    ■ Tell clients to reduce setting on water heater to no higher than 120° F.

    ■ Reinforce to clients to avoid sun exposure between 10 a.m. and 4 p.m., use sun block, and wear protective clothing.

    ■ Instruct clients to avoid using tanning beds.

    ■ Encourage clients to avoid smoking in bed and smoking when under the influence of alcohol or sedating medications.

  ○ Client Outcomes

    ■ The client remains free of complications.

    ■ The client is able to perform ADLs.

    ■ The client demonstrates wound care.

Complications

- Airway Injury

  o Thermal injuries to the airway may result from steam or chemical inhalation, aspiration of scalding liquid, and explosion while breathing. If the injury took place in an enclosed space, carbon monoxide poisoning should be suspected.

  o Clinical manifestations may be delayed for 24 to 48 hr.

  o Signs and symptoms include progressive hoarseness, brassy cough, difficulty swallowing, drooling, increased secretions, adventitious breath sounds, and expiratory sounds that include audible wheezes, crowing, and stridor.

  o Nursing Actions

    ▪ Maintain airway and ventilation, and provide oxygen as prescribed.

  o Client Education

    ▪ Educate clients and families about airway management, such as deep breathing, coughing, and elevating the head of the bed.

- Wound Infections

  o Nursing Actions

    ▪ Observe for discoloration, edema, odor, and drainage.

    ▪ Observe for fluctuations in temperature and heart rate.

    ▪ Obtain wound culture.

    ▪ Administer antibiotics as prescribed.

    ▪ Monitor laboratory results, observing for anemia and infection.

    ▪ Maintain surgical aseptic technique with dressing changes.

  o Client Education

    ▪ Educate clients and families on the importance of infection control.

Ⓐ **APPLICATION EXERCISES**

1. A nurse in a provider's office is collecting data from a client who has severe sunburn. Which of the following is the proper classification of this burn?

   A. Superficial

   B. Superficial partial-thickness

   C. Deep partial-thickness

   D. Full-thickness

2. A nurse is caring for a client who was admitted 24 hr ago with full thickness burns to 50% of his body. Which of the following are expected findings for this client? (Select all that apply.)

   _____ Hypertension

   _____ Bradycardia

   _____ Hyperkalemia

   _____ Hyponatremia

   _____ Decreased hematocrit

Scenario: A nurse is caring for a client who is to receive fentanyl (Sublimaze) for pain. The client was admitted to the hospital 24 hr ago with deep partial-thickness and full-thickness burns over 70% of his body.

3. Which of the following routes should be used for medication administration?

   A. Subcutaneous

   B. Intramuscular

   C. Intravenous

   D. Intraosseous

4. The nurse should implement which of the following interventions to prevent infection for the client? (Select all the apply.)

   _____ Decrease protein intake.

   _____ Decrease caloric intake.

   _____ Restrict number of visitors.

   _____ Restrict live flowers and plants.

   _____ Administer tetanus toxoid if indicated.

   _____ Apply topical antimicrobials.

   _____ Use client-designated equipment.

5. A nurse is caring for a client who sustained burns to 35% of his total body surface area. Of the burns, 20% are full-thickness. The burns are on the client's arms, face, neck, and shoulders. The client's voice seems hoarse, and he is wheezing with a brassy cough. The nurse recognizes that this data indicates an _____.

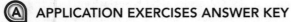

APPLICATION EXERCISES ANSWER KEY

1. A nurse in a provider's office is collecting data from a client who has severe sunburn. Which of the following is the proper classification of this burn?

    A. Superficial

    B. Superficial partial-thickness

    C. Deep partial-thickness

    D. Full-thickness

    Sunburn results in a superficial burn. A superficial partial-thickness burn can be caused by a flame or burn scald; a deep partial-thickness or full-thickness burn can be caused by grease or tar. Full thickness burns are caused by prolonged exposure to heat, chemicals, or electricity.

    NCLEX® Connection: Physiological Adaptation, Pathophysiology

2. A nurse is caring for a client who was admitted 24 hr ago with full thickness burns to 50% of his body. Which of the following are expected findings for this client? (Select all that apply.)

    _____ Hypertension

    _____ Bradycardia

    __X__ **Hyperkalemia**

    __X__ **Hyponatremia**

    _____ Decreased hematocrit

    A client who has partial-thickness and full-thickness burns to 40% of his body can experience shock. Immediately after the burn injury, fluids shift from the intracellular space into the interstitial space. Fluid leaks from the capillaries at the site of the burn and throughout the body. Due to the loss of fluids in the intracellular space and the intravascular space, the client experiences hypovolemia. In response to shock, the client develops hypotension and tachycardia. Leakage of fluid from the intracellular space causes hyperkalemia. Sodium is retained in the interstitial space, leading to hyponatremia. Due to hypovolemia, hematocrit is elevated.

    NCLEX® Connection: Physiological Adaptation, Fluid and Electrolyte Imbalances

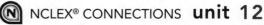

UNIT 12: NURSING CARE OF CLIENTS WiTH ENDOCRINE DISORDERS

- Endocrine Diagnostic Procedures
- Posterior Pituitary Disorders
- Thyroid Disorders
- Adrenal Disorders
- Diabetes Management

NCLEX® CONNECTIONS

When reviewing the chapters in this section, keep in mind the relevant sections of the NCLEX® outline, in particular:

CLIENT NEEDS: PHARMACOLOGICAL THERAPIES	CLIENT NEEDS: REDUCTION OF RISK POTENTIAL	CLIENT NEEDS: PHYSIOLOGICAL ADAPTATION
Relevant topics/tasks include:	Relevant topics/tasks include:	Relevant topics/tasks include:
• Adverse Effects/ Contraindications/Side Effects/Interactions	• Changes/Abnormalities in Vital Signs	• Alterations in Body Systems
○ Reinforce client teaching on possible effects of medications.	○ Compare vital signs to client baseline vital signs.	○ Provide care to correct client alteration in body system.
• Dosage Calculation	• Laboratory Values	• Fluid and Electrolyte Imbalances
○ Perform calculations needed for medication administration.	○ Compare client laboratory values to normal laboratory values.	○ Provide interventions to restore client fluid and/ or electrolyte balance.
• Medication Administration	• Therapeutic Procedures	• Medical Emergencies
○ Mix client medication from two vials as necessary.	○ Reinforce client teaching on treatments and procedures.	○ Notify primary health care provider about client unexpected response/emergency situation.

Overview

- The function of the endocrine system is evaluated primarily by using laboratory tests. These tests vary according to the organ or system involved.

- Many of these tests are blood tests used to determine an excess or lack of a particular hormone in the body. Some tests are used to stimulate a reaction in the body that will facilitate diagnosis of a particular disorder.

- Endocrine diagnostic procedures that nurses should be knowledgeable about include those used to diagnose disorders of the:

  o   Posterior pituitary gland

  o   Adrenal cortex

  o   Adrenal medulla

  o   Pancreas

  o   Thyroid and anterior pituitary glands

Posterior Pituitary Gland

- The posterior pituitary gland secretes the hormone vasopressin (antidiuretic hormone [ADH]). ADH increases permeability of the renal distal tubules, causing the kidneys to reabsorb water.

  o   A deficiency of ADH causes diabetes insipidus (DI), which is characterized by the excretion of a large quantity of dilute urine.

  o   Excessive secretion of ADH causes the syndrome of inappropriate antidiuretic hormone (SIADH). In SIADH, the kidneys retain water, urine becomes concentrated, output drops, and extracellular fluid volume is increased.

- Water deprivation test

  o   Easy and reliable. Dehydration is induced by withholding fluids. Urine output is measured and tested hourly.

  o   Indications

    ▪   This test is performed to diagnose DI.

- ○ Interpretation of Findings
  - ■ The test is positive for DI if the kidneys are unable to concentrate urine despite increased plasma osmolality.
    - □ Nursing Actions
      - ▸ Obtain baseline weight, vital signs, serum electrolytes and serum osmolarity, and urine-specific gravity and urine osmolarity.
      - ▸ Monitor vital signs, urine-specific gravity, and urine osmolarity hourly.
      - ▸ Monitor for severe dehydration.
        - ▹ Early indications may be orthostatic hypotension, tachycardia, and dizziness. The nurse should be prepared to discontinue the test if these indicators develop.
    - □ Client Education
      - ▸ Explain the test procedure to clients.
      - ▸ Advise clients to notify the nurse of any dizziness, headache, or nausea.
- ● Serum ADH, serum and urine electrolytes, and urine-specific gravity
  - ○ Indications
    - ■ These tests are performed to diagnose SIADH.

TEST	NORMAL REFERENCE RANGE	INTERPRETATION OF FINDINGS	NURSING ACTIONS
Serum ADH	• 0 to 4.7 pg/mL	• Increased serum ADH is expected with SIADH.	• Clients should fast and avoid stress for 12 hr prior to the test. • Some medications can interfere with the test. Review medications with the provider. • Blood is drawn and then transported to the laboratory within 10 min.
Serum electrolytes	• Sodium – 136 to 145 mEq/L • Potassium – 3.5 to 5.0 mEq/L • Chloride – 98 to 106 mEq/L • Magnesium – 1.3 to 2.1 mEq/L	• Low serum sodium is expected with SIADH.	• No pre- or postprocedure care required – samples of blood are analyzed for electrolyte components.

TEST	NORMAL REFERENCE RANGE	INTERPRETATION OF FINDINGS	NURSING ACTIONS
Urine electrolytes	• Urine sodium – 75 to 200 mEq/day • Urine potassium – 26 to123 mEq/day (intake dependent) • Urine chloride – 110 to 250 mEq/24 hr	• High urine sodium is expected with SIADH.	• No pre- or postprocedure care is required – samples of urine are analyzed for electrolyte components.
Urine-specific gravity	• 1.010 to 1.025	• The urine sample is analyzed for specific gravity. • A decrease in urine output and an increase in urine-specific gravity occur as a result of excess production of ADH.	• This test is usually performed in a laboratory, but can be done in the clinical unit using a calibrated hydrometer or a temperature-compensated refractometer.

Adrenal Cortex

- Cushing's disease and Cushing's syndrome (hypercortisolism) are characterized by a hyperfunctioning adrenal cortex and an excess production of cortisol. Addison's disease is characterized by hypofunctioning of the adrenal cortex and a consequent lack of adequate amounts of serum cortisol.

  o A CT scan and/or an MRI can be performed to determine if there is atrophy of the adrenal glands causing hypofunction.

- Dexamethasone suppression test

  o This test is performed to determine if dexamethasone, which is a steroid similar to cortisol, has an effect on cortisol levels. Typically, clients take a low or high dose of dexamethasone by mouth, and blood is drawn the next morning to determine if cortisol is present.

    ▪ A low dose of dexamethasone (Decadron) is given to screen a client for Cushing's disease; high doses are given to determine the cause of the disease.

    ▪ Medications that can affect the outcome of the test results are withheld and stress is reduced prior to and during testing.

  o Indications

    ▪ Cushing's disease

  o Interpretation of Findings

    ▪ When decreased amounts of ACTH are produced by the pituitary gland, decreased amounts of cortisol are released by the adrenal glands.

    ▪ When dexamethasone is given to clients who have Cushing's disease, there is no decrease in the production of ACTH and cortisol.

- Plasma and salivary cortisol, 24-hr urine for cortisol, serum ACTH, and ACTH stimulation tests
  - Indications
    - To diagnose Cushing's disease, Cushing's syndrome, and Addison's disease

TEST	EXPECTED REFERENCE RANGE	INTERPRETATION OF FINDINGS	NURSING ACTIONS
Plasma cortisol	This test varies according to the time of day. Since it has a diurnal pattern, higher levels are present in the early morning, and the lowest levels occur around midnight, or 3 to 5 hr after the onset of sleep.	Diurnal variations are not seen in a client who has Cushing's syndrome.	• Plasma cortisol is usually collected at midnight.
Salivary cortisol	A typical salivary cortisol value at midnight is less than 2.0 ng/mL.	Higher levels indicate hypercortisolism.	• Salivary cortisol is usually collected at midnight. • A sample of saliva is obtained by placing a salivary cushion pad inside the client's cheek, directly over the salivary gland.

Urinary cortisol	10 to 100 mcg/day	Higher levels indicate hypercortisolism.	• Urinary cortisol is measured during 24-hr urine collection.
			  ○ Clients empty the bladder and then collect all urine excreted during the next 24-hr period.
			  ○ The urine must be kept in a jug with boric acid added and kept on ice.
			  ○ If clients are receiving spironolactone, this should be held for 7 days prior to the test.

Serum ACTH	Typical early morning values are from 25 to 200 pg/mL and early evening values are usually from 0 to 50 pg/mL.	ACTH may be elevated with Addison's disease or decreased with Cushing's disease.	• Serum ACTH is most accurate if performed in the morning.
ACTH stimulation test	If no increase in cortisol occurs after administration of ACTH, the test is positive for Addison's disease or hypocortisolism.	ACTH stimulation test determines the functioning of the pituitary gland in relation to stimulating the secretion of adrenal hormones of cortisol.	• Two consecutive collections of 24-hr urine are used, one prior to and one after the administration of ACTH.

Adrenal Medulla

- Disorders of the adrenal medulla can result in the hypersecretion of catecholamines, resulting in stimulation of a sympathetic response, such as tachycardia, hypertension, and diaphoresis.

- VMA testing

  - VMA testing is a 24-hr urine collection for VMA, a breakdown product of catecholamines. Analysis of other urinary catecholamines may also be measured, such as dopamine and normetanephrine.

  - Indications

    - Diagnosis of pheochromocytoma

  - Interpretation of Findings

    - Expected VMA is 2 to 7 mg/24 hr.

    - High VMA levels at rest indicate pheochromocytoma.

  - Preprocedure

    - Nursing Actions

      □ Instruct clients regarding 24-hr urine collection. Urine is collected for 24 hr (in a container with a preservative) beginning and ending with an empty bladder.

    - Client Education

      □ The following may be restricted for 2 to 3 days before the test: caffeine, vanilla, bananas, and chocolate. Clients may also be asked to withhold aspirin and antihypertensive medications.

      □ Instruct clients to maintain a moderate level of activity.

- Clonidine suppression test

  - The client's plasma catecholamines levels are taken prior to and 3 hr after administration of clonidine (Catapres).

  - Indications

    - Diagnosis of pheochromocytoma

  - Interpretation of Findings

    - If a client does not have a pheochromocytoma, clonidine suppresses catecholamine release and decreases the serum level of catecholamines (decreases blood pressure).

    - If clients have a pheochromocytoma, the clonidine has no effect (no decreased blood pressure).

- Phentolamine blocking test

  - Phentolamine (Regitine), an alpha blocker, is administered to clients.

○ Indications

■ Diagnosis of pheochromocytoma

○ Interpretation of Findings

■ A rapid decrease in systolic blood pressure of ≥ 35 mm Hg and diastolic blood pressure of ≥ 25 mm Hg with the administration of phentolamine is diagnostic for pheochromocytoma.

○ Intraprocedure

■ Nursing Actions

□ Monitor the client's blood pressure.

Pancreas

- Dysfunction of the beta cells of the islets of Langerhans of the pancreas can lead to an absolute or relative deficiency of insulin.

- Fasting blood glucose, oral glucose tolerance testing, and glycosylated hemoglobin (HbA1c)

○ Indications

■ To diagnose type 1 and type 2 diabetes mellitus.

TEST	EXPECTED REFERENCE RANGE	INTERPRETATION OF FINDINGS	NURSING ACTIONS
Fasting blood glucose	<110 mg/dL	• This test is done to determine the client's blood glucose level when no foods or fluids (other than water) have been consumed during the previous 8 hr.	• Ensure that clients have fasted (no food or drink other than water) for the 8 hr prior to the blood draw. • Antidiabetic medications should be postponed until after the blood is drawn.
Oral glucose tolerance test	<140 mg/dL	• This test is done to determine the client's ability to metabolize a standard amount of glucose.	• Instruct clients to consume a balanced diet for the 3 days prior to the test and fast for the 10 to 12 hr prior to the test. • A fasting blood glucose level is drawn at start of the test. • Clients are then instructed to consume a specified amount of glucose. • Blood glucose levels are drawn every 30 min for 2 hr. Clients must be checked for hypoglycemia throughout the procedure.

TEST	EXPECTED REFERENCE RANGE	INTERPRETATION OF FINDINGS	NURSING ACTIONS
HbA1c	4% to 6% expected range greater than 8% indicates poor control of diabetes mellitus	• HbA1c is the best indicator of an average blood glucose level for the past 120 days. • This test assists in evaluating treatment effectiveness and adherence with the diet plan, medication regimen, and exercise schedule.	• No pre- or postprocedure care is required. The test requires a random blood sample obtained by a laboratory.

Thyroid and Anterior Pituitary Gland

- The anterior pituitary gland secretes thyroid stimulating hormone (TSH). Hyposecretion of TSH can lead to secondary hypothyroidism, and hypersecretion of TSH can cause secondary hyperthyroidism.

- Ultrasounds or scans can also be performed to determine the size, shape, and presence of nodules and masses on these glands.

- Serum triiodothyronine (T_3), serum thyroxine (T_4), serum thyroid stimulating hormone (TSH) stimulation test, serum thyrotropin-releasing hormone (TRH) stimulation test, and measurement of radioactive iodine uptake (RAIU)

  ○ Indications

    ▪ To diagnose disorders of the thyroid gland.

TEST	EXPECTED REFERENCE RANGE	INTERPRETATION OF FINDINGS	NURSING ACTIONS
T_3 T_4	70 to 205 ng/dL 4.0 to 12.0 mcg/dL	• Low and high levels of each indicate hypothyroidism and hyperthyroidism respectively; a high level of T_3 is more diagnostic of hyperthyroidism than is T_4.	• No pre- or postprocedure care is required for either test; the laboratory requires a random blood sample.

UNIT 12	NURSING CARE OF CLIENTS WITH ENDOCRINE DISORDERS
Chapter 75	Posterior Pituitary Disorders

Ⓞ Overview

- The posterior pituitary gland secretes the hormone vasopressin (antidiuretic hormone [ADH]).

  ○ Vasopressin increases permeability of the renal distal tubules, causing the kidneys to reabsorb water.

  ○ A deficiency of ADH causes diabetes insipidus (DI).

    ▪ Diabetes insipidus is characterized by the excretion of a large quantity of diluted urine.

  ○ Excessive secretion of ADH causes the syndrome of inappropriate antidiuretic hormone (SIADH).

    ▪ In SIADH, the kidneys retain water, urine output drops, and extracellular fluid volume is increased.

- Posterior pituitary disorders result in fluid and electrolyte imbalances.

DIABETES INSIPIDUS

Ⓞ Overview

- DI results from a deficiency of ADH, which is secreted by the posterior lobe of the pituitary gland (neurohypophysis).

- Decreased ADH reduces the ability of collecting and distal renal tubules in the kidneys to concentrate urine, resulting in excessive dilute urine, excessive thirst, and excessive fluid intake.

- Types of DI:

  ○ Neurogenic (also known as central or primary) – Caused by damage to the hypothalamus or pituitary gland from trauma, irradiation, or cranial surgery

  ○ Nephrogenic – Inherited; renal tubules do not react to ADH

  ○ Drug-induced – Lithium carbonate (Lithobid) or demeclocycline (Declomycin) can alter the way the kidneys respond to ADH.

Data Collection

- Risk Factors

    o Clients who have a head injury, a tumor or lesion, surgery near or around the pituitary gland, or an infection (meningitis, encephalitis)

    o Clients who are taking lithium carbonate (Lithobid) or demeclocycline (Declomycin)

    o Older adult clients are at higher risk for dehydration due to lower water content of the body, decreased thirst response, decreased ability of the kidneys to concentrate urine, increased use of diuretics, and swallowing difficulties or poor food intake.

- Subjective Data

    o Polyuria (abrupt onset of excessive urination, urinary output of 5 to 20 L/day of dilute urine)

    o Polydipsia (excessive thirst, consumption of 4 to 30 L/day)

    o Nocturia

    o Fatigue

    o Dehydration, as evidenced by extreme thirst, weight loss, muscle weakness, headache, tachycardia, hypotension, poor skin turgor, dry mucous membranes, constipation, and dizziness

- Objective Data

    o Physical Findings

    o Laboratory Tests

    - Urine chemistry – Think DILUTE.
        - Decreased urine specific gravity (less than 1.005)
        - Decreased urine osmolality (less than 300 mOsm/L)
        - Decreased urine pH
        - Decreased urine sodium
        - Decreased urine potassium
        - As urine volume increases, urine osmolality decreases.

    - Serum chemistry – Think CONCENTRATED.
        - Increased serum osmolality (greater than 300 mOsm/L)
        - Increased serum sodium
        - Increased serum potassium
        - As serum volume decreases, the serum osmolality increases.

    - Radioimmunoassay – Decreased ADH

- o Diagnostic Procedures
  - Water deprivation test
    - □ Easy and reliable. Dehydration is induced by withholding fluids. Urine output is measured and tested hourly.
    - □ The test is positive for DI if the kidneys are unable to concentrate urine despite increased plasma osmolarity.
  - Vasopressin test
    - □ A subcutaneous injection of vasopressin produces a urine output with an increased specific gravity if clients have central DI. This helps differentiate central from nephrogenic DI.

Collaborative Care

- Nursing Care

  - o Monitor vital signs, urinary output, central venous pressure, I&O, specific gravity, and laboratory studies (potassium, sodium, BUN, creatinine, specific gravity, osmolarity).

  - o Weigh clients daily.

  - o Promote the prescribed diet (regular diet with restriction of foods that exert a diuretic effect, such as caffeine).

  - o Monitor clients receiving IV therapy – I&O must be matched to prevent dehydration and electrolyte replacement.

  - o Promote safety – keep bedside rails up and provide assistance with walking if clients are dizzy or have muscle weakness. Make sure clients have easy access to a bathroom or bedpan and answer the call lights promptly.

  - o Add bulk foods and fruit juices to the diet if constipation develops. Clients may require a mild laxative.

  - o Check skin turgor and mucous membranes.

  - o Provide meticulous skin and mouth care and apply a lubricant to cracked or sore lips. Use a soft toothbrush and mild mouthwash to avoid trauma to the oral mucosa. Use alcohol-free skin care products and apply emollient lotion after baths.

  - o Encourage clients to drink fluids in response to thirst.

  - o Administer medications as prescribed.

- Medications

  - o ADH replacement agents – Desmopressin acetate (DDAVP) or aqueous vasopressin (Pitressin) administered intranasally, orally, or parenterally

    - Used as a synthetic posterior pituitary hormone that causes an increase in water absorption from kidneys and a decrease in urine output

- Nursing Considerations
  - Monitor vital signs, urinary output, central venous pressure, I&O, specific gravity, and laboratory studies (potassium, sodium, BUN, creatinine, specific gravity, osmolarity).
  - Monitor blood pressure.
  - Dose may need to be adjusted to urine output.
- Client Education
  - For an intranasal dose, teach clients to clear nasal passage and sit upright prior to nasal inhalation.
  - Instruct clients to monitor weight daily and notify the provider of a gain greater than 0.9 kg (2 lb) in 24 hr.
  - Instruct clients to restrict fluids if directed and notify the provider of headache or confusion.

○ ADH stimulants – Carbamazepine (Tegretol)

- Anticonvulsants stimulate release of ADH. They may be effective in partial central diabetes insipidus.
- Nursing Considerations
  - Monitor vital signs, urinary output, central venous pressure, I&O, specific gravity, and laboratory studies (potassium, sodium, BUN, creatinine, specific gravity, osmolarity).
  - Monitor blood pressure.
  - Monitor for dizziness or drowsiness related to the medication.
  - Monitor for signs of thrombocytopenia (sore throat, bruising, fever).
- Client Education
  - Advise clients to:
    - Take the medication with food to reduce gastric distress.
    - Use caution when driving or operating heavy machinery until effects of the medication are established.
    - Notify the provider of sore throat, fever, or bleeding.

○ Vasopressin (Pitressin)

- Posterior pituitary hormone that causes an increase in water absorption from kidneys and a decrease in urine output
- Nursing Considerations
  - Give cautiously to clients who have coronary artery disease because the medication can cause vasoconstriction.
  - Monitor vital signs, urinary output, central venous pressure, I&O, specific gravity, and laboratory studies (potassium, sodium, BUN, creatinine, specific gravity, osmolarity).

□ Monitor blood pressure.

□ Monitor for headache, confusion, or other signs of water intoxication.

- Client Education

  □ Educate clients regarding lifelong vasopressin therapy, daily weights, and the importance of reporting weight gain, polyuria, and polydipsia to the provider.

  □ Instruct clients to restrict fluids if directed, and notify the provider of headache or confusion.

- Interdisciplinary Care

  ○ Recognize the need for a referral for home health services for fluid, medication, and dietary management.

- Care After Discharge

  ○ Client Education

    - Instruct clients to weigh daily, eat a diet that is high in fiber, wear a medical alert wristband, and monitor fluid intake.

    - Reinforce to clients to monitor for signs of dehydration (weight loss; dry, cracked lips; confusion; weakness).

    - Advise clients to restrict fluids if instructed to prevent water intoxication, and avoid consumption of alcohol.

- Client Outcomes

  ○ The client will establish and maintain fluid and electrolyte balance through medication and fluid management.

Complications

- Untreated diabetes insipidus can produce hypovolemia, hyperosmolarity, hypernatremia, circulatory collapse, unconsciousness, central nervous system damage, and seizures.

  ○ Excessive urine output causing severe dehydration can lead to these complications.

  ○ Nursing Actions

    - Monitor fluid balance and prevent dehydration with providing proper fluid intake.

  ○ Client Education

    - Advise clients to seek early medical attention for any sign of diabetes insipidus and follow care instructions.

SYNDROME OF INAPPROPRIATE ANTIDIURETIC HORMONE (SIADH)

Overview

- Syndrome of inappropriate antidiuretic hormone (SIADH) is an excessive release of ADH, also known as vasopressin, secreted by the posterior lobe of the pituitary gland (neurohypophysis).

- Excess ADH leads to renal reabsorption of water and suppression of the renin-angiotensin mechanism, which causes renal excretion of sodium leading to water intoxication, cellular edema, and dilutional hyponatremia. Fluid shifts within compartments cause decreased serum osmolarity.

Data Collection

- Risk Factors

  - Conditions that stimulate the hypothalamus to hypersecrete ADH include malignant tumors (the most common cause is oat-cell lung cancer), increasing intrathoracic pressure (such as with positive pressure ventilation), head injury, meningitis, cardiovascular accident, medications (alcohol, lithium carbonate, phenytoin), trauma, pain, and stress.

  - Diuretics are sometimes used to treat conditions such as heart failure. Sodium losses due to diuretic use can further contribute to the problems caused by SIADH. A thorough client history and medication review can help alert nurses to the possibility of SIADH.

- Subjective Data

  - Early symptoms of SIADH include headache, weakness, anorexia, muscle cramps, and weight gain (without edema because water, not sodium, is retained).

  - As the serum sodium level decreases, clients experience personality changes, hostility, sluggish deep tendon reflexes, nausea, vomiting, diarrhea, and oliguria.

- Objective Data

  - Physical Findings

    - Manifestations of fluid volume excess can include tachycardia, hypertension, crackles in lungs, distended neck veins, and taut skin. Intake is greater than output.

    - Confusion, lethargy, and Cheyne-Stokes respirations indicate impending crisis. If the serum sodium level drops further, seizures, coma, and death may occur.

○ Laboratory Tests

- Urine chemistry – Think CONCENTRATED.

  □ Increased urine sodium

  □ Increased urine osmolarity

  □ As urine volume decreases, urine osmolarity increases.

- Blood chemistry – Think DILUTE.

  □ Decreased serum sodium

  □ Decreased serum osmolarity (less than 270 mEq/L)

  □ As serum volume increases, serum osmolarity decreases.

  □ Radioimmunoassay – Increased ADH

Collaborative Care

- Nursing Care

  ○ Restrict oral fluids to 500 to 1,000 mL/day to prevent further hemodilution (first priority). During fluid restriction, provide comfort measures for thirst, including mouth care, ice chips, lozenges, and staggered water intake.

  ○ Flush all enteral and gastric tubes with 0.9% sodium chloride, instead of water to replace sodium and prevent further hemodilution.

  ○ Record accurate I&O. Report decreased urine output.

  ○ Monitor vital signs for increased blood pressure, tachycardia, and hypothermia.

  ○ Monitor for decreased serum sodium/osmolarity and elevated urine sodium/osmolarity.

  ○ Weigh daily. A weight gain of 0.9 kg (2 lb) indicates a gain of 1 L of fluid.

  ○ Report altered mental status (headache, confusion, lethargy, seizures, coma).

  ○ Reduce environmental stimuli and reposition clients as needed.

  ○ Provide a safe environment for clients who have altered levels of consciousness. Initiate seizure precautions.

  ○ Monitor clients for signs and symptoms of heart failure, which can occur from fluid overload. Administer loop diuretics as indicated.

- Medications

  ○ Demeclocycline (Declomycin)

    - Tetracycline derivative

    - Can cause drug-induced diabetes insipidus

- Nursing Considerations
  - Monitor for effective treatment, such as increased serum sodium/osmolarity and decreased urine sodium osmolarity.
- Client Education
  - Advise clients:
    - That it may take a week to see results.
    - To monitor for signs of a yeast infection, such as a white, cheese-like film inside the mouth.
  - Have clients rinse toothbrush with a diluted bleach solution (10%) and increase consumption of yogurt.
- Lithium (Eskalith)
  - Used to block the renal response to ADH
  - Can induce DI
  - Nursing Considerations
    - Monitor:
      - For adverse effects (lithium toxicity, nausea, diarrhea, tremors, ataxia).
      - ECG for dysrhythmias.
      - For effective treatment (increased serum sodium/osmolarity, decreased urine sodium/osmolarity).
  - Client Education
    - Advise clients to:
      - Monitor for symptoms of lithium toxicity.
      - Take the medication with food.
      - Allow 1 to 3 weeks to see effects.
- Furosemide (Lasix)
  - A loop diuretic is used to increase water excretion from kidneys.
  - Nursing Considerations
    - Use with caution.
    - Causes sodium excretion and can worsen hyponatremia
  - Client Education
    - Advise clients to:
      - Change positions slowly in case of orthostatic hypotension.
      - Notify the provider of signs of hyponatremia, such as nausea, decreased appetite, and vomiting.

- Interdisciplinary Care

  ○ Request referral for home health services for fluid, medication, and dietary management.

- Therapeutic Procedures

  ○ Hypertonic IV fluid

    ■ The goal of hypertonic saline therapy is to elevate the sodium level enough to alleviate signs of neurologic compromise/not to raise the level to normal.

    ■ Nursing Actions

      □ In severe hyponatremia/water intoxication, administration of 200 to 300 mL of hypertonic IV fluid (3% to 5% sodium chloride) is indicated.

      □ Monitor for fluid overload and heart failure (distended neck veins, crackles in lungs).

    ■ Client Education

      □ Include information about medications with discharge instructions.

      □ Instruct clients to wear a medical alert wristband and restrict fluid intake.

      □ Instruct clients to monitor weight every day, keep a daily record, and report an increase of 0.9 kg (2 lb) or more in a day to the provider.

      □ Encourage client to avoid alcohol.

      □ Advise clients to notify the provider regarding:

        ‣ Signs of hypervolemia and heart failure (weight gain, difficulty breathing, shortness of breath).

        ‣ Neurological changes (tremors, disorientation), which can lead to seizures.

        ‣ Signs of hyponatremia (nausea, vomiting, decreased appetite).

- Client Outcomes

  ○ The client will establish and maintain fluid and electrolyte balance through medication and fluid management.

Complications

- Water intoxication, cerebral edema, and severe hyponatremia

  ○ Without prompt treatment, SIADH can lead to these complications and result in coma or death.

- ○ Nursing Actions
  - ▪ Monitor for early signs of water intoxication, such as lung crackles, distended neck veins, and changes in neurological state (twitching, disorientation).
  - ▪ Initiate seizure precautions.
  - ▪ Monitor serum sodium level.
- ○ Client Education
  - ▪ Instruct clients and family about fluid restrictions and offer information about the condition and treatment.
  - ▪ Provide support to ease the client's fear about the disease.

- Central pontine myelinolysis (CPM)

  - ○ Treatment for SIADH can result in CPM, a condition characterized by nerve damage that is caused by the destruction of the myelin sheath in the brainstem (pons). The most common cause is a rapid change in sodium levels in the body. This most commonly occurs when a client is being treated for hyponatremia and the levels rise too fast.

  - ○ Nursing Actions
    - ▪ Monitor serum osmolarity and sodium every 2 to 4 hr while receiving hypertonic saline or loop diuretics.
    - ▪ Report any deterioration in neurologic status immediately.

  - ○ Client Education
    - ▪ Inform clients and their families about the condition.
    - ▪ Explain all procedures and information about medication and treatment.

- Subjective and Objective Data

  o Nervousness, irritability, hyperactivity, emotional lability, and decreased attention span

  o Weakness, easy fatigability, and exercise intolerance

  o Heat intolerance

  o Weight change (usually loss) and increased appetite

  o Insomnia and interrupted sleep

  o Frequent stools and diarrhea

  o Menstrual irregularities and decreased libido

  o Warm, sweaty, flushed skin with velvety-smooth texture

  o Tremor, hyperkinesias, and hyperreflexia

  o Vision changes, exophthalmos, retracted eye lids, and staring gaze

  (M) View Media Supplement: Exophthalmos (Image)

  o Hair loss

  o Goiter

  o Bruit auscultated over the thyroid gland

  o Elevated systolic blood pressure, widened pulse pressure, and S_3 heart sound

  o Tachycardia and dysrhythmias

  o Findings in older adult clients are often more subtle than those in younger clients.

  o Occasionally an older adult client who has hyperthyroidism will demonstrate apathy or withdrawal instead of the more typical hypermetabolic state.

  o Older adult clients who have hyperthyroidism often present with heart failure and atrial fibrillation.

  o Laboratory Tests

    ▪ Serum TSH test – Decreased in the presence of Graves' disease (can be elevated in secondary or tertiary hyperthyroidism)

    ▪ Free thyroxine index (FTI) and T_3 – Elevated in the presence of disease

    ▪ Thyrotropin-releasing hormone (TRH) stimulation test – Failure of expected rise in TSH

  o Diagnostic Procedures

    ▪ Radioiodine (^{123}I) uptake and thyroid scan

      □ Clarifies size of gland and detects presence of hot or cold nodules

- ▪ Nursing Actions
  - ▫ Confirm that clients are not pregnant prior to the scan.
  - ▫ Take a medication history to determine the use of iodides.
  - ▫ Recent use of contrast media and oral contraceptives can cause falsely elevated serum thyroid hormone levels.
  - ▫ Severe illness; malnutrition; and the use of aspirin, corticosteroids, and phenytoin sodium can cause a false decrease in serum thyroid hormone levels.
  - ▫ Inform the provider if clients received any iodine contrast within 4 weeks of test.
- ▪ Client Education
  - ▫ Advise clients to avoid foods high in iodine for 1 week prior to the test.
  - ▫ Suggest that clients use noniodized salt, avoid fish and shellfish, reduce milk intake, and avoid canned fruits and vegetables.

Collaborative Care

- • Nursing Care
  - ○ Minimize the client's energy expenditure by assisting with activities as needed and by encouraging clients to alternate periods of activity with rest.
  - ○ Promote a calm environment.
  - ○ Observe the client's mental status and decision-making ability. Intervene as needed to ensure safety.
  - ○ Monitor the client's nutritional status. Provide increased calories, protein, and other nutritional support as necessary.
  - ○ Provide eye protection (patches, eye lubricant, tape to close eyelids) for a client who has exophthalmos.
  - ○ Administer antithyroid medications as prescribed.
  - ○ Prepare clients for a total/subtotal thyroidectomy if they are unresponsive to antithyroid medications or have an airway-obstructing goiter.
- • Medications
  - ○ Propylthiouracil (PTU) or methimazole (Tapazole)
    - ▪ Antihyperthyroid medications that act by blocking thyroid hormone synthesis and reducing thyroid hormone level
    - ▪ Nursing Considerations
      - ▫ Monitor for signs of hypothyroidism, such as intolerance to cold, edema, bradycardia, increase in weight, or depression.
      - ▫ Monitor CBC for leukopenia or thrombocytopenia.

- Client Education
  - Advise clients to:
    - ▸ Take the medication in divided doses at regular intervals to maintain an even therapeutic medication level.
    - ▸ Take the medication with meals.
    - ▸ Report fever, sore throat, or bruising.
    - ▸ Report any sign of jaundice (yellowing of skin or eyes, darkening of urine).
    - ▸ Follow the provider's instructions about dietary intake of iodine.
  - Propranolol (Inderal)
    - Beta-adrenergic blocker – Treats sympathetic nervous system effects (tachycardia, palpitations)
    - Nursing Considerations
      - Monitor blood pressure, heart rate, and ECG.
    - Client Education
      - Advise clients to take the dose with meals to increase absorption.
      - Reinforce to clients to check apical pulse prior to each dosage. If pulse is less than 50/min, hold the dose and notify the provider.
  - Saturated solution of potassium iodide (SSKI)
    - Iodine-containing medications – Inhibit the release of stored thyroid hormone and retard hormone synthesis
    - Nursing Considerations
      - These medications are for short-term use only.
      - Give 1 hr after an antithyroid medication.
      - Use of these medications is contraindicated in pregnancy.
    - Client Education
      - Instruct clients to notify the provider of fever, sore throat, or mouth ulcers.
- Interdisciplinary Care
  - Interdisciplinary care may involve an endocrinologist and a radiologist.
- Therapeutic Procedures
  - Radioactive iodine therapy – Radioactive iodine is taken up by the thyroid and destroys some of the hormone-producing cells.

- Nursing Actions
  - Radioactive iodine therapy is contraindicated in women who are pregnant.
  - Monitor for symptoms of hypothyroidism, such as edema, intolerance to cold, bradycardia, increase in weight, or depression.
- Client Education
  - Advise clients:
    - That the effects of therapy may not be evident for 6 to 8 weeks.
    - To continue to take the medication as directed.
    - To stay away from infants or small children for 2 to 4 days and to avoid becoming pregnant for 6 months following therapy.

- Surgical Interventions
  - Total or subtotal thyroidectomy
    - A thyroidectomy is the surgical removal of part or all of the thyroid gland.
      - A subtotal thyroidectomy can be performed for the treatment of hyperthyroidism when medication therapy fails or radiation therapy is contraindicated. After surgery, the remaining thyroid tissue usually supplies enough thyroid hormone for normal function.
      - A total thyroidectomy can be performed for certain types of thyroid cancers. Lifelong thyroid replacement therapy is required for clients who have total thyroidectomies.
    - Nursing Actions
      - Preprocedure
        - Explain the purpose of the thyroidectomy to clients.
        - Tell clients:
          - There will be an incision in the neck, a dressing, and possibly a drain in place.
          - Some hoarseness and a sore throat from intubation and anesthesia may be experienced.
        - Ensure that clients have adhered to the preoperative medication regimen.
          - Propylthiouracil or methimazole 4 to 6 weeks before surgery
          - Iodine for 10 to 14 days before surgery to reduce the gland's size and prevent excess bleeding
          - Propranolol (Inderal) to block adrenergic effects

- ☐ Postprocedure
  - ▸ Keep clients in a high-Fowler's position to promote venous return from the head and neck and to decrease oozing into the incision.
  - ▸ Check for laryngeal nerve damage by asking clients to speak as soon as they awaken from anesthesia.
  - ▸ Administer a mild analgesic as prescribed.
  - ▸ Show clients how to change positions while supporting the back of the their neck.
  - ▸ Assist clients to cough and deep breathe while supporting the neck.
  - ▸ Inspect the surgical dressing for bleeding, especially at the back of the neck, and change the dressing as directed.
  - ▸ Expect about 50 mL of drainage in the first 24 hr.
  - ▸ If no drainage is found, check for drain kinking or the need to reestablish suction.
  - ▸ Expect only scant drainage after 24 hr.
  - ▸ If no drain is in place, prepare clients for discharge the day following surgery as indicated. However, if a drain is in place, the provider will usually remove it, along with half of the surgical clips, on the second day after surgery. The remaining clips are removed the following day before discharge.
  - ▸ Support the client's head and neck with pillows or sandbags. If the client needs to be transferred from a stretcher to the bed, support the client's head and neck in good body alignment.
- ■ Client Education
  - ☐ Advise clients:
    - ▸ To be careful of the incisional drain if applicable.
    - ▸ That their voice will be hoarse and to expect some pain.
    - ▸ To notify the nurse of any tingling sensation of the mouth, tingling of the distal extremities, or muscle twitching.
    - ▸ That they will be asked to try to talk at intervals to check for nerve damage.
    - ▸ To notify the provider of incisional drainage, swelling, or redness that may indicate infection.
    - ▸ To take all medications as directed.
    - ▸ Who have had a total thyroidectomy that lifelong thyroid replacement medications will be required.
    - ▸ To keep all follow-up appointments.
    - ▸ To notify the provider of fever, increased restlessness, palpitations, or chest pain.

- Care After Discharge
  - Client Education
    - Advise clients to:
      - □ Take all medications as directed.
      - □ Keep all follow-up appointments.
      - □ Try to avoid stress and get rest as needed.
      - □ Notify the provider of fever, increased restlessness, palpitations, or chest pain.
- Client Outcomes
  - The client will be able to get adequate sleep.
  - The client will achieve and maintain appropriate weight and nutrition.
  - The client will maintain a normal blood pressure and heart rate within the normal reference range.
  - The client will be free of complications of hyperthyroidism.

Complications

- Thyroid Storm
  - Also known as thyrotoxic crisis, thyroid storm results from a sudden surge of large amounts of thyroid hormones into the bloodstream, causing an even greater increase in body metabolism. This is a medical emergency with a high mortality rate.
  - Precipitating factors include infection, trauma, and emotional stress, all of which increase demands on body metabolism. It can also occur following a subtotal thyroidectomy as a result of manipulation of the gland during surgery.
  - Findings are hyperthermia, hypertension, delirium, vomiting, abdominal pain, hyperglycemia, and tachydysrhythmias.
  - Nursing Actions
    - Maintain a patent airway.
    - Provide continuous cardiac monitoring for dysrhythmias.
    - Administer acetaminophen to decrease the client's temperature.
      - □ Caution – Aspirin is contraindicated because it releases thyroxine from protein-binding sites and increases free thyroxine levels.
    - Provide cool sponge baths or apply ice packs to the client's axilla and groin areas to decrease fever. If fever continues, obtain a prescription for a cooling blanket for hyperthermia.
    - Administer propylthiouracil to prevent further synthesis and release of thyroid hormones.
    - Administer propranolol to block sympathetic nervous system effects.

- Monitor administration of IV fluid replacement.

- Administer sodium iodide as prescribed, 1 hr after administering PTU.

- Administer small doses of insulin as prescribed to control hyperglycemia. Hyperglycemia can occur because of the hypermetabolic state.

- Administer supplemental O_2 to meet increased oxygen demands.

   ○ Client Education

- Provide clients and their families with support and information about the client's condition and all procedures. Advise clients to notify their health care provider of fever, increased restlessness, palpitations, or chest pain.

● Airway Obstruction (following thyroidectomy)

   ○ Hemorrhage, tracheal collapse, tracheal mucus accumulation, laryngeal edema, and vocal cord paralysis can cause respiratory obstruction, with sudden stridor and restlessness.

   ○ Nursing Actions

- Keep a tracheostomy tray and suction equipment at the bedside at all times during the immediate recovery period.

- Maintain the bed in a high-Fowler's position to decrease edema and swelling of the neck.

- Notify the provider immediately if clients report that the dressing feels tight.

- Listen at the client's neck for respiratory stridor.

- Provide humidified air.

- Medicate as prescribed to reduce swelling.

   ○ Client Education

- Instruct clients to notify the nurse of tightness or difficulty breathing.

● Hypocalcemia and Tetany (following thyroidectomy)

   ○ Damage to a parathyroid gland causes hypocalcemia and tetany.

   ○ Nursing Actions

- Monitor for signs of hypocalcemia (tingling of the fingers and toes, carpopedal spasms, convulsions).

- Test for Chvostek's and Trousseau's signs, which are indicators of neuromuscular irritability from hypocalcemia.

- Maintain seizure precautions.

- Assist with emergency care.

      □ Have IV calcium gluconate available for emergency administration.

□ Keep emergency equipment near the bedside.

▸ Monitor clients for signs of hypocalcemia, such as tingling, muscle twitching, and numbness of mouth or distal extremities.

▸ Advise clients to report any muscle twitching or tingling sensation of the mouth or distal extremities.

○ Client Education

■ Advise clients to notify the nurse of any tingling sensation of the mouth, tingling of distal extremities, or muscle twitching.

- Nerve Damage (following thyroidectomy)

○ Nerve damage can lead to vocal cord paralysis and vocal disturbances.

○ Incisional damage or swelling can cause nerve damage.

○ Nursing Actions

■ Inform clients that they will be hoarse, they will be able to speak only rarely, and they will need to rest their voice for several days.

■ After the procedure, monitor the client's ability to speak with each measurement of vital signs.

■ Check the client's voice tone and quality and compare it to the preoperative voice.

○ Client Education

■ Remind clients that they will be asked to try to talk at intervals to check for nerve damage. Advise clients that a hoarse voice is not typically permanent.

HYPOTHYROIDISM

Overview

- Classifications of hypothyroidism by etiology

○ Primary – Primary hypothyroidism stems from dysfunction of the thyroid gland. This is the most common type of hypothyroidism and is caused by disease (autoimmune thyroiditis – Hashimoto's disease) or loss of the thyroid gland (iodine deficiency, surgical removal of the gland).

○ Secondary – Secondary hypothyroidism is caused by failure of the anterior pituitary gland to stimulate the thyroid gland or failure of the target tissues to respond to the thyroid hormones (pituitary tumors).

○ Tertiary – Tertiary hypothyroidism is caused by failure of the hypothalamus to produce thyroid-releasing factor.

- Hypothyroidism is also classified by age of onset.

  ○ Cretinism – Cretinism is a state of severe hypothyroidism found in infants. When infants do not produce normal amounts of thyroid hormones, their central nervous system development and skeletal maturation are altered, resulting in mental retardation, and/or impaired physical growth.

  ○ Juvenile hypothyroidism – Juvenile hypothyroidism is most often caused by chronic autoimmune thyroiditis and affects the growth and sexual maturation of the child. Signs and symptoms are similar to adult hypothyroidism, and the treatment reverses most of the clinical manifestations of the disease.

  ○ Adult hypothyroidism

  ○ Because older adult clients who have hypothyroidism can have confusing signs and symptoms that mimic the aging process, hypothyroidism is often undiagnosed in older adult clients, which can lead to potentially serious side effects from medications (sedatives, opiates, anesthetics).

Data Collection

- Risk Factors

  ○ The disorder is most prevalent in women, with the incidence rising significantly in people who are 40 to 50 years of age.

  ○ Use of medications (lithium [Eskalith], amiodarone)

  ○ Inadequate intake of iodine

- Subjective and Objective Data

  ○ Hypothyroidism is often characterized by vague and varied symptoms that develop slowly over time.

  ○ Early findings

    ▪ Fatigue

    ▪ Intolerance to cold

    ▪ Decreased bowel motility

    ▪ Weight gain

    ▪ Pale skin

    ▪ Thin, brittle fingernails

    ▪ Depression

    ▪ Thinning hair

    ▪ Joint and/or muscle pain

  ○ Late findings

    ▪ Slow thought processes and speech

    ▪ Thickening of the skin

- ■ Thinning of hair on the eyebrows
- ■ Dry, flaky skin
- ■ Swelling in face, hands, and feet (myxedema [non-pitting, mucinous edema])

ⓜ View Media Supplement: Myxedema (Image)

- ■ Decreased acuity of taste and smell
- ■ Hoarse, raspy speech
- ■ Abnormal menstrual periods and decreased libido
- ○ Laboratory Tests

LABORATORY TEST	EXPECTED RESULTS WITH HYPOTHYROIDISM
T_3	Decreased
Serum thyroid-stimulating hormone (TSH)	• Elevates with primary hypothyroidism • Decreases with secondary hypothyroidism
Free thyroxine index (FTI) and thyroxine (T_4) levels	Decreased
Serum cholesterol	Elevated
CBC	Anemia

- ○ Diagnostic Procedures
  - ■ Skull x-ray, magnetic resonance imaging (MRI), and computed tomography (CT) scans
    - □ These procedures can help locate pituitary or hypothalamic lesions that may be the underlying cause of hypothyroidism.
  - ■ Radioisotope (^{131}I) scan and uptake
    - □ Results will be less than 10% in a 24-hr period. In secondary hypothyroidism, intake increases with administration of exogenous TSH.
  - ■ ECG
    - □ Sinus bradycardia and flat or inverted T waves

Collaborative Care

- • Nursing Care

  - ○ Monitor for cardiovascular changes (low blood pressure, bradycardia, dysrhythmias).
  - ○ If the client's mental status is compromised, orient periodically and provide safety measures.
  - ○ Increase the client's activity level gradually, and provide frequent rest periods to avoid fatigue and decrease myocardial oxygen demands.

- ○ Apply antiembolism stockings and elevate the client's legs to promote venous return.

- ○ Encourage clients to cough and breathe deeply to prevent pulmonary complications.

- ○ Provide a low-calorie, high-bulk diet, and encourage activity to help prevent constipation and promote weight loss. Administer cathartics and stool softeners as needed. Avoid fiber laxatives, which interfere with absorption of levothyroxine.

- ○ Provide meticulous skin care. Turn and reposition clients every 2 hr. Use alcohol-free skin care products and an emollient lotion after bathing.

- ○ Provide extra clothing and blankets, and keep room warm for clients with decreased cold tolerance.

- ○ Encourage clients to verbalize feelings and fears about changes in body image. Provide reassurance that most of the physical manifestations are reversible, but take time.

- ○ Use caution due to alteration in metabolism.

  - ■ CNS depressants (barbiturates or sedatives) are contraindicated or given at a significantly decreased dose.

  - ■ External warming measures are contraindicated because they can produce vasodilatation and vascular collapse.

- • Medications

  - ○ Thyroid hormone replacement therapy – levothyroxine (Synthroid)

    - ■ Thyroid hormone replacement therapy is a treatment of choice.

    - ■ It increases the effects of warfarin (Coumadin) and can increase the need for insulin and digoxin (Lanoxin).

    - ■ Use caution when starting thyroid hormone replacement with older adult clients and those who have coronary artery disease to avoid coronary ischemia because of increased oxygen demands of the heart. It is preferable to start with much lower doses and increase gradually, taking 1 to 2 months to reach full replacement doses.

    - ■ Nursing Considerations

      - □ Monitor for cardiovascular compromise (chest pain, palpitations, rapid heart rate, shortness of breath) during early thyroid therapy.

      - □ Check apical pulse and blood pressure prior to administering.

    - ■ Client Education

      - □ Instruct clients that treatment begins slowly and the dosage is increased every 2 to 3 weeks until the desired response is obtained. Serum TSH will need to be drawn at scheduled times to ensure appropriate dosage.

      - □ Instruct clients to monitor for and report signs and symptoms of hyperthyroidism (irritability, tremors, tachycardia, palpitations, heat intolerance).

      - □ Inform clients that the treatment is considered to be lifelong, requiring ongoing medical assessment of thyroid function.

- Interdisciplinary Care

  o Request a referral for home health services to visit clients and assess for side effects during the first few weeks of therapy.

- Client Outcomes

  o The client's TSH will return to the expected reference range.

Complications

- Myxedema Coma

  o Myxedema coma is a life-threatening condition that occurs when hypothyroidism is untreated or when a stressor, such as infection, affects an individual who has hypothyroidism. Clients who have been taking levothyroxine sodium and suddenly stop the medication are also at risk.

  o Clients who have myxedema coma experience:

    - Significantly depressed respirations (hypoxia, hypercapnia)

    - Decreased cardiac output

    - Worsening cerebral hypoxia

    - Stupor

    - Hypothermia

    - Bradycardia

    - Hypotension

    - Hypoglycemia

    - Hyponatremia

  o Nursing Actions

    - Maintain airway patency with ventilatory support if necessary.

    - Monitor IV fluid replacement.

    - Provide continuous ECG monitoring.

    - Monitor ABGs for hypoxia and metabolic acidosis.

    - Warm clients with blankets.

    - Monitor the client's body temperature until stable.

    - Assist with clients receiving large doses of levothyroxine (Synthroid) IV. Monitor vital signs because rapid correction of hypothyroidism can cause adverse cardiac effects.

    - Monitor I&O and daily weights.

    - Administer corticosteroids as prescribed.

    - Check for possible sources of infection (blood, sputum, urine), which may have precipitated the coma. Treat any underlying illness.

Ⓐ APPLICATION EXERCISES

Scenario: A 35-year-old client visits the outpatient clinic with symptoms of insomnia, anxiety, and feeling as though her heart is "racing." The client has lost 6.7 kg (14.7 lb) over the past 3 weeks without dieting. Vital signs are: BP 152/92 mm Hg, pulse 122/min, and respirations 24/min. She also reports not being able to tolerate the heat and a decrease in her menstrual flow. The provider suspects Graves' disease.

1. Which of the following laboratory test results should the nurse expect?

   A. Decreased T_3

   B. Decreased FTI

   C. Decreased TSH

   D. Decreased TSH-RAb

2. The client is diagnosed with hyperthyroidism. Which of the following clinical manifestations of hyperthyroidism should the nurse expect to find? (Select all that apply.)

   _____ Excessive sweating

   _____ Tremors

   _____ Gastric hypermotility

   _____ Increased white blood cell count

   _____ Hypothermia

   _____ Photophobia

   _____ Exophthalmus

3. The provider prescribes medication for the client's hyperthyroidism. Which of the following medications blocks the synthesis of thyroid hormone?

   A. Propylthiouracil (PTU)

   B. Metoprolol (Lopressor)

   C. Amoxicillin (Amoxil)

   D. Docusate sodium (Colace)

4. A nurse on the surgical unit is preparing to care for a client 12 hr post-total thyroidectomy. Which of the following interventions should the nurse anticipate implementing? (Select all that apply.)

   _____ Restrict the client from speaking.

   _____ Monitor vital signs every 4 hr.

   _____ Keep the client in a high-Fowler's position.

   _____ Administer mild analgesics as prescribed.

   _____ Support the neck while client coughs and deep breathes every 2 hr.

Scenario: A 32-year-old client visits the outpatient clinic for symptoms of fatigue, cold intolerance, dry scaly skin, hoarseness, weight gain, and fluid retention. Based on these symptoms, thyroid studies are performed and reveal an elevated thyroid stimulating hormone (TSH) and decreased T_3 and T_4 levels. The provider prescribes levothyroxine sodium (Synthroid) 0.1 mg by mouth daily and instructs the client to return to the clinic in 1 month to have a TSH drawn.

5. A nurse caring for the client recognizes that the client's TSH is a reliable indicator of the efficacy of the levothyroxine sodium because the TSH will

    A. have a value of zero when an euthyroid state is re-established.

    B. return to its expected reference range when an euthyroid state is re-established.

    C. increase above its expected reference range when a therapeutic medication level is reached.

    D. decrease below its expected reference range when a therapeutic medication level is reached.

6. Which of the following should the nurse reinforce in regard to taking levothyroxine? (Select all that apply.)

    _____ Use fiber laxatives for constipation.

    _____ Expect to take this medication for 3 to 6 months.

    _____ Return to clinic for follow-up laboratory tests of serum TSH.

    _____ Take medication 30 min before bedtime.

    _____ Side effects such as nervousness, heat intolerance, and diarrhea.

(A) APPLICATION EXERCISES ANSWER KEY

Scenario: A 35-year-old client visits the outpatient clinic with symptoms of insomnia, anxiety, and feeling as though her heart is "racing." The client has lost 6.7 kg (14.7 lb) over the past 3 weeks without dieting. Vital signs are: BP 152/92 mm Hg, pulse 122/min, and respirations 24/min. She also reports not being able to tolerate the heat and a decrease in her menstrual flow. The provider suspects Graves' disease.

1. Which of the following laboratory test results should the nurse expect?

    A. Decreased T_3

    B. Decreased FTI

    C. Decreased TSH

    D. Decreased TSH-RAb

    A client who has Graves' disease will have a decreased TSH due to elevated serum thyroid hormone. T_3, FTI, and TSH-RAb will all be elevated.

(N) NCLEX® Connection: Reduction of Risk Potential, Laboratory Values

2. The client is diagnosed with hyperthyroidism. Which of the following clinical manifestations of hyperthyroidism should the nurse expect to find? (Select all that apply.)

__X__	**Excessive sweating**
__X__	**Tremors**
__X__	**Gastric hypermotility**
_____	Increased white blood cell count
_____	Hypothermia
__X__	**Photophobia**
__X__	**Exophthalmus**

    Excessive sweating, tremors, gastric hypermotility, photophobia, and exophthalmus are findings consistent with hyperthyroidism. Increased white blood cell count and hypothermia are not expected findings of hypothyroidism.

(N) NCLEX® Connection: Physiological Adaptations, Basic Pathophysiology

3. The provider prescribes medication for the client's hyperthyroidism. Which of the following medications blocks the synthesis of thyroid hormone?

    A. Propylthiouracil (PTU)

    B. Metoprolol (Lopressor)

    C. Amoxicillin (Amoxil)

    D. Docusate sodium (Colace)

    Propylthiouracil blocks the synthesis of thyroid hormone. The other medications do not affect thyroid hormone synthesis.

 NCLEX® Connection: Pharmacological Therapies, Expected Actions/Outcomes

---

4. A nurse on the surgical unit is preparing to care for a client 12 hr post-total thyroidectomy. Which of the following interventions should the nurse anticipate implementing? (Select all that apply.)

_____	Restrict the client from speaking.
__X__	**Monitor vital signs every 4 hr.**
__X__	**Keep the client in a high-Fowler's position.**
__X__	**Administer mild analgesics as prescribed.**
__X__	**Support the neck while client coughs and deep breathes every 2 hr.**

    The appropriate interventions include monitoring of vital signs every 4 hr, keeping the client in a high-Fowler's position, administering mild analgesics, and supporting the neck while the client coughs and breathes deep. The nurse should ask the client to speak in order to monitor for laryngeal nerve damage.

 NCLEX® Connection: Reduction of Risk Potential, Potential for Complications from Surgical Procedures and Health Alterations

Scenario: A 32-year-old client visits the outpatient clinic for symptoms of fatigue, cold intolerance, dry scaly skin, hoarseness, weight gain, and fluid retention. Based on these symptoms, thyroid studies are performed and reveal an elevated thyroid stimulating hormone (TSH) and decreased T_3 and T_4 levels. The provider prescribes levothyroxine sodium (Synthroid) 0.1 mg by mouth daily and instructs the client to return to the clinic in 1 month to have a TSH drawn.

5. A nurse caring for the client recognizes that the client's TSH is a reliable indicator of the efficacy of the levothyroxine sodium because the TSH will

    A. have a value of zero when an euthyroid state is re-established.

    B. return to its expected reference range when an euthyroid state is re-established.

    C. increase above its expected reference range when a therapeutic medication level is reached.

    D. decrease below its expected reference range when a therapeutic medication level is reached.

    The TSH will return to is normal reference range when the level of T_4 is re-established and an euthyroid state exists.

    (N) NCLEX® Connection: Reduction of Risk Potential, Laboratory Values

6. Which of the following should the nurse reinforce in regard to taking levothyroxine? (Select all that apply.)

    _____ Use fiber laxatives for constipation.

    _____ Expect to take this medication for 3 to 6 months.

    __X__ **Return to clinic for follow-up laboratory tests of serum TSH.**

    _____ Take medication 30 min before bedtime.

    __X__ **Side effects such as nervousness, heat intolerance, and diarrhea.**

    The client will need to return to the clinic for follow-up laboratory tests of serum TSH because the dose of levothyroxine will also be monitored by the TSH level to avoid dosages that are too high or low. Clients should report nervousness, heat intolerance, and diarrhea, because a decrease in dosage may be indicated. Fiber laxatives should not be recommended as they can interfere with the absorption of levothyroxine. Levothyroxine replaces a hormone that is usually produced by the thyroid gland and will probably need to be taken for the rest of the client's life. Medication is best absorbed on an empty stomach; morning is preferred because evening doses can cause insomnia.

    (N) NCLEX® Connection: Pharmacological Therapies, Adverse Effects/Contraindications/Side Effects/Interactions

UNIT 12	NURSING CARE OF CLIENTS WITH ENDOCRINE DISORDERS
Chapter 77	Adrenal Disorders

Overview

- The adrenal cortex produces:

  o Mineralocorticoids – Aldosterone (increases sodium absorption, causes potassium excretion in the kidney)

  o Glucocorticoids – Cortisol (affects glucose, protein, and fat metabolism; the body's response to stress, and the body's immune function)

  o Sex hormones – Androgens and estrogens

- Disorders of the adrenal gland include Cushing's disease, Cushing's syndrome, Addison's disease, and pheochromocytoma.

CUSHING'S DISEASE AND CUSHING'S SYNDROME

Overview

- Pituitary Cushing's results from oversecretion of adrenocorticotropic hormone (ACTH), which results in excess stimulation of the adrenal cortex (usually bilaterally) and secretion of adrenal cortex hormones.

- Adrenal Cushing's disease results from a disorder of the adrenal cortex and is usually unilateral.

- Cushing's syndrome is the disease process or the signs and symptoms that are seen with prolonged exposure to the glucocorticoid hormones.

Data Collection

- Risk Factors

  o Endogenous causes of increased cortisol (Cushing's disease)

    ▪ Adrenal hyperplasia

    ▪ Adrenocortical carcinoma

    ▪ Carcinomas of the lung, gastrointestinal (GI) tract, or pancreas (These tumors can secrete ACTH.)

    ▪ Pituitary carcinoma that secretes ACTH

- o Exogenous causes of increased cortisol (Cushing's syndrome) include the therapeutic use of glucocorticoids for:
  - Organ transplant
  - Chemotherapy
  - Autoimmune diseases
  - Asthma
  - Allergies
  - Chronic inflammatory diseases
- Subjective Data
  - o Weakness
  - o Fatigue
  - o Back and joint pain
  - o Altered emotional state (may include irritability or depression)
- Objective Data
  - o Physical Findings
    - Evidence of decreased immune function and decreased inflammatory response (increased incidence of infections without the accompanying fever, swelling, drainage, and redness)
    - Thin, fragile skin
    - Bruising and petechiae (fragile blood vessels)
    - Hypertension (sodium and water retention)
    - Tachycardia
    - Weight gain
    - Dependent edema – Changes in fat distribution, including the characteristic fat distribution of moon face, truncal obesity, and fat collection on the back of the neck (buffalo hump)

       View Media Supplement: Moon Face (Image)

    - Fractures (osteoporosis)
    - Muscle wasting (particularly in the extremities)
    - Impaired glucose tolerance
    - Hirsutism (abnormal or excessive hair growth)
    - Acne
    - Red cheeks

- ■ Striae (reddened lines on abdomen and thighs)
- ■ Emotional lability
- ○ Laboratory Tests
  - ■ Elevated plasma cortisol levels in the absence of acute illness or stress are diagnostic for Cushing's disease/syndrome. Urine cortisol levels (24-hr urine collection) contain elevated levels of free cortisol.
  - ■ Plasma ACTH levels
    - □ Hypersecretion of ACTH by the anterior pituitary results in elevated ACTH levels.
    - □ Disorder of the adrenal cortex or medication therapy results in decreased ACTH levels.
  - ■ Serum potassium and calcium levels – Decreased
  - ■ Serum glucose level – Increased
  - ■ Serum sodium level – Increased
  - ■ Lymphocytes – Decreased
  - ■ Dexamethasone suppression tests – Tests vary in length and amount of dexamethasone administered. Twenty-four hr urine collections reveal suppression of cortisol excretion in clients without Cushing's disease. Nonsuppression of cortisol excretion is indicative of Cushing's disease. Medications are withheld and stress is reduced prior to and during testing. False positive results can occur in clients who have acute illness and alcoholism.
- ○ Diagnostic Procedures
  - ■ X-ray, MRI, and CT scans can be performed to identify lesions of the pituitary gland, adrenal gland, lung, gastrointestinal tract, or pancreas.
  - ■ Radiological imaging can be performed to determine the source of adrenal insufficiency (tumor, adrenal atrophy).

Collaborative Care

- • Nursing Care
  - ○ Dietary alterations – Decrease sodium intake and increase intake of potassium, protein, and calcium.
  - ○ Monitor I&O.
  - ○ Obtain daily weight.
  - ○ Monitor for signs of hypervolemia (edema, distended neck veins, shortness of breath, presence of adventitious breath sounds).
  - ○ Maintain a safe environment to minimize the risk of pathological fractures and skin trauma.
  - ○ Prevent infection by performing frequent hand hygiene.

- o Encourage physical activity within the client's limitations.

- o Provide meticulous skin care.

- o Monitor for and protect against skin breakdown and infection.

- Medications

  - o Treatment is dependent upon the cause. For Cushing's syndrome, tapering off glucocorticoids or managing the symptoms may be necessary.

  - o Aminoglutethimide (Cytadren)

    - Adrenal corticosteroid inhibitor

    - Aminoglutethimide decreases adrenal hormone synthesis to provide short-term symptom relief for clients who have Cushing's syndrome.

  - o Ketoconazole (Nizoral)

    - Adrenal corticosteroid inhibitor

    - Ketoconazole is an antifungal agent that when taken in high dosages inhibits adrenal corticosteroid synthesis.

    - Nursing Considerations

      - □ Use temporarily until surgery or other treatment is finished, usually no more than 3 months.

      - □ Monitor blood pressure for hypotension. (Aminoglutethimide)

      - □ Monitor liver enzymes and monitor for signs of liver toxicity (yellow sclera, dark-colored urine). (Ketoconazole)

      - □ Monitor fluids and electrolytes for clients who have gastric effects.

    - Client Education

      - □ Advise clients not to drive or operate machinery until medication effects are known.

      - □ Advise clients that the medication can cause nausea, drowsiness, dizziness, or rash.

      - □ Advise clients that relief is temporary. Symptoms will return if medication is discontinued.

      - □ Inform clients that the medication can be taken with food to relieve gastric effects.

- Interdisciplinary Care

  - o Request a referral for nutritional services to educate clients regarding the need for fluid restriction and appropriate food choices that would be part of a low-sodium, high-protein diet.

- Therapeutic Procedures

  - o Chemotherapy with cytotoxic agents for Cushing's disease caused by a tumor

- Nursing Actions
  - Monitor for adverse effects (thrombocytopenia or nausea and vomiting, depending on the chemotherapeutic agent).
  - Monitor WBC, absolute neutrophil count, platelet count, hemoglobin, and hematocrit.
  - Check clients for bruising and bleeding gums.
  - Administer an antiemetic as prescribed.
- Client Education
  - Instruct clients to avoid crowds and contact with individuals who are infected.
  - Advise clients to monitor for and report signs of bleeding (tarry stools or coffee-ground emesis).
  - Advise clients that alopecia can occur.

○ Radiation Therapy

- Nursing Actions
  - Provide skin care and check for skin damage.
- Client Education
  - Advise clients to:
    - ▶ Avoid removing radiation markings.
    - ▶ Avoid applying lotions other than those prescribed by the radiologist to affected areas.
    - ▶ Avoid exposing irradiated areas to sun.
    - ▶ Expect fatigue and altered taste due to radiation.

- Surgical Interventions

  ○ Hypophysectomy

  - Surgical removal of the pituitary gland (depending on the cause of Cushing's disease)
  - Nursing Actions
    - Monitor and correct electrolyte imbalances, especially sodium, potassium, and chloride.
    - Monitor daily weights and I&O.
    - Monitor and report serum glucose levels.
    - Monitor ECG.
    - Protect clients from developing an infection by using good hand hygiene and avoiding contact with individuals who have infections. Use caution to prevent a fracture by providing assistance getting out of bed and raising side rails.

- ☐ Monitor for bleeding. Monitor nasal drainage for a possible cerebral spinal fluid (CSF) leak. Assess drainage for the presence of glucose or a halo sign (yellow on the edge and clear in the middle), which may indicate CSF.

- ☐ Monitor neurologic condition every hour for the first 24 hr and then every 4 hr.

- ☐ Administer glucocorticoids as prescribed to prevent an abrupt drop in cortisol level.

- ☐ Administer stool softeners as prescribed to prevent straining.

- ■ Client Education

  - ☐ Advise clients to use caution preoperatively to prevent infection or fractures.

  - ☐ Advise clients that they may have nasal packing following a transsphenoidal hypophysectomy. A drip pad will be placed under the nose for bloody drainage. Instruct clients to breathe through the mouth. Advise clients to avoid coughing, blowing their nose, or sneezing.

  - ☐ Instruct clients to avoid bending over and straining to prevent increased intracranial pressure.

  - ☐ Advise clients to notify the provider of sweet-tasting drainage, drainage that makes a halo (yellow on the edge and clear in the middle), or clear drainage from the nose, which may indicate CSF leak. Another indication may be a headache.

- ○ Adrenalectomy

  - ■ Surgical removal of the adrenal gland (can be unilateral [one gland] or bilateral [both glands]).

  - ■ Nursing Actions

    - ☐ Provide postoperative care to prevent complications including hypotension and hypovolemia due to the sudden decrease in catecholamines.

    - ☐ Provide glucocorticoid and hormone replacement as needed.

    - ☐ Monitor for adrenal crisis due to an abrupt drop in cortisol level. Findings can include hypotension, tachycardia, tachypnea, nausea, and headache.

    - ☐ Slowly introduce foods.

  - ■ Client Education

    - ☐ Reinforce to clients about postoperative pain management, deep breathing, and anti-embolism care.

    - ☐ Advise clients of the need to take glucocorticoids, mineralocorticoids, and hormone replacements.

    - ☐ If a bilateral adrenalectomy is performed, lifelong glucocorticoid and mineralocorticoid replacement is required.

    - ☐ If a unilateral adrenalectomy is performed, glucocorticoid supplementation may be needed until the remaining gland is able to produce enough hormones.

- Care After Discharge
  - Client Education
    - Advise clients to take prescribed medications as instructed and monitor for adverse reactions. Advise the client that medication therapy may be lifelong.
    - Advise clients to eat foods high in calcium and vitamin D. The client should not use alcohol or caffeine. Advise clients to monitor for signs of gastric bleeding (coffee-ground emesis or black, tarry stools).
    - Advise clients to avoid infection by using good hygiene and avoiding crowds or individuals who are infected.
    - Advise clients that residual muscle weakness may be present and home assistance may be needed.
    - Instruct clients to monitor weight every day and report weight gain.
- Client Outcomes
  - The client will maintain adequate nutritional intake.
  - The client will maintain a constant weight with balanced fluid I&O.
  - The client will be free of pain.
  - The client will be free of infection or fracture.

Complications

- Risk for bone fractures due to hypocalcemia
  - Nursing Actions
    - Use caution when moving the client.
    - Provide assistance when ambulating.
    - Clear floors to prevent falls.
  - Client Education
    - Encourage a diet high in calcium and vitamin D.
    - Reinforce to clients about dangerous activities that should be avoided.
- Risk for infection due to immunosuppression
  - Immunosuppression and reduced inflammatory response occur due to elevated glucocorticoid levels.
  - Nursing Actions
    - Monitor for subtle signs of infection (fatigue, fever, localized swelling, or redness).

- ○ Client Education

  - ■ Instruct clients about measures to minimize exposure to infectious organisms (avoid ill people and crowds, use good hand hygiene).

  - ■ Report signs of infection to the provider (fever, sore throat, foul-smelling wound drainage, urinary urgency, frequency or burning on urination).

- Risk for adrenal crisis (also known as acute adrenal insufficiency)

  - ○ Sudden drop in corticosteroids due to sudden withdrawal of medication or tumor removal

  - ○ Can develop with abrupt withdrawal of steroid medication

  - ○ Nursing Actions

    - ■ Monitor for hypotension, hyperkalemia, abdominal pain, weakness, and weight loss.

    - ■ Administer glucocorticoids for acute adrenal insufficiency.

  - ○ Client Education

    - ■ Instruct clients to gradually taper the medication.

    - ■ During times of stress, additional glucocorticoids may be needed to prevent adrenal crisis.

ADDISON'S DISEASE

Overview

- Addison's disease is an adrenocortical insufficiency. It is caused by damage or dysfunction of the adrenal cortex. The adrenal cortex produces mineralocorticoids and glucocorticoids.

  - ○ With Addison's disease, the production of mineralocorticoids and glucocorticoids is diminished, resulting in decreased aldosterone and cortisol.

  - ○ Older adult clients are less able to tolerate the complications of Addison's disease and adrenal crisis and will need more frequent monitoring.

Data Collection

- Risk Factors

  - ○ Causes of primary Addison's disease:

    - ■ Idiopathic autoimmune dysfunction (majority of cases)

    - ■ Tuberculosis

    - ■ Histoplasmosis

    - ■ Adrenalectomy

    - ■ Cancer

- o Causes of secondary Addison's disease:
  - Steroid withdrawal
  - Hypophysectomy
  - Pituitary neoplasm
- Subjective and Objective Data
  - o Physical Findings
    - Signs and symptoms of chronic Addison's disease develop slowly.
      - □ Hyperpigmentation
      - □ Weakness and fatigue
      - □ Nausea and vomiting
      - □ Dizziness with orthostatic hypotension
      - □ Severe hypotension (adrenal crisis)
      - □ Dehydration
      - □ Hyponatremia
      - □ Hyperkalemia
      - □ Hypoglycemia
      - □ Hypercalcemia
  - o Laboratory Tests
    - Serum electrolytes – Increased potassium, decreased sodium, and increased calcium
    - BUN and creatinine – Increased
    - Serum glucose – Decreased
    - Serum cortisol – Decreased
    - Adrenocorticotropic hormone (ACTH) stimulation test – ACTH is infused, and the cortisol response is measured. With primary adrenal insufficiency, plasma cortisol levels do not rise.
  - o Diagnostic Procedures
    - ECG
      - □ Used to assess for ECG changes or dysrhythmias associated with electrolyte imbalance
      - □ Nursing Actions
        - ▸ Apply electrodes using conductive gel.
      - □ Client Education
        - ▸ Explain all procedures to clients.
    - X-ray, MRI, and CT scans
      - □ Radiological imaging to determine source of adrenal insufficiency (tumor or adrenal atrophy)

Collaborative Care

- Nursing Care

  - Monitor clients for fluid deficits and hyponatremia. Observe for signs and symptoms of dehydration. Obtain orthostatic vital signs.

  - Monitor clients receiving hydrocortisone boluses and a continuous infusion or periodic boluses.

  - Monitor for and treat hyperkalemia:

    - Obtain a serum potassium and ECG.

    - Administer sodium polystyrene sulfonate (Kayexalate), insulin, calcium, glucose, and sodium bicarbonate as prescribed.

  - Monitor for and treat hypoglycemia:

    - Perform frequent checks of the client's neurologic status, monitor for signs and symptoms of hypoglycemia, and check serum glucose.

    - Administer food and/or supplemental glucose.

  - Maintain a safe environment:

    - Provide assistance ambulating.

    - Raise side rails.

    - Prevent falls by keeping floors clear.

- Medications

  - Hydrocortisone (Cortef), prednisone (Deltasone), and cortisone (Cortisone)

    - Glucocorticoid is used as an adrenocorticoid replacement for adrenal insufficiency and as an anti-inflammatory.

    - Nursing Considerations

      □ Monitor weight, blood pressure, and electrolytes.

      □ Increase dosage during periods of stress or illness if necessary.

      □ Taper dose if discontinuing to avoid adrenal crisis.

      □ Give with food to reduce gastric effects.

    - Client Education

      □ Advise clients to:

        ‣ Take medication as directed.

        ‣ Avoid discontinuing the medication abruptly.

        ‣ Report symptoms of Cushing's syndrome (round face, edema, weight gain).

        ‣ Take the medications with food to avoid GI upset.

        ‣ Report symptoms of adrenal insufficiency (fever, fatigue, muscle weakness, anorexia).

- ○ Fludrocortisone (Florinef)
  - ■ Fludrocortisone is a mineralocorticoid used as a replacement in adrenal insufficiency.
  - ■ Nursing Considerations
    - □ Monitor weight, blood pressure (hypertension), and electrolytes.
    - □ Dosage may need to be increased during periods of stress or illness.
  - ■ Client Education
    - □ Advise clients to take the medication as directed.
    - □ Warn the client to expect mild peripheral edema.
- • Interdisciplinary Care
  - ○ Request a referral for home assistance for fluid, medication, and dietary management as needed.
- • Care After Discharge
  - ○ Client Education
    - ■ Advise clients to:
      - □ Take prescribed medications as instructed and monitor for adverse reactions.
      - □ Avoid using alcohol and caffeine.
      - □ Monitor for and report signs of gastric bleeding (tarry, black stool, coffee-ground emesis).
      - □ Monitor for hypoglycemia (diaphoresis, shaking, tachycardia, headache).
      - □ Report symptoms of adrenal insufficiency (fever, fatigue, muscle weakness, dizziness, anorexia).
      - □ Instruct clients who have Addison's disease to increase corticosteroid doses as directed by a provider, during times of stress.
    - ■ Inform clients that medication therapy may be lifelong.
- • Client Outcomes
  - ○ The client will maintain balanced electrolytes and glucose levels.
  - ○ The client will maintain a normal blood pressure with balanced fluid intake and output.

Complications

- • Addisonian Crisis (also known as adrenal crisis or acute adrenal insufficiency) has a rapid onset. It is a medical emergency.
  - ○ Addisonian crisis occurs when there is an acute drop in adrenocorticoids due to sudden discontinuation of glucocorticoid medications or when induced by severe trauma, infection, or stress. Signs and symptoms of adrenal crisis develop rapidly.

- ○ Nursing Actions
  - Monitor clients receiving IV fluid replacements.
  - Monitor ECG and electrolytes.
  - Monitor vital signs.
  - Administer adrenocorticoids as prescribed.
- ○ Client Education
  - Advise clients to:
    - □ Notify the provider of any infection, trauma, or stress that can increase the need for adrenocorticoids.
    - □ Take the medication as directed.
    - □ Not discontinue their medication abruptly.

- Hypoglycemia
  - ○ Insufficient glucocorticoid production causes increased insulin sensitivity and decreased glycogen, which leads to hypoglycemia.
  - ○ Nursing Actions
    - Monitor glucose levels.
  - ○ Client Education
    - Advise clients to monitor for hypoglycemia.
      - □ Symptoms can include diaphoresis, shaking, tachycardia, and headache.
    - Instruct clients to have a 15-gram carbohydrate snack readily available.

- Hyperkalemia/Hyponatremia
  - ○ Decrease in aldosterone levels can cause increased excretion of sodium and decreased excretion of potassium.
  - ○ Nursing Actions
    - Monitor electrolytes and ECG.
  - ○ Client Education
    - Advise clients to take the medications as directed.
    - Instruct clients to report signs of hyperkalemia (nausea, cardiac palpitations/missed beat).

PHEOCHROMOCYTOMA

Overview

- Pheochromocytoma is a tumor that produces and stores catecholamines (epinephrine and norepinephrine). The excess epinephrine and norepinephrine produce sympathetic nervous system effects.

- If the catecholamine surge of a pheochromocytoma is recognized promptly and treated appropriately, it is potentially curable. If the diagnosis is missed, the client may suffer severe cardiac and neurologic damage.

- The cause of pheochromocytomas is not known.

Data Collection

- Risk Factors

  o Occurs more often in clients with

    ▪ Neurofibromatosis

    ▪ Multiple endocrine neoplasia syndromes

    ▪ Age between 40 and 60 years

  o Precipitating causes of a catecholamine surge by a pheochromocytoma

    ▪ Anesthesia

    ▪ Opiates and opiate antagonists (naloxone)

    ▪ Dopamine antagonists (droperidol, phenothiazines)

    ▪ Medications that inhibit catecholamine reuptake (tricyclic antidepressants)

    ▪ Childbirth

    ▪ Radiographic contrast media

    ▪ Foods high in tyramine (wine, aged cheese)

    ▪ Increases in intra-abdominal pressure (abdominal palpation) can cause a hypertensive episode

    ▪ Older adult clients may be less able to tolerate elevations in blood pressure caused by pheochromocytomas.

- Subjective and Objective Data

  o Pain in chest/abdomen accompanied by nausea and vomiting

  o Hypertension

  o Headache

  o Palpitations

  o Diaphoresis

○ Heat intolerance

○ Tremors

○ Apprehension

○ Laboratory Tests

- Vanillylmandelic acid (VMA) testing – 24-hr urine collection for VMA, a breakdown product of catecholamines

  □ A normal VMA level is 2 to 7 mg/24 hr. High levels at rest indicate a pheochromocytoma.

○ Diagnostic Procedures

- Clonidine suppression test

  □ If a client does not have a pheochromocytoma, clonidine (Catapres) suppresses catecholamine release and decreases the serum level of catecholamines (decreased blood pressure). If the client does have a pheochromocytoma, the clonidine has no effect (no decreased blood pressure).

- Administration of phentolamine (Regitine)

  □ Phentolamine is used to control hypertensive crisis. A rapid decrease in systolic blood pressure of 35 mm Hg or greater and a diastolic blood pressure of 25 mm Hg or greater with the administration of phentolamine (Regitine), an alpha blocker, is diagnostic.

Collaborative Care

- Nursing Care

  ○ Do not palpate the abdomen. This can cause catecholamine release, which can lead to a hypertensive crisis.

  ○ Monitor ECG changes and fluid and electrolyte laboratory values.

  ○ Monitor blood glucose levels closely.

- Medications

  ○ Alpha adrenergic blockers – Prazosin (Minipress) and phenoxybenzamine (Dibenzyline)

    - Given before surgery to regulate hypertension

    - Nursing Considerations

      □ Always obtain the client's blood pressure before administering.

      □ Start with a low dose of medication.

      □ Watch for orthostatic hypotension.

      □ Monitor blood pressure 2 hr after administering the initial dose.

- Client Education
  - Instruct clients to change positions slowly and notify the nurse if feelings of lightheadedness occur.
  - Have clients take the medication with food.
  - Beta blockers – Metoprolol (Lopressor)
    - Given before surgery to regulate hypertension
    - Nursing Considerations
      - Always obtain the client's blood pressure and pulse before administering.
      - Watch for bradycardia (heart rate less than 60/min). If bradycardia occurs, hold medication and notify the provider.
      - Watch for orthostatic hypotension.
      - Use cautiously with clients who have diabetes mellitus.
    - Client Education
      - Provide clients with knowledge about the disease, the reasons for the diagnostic tests, the need for yearly testing of metanephrine, the need to monitor blood pressure, and the symptoms of high blood pressure.
      - Instruct clients to change positions slowly and notify the nurse if feelings of light-headedness occur.
      - Have the client take the medication with food.
  - Glucocorticoids – Prednisone (Deltasone)
    - Given after surgery for adrenal suppression, to replace a drop in cortisol levels

- Interdisciplinary Care
  - Endocrinology services may be consulted to manage adrenal disease.

- Surgical Interventions
  - Unilateral or bilateral adrenalectomy surgery (the removal of one or both adrenal glands to excise the tumor) is the preferred therapeutic procedure.

- Care After Discharge
  - Request a referral for home health services, which may be indicated regarding incision care, medication regimen, and blood pressure follow-up.
  - Client Education
    - Demonstrate how to properly take blood pressure and interpret readings.
    - Promote good hand hygiene to prevent infection.
    - Encourage clients to check skin daily for skin breakdown and sensitivity.
    - Advise clients to check weight daily and keep a daily record to monitor for fluid excess.

- Advise clients to notify the provider if there is a weight gain of 3 lbs or more in a week.

- Encourage clients to wear a medical identification bracelet.

- Promote a diet rich in vitamins, calories, and minerals.

- Encourage smoking cessation, if the client smokes.

- Encourage clients to avoid caffeinated beverages.

- Client Outcomes

  o The client will maintain baseline blood pressure.

  o The client will maintain a weight that is within 10% of his ideal body weight.

  o The client will maintain a diet regimen high in vitamins, calories, and minerals.

  o The client will take medications as prescribed.

Complications

- Hypertensive Crisis

  o This is the most significant complication of a pheochromocytoma.

  o Nursing Actions

    - Monitor clients receiving alpha blockers as prescribed (phentolamine IV, phenoxybenzamine).

APPLICATION EXERCISES

1. A client who has Cushing's disease is at risk for developing which of the following? (Select all that apply.)

    _____ Dysphagia

    _____ Renal failure

    _____ Infection

    _____ Gastric ulcer

    _____ Bone fractures

    _____ Skin breakdown

    _____ Decreased muscle mass

2. A client who has Cushing's disease has excessive cortisol levels. Which of the following is the highest priority data to collect?

    A. Heart rate

    B. Daily weights

    C. Respiratory rate

    D. Check for edema

3. A client who has Cushing's disease is at risk for bone fractures. Which of the following should be reinforced to help reduce the risk for bone fractures at home? (Select all that apply.)

    _____ Cushion floor with throw rugs.

    _____ Install grab bars in the shower.

    _____ Eat a diet high in calcium.

    _____ Avoid exposure to the sun.

    _____ Use cane or walker when ambulating.

4. A nurse is caring for a client who has Addison's disease and has been prescribed prednisone (Deltasone) by the provider. Which of the following instructions should the nurse reinforce? (Select all that apply.)

    _____ Eat a low-sodium diet.

    _____ Take medication on an empty stomach.

    _____ Do not discontinue medication suddenly.

    _____ Notify the provider of any illness or stress.

    _____ Report any symptoms of weakness or dizziness.

UNIT 12	NURSING CARE OF CLIENTS WITH ENDOCRINE DISORDERS
Chapter 78	Diabetes Management

Overview

- Diabetes mellitus is characterized by chronic hyperglycemia due to inadequate insulin secretion and/or the effectiveness of endogenous insulin (insulin resistance).

- Diabetes mellitus is a contributing factor to development of cardiovascular disease, hypertension, renal failure, blindness, and stroke as individuals age.

Data Collection

- Risk Factors

  o Genetics may predispose an individual to the occurrence of type 1 or type 2 diabetes mellitus.

  o Toxins and viruses can predispose an individual to diabetes mellitus by destroying the beta cells of the islets of Langerhans in the pancreas, leading to type 1 diabetes mellitus.

  o Obesity, physical inactivity, high triglycerides (greater than 250 mg/dL), and hypertension may lead to the development of insulin resistance and type 2 diabetes.

  o Secondary causes of diabetes include pancreatitis and Cushing's syndrome.

  o Because of the deterioration of the function of all organs, older adult clients are at risk for:

    ▪ Kidney and liver dysfunction leading to altered urinary output and altered metabolism of medications.

    ▪ Vision alterations (yellowing of lens, decreased ability of depth perception, cataracts), as well as eye changes, may be related to diabetic retinopathy.

- Subjective and Objective Data

  o Blood glucose – Level less than 70 mg/dL; rapid onset

AUTONOMIC NERVOUS SYSTEM RESPONSES – RAPID ONSET	IMPAIRED CEREBRAL FUNCTION – GRADUAL ONSET
• Hunger, lightheadedness, and shakiness • Anxiety, nervousness, and irritability • Pale, cool skin • Diaphoresis • Respirations may be unchanged or shallow • Irritability • Tachycardia and palpitations	• Strange or unusual feelings • Decreased level of consciousness • Difficulty in thinking and inability to concentrate • Change in emotional behavior • Slurred speech • Headache and blurred vision • Seizures leading to coma

- ■ Hyperglycemia – Blood glucose level usually greater than 250 mg/dL; gradual onset

- ■ Mental status varies from alertness to stupor

- ■ Thirst

- ■ Frequent urination

- ■ Nausea and vomiting

- ■ Skin that is warm, dry, and flushed with poor turgor

- ■ Dry mucous membranes

- ■ Soft eyeballs

- ■ Weakness

- ■ Rapid, weak pulse and hypotension

- ■ Rapid, deep respirations (Kussmaul respirations, with acetone/fruity odor due to ketones)

  - ○ Laboratory Tests

    - ■ Diagnostic criteria for diabetes include two of the following findings (on separate days)

      - □ Symptoms of diabetes plus casual plasma glucose concentration of greater than 200 mg/dL (without regard to time since last meal)

      - □ Fasting blood glucose greater than 126 mg/dL

      - □ Two-hour glucose greater than 200 mg/dL with an oral glucose tolerance test

    - ■ Fasting blood glucose

      - □ Nursing Actions

        - ▸ Postpone administration of antidiabetic medication until after the level is drawn.

      - □ Client Education

        - ▸ Ensure that clients have fasted (no food or drink other than water) for the 8 hr prior to the blood draw.

- Oral glucose tolerance test
  - Obtain a blood sample to determine a fasting blood glucose level at the start of the test.
  - Instruct clients to consume a specified amount of glucose.
  - Obtain a blood sample for blood glucose levels every 30 min for 2 hr.
  - Monitor clients for hypoglycemia throughout the procedure.
  - Client Education
    - Instruct the client to consume a balanced diet for 3 days prior to the test. Then, instruct the client to fast for 10 to 12 hr prior to the test.
- Glycosylated hemoglobin (HbA1c)
  - The expected reference range is 4% to 6%, but an acceptable target for clients who have diabetes may be 6.5% to 8%, with a target goal of less than 7%. HbA1c is the best indicator of the average blood glucose level for the past 120 days. It assists in evaluating treatment effectiveness and adherence.

- Diagnostic Procedures
  - Self-monitored blood glucose (SMBG)
    - Nursing Actions
      - Instruct clients in the proper procedure for blood sample collection and use of a glucose meter. Supplemental short-acting insulin can be prescribed for elevated pre-meal glucose levels.
    - Client Education
      - Instruct clients to check the accuracy of the strips with the control solution provided.
      - Advise clients to keep a record of the SMBG that includes time, date, serum glucose level, insulin dose, food intake, and other events that may alter glucose metabolism, such as activity level or illness.

Collaborative Care

- Nursing Care
  - Monitor:
    - Blood glucose levels and factors affecting levels (other medications).
    - I&O and weight.
    - Skin integrity and healing status of any wounds (feet and folds of the skin should be monitored closely).
    - Sensory alterations (tingling, numbness).
    - Visual alterations.
    - Presence of recurrent infections.

- Dietary practices.
- Exercise patterns.
- The client's self-monitoring blood glucose skill proficiency.
- The client's self-medication administration proficiency.

○ Reinforce proper foot care.

- Inspect feet daily and use a mirror to check the bottom of the feet, as needed.
- Wash feet daily with mild soap and warm water.
- Pat feet dry gently, especially between the toes.
- Use mild foot powder (powder with cornstarch) on sweaty feet.
- Do not use commercial remedies for the removal of calluses or corns.
- Consult a podiatrist.
- Perform nail care after a bath/shower.
- Separate overlapping toes with cotton or lamb's wool.
- Avoid open-toe, open-heel shoes. Leather shoes are preferred to plastic ones. Wear shoes that fit correctly. Wear slippers with soles. Do not go barefoot. Shake out shoes before putting them on.
- Wear clean, absorbent socks or stockings that are made of cotton or wool and have not been mended.
- Do not use hot water bottles or heating pads to warm feet. Wear socks for warmth.
- Avoid prolonged sitting, standing, and crossing of legs.

○ Follow agency policies for nail care. Some protocols allow for trimming toenails straight across with clippers and filing edges with an emery board or nail file. If clippers or scissors are contraindicated, clients should file the nails straight across.

○ Instruct clients to cleanse cuts with warm water and mild soap, gently dry, and apply a dry dressing. Instruct clients to monitor healing and to seek intervention promptly.

○ Provide nutritional guidelines.

- Plan meals to achieve appropriate timing of food intake, activity, onset, and peak of insulin. Calories and food composition should be similar each day.
- Eat at regular intervals and do not skip meals.
- Count grams of carbohydrates consumed.
- Recognize that 15 g of carbohydrates are equal to 1 carbohydrate exchange.
- Restrict calories and increase physical activity as appropriate to facilitate weight loss (for clients who are obese) or to prevent obesity.
- Include fiber in the diet to increase carbohydrate metabolism and to help control cholesterol levels.

- Use artificial sweeteners.
- Keep fat content below 30% of the total caloric intake.

○ Instruct clients in appropriate techniques for SMBG, including obtaining blood samples, recording and responding to results, and correctly handling supplies and equipment.

○ Instruct clients in guidelines to follow when sick.

- Monitor blood glucose every 3 to 4 hr.
- Continue to take insulin or oral antidiabetic agents.
- Consume 4 oz of sugar-free, non-caffeinated liquid every 0.5 hr to prevent dehydration.
- Meet carbohydrate needs through soft food if possible. If not, consume liquids equal to usual carbohydrate content.
- Test urine for ketones and report to provider if they are abnormal (the level should be negative to small).
- Rest.
- Call the provider if:
  □ Blood glucose is greater than 240 mg/dL.
  □ Fever is greater than 38.9° C (102° F), does not respond to acetaminophen, or lasts more than 12 hr.
  □ Feeling disoriented or confused.
  □ Experiencing rapid breathing.
  □ Vomiting occurs more than once.
  □ Diarrhea occurs more than five times or for longer than 24 hr.
  □ Unable to tolerate liquids.
  □ Illness lasts longer than 2 days.

○ Advise clients to eat at regular intervals, avoid alcohol intake, and adjust insulin to exercise and diet to avoid hypoglycemia.

○ Instruct clients what to do if they experience signs and symptoms of hypoglycemia (hunger, lightheadedness, shakiness, anxiety, nervousness, irritability, pallor, diaphoresis, palpitations, drowsiness, headache, dizziness, confusion).

- Check blood glucose level.
- Follow guidelines outlined by the provider/diabetes educator. Guidelines may include:
  □ Treat with 15 to 20 g carbohydrates.
    ▸ Examples – 4 oz orange juice, 2 oz grape juice, 8 oz milk, glucose tablets per manufacturer's suggestion to equal 15 g

- ☐ Recheck blood glucose in 15 min.
- ☐ If still low (less than 70 mg/dL), give 15 to 20 g more of carbohydrates.
- ☐ Recheck blood glucose in 15 min.
- ☐ If blood glucose is within normal limits, take 7 g protein (if the next meal is more than an hour away).
  - ▸ Example – 1 oz of cheese (1 string cheese), 2 tablespoons of peanut butter, or 8 oz of milk
- ■ Instruct family members to administer glucagon SC or IM (repeat in 10 min if still unconscious) if the client is unconscious or unable to swallow and to notify the provider.
- ○ Instruct clients regarding signs and symptoms of hyperglycemia (hot, dry skin and fruity breath) and measures to take in response to hyperglycemia.
  - ■ Encourage oral fluid intake.
  - ■ Administer insulin as prescribed.
  - ■ Restrict exercise when blood glucose levels are greater than 250 mg/dL.
  - ■ Test urine for ketones and report if abnormal.
  - ■ Consult the provider if symptoms progress.
- ○ Instruct clients to wear a medical identification wristband.

- ● Medications
  - ○ Clients who have type 1 diabetes are on an insulin regimen that frequently consists of more than one type of insulin (rapid, short, intermediate, and long acting). Insulin given in this manner is administered one or more times per day and based on a client's blood glucose level. Some clients who have type 2 diabetes or women who have gestational diabetes may require insulin if glycemic control is unable to be obtained with diet, exercise, and oral hypoglycemics.
  - ○ Some clients are placed on an insulin pump, which is a small pump that is worn externally, contains insulin, and delivers insulin as programmed via a needle inserted into the subcutaneous tissue. The needle should be changed at least every 3 days.

 View Media Supplement: Insulin Pump (Image)

  - ○ Clients who have type 2 diabetes can usually regulate their blood glucose with diet and exercise, but may also need pharmacological intervention.

TYPE	TRADE NAME	ONSET	PEAK	DURATION
Rapid acting	Insulin lispro (Humalog)	Less than 15 min	0.5 to 1 hr	3 to 4 hr
Short acting	Regular insulin (Humulin R)	0.5 to 1 hr	2 to 3 hr	5 to 7 hr
Intermediate acting	NPH insulin (Humulin N)	1 to 2 hr	4 to 12 hr	18 to 24 hr
Long acting	Insulin glargine (Lantus)	1 hr	none	10.4 to 24 hr

- Nursing Considerations
  - Observe clients performing self-administration of insulin and offer additional instruction as indicated.
- Client Education
  - Provide information regarding oral antidiabetic medications.
    - Administer as prescribed (for example, 30 min before first main meal for most oral blood glucose lowering agents or with the first bite of each main meal for alpha-glucosidase inhibitors).
    - Avoid alcohol with sulfonylurea agents (disulfiram-like reaction).
    - Monitor renal function (biguanides).
    - Monitor liver function (thiazolidinediones and alpha-glucosidase inhibitors).
    - Advise women of childbearing age taking thiazolidinediones that additional contraception methods may be needed, because these medications reduce the blood levels of some oral contraceptives.
  - Provide information regarding self-administration of insulin.
    - Rotate injection sites (prevent lipohypertrophy) within one anatomic site (to prevent day-to-day changes in absorption rates).
    - Do not mix insulin glargine (Lantus) with other insulins due to incompatibility.

 View Media Supplement: Insulin SQ Injection Sites (Image)

    - Inject at a 90° angle (45° angle if thin). Aspiration for blood is not necessary.
    - When mixing a rapid- or short-acting insulin with a longer-acting insulin, draw up the shorter-acting insulin into the syringe first and then the longer-acting insulin (this reduces the risk of introducing the longer-acting insulin into the shorter-acting insulin vial).
- Oral hypoglycemics
  - Biguanides – Metformin HCL (Glucophage)
    - Reduces the production of glucose through suppression of gluconeogenesis
    - Nursing Considerations
      - Monitor significance of gastrointestinal (GI) effects (anorexia, nausea, vomiting).
      - Monitor for lactic acidosis, especially in clients who have renal insufficiency or liver dysfunction.

- ☐ Client Education
  - ▸ Instruct clients:
    - ▹ To take vitamin B_{12} and folic acid supplements.
    - ▹ To contact the provider if signs of lactic acidosis (myalgia, sluggishness, somnolence, hyperventilation) are experienced.
    - ▹ That this medication can be taken during pregnancy for gestational diabetes.

- ■ Sulfonylureas – Tolbutamide (Orinase), chlorpropamide (Diabinese), and glyburide (DiaBeta, Micronase)
  - ☐ Stimulates insulin release from the pancreas
  - ☐ Nursing Considerations
    - ▸ Monitor for hypoglycemia. Beta blockers can mask tachycardia typically seen during hypoglycemia. Provide instruction regarding symptoms of hypoglycemia accordingly.
  - ☐ Client Education
    - ▸ Instruct clients to avoid:
      - ▹ During pregnancy.
      - ▹ Alcohol due to disulfiram effect.

- ■ Meglitinides – Repaglinide (Prandin) and nateglinide (Starlix)
  - ☐ Stimulates insulin release from pancreas
  - ☐ Nursing Considerations
    - ▸ Monitor for hypoglycemia.
    - ▸ Do not administer with gemfibrozil (Lopid).
  - ☐ Client Education
    - ▸ Instruct the client to take before meals exactly as prescribed, usually within 30 min, and to not take the medication if the meal is skipped.

- ■ Thiazolidinediones – Rosiglitazone (Avandia) and pioglitazone (Actos)
  - ☐ Increase cellular response to insulin by decreasing insulin resistance
  - ☐ Nursing Considerations
    - ▸ Monitor for fluid retention, especially in clients who have a history of heart failure.
    - ▸ Monitor the client's LDL and triglycerides for elevations.
  - ☐ Client Education
    - ▸ Instruct clients to have serum alanine aminotransferase (ALT) checked every 6 months after baseline.

- Alpha-Glucosidase Inhibitors – Acarbose (Precose) and miglitol (Glyset)
  - Slows carbohydrate absorption and digestion
  - Nursing Considerations
    - Monitor for iron deficiency anemia (hemoglobin and iron levels).
  - Client Education
    - Instruct clients to take with first bite of each meal.
    - Alert clients regarding GI discomfort, which is common with these medications (abdominal distention, cramps, excessive gas, diarrhea).
    - Instruct clients to have liver function tests performed every 3 months or as prescribed.
    - Instruct clients to report jaundice immediately.
- Gliptins – Sitagliptin (Januvia)
  - Augments naturally occurring incretin hormones, which promote release of insulin and decrease secretion of glucagon
  - Nursing Considerations
    - These medications have very few side effects, but upper respiratory symptoms (nasal and throat inflammation) may be present.
  - Client Education
    - Instruct clients to report persistent upper respiratory symptoms.

- Supplemental medications
  - Pramlintide (Symlin)
    - Pramlintide mimics the actions of the naturally occurring peptide hormone amylin, resulting in reduction of postprandial glucose levels from decreased gastric emptying time and inhibition of secretion of glucagon. There is also an increase in the sensation of satiety, which helps decrease caloric intake.

- Nursing Considerations
  - Supplemental glucose control for clients with type 1 or type 2 diabetes
    - Use in conjunction with insulin or an oral hypoglycemic agent, usually metformin or a sulfonylurea.

- Client Education
  - Instruct clients to administer subcutaneously prior to meals, using the thigh or abdomen.
    - Instruct clients to keep unopened vials in the refrigerator and not to freeze. Opened vials can be kept cool or at room temperature, but should be discarded after 28 days. Keep vials out of direct sunlight.
    - Instruct clients not to mix medication with insulin in the same syringe.

- Exenatide (Byetta)
  - Mimics the effects of naturally occurring glucagon-like peptide-1, and thereby promotes release of insulin, decreases secretion of glucagon, and slows gastric emptying. Fasting and postprandial blood glucose levels are lowered.
  - Nursing Considerations
    - Supplemental glucose control for clients with type 2 diabetes
      - Can be used in conjunction with an oral hypoglycemic agent, usually metformin or a sulfonylurea.
  - Client Education
    - Instruct clients:
      - That this medication is supplied in prefilled injector pens.
      - To administer subcutaneously in the thigh, abdomen, or upper arms.
      - To give injection within 60 min before the morning and evening meal. Never administer after a meal.
      - To keep the injection pen in the refrigerator and to discard after 30 days.
- Interdisciplinary Care
  - Request a referral to a diabetes educator for comprehensive education in diabetes management.
- Care After Discharge
  - Client Education
    - Reinforce to clients:
      - That exercise and good nutrition are necessary for controlling diabetes.
      - How to monitor blood glucose levels.
      - The importance of diligent foot and skin care.
- Client Outcomes
  - The client will:
    - Have blood glucose levels within an acceptable range.
    - Be able to self-administer insulin.
    - Be able to monitor for complications and intervene as necessary.

Complications

- Cardiovascular and cerebrovascular disease

  o Hypertension, myocardial infarction, and stroke

  o Nursing Actions

    ▪ Monitor blood pressure.

  o Client Education

    ▪ Encourage clients to:

      □ Have cholesterol (HDL, LDL, and triglycerides) checked yearly along with blood pressure and have HbA1c levels checked every 3 months.

      □ Participate in regular physical activity.

      □ Follow a dietary plan that includes low-fat meals that are high in fruits, vegetables, and whole grain foods.

    ▪ Remind clients to report shortness of breath, headaches (persistent and transient), numbness in distal extremities, swelling of feet, infrequent urination, and changes in vision.

- Impaired vision and blindness

  o Caused by diabetic retinopathy

  o Client Education

    ▪ Encourage:

      □ Yearly eye exams to ensure the health of the eyes and to protect vision.

      □ Clients to inspect feet daily and to use a mirror to assess the bottom of the feet, as needed.

- Foot injury

  o Caused by sensory neuropathy, ischemia, and infection

  o Nursing Actions

    ▪ Monitor blood glucose levels.

    ▪ Provide foot care.

  o Client Education

    ▪ Encourage annual exams by a podiatrist.

    ▪ Instruct the client to examine feet daily.

    ▪ Provide foot care instructions.

- Renal failure

  o Damage to the kidneys from prolonged elevated blood glucose levels and dehydration

- o Nursing Actions

  - ▪ Monitor hydration and renal function (I&O, creatinine levels).

  - ▪ Report an hourly output of less than 30 mL/hr.

  - ▪ Monitor blood pressure.

- o Client Education

  - ▪ Encourage yearly urine analysis, BUN, and creatinine clearance.

  - ▪ Encourage the client to avoid soda, alcohol, and toxic levels of acetaminophen.

  - ▪ Teach the client to consume 2 to 3 L of fluid per day from food and beverage sources and to drink an adequate amount of water.

  - ▪ Tell the client to report decrease in urine output to the provider.

View Media Supplement:
- Diabetic Retinopathy (Image)
- Diabetic Foot Ulcers (Images)

- Diabetic ketoacidosis (DKA) is an acute, life-threatening condition characterized by hyperglycemia (greater than 300 mg/dL) resulting in the breakdown of body fat for energy and an accumulation of ketones in the blood and urine. The onset is rapid, and the mortality rate of DKA is 1% to 10%.

- Hyperglycemic-hyperosmolar state (HHS) is an acute, life-threatening condition characterized by profound hyperglycemia (greater than 600 mg/dL), dehydration, and an absence of ketosis. The onset generally occurs over several days, and the mortality rate of HHS is up to 15% or more.

- Nursing Actions

  - o Monitor clients receiving IV fluid and electrolyte replacement.

  - o Provide rapid isotonic fluid (0.9% sodium chloride) replacement to maintain perfusion to vital organs. Monitor the client for evidence of fluid volume excess due to the need for large quantities of fluid.

  - o Follow with a hypotonic fluid (0.45% sodium chloride) to continue replacing losses to total body fluid.

  - o When serum glucose levels approach 250 mg/dL, add glucose to IV fluids to minimize the risk of cerebral edema associated with drastic changes in serum osmolality.

  - o Monitor clients receiving Regular insulin (Humulin R) 0.1 unit/kg as an IV bolus dose and then follow with a continuous IV infusion of Regular insulin at 0.1 unit/kg/hr.

  - o Monitor glucose levels hourly.

  - o Monitor serum potassium levels. Potassium levels will initially be elevated with insulin therapy, but potassium will shift into cells and the client will need to be monitored for hypokalemia.

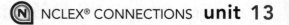

UNIT 13: NURSING CARE OF CLIENTS WITH IMMUNE SYSTEM AND INFECTIOUS DISORDERS

- Immune and Infectious Disorders Diagnostic Procedures
- HIV/AIDS
- Autoimmune Disorders
- Immunizations
- Bacterial, Viral, Fungal, and Parasitic Infections
- General Principles of Cancer
- Cancer Treatment Options
- Pain Management for Clients with Cancer

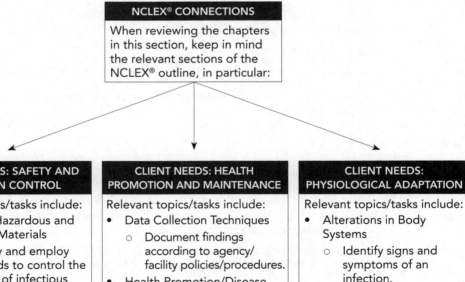

NCLEX® CONNECTIONS

When reviewing the chapters in this section, keep in mind the relevant sections of the NCLEX® outline, in particular:

CLIENT NEEDS: SAFETY AND INFECTION CONTROL

Relevant topics/tasks include:
- Handling Hazardous and Infectious Materials
  - Identify and employ methods to control the spread of infectious agents.
- Standard Precautions/Transmission-Based Precautions/Surgical Asepsis
  - Identify communicable diseases and modes of transmission.

CLIENT NEEDS: HEALTH PROMOTION AND MAINTENANCE

Relevant topics/tasks include:
- Data Collection Techniques
  - Document findings according to agency/facility policies/procedures.
- Health Promotion/Disease Prevention
  - Gather data on client health history and risk for disease.
- Lifestyle Choices
  - Identify client lifestyle practices that may have an impact on health.

CLIENT NEEDS: PHYSIOLOGICAL ADAPTATION

Relevant topics/tasks include:
- Alterations in Body Systems
  - Identify signs and symptoms of an infection.
- Basic Pathophysiology
  - Consider general principles of client disease process when providing care.

UNIT 13	NURSING CARE OF CLIENTS WITH IMMUNE SYSTEM AND INFECTIOUS DISORDERS
Chapter 79	Immune and Infectious Disorders Diagnostic Procedures

Overview

- Diagnostic procedures for immune and infectious disorders involve identification of pathogenic micro-organisms. The most accurate and definitive way to identify micro-organisms and cell characteristics is by examining blood, body fluids, and tissue samples under a microscope.

- Immune and infectious disorders diagnostic procedures that nurses should be knowledgeable about include:

  o Culture and sensitivity

  o Serum WBC count with differential

  o Radioallergosorbent test

  o Skin testing for allergens

- Effective treatment of infectious disease begins with identification of the pathogenic micro-organism.

Culture and Sensitivity

- Culture refers to isolation of the pathogen on culture media.

- Sensitivity refers to the effect that antimicrobial agents have on the micro-organism.

  o If the micro-organism is killed by the antimicrobial, the microbe is considered to be sensitive to that medication.

  o If tolerable levels of the medication are unable to kill the microbe, the microbe is considered to be resistant to that medication.

- A culture and sensitivity can be done on a sample of purulent drainage, urine, sputum, and other body fluids.

- Cultures should be done prior to initiating antimicrobial therapy.

- Indications

  o Evidence of an infection may include an area that is raised, reddened, edematous, and/or warm. There may be purulent drainage and/or fever.

- Interpretation of Findings

  o The microbe responsible for the infection is identified in the culture, and the antimicrobials that are sensitive to that microbe are listed.

  o Heavy growth of greater than 100,000 colonies definitively diagnoses an infection. Negative results are less than 10,000 colonies.

  o Indeterminate results are 10,000 to 100,000 colonies.

  o Appropriate medications are those with 3 to 4 degrees of sensitivity.

- Preprocedure

  o Nursing Actions

    ▪ Use standard precautions when collecting and handling specimens.

    ▪ Most specimens will be collected by the nurse.

  o Client Education

    ▪ Encourage clients to wash hands frequently.

    ▪ Clients should notify the nurse when a sample is available for collection (urine specimen).

- Intraprocedure

  o Nursing Actions

    ▪ Ensure a sufficient quantity of a specimen is collected and placed in the appropriate sterile container. Culturette tubes are also available and contain a sterile cotton-tipped applicator and a fixative that is released after the infectious exudate is applied to the applicator and inserted in the tube.

    ▪ Label the specimen and deliver it to the laboratory promptly for appropriate storage and analysis. Check facility protocol regarding the timeframe in which cultures should be delivered to the laboratory.

- Postprocedure

  o Nursing Actions

    ▪ Results of culture and sensitivity tests are usually available preliminarily within 24 to 48 hr, with final results in 72 hr.

    ▪ If culture and sensitivity results reveal that the cultured organism is not sensitive to currently prescribed antimicrobial agents, it is the nurse's responsibility to report the results to the provider before administering subsequent doses of an ineffective antimicrobial.

      □ Ideally, antimicrobial therapy should not begin until after the specimen for culture and sensitivity has been collected. Providers may prescribe a broad-spectrum antibiotic until laboratory findings are reviewed.

White Blood Cells

- WBCs, or leukocytes, stimulate the inflammatory response and offer protection against various types of infection and foreign antigens.

- There are five types of WBCs. Laboratory analysis of these various types of circulating WBCs is called the differential. The differential on the laboratory report is listed so the percentages of cells equal 100%. This number is arrived at by counting the number of each type of cell in a representative sample of 100 WBCs and multiplying it by 100. If the percent of one type of cell increases, the percents of other types decrease accordingly.

- Interpretation of Findings

    Ⓖ

    - The normal reference range for WBCs is 5,000 to 10,000/mm³. A healthy older adult can have a range of 3,000 to 9,000/mm³.

    - A total WBC count less than 4,300/mm³ is called leukopenia. It may indicate a compromised inflammatory response or viral infection.

    - A count greater than 10,000/mm³ is called leukocytosis. It may indicate an inflammatory response to a pathogen or a disease process.

    - A neutrophil count less than 2,000/mm³ is called neutropenia. Neutropenia occurs in clients who are immunocompromised, are undergoing chemotherapy, or have a process that reduces the production of neutrophils. A client who has neutropenia is at an increased risk for infection.

        - Clients who have neutropenia may also have an absolute neutrophil count (ANC) calculated by multiplying the total WBC count by the summed number of neutrophils and bands and then dividing by 100. Neutropenic precautions (a private room; designated equipment; restricted exposure to live plants, ingestion of fresh fruits, and vegetables) will be instituted if the client's ANC is 1.0 or less.

        - An increase in "banded" or immature neutrophils indicates an infectious process is present and is called a "left shift." This occurs in response to an increased production of neutrophils in response to the infection, allowing the release of some before full maturity is reached.

PERCENT OF CIRCULATING WBCS	INCREASED IN RELATION TO:	DECREASED IN RELATION TO:	ADDITIONAL INFORMATION
Neutrophils			
55% to 75%	• Acute bacterial infections • Fungal infections	• Sepsis • Radiation therapy, aplastic anemia, chemotherapy, and influenza	• The majority of neutrophils are segmented (mature) with a lesser amount being banded (not fully mature). • Immature neutrophils should not be found in the blood.

PERCENT OF CIRCULATING WBCS	INCREASED IN RELATION TO:	DECREASED IN RELATION TO:	ADDITIONAL INFORMATION
Lymphocytes (T cells and B cells)			
20% to 40%	• Chronic bacterial or viral infection • Viruses (mononucleosis, mumps, and measles) • Bacteria (hepatitis) • Lymphocytic leukemia, multiple myeloma	• Leukemia • Sepsis	• T-lymphocytes initiate cell-mediated immunity. • B-lymphocytes initiate humoral immunity.
Monocytes			
2% to 8%	• Chronic inflammation • Protozoal infections • Tuberculosis • Viral infections (mononucleosis, mumps, and measles)	• Corticosteroids	
Eosinophils			
1% to 4%	• Allergic reactions • Parasitic infections • Chronic inflammation • Hodgkin's disease	• Stress • Corticosteroids	
Basophils			
0.5% to 1%	• Leukemia	• Acute allergic/hypersensitivity reaction • Hyperthyroidism	

Radioallergosorbent Test

- A radioallergosorbent test (RAST) is done on a sample of a client's blood to determine sensitivity to various allergens. It can be done in conjunction with skin testing or as an alternative when the risk of a hypersensitivity reaction to an allergen exists.

- The advantage to RAST testing is that it will not precipitate a dangerous allergic reaction in clients and is quicker to administer.

- The disadvantage to RAST testing is that it is available for fewer antigens, may be less sensitive than skin testing, and is more expensive.

- Indications

  o Potential Diagnoses

    ▪ Suspected environmental and food allergies

○ Client Presentation

- Report of hypersensitivity reactions

- Presence of hives, asthma, and/or gastrointestinal dysfunction

- Interpretation of Findings

  ○ During the test, various radiolabeled allergens are exposed to the client's blood and the amount of the client's immunoglobulin E (IgE) that is attracted to each specific allergen is measured according to standardized values. If an allergen is not attracted, this is considered a negative result. If a client's IgE is attracted to an allergen, the amount is measured on a scale of 1 to 5 with the higher number indicating a higher level from sensitivity.

- Intraprocedure

  ○ Nursing Actions

  - Draw a blood sample.

- Postprocedure

  ○ Nursing Actions

  - Inform clients of when to expect results (usually takes at least a week).

Skin Testing for Allergens

- Skin testing for allergens involves the use of intradermal injections or scratching the superficial layer (scratch or prick test) of the skin with small amounts of suspected allergens.

- Intradermal testing runs a higher risk of hypersensitivity reactions and is usually done if the scratch test is inconclusive.

- Indications

  ○ Potential Diagnoses

  - Suspected environmental and food allergies

  ○ Client Presentation

  - Presence of hives, asthma, and/or gastrointestinal dysfunction

- Interpretation of Findings

  ○ Allergens that provoke a localized reaction (wheal and flare) are considered a positive reaction to that allergen.

  ○ The larger the reaction, the stronger the allergy.

- Preprocedure

  o Nursing Actions

    ▪ Prepare the client's skin for application of various allergens using soap and water (client's back or forearm are usually sites for testing).

    ▪ Alcohol may be used to remove oil from the client's skin.

    ▪ Have equipment and medication available for a possible anaphylaxis reaction.

  o Client Education

    ▪ Instruct clients to avoid taking corticosteroids and antihistamines 5 days prior to the testing.

- Intraprocedure

  o Nursing Actions

    ▪ The client's skin is scratched or pricked with a needle after application of a drop of an allergen.

    ▪ Standard pattern of application should be used so identification of the allergen can be done according to the location of the reaction.

    ▪ Application of saline (negative control reaction) and histamine (positive control for reaction) should be done as a baseline for expected reactions.

    ▪ An assessment of reactions is done after 15 to 20 min.

- Postprocedure

  o Nursing Actions

    ▪ Assess the client's skin for areas of reaction and document the allergen that is responsible.

    ▪ Remove all solutions from the client's skin.

    ▪ Inform clients when results will be available.

    ▪ Recommend an antihistamine or topical corticosteroid if clients experience itching secondary to the testing.

  o Client Education

    ▪ Teach desensitizing options and avoidance therapies to clients related to identifying allergens.

    ▪ Advise clients to follow a special diet that eliminates allergens (gluten-free).

(A) APPLICATION EXERCISES

1. A nurse is caring for a client who was admitted to a hospital with a neutrophil count of 1,100/mm³. Which of the following interventions should the nurse use?

    A. Assign the client to a semi-private room.

    B. Allow live plants in the client's room.

    C. Offer the client fresh fruits and vegetables.

    D. Use designated equipment with the client.

2. A nurse is preparing a client who has suspected allergies for a radioallergosorbent test (RAST). Which of the following client statements reveals the need for further reinforcement of teaching?

    A. "It is more expensive than a scratch test."

    B. "This test is done on a sample of my blood."

    C. "I won't have any allergic reaction to the test."

    D. "It tests many more allergens than a scratch test."

3. A nurse is preparing to administer a scratch test on a client who is suspected of having multiple food and environmental allergies. Which of the following actions should the nurse perform prior to beginning the procedure? (Select all that apply.)

    _____ Tell client to expect itching at one site.

    _____ Obtain emergency resuscitation equipment and medication.

    _____ Ask client about previous reactions to allergens.

    _____ Cleanse client's skin with povidone-iodine (Betadine).

    _____ Ask client about medications taken over the past several days.

APPLICATION EXERCISES ANSWER KEY

1. A nurse is caring for a client who was admitted to a hospital with a neutrophil count of 1,100/mm³. Which of the following interventions should the nurse use?

   A. Assign the client to a semi-private room.

   B. Allow live plants in the client's room.

   C. Offer the client fresh fruits and vegetables.

   D. Use designated equipment with the client.

   Neutropenia, defined as a neutrophil count less than 2,000/mm³, increases the client's risk for infections. Using designated equipment decreases the risk of infection. Assigning the client to a semi-private room increases the client's risk of exposure. Allowing live plants and offering the client fresh fruits and vegetables can expose the client to harmful bacteria and should be avoided.

    NCLEX® Connection: Physiological Adaptations, Basic Pathophysiology

2. A nurse is preparing a client who has suspected allergies for a radioallergosorbent test (RAST). Which of the following client statements reveals the need for further reinforcement of teaching?

   A. "It is more expensive than a scratch test."

   B. "This test is done on a sample of my blood."

   C. "I won't have any allergic reaction to the test."

   D. "It tests many more allergens than a scratch test."

   A radioallergosorbent test (RAST) is more expensive than a scratch test. A sample of blood is used for the test, which decreases the chance of having an allergic reaction. The limitation of RAST is it tests fewer allergens than a scratch test.

    NCLEX® Connection: Reduction of Risk Potential, Diagnostic Tests

3. A nurse is preparing to administer a scratch test on a client who is suspected of having multiple food and environmental allergies. Which of the following actions should the nurse perform prior to beginning the procedure? (Select all that apply.)

       X   **Tell client to expect itching at one site.**

       X   **Obtain emergency resuscitation equipment and medication.**

       X   **Ask client about previous reactions to allergens.**

             Cleanse client's skin with povidone-iodine (Betadine).

       X   **Ask client about medications taken over the past several days.**

    Because histamine will be applied as a control site, the client will experience itching at this site. Emergency equipment and medication should be available even if the client denies such type of reaction. The nurse should ask if the client has had any previous reactions to allergens that could indicate an increased risk of an anaphylactic reaction. The client should be asked if any antihistamines or corticosteroids were taken within 5 days of testing due to their ability to suppress reactions. The nurse should use soap and water to cleanse the skin, not povidone iodine, which could interfere with an allergen and elicit a response.

     NCLEX® Connection: Reduction of Risk Potential, Potential for Complications of Diagnostic Tests/Treatments/Procedures

UNIT 13   NURSING CARE OF CLIENTS WITH IMMUNE SYSTEM AND
            INFECTIOUS DISORDERS

Chapter 80   HIV/AIDS

Overview

- Human immunodeficiency virus (HIV) is a retrovirus that is transmitted through blood and body fluids (semen, vaginal secretions).

- HIV targets CD4+ lymphocytes, also known as T-cells or T-lymphocytes.

  o T-cells work in concert with B-lymphocytes. Both are part of specific acquired (adaptive) immunity.

  o HIV integrates its RNA into host cell DNA through reverse transcriptase, reshaping the host's immune system.

- Clients who are HIV positive are at greatest risk for opportunistic infections from protozoan, viral, bacterial, and fungal pathogens. These pathogens are from the normal environment, but normal immune function prevents infections from developing. Clients who are HIV positive develop opportunistic infections due to extreme immune suppression.

Data Collection

- Risk Factors

  o Unprotected sex (vaginal, anal, oral)

  o Multiple sex partners

  o Occupational exposure (health care workers)

  o Perinatal exposure

  o Blood transfusions (not a significant source of infection in the U.S.)

  o Intravenous drug use with a contaminated needle

  o HIV infection may go undiagnosed in older adult clients due to the similarity of its manifestations to other illnesses that are common in this age group.

  o Older adults are more susceptible to fluid and electrolyte imbalances, malnutrition, skin alterations, and wasting syndrome than younger adults.

  o Older women experience vaginal dryness and thinning of the vaginal wall, increasing their susceptibility to HIV infection.

- Subjective Data

  o Chills

  o Anorexia, nausea, and weight loss

  o Weakness and fatigue

  o Headache

  o Night sweats

- Objective Data

  o Physical Findings and Laboratory Data

    ▪ A confirmed case classification meets the laboratory criteria for a diagnosis of HIV infection and one of the four HIV infection stages (stage 1, stage 2, stage 3, or unknown).

STAGE	DEFINING CONDITIONS	CD4+ T-LYMPHOCYTE COUNT	CD4+ T-LYMPHOCYTE PERCENTAGE OF TOTAL LYMPHOCYTES
Stage 1	• None	500 cells/mEq/L or more	29 or more
Stage 2	• None	200 to 499 cells/mEq/L	14 to 28
Stage 3 (AIDS)*	• Candidiasis of the esophagus, bronchi, trachea, or lungs • Herpes simplex – Chronic ulcers (of more than 1 month's duration) • HIV-related encephalopathy • Disseminated or extrapulmonary histoplasmosis • Kaposi's sarcoma • Burkitt's lymphoma • Mycobacterium tuberculosis of any site • *Pneumocystis jiroveci* pneumonia • Recurrent pneumonia • Progressive multifocal leukoencephalopathy • Recurrent *Salmonella septicemia* • Wasting syndrome attributed to HIV	Less than 200 cells/mEq/L	Less than 14
Stage unknown	• No information available	No information available	No information available

*Documentation of an AIDS-defining condition supersedes a CD4+ T-lymphocyte count of 200 cells/mEq/L or more and a CD4+ T-lymphocyte percentage of total lymphocytes of more than 14.

Source: Human Immunodeficiency Virus Infection (HIV) (retrieved 3/18/10 from http://www.cdc.gov). To read more about HIV, go to the Web site of the Centers for Disease Control and Prevention (http://www.cdc.gov).

- CBC and differential – Abnormal (anemia, thrombocytopenia, leukopenia)
- Platelet Count – Decreased, less than 150,000/mm³

○ Diagnostic Procedures

- Laboratory criteria for diagnosis
    - □ Positive result from an HIV antibody screening test (reactive enzyme immunoassay [EIA]) confirmed by a positive result from a supplemental HIV antibody test (Western blot or indirect immunofluorescence assay test)
    - □ Positive result or report of a detectable quantity from any of the following HIV virologic (non-antibody) tests:
        - ▸ HIV nucleic acid (DNA or RNA) detection test (polymerase chain reaction [PCR])
        - ▸ HIV p24 antigen test, including neutralization assay
        - ▸ HIV isolation (viral culture)
- Liver profile, biopsies, and testing of stool for parasites
    - □ Nursing Actions
        - ▸ Prepare clients for the test.
    - □ Client Education
        - ▸ Inform clients about the details of the test (length and what to expect).
- Brain or lung MRI or CT scan
    - □ Detailed image of the brain or lung to detect abnormalities
    - □ Nursing Actions
        - ▸ Prepare clients for the procedure.
    - □ Client Education
        - ▸ Inform clients about the length of time the test takes (sometimes up to 1 hr).

Collaborative Care

- Nursing Care

    ○ Monitor fluid intake/urinary output.

    ○ Obtain daily weights to monitor weight loss.

    ○ Encourage a balanced diet that is high in calories and protein. Obtain the client's preferred food and beverages. Give nutritional supplements.

    ○ Monitor clients receiving TPN.

    ○ Protect/prevent infection using standard precautions.

    ○ Encourage deep breathing and coughing.

- o Maintain good hand hygiene.

- o Remind clients to avoid individuals who have colds/infections/viruses.

- o Encourage immunizations with killed viruses, to include pneumococcal vaccine (PCV) and yearly seasonal influenza vaccine.

- o Monitor for signs of opportunistic infections.

- Provide for good oral care and report abnormalities for treatment.

- Keep the client's skin clean and dry.

- Provide nonpharmacological methods of pain relief.

- o Monitor clients for pain and provide adequate pain management. Use of medications may include nonsteroidal anti-inflammatory drugs (NSAIDs), acetaminophen (Tylenol), opioids, and muscle relaxants.

- Encourage activity alternated with rest periods.

- Administer supplemental oxygen as needed.

- Medications

- o Highly active antiretroviral therapy (HAART) involves using three to four HIV medications in combination with other antiretroviral medications to reduce medication resistance, adverse effects, and dosages.

  - ▪ Entry/infusion inhibitors – Enfuvirtide (Fuzeon)

    - □ Helps to decrease the amount of virus in the body and limit its spread

  - ▪ Nucleoside reverse transcriptase inhibitors (NRTIs) – Zidovudine (Retrovir)

    - □ Interfere with the virus's ability to convert RNA into DNA

  - ▪ Non-nucleoside reverse transcriptase inhibitors (NNRTIs) – Delavirdine (Rescriptor) and efavirenz (Sustiva)

    - □ Inhibit viral replication in cells

  - ▪ Protease inhibitors – Amprenavir (Agenerase), nelfinavir (Viracept), saquinavir (Invirase), and indinavir (Crixivan)

    - □ Inhibit an enzyme needed for the virus to replicate

  - ▪ Antineoplastic medication – Interleukin (Interferon)

    - □ Immunostimulant that enhances the immune response and reduces the production of cancer cells (used commonly with Kaposi's sarcoma)

- o Nursing Considerations

  - ▪ Monitor laboratory results (CBC, WBC, liver function tests). Antiretroviral medications may increase alanine aminotransferase (ALT), aspartate aminotransferase (AST), bilirubin, mean corpuscular volume (MCV), high-density lipoproteins (HDLs), total cholesterol, and triglycerides.

- o Client Education
  - Reinforce to clients about the side effects of the medications and ways to decrease the severity of the side effects.
  - Reinforce to clients about the need to take medications on a regular schedule and to not miss doses.
  - Encourage clients to inform the provider of use of vitamins, herbal products, and shark cartilage that are being used to alleviate the symptoms of HIV. These can alter the effects of the prescribed medications.

- Interdisciplinary Care
  - o Request respiratory services to improve respiratory status and provide oxygen.
  - o Request nutritional services for dietary counseling and delivery of meals.
  - o Request physical therapy for assistance with ADLs.
  - o Request home health services for assistance with IVs, dressing changes, and total parenteral nutrition (TPN).

- Request a referral for hospice services if indicated.

- Care After Discharge
  - o Client Education
    - Inform clients how the virus is transmitted and ways to prevent infection.
    - Encourage clients to maintain up-to-date immunizations, including yearly seasonal influenza and pneumococcal polysaccharide vaccine (PPSV).
    - Suggest participation in support group.
    - Instruct clients to practice good hygiene, frequent hand hygiene, and to avoid crowded areas and people with colds or flu viruses.
    - Encourage clients to avoid raw fruits and vegetables.
    - Instruct clients to avoid cleaning pet litter boxes to reduce the risk of toxoplasmosis.
    - Reinforce client teaching regarding:
      - □ Transmission, infection control measures, and safe sex practices.
      - □ The importance of maintaining a well-balanced diet.
      - □ Self-administration of prescribed medications and potential side effects.
      - □ Signs/symptoms that need to be reported immediately (infection).
    - Instruct the client about the need for frequent follow-up monitoring of CD4+ and viral load counts.
    - Assist clients with identifying primary support systems and to use constructive coping mechanisms.

- Client Outcomes

  o The client will have adequate gas exchange.

  o The client will be free from pain.

  o The client will be able to maintain a weight within 10% of ideal body weight.

  o The client will adhere to the prescribed medication regimen.

Complications

- Opportunistic infections

  o Bacterial diseases (tuberculosis, bacterial pneumonia, and septicemia [blood poisoning])

  o HIV-associated malignancies (Kaposi's sarcoma, lymphoma, and squamous cell carcinoma)

  o Viral diseases (those caused by cytomegalovirus, herpes simplex, and herpes zoster virus)

  o Fungal diseases (PCP, candidiasis, cryptococcosis, and penicilliosis)

  o Protozoal diseases (toxoplasmosis, microsporidiosis, cryptosporidiosis, isosporiasis, and leishmaniasis)

  o Nursing Actions

    ▪ Implement and maintain anti-retroviral medication therapy as prescribed.

    ▪ Administer antineoplastics, antibiotics, analgesics, antifungals, and antidiarrheals as prescribed.

    ▪ Administer appetite stimulants (to enhance nutrition).

    ▪ Monitor for skin breakdown.

    ▪ Maintain fluid intake.

    ▪ Maintain nutrition.

  o Client Education

    ▪ Reinforce to clients to report signs of infection immediately to the provider.

(A) APPLICATION EXERCISES

Scenario: A client visits an outpatient clinic and reports night sweats and fatigue. He states he has a cough, has been nauseated, and is having abdominal pain and frequent diarrhea. His temperature is 38.1° C (100.6° F) orally. He states he has Human Immunodeficiency Virus (HIV), but his monogamous partner for many years does not have HIV.

1. Which of the following stages of the infection is the client experiencing?

    A. Stage 1
    B. Stage 2
    C. Stage 3
    D. Stage 4

2. Which of the following client statements reveals the need for reinforcement of teaching? (Select all that apply.)

    _____ "If I have AIDS, then I also have HIV."
    _____ "If I have HIV, then I also have AIDS."
    _____ "I can only transmit HIV in Stage 1 and Stage 2."
    _____ "AIDS means I have a positive HIV test and a CD4-T-cell count less than 200 cells/mm³."
    _____ "I was most infectious right after I got HIV."

3. Preventing the spread of HIV to his monogamous partner is important. Which of the following is considered safe sex practice? (Select all that apply.)

    _____ Only have sex with your partner.
    _____ Reuse condoms only once with that partner.
    _____ Use natural membrane condoms.
    _____ Make sure condom is correct size.
    _____ Use petroleum jelly for lubricant.
    _____ Leave space at the end of the condom for the semen.

4. A nurse is caring for a client who was recently admitted with encephalitis. In reviewing the chart, the nurse recognizes the client is being evaluated for HIV based on the results of which of the following laboratory tests?

    A. Western blot
    B. Platelet count
    C. Liver biopsy
    D. Differential

(A) APPLICATION EXERCISES ANSWER KEY

Scenario: A client visits an outpatient clinic and reports night sweats and fatigue. He states he has a cough, has been nauseated, and is having abdominal pain and frequent diarrhea. His temperature is 38.1° C (100.6° F) orally. He states he has Human Immunodeficiency Virus (HIV), but his monogamous partner for many years does not have HIV.

1. Which of the following stages of the infection is the client experiencing?

    A. Stage 1

    B. Stage 2

    C. Stage 3

    D. Stage 4

    The client has AIDS, which is the third and last stage of the infection. The client is symptomatic (cough, fever, diarrhea), which indicates his immune system is significantly deficient and he is no longer able to fight off opportunistic infections. There are only three stages in categorizing the stages of AIDS.

 NCLEX® Connection: Health Promotion and Maintenance, Developmental Stages and Transitions

2. Which of the following client statements reveals the need for reinforcement of teaching? (Select all that apply.)

    _____ "If I have AIDS, then I also have HIV."

    __X__ **"If I have HIV, then I also have AIDS."**

    __X__ **"I can only transmit HIV in Stage 1 and Stage 2."**

    _____ "AIDS means I have a positive HIV test and a CD4-T-cell count less than 200 cells/mm³."

    _____ "I was most infectious right after I got HIV."

    Everyone who has AIDS has the HIV infection, but not everyone with the HIV infection has AIDS. HIV can be transmitted during any stage of the infection, but is more likely to spread right after being recently infected. A diagnosis of AIDS is made when the client has the HIV infection and a CD4-T-cell count less than 200 cells/mm³.

 NCLEX® Connection: Physiological Adaptations, Alterations in Body Systems

3. Preventing the spread of HIV to his monogamous partner is important. Which of the following is considered safe sex practice? (Select all that apply.)

   X   **Only have sex with your partner.**

           Reuse condoms only once with that partner.

           Use natural membrane condoms.

   X   **Make sure condom is correct size.**

           Use petroleum jelly for lubricant.

   X   **Leave space at the end of the condom for the semen.**

Having sex just with his monogamous partner, making sure the condom fits appropriately, and leaving space at the end of the condom for semen are all safe sex practices. Condoms should be discarded after use. Latex condoms, as opposed to natural membrane condoms, provide more protection. Use water-based lubricants because petroleum lubricants can damage the condom.

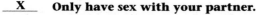 NCLEX® Connection: Health Promotion and Maintenance, Lifestyle Choices

---

4. A nurse is caring for a client who was recently admitted with encephalitis. In reviewing the chart, the nurse recognizes the client is being evaluated for HIV based on the results of which of the following laboratory tests?

A. Western blot

B. Platelet count

C. Liver biopsy

D. Differential

The Western blot test is a supplemental HIV antibody test used to confirm a diagnosis of HIV. A platelet count, liver biopsy, and differential are useful in evaluating the physiological status of the client, but do not confirm a suspected diagnosis of HIV.

NCLEX® Connection: Physiological Adaptations, Alterations in Body Systems

UNIT 13	NURSING CARE OF CLIENTS WITH IMMUNE SYSTEM AND INFECTIOUS DISORDERS
Chapter 81	Autoimmune Disorders

Overview

- In autoimmune disorders, small antigens may bond with healthy tissue. The body then produces antibodies that attack the healthy tissue. This can be triggered by toxins, medications, bacteria, and/or viruses.

- Control of symptoms and decrease in number of exacerbations is the goal of treatment, because there is no cure for autoimmune disorders.

- Occurrence of autoimmune disorders increases with age.

- Autoimmune disorders discussed in this chapter include systemic lupus erythematosus (SLE) and rheumatoid arthritis. Other autoimmune disorders include vasculitis, multiple sclerosis, scleroderma (including Raynaud's phenomenon), and psoriasis.

SYSTEMIC LUPUS ERYTHEMATOSUS

Overview

- Systemic lupus erythematosus (SLE) is an autoimmune disorder in which an atypical immune response results in chronic inflammation and destruction of healthy tissue.

- SLE varies in severity and progression. It is generally characterized by periods of exacerbations (flare-ups) and remissions.

- SLE classifications include:

  ○ Discoid SLE primarily affects the skin. It is characterized by an erythematosus butterfly rash over the nose and cheeks and is generally self-limiting.

  ○ Systemic SLE affects the connective tissues of multiple organ systems and can lead to major organ failure.

  ○ Lupus-like syndrome, which is transient and is caused by some medications (procainamide [Pronestyl], hydralazine, infliximab [Remicade]). Symptoms resolve when the medication is discontinued, and it does not cause renal or neurologic disease.

- SLE can be difficult to diagnose because of the vagueness of early symptoms.

Data Collection

- Risk Factors

  - Females between the ages of 15 and 40 are at risk.

  - African American, Asian, or Native American descent are predisposed.

  - The incidence of lupus declines in women following menopause, but remains steady in men.

  - Diagnosis of SLE may be delayed in older adult clients because many of the clinical manifestations mimic other disorders or may be associated with reports common to the normal aging process.

    - Joint pain and swelling can significantly limit ADLs in older adult clients who have comorbidities.

    - Older adult clients are at an increased risk for fractures if corticosteroid therapy is used.

- Subjective Data

  - Fatigue/malaise

  - Alopecia

  - Anorexia/weight loss

  - Depression

- Objective Data

  - Physical Findings

    - Fever (also a major symptom of exacerbation)

    - Findings consistent with organ involvement (kidney, heart, lungs, and vasculature)

      - Decreased urine output (renal compromise)

      - Hypertension and edema (renal compromise)

      - Diminished breath sounds (pleural effusion)

      - Tachycardia and sharp inspiratory chest pain (pericarditis)

      - Rubor, pallor, and cyanosis of hands/feet (vasculitis/vasospasm in response to cold/stress, Raynaud's phenomenon)

    - Joint pain, swelling, and tenderness (joint and connective tissue involvement)

      - Changes in mental status that indicate neurologic involvement (psychoses, paresis, seizures)

    - Anemia

    - Lymphadenopathy

- Butterfly rash on face

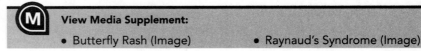

View Media Supplement:
- Butterfly Rash (Image)
- Raynaud's Syndrome (Image)

- o Laboratory Tests
  - Autoantibodies
    - □ Antinuclear antibody (ANA) titer (antibody produced against one's own DNA) – Positive ANA titer in 90% of clients who have lupus (normal is negative ANA titer at 1:20 dilution)
  - Anti-DNA – Positive (not specific for SLE, but positive in the vast majority of clients who have SLE)
  - Extractible nuclear antibodies (ENAs) specific for selected parts of a cell's nucleus
    - □ Anti-Smith – Positive (highly specific for SLE)
    - □ Anti-RO – Positive
    - □ Anti-LA – Positive
    - □ Anti-RNP – Positive
    - □ Anti-phospholipids – Positive
  - Serum complement (C3, C4) – Decreased
    - □ The complement system is made up of proteins (there are nine major complement proteins). These proteins work with the immune system and play a role in the development of inflammation. C3 and C4 are diagnostic for SLE because they decrease due to depletion secondary to an exaggerated inflammatory response.
  - BUN and serum creatinine – Elevated (with renal involvement)
  - Urinalysis – Positive for protein and RBCs (renal involvement)
  - CBC – Pancytopenia

Collaborative Care

- Nursing Care

  - o Monitor

  - o Provide small, frequent meals if anorexia is a concern. Offer between-meal supplements.

  - o Encourage clients to limit salt intake to prevent fluid retention secondary to steroid therapy.

  - o Provide emotional support to clients and their families.

- Medications
  - NSAIDs
    - Used to reduce inflammation
    - Nursing Considerations
      - NSAIDs are contraindicated for clients who have renal compromise.
      - Monitor for NSAID-induced hepatitis.
  - Corticosteroids
    - Used for immunosuppression and to reduce inflammation
    - Nursing Considerations
      - Monitor weight (fluid retention), blood pressure (hypertension), and urine output (renal dysfunction).
    - Client Education
      - Reinforce to clients not to stop taking steroids or decrease the dose abruptly.
      - Reinforce to clients to use alternate day dosing if prescribed.
      - Reinforce to clients to avoid crowds and people who are ill due to increased risk of infection.
      - Reinforce to clients to report signs of infection or impaired healing.
  - Immunosuppressant agents – Methotrexate (Rheumatrex) and azathioprine (Imuran)
    - Used to suppress the immune response
    - Nursing Considerations
      - Monitor for toxic effects (bone marrow suppression, increased liver enzymes).
  - Antimalarial – Hydroxychloroquine (Plaquenil)
    - Used for suppression of synovitis, fever, and fatigue
    - Nursing Considerations
      - Encourage frequent eye examinations.
- Interdisciplinary Care
  - Discuss referral for physical and occupational therapy for strengthening exercises and adaptive devices as needed.
- Care After Discharge
  - Client Education
    - Reinforce teaching to clients regarding the need to:
      - Avoid UV and sun exposure. Clients should use sunscreen when outside and exposed to sunlight.
      - Use mild protein shampoo and avoid harsh hair treatments.

       ☐ Use steroid creams for skin rash.

       ☐ Report peripheral and periorbital edema promptly.

       ☐ Report signs/symptoms of infection related to immunosuppression.

       ☐ Avoid crowds and individuals who are sick, because illness can precipitate an exacerbation.

- Client Outcomes

   ○ The client's laboratory values will indicate a decrease in immune and inflammatory response.

   ○ The client will have extended periods of remission from the disease.

Complications

- Lupus nephritis (renal failure/glomerulonephritis)

   ○ Clients whose SLE is unable to be managed with immunosuppressants and corticosteroids may experience renal failure secondary to glomerulonephritis. This is a major cause of death, and a renal transplant may be necessary.

   ○ Nursing Actions

      ■ Monitor for periorbital and lower extremity swelling and hypertension. Monitor the client's renal status closely (creatinine, BUN).

   ○ Client Education

      ■ Reinforce to clients the importance of taking immunosuppressants and corticosteroids as prescribed.

      ■ Reinforce to clients the significance of avoiding stress and illness.

- Pericarditis and myocarditis

   ○ Inflammation of the heart, its vessels, and the surrounding sac can occur secondary to SLE.

   ○ Nursing Actions

      ■ Monitor for chest pain, fatigue, arrhythmias, and fever.

   ○ Client Education

      ■ Reinforce instructions to:

         ☐ Take immunosuppressants and corticosteroids as prescribed.

         ☐ Avoid stress and illness.

         ☐ Report chest pain to the provider.

RHEUMATOID ARTHRITIS

Overview

- Rheumatoid arthritis (RA) is a chronic, progressive inflammatory disease that can affect tissues and organs, but principally attacks the joints producing an inflammatory synovitis. It involves joints bilaterally and symmetrically, and it typically affects several joints at one time.

- RA is an autoimmune disease that is precipitated by WBCs attacking synovial tissue. The WBCs cause the synovial tissue to become inflamed and thickened. The inflammation can extend to the cartilage, bone, tendons, and ligaments that surround the joint. Joint deformity may result from these changes, decreasing the joint's range of motion and function.

- RA is also a systemic disease that can affect any connective tissue in the body. Common structures that are affected are the blood vessels, pleura surrounding the lungs, and pericardium. Iritis and scleritis can also develop in the eyes.

- The natural course of the disease is one of exacerbations and remissions.

Data Collection

- Risk Factors

  - Female gender

  - Age 20 to 50 years

  - Genetic predisposition

  - Epstein-Barr virus

  - Stress

  - Early signs of RA (fatigue, joint discomfort) are vague and may be attributed to other disorders in older adult clients.

  - Joint pain and dysfunction may have a greater effect on older adult clients than on younger adult clients, due to the presence of other chronic conditions.

  - Older adult clients may be less able to overcome and/or cope with joint pain/deformity.

- Subjective Data

  - Pain at rest and with movement

  - Morning stiffness

  - Pleuritic pain (pain upon inspiration)

  - Xerostomia (dry mouth)

  - Anorexia/weight loss

- o Fatigue
- o Paresthesias
- o Recent illness/stressor
- Objective Data
  - o Clinical findings depend on the area affected by the disease process.
  - o Joint swelling and deformity
    - Finger, hand, wrist, knee, and foot joints are generally affected.
    - Finger joints affected are the proximal interphalangeal and metacarpophalangeal joints.
    - Joints may become deformed merely by completing ADLs.
    - Ulnar deviation, swan neck, and boutonnière deformities are common in the fingers.

(M) View Media Supplement: Ulnar Deviation of the Hand (Image)

  - o Subcutaneous nodules
  - o Fever (generally low grade)
  - o Muscle weakness/atrophy
  - o Reddened sclera and/or abnormal shape of pupils
  - o Laboratory Tests
    - Anti-CCP antibodies – Positive
      - □ This test detects antibodies to cyclic citrullinated peptide. The result is positive in most people who have rheumatoid arthritis, even years before symptoms develop. The test is more sensitive for RA than rheumatoid factor (RF) antibodies.
    - RF antibody
      - □ Diagnostic level for rheumatoid arthritis is 1:40 to 1:60 (normal 1:20 or less).
      - □ High titers correlate with severe disease.
      - □ Other autoimmune diseases can also increase RF antibody.
    - Erythrocyte sedimentation rate (ESR) – Elevated
      - □ The increase is associated with inflammation or infection in the body.
      - □ 20 to 40 mm/hr is mild inflammation.
      - □ 40 to 70 mm/hr is moderate inflammation.
      - □ 70 to 150 mm/hr is severe inflammation.
      - □ Other autoimmune diseases can also increase ESR.

- C-reactive protein (may be done in place of ESR) – Positive
  - This test is useful for diagnosing disease or monitoring disease activity, and for monitoring the response to anti-inflammatory therapy.
- Antinuclear antibody (ANA) titer (antibody produced against one's own DNA)
  - A positive ANA titer is associated with RA (it is normally negative at 1:20 dilution).
  - Other autoimmune diseases can also increase ANA.
- Elevated WBCs
  - WBC count may be elevated during an exacerbation secondary to the inflammatory response.

- ○ Diagnostic Procedures
  - Arthrocentesis
    - Synovial fluid aspiration by needle
    - With RA, increased WBCs and RF are present in fluid.
    - Nursing Actions
      - ▸ Monitor for bleeding or a synovial fluid leak from the needle biopsy site.
    - Client Education
      - ▸ Reinforce instructions to take acetaminophen (Tylenol) for pain.
  - X-ray
    - X-rays are used to determine the degree of joint destruction and monitor its progression. They may provide adequate visualization and negate the need for more expensive radiologic tests (CTs and MRIs).
    - Nursing Actions
      - ▸ Assist clients into position.
    - Client Education
      - ▸ Instruct clients about the need to minimize movement during the procedure.

Collaborative Care

- Nursing Care
  - ○ Apply heat or cold to the affected areas as indicated based on client response.
    - Morning stiffness (hot shower)
    - Pain in hands/fingers (heated paraffin)
    - Edema (cold therapy)

- o Assist with and encourage physical activity to maintain joint mobility (within the capabilities of clients).

- o Monitor clients for signs/symptoms of fatigue.

- o Reinforce client teaching about measures to:

  - Maximize functional activity.

  - Minimize pain.

  - Conserve energy (space activities, take rest periods).

- o Provide a safe environment.

  - Facilitate the use of assistive devices.

  - Remove unnecessary equipment/supplies.

- o Encourage clients to use progressive muscle relaxation.

- o Administer medications as prescribed.

- o Monitor for medication effectiveness (reduced pain, increased mobility).

- Medications

  - o NSAIDs

    - NSAIDs provide analgesic, antipyretic, and anti-inflammatory effects. NSAIDs can cause considerable gastrointestinal (GI) distress.

    - Nursing Considerations

      - □ Request a concurrent prescription for a GI acid-lowering agent (H2 receptor blocker, proton pump inhibitor) if GI distress reported.

      - □ Monitor for fluid retention, hypertension, and renal dysfunction.

    - Client Education

      - □ Reinforce teaching to:

        - ▸ Take the medication with food or with a full glass of water or milk. If taking routinely, instruct clients to observe for GI bleeding (coffee ground emesis; dark, tarry stools) and to report to provider.

        - ▸ Avoid alcohol, which can increase risk of GI complications.

  - o Corticosteroids

    - Corticosteroids (Prednisone) are strong anti-inflammatory medications that can be given for acute exacerbations or advanced forms of the disease. They are not given for long-term therapy due to significant side effects (osteoporosis, cataracts).

  - o Disease modifying anti-rheumatic drugs (DMARDs)

    - DMARDs work in a variety of ways to slow the progression of RA and suppress the immune system's reaction to RA that causes pain and inflammation. Relief of symptoms may not occur for several weeks.

    - Antimalarial agent – Hydroxychloroquine (Plaquenil)

- ■ Antibiotic – Minocycline (Minocin)

- ■ Sulfonamide – Sulfasalazine (Azulfidine)

- ■ Biologic response modifiers – Etanercept (Enbrel), infliximab (Remicade), adalimumab (Humira), and chelator penicillamine (Cuprimine)

- ■ Cytotoxic medications – Methotrexate (Rheumatrex), leflunomide (Arava), cyclophosphamide (Cytoxan), and azathioprine (Imuran)

- Interdisciplinary Care

  - o Discuss referral to support groups as appropriate.

  - o Discuss referral to occupational therapy for adaptive devices that can facilitate carrying out ADLs and prevent deformities.

  - o Discuss referral for a home health aide for assistance with ADLs.

- Therapeutic Procedures

  - o Plasmapheresis

    - ■ Removes circulating antibodies from plasma, decreasing attacks on the client's tissues

  - o May be done for a severe, life-threatening exacerbation

- Surgical Interventions

  - o Total joint arthroplasty

    - ■ May be done for a severely deformed joint that has not responded to medication therapy

- Care After Discharge

  - o Client Education

    - ■ Encourage clients to use adaptive devices that prevent development of deformity of inflamed joints during ADLs.

    - ■ Encourage clients to continue using affected joints and ambulating to maintain function and range of motion.

    - ■ Inform clients of signs/symptoms that need to be reported immediately (fever, infection, pain upon inspiration, pain in the substernal area of the chest).

- Client Outcomes

  - o The client will maintain highest functional range of motion of joints.

  - o The client's pain will be managed so that ADLs can be comfortably carried out.

  - o The client will use adaptive devices so that ADLs can be independently carried out and deformities prevented.

Complications

- Sjögren's syndrome (triad of symptoms – dry eyes, dry mouth, and dry vagina)
  - ○ Caused by obstruction of secretory ducts and glands
  - ○ Nursing Actions
    - ■ Provide clients with eye drops and artificial saliva, and recommend vaginal lubricants as needed.
    - ■ Provide fluids with meals.
- Secondary osteoporosis
  - ○ Immobilization caused by arthritis can contribute to the development of osteoporosis.
  - ○ Nursing Actions
    - ■ Encourage weight-bearing exercises as tolerated.
- Vasculitis (organ ischemia)
  - ○ Inflammation of arteries can disrupt blood flow, causing ischemia. Smaller arteries in the skin, eyes, and brain are most commonly affected in RA.
  - ○ Nursing Actions
    - ■ Monitor for skin lesions, decrease in vision, and symptoms of cognitive dysfunction.

Ⓐ APPLICATION EXERCISES

Scenario: A 32-year-old client is experiencing an exacerbation of systemic lupus erythematosus (SLE). She reports fatigue, joint tenderness, and anorexia. Her knees are swollen, she has an oral temperature of 38.2° C (100.8° F), and her blood pressure is 152/90 mm Hg. Renal compromise is suspected.

1. Based on the client's data, which of the following abnormal laboratory findings should the nurse anticipate? (Select all that apply.)

    _____ Decreased serum complement C3

    _____ Positive ANA

    _____ 2+ urine protein

    _____ Elevated BUN

    _____ Increased hematocrit

    _____ Positive Anti-DNA

    _____ Positive Anti-Smith

    _____ Increased hemoglobin

    _____ Decreased WBC count

2. Which of the following should the nurse reinforce when instructing the client about self-care? (Select all that apply.)

    _____ Avoid sun exposure.

    _____ Avoid harsh hair treatments.

    _____ Report peripheral edema to the provider.

    _____ Avoid the use of steroid creams for skin rash.

    _____ Avoid crowds and individuals who are sick.

    _____ Do not notify the provider of a productive cough unless a fever is present.

3. A 49-year-old client visits the outpatient clinic due to an exacerbation of her rheumatoid arthritis (RA). She is experiencing increased joint tenderness and swelling. She has subcutaneous nodules in the metacarpophalangeal and distal interphalangeal joints of her hands bilaterally. Which of the following further data is essential in order to implement care for the client? (Select all that apply.)

    _____ Pain status

    _____ Blood pressure

    _____ Temperature

    _____ Range of motion

    _____ History of recent illness

    _____ Date of original diagnosis

    _____ Family members who have the disease

(A) APPLICATION EXERCISES ANSWER KEY

Scenario: A 32-year-old client is experiencing an exacerbation of systemic lupus erythematosus (SLE). She reports fatigue, joint tenderness, and anorexia. Her knees are swollen, she has an oral temperature of 38.2° C (100.8° F), and her blood pressure is 152/90 mm Hg. Renal compromise is suspected.

1. Based on the client's data, which of the following abnormal laboratory findings should the nurse anticipate? (Select all that apply.)

   __X__ **Decreased serum complement C3**

   __X__ **Positive ANA**

   __X__ **2+ urine protein**

   __X__ **Elevated BUN**

   _____ Increased hematocrit

   __X__ **Positive Anti-DNA**

   __X__ **Positive Anti-Smith**

   _____ Increased hemoglobin

   _____ Decreased WBC count

   Decreased serum complement C3, positive ANA titer, positive Anti-DNA, and positive Anti-Smith are expected findings with SLE. Urine protein and elevated BUN provide information regarding renal involvement. An increased hematocrit and hemoglobin and decreased WBC count are not expected.

    NCLEX® Connection: Reduction of Risk Potential, Laboratory Values

2. Which of the following should the nurse reinforce when instructing the client about self-care? (Select all that apply.)

   __X__ **Avoid sun exposure.**

   __X__ **Avoid harsh hair treatments.**

   __X__ **Report peripheral edema to the provider.**

   _____ Avoid the use of steroid creams for skin rash.

   __X__ **Avoid crowds and individuals who are sick.**

   _____ Do not notify the provider of a productive cough unless a fever is present.

   Clients who have SLE should avoid sun exposure, harsh hair treatments such as permanent waves, report peripheral and periorbital edema to the provider, and avoid crowds and individuals who are sick. Steroid creams should be used for skin rashes. And the client should report a productive cough even if fever is not present.

   (N) NCLEX® Connection: Reduction of Risk Potential, Potential for Alterations in Body Systems

3. A 49-year-old client visits the outpatient clinic due to an exacerbation of her rheumatoid arthritis (RA). She is experiencing increased joint tenderness and swelling. She has subcutaneous nodules in the metacarpophalangeal and distal interphalangeal joints of her hands bilaterally. Which of the following further data is essential in order to implement care for the client? (Select all that apply.)

X	**Pain status**
X	**Blood pressure**
X	**Temperature**
X	**Range of motion**
X	**History of recent illness**
	Date of original diagnosis
	Family members who have the disease

    Baselines regarding pain status and range of motion are needed for evaluation of intervention effectiveness. Determination of whether or not the client's disease is manifesting with a low-grade fever and identification of exacerbating factors, such as a recent illness, are important to developing a comprehensive plan of care. Blood pressure variations are not usually a component of RA, but may be affected by medications the client is currently taking. Information about family members who have RA and date of original diagnosis will not provide additional data helpful for development of the client's plan of care.

    NCLEX® Connection: Physiological Adaptations, Basic Pathophysiology

UNIT 13	NURSING CARE OF CLIENTS WITH IMMUNE SYSTEM AND INFECTIOUS DISORDERS

Chapter 82   Immunizations

Overview

- Administration of a vaccine causes production of antibodies that prevent illness from a specific microbe.

- Active-natural immunity develops when the body produces antibodies in response to exposure to a live pathogen. Active-artificial immunity develops when a vaccine is given and the body produces antibodies in response to exposure to a killed or attenuated virus.

- Passive-natural occurs when antibodies are passed from the mother to the fetus/newborn through the placenta and then breastfeeding. Passive-artificial immunity occurs after antibodies in the form of immune globulins are administered to an individual who requires immediate protection against a disease where exposure has already occurred.

- Vaccines may be made from killed viruses or live, attenuated (or weakened) viruses.

Medication Classification: Vaccinations

- The 2010 Centers for Disease Control and Prevention (CDC) vaccination recommendations for adults 18 years and older (go to www.cdc.gov for updates):

  o Tetanus diphtheria (Td) booster – Give booster every 10 years. For adults 19 to 64 years of age who did not receive a dose of the tetanus diphtheria, pertussis (Tdap) vaccine previously, substitute one dose with Tdap.

  o Measles, mumps, and rubella vaccine (MMR) – Give one to two doses at ages 19 to 49.

  o Varicella vaccine – Give two doses to adults who do not have evidence of a previous infection. A second dose should be given to adults who have had only one previous dose.

  o Pneumococcal polysaccharide vaccine (PPSV) – Vaccinate adults who are immunocompromised, who have a chronic disease, who smoke cigarettes, or who live in a long-term care facility. CDC guidelines should be followed for revaccination. Give one dose to adults older than 65 years of age who have not previously been vaccinated nor have history of disease.

  o Hepatitis A – Two doses for high-risk individuals

  o Hepatitis B – Three doses for high-risk individuals

- o Seasonal influenza vaccine – Give one dose annually. Recommended for all adults older than 50; health care providers, including those who care for young children; individuals who have chronic medical conditions such as cerebral palsy, asthma, and diabetes mellitus; individuals who are immunocompromised; and individuals living in long-term care settings. Note that the live attenuated influenza vaccine (LAIV), given as a nasal spray, is only indicated for adults under age 50 or for those who are not pregnant or immunocompromised.

- o Meningococcal conjugate vaccine (MCV4) – Given to students entering college and living in college dormitories, if not previously immunized. Meningococcal polysaccharide vaccine (MPSV4) is recommended for adults older than 56 years of age. Revaccination may be recommended after 5 years for adults at high risk for infection, such as adults without a spleen, military recruits, or adults traveling to a country that is hyperendemic or epidemic.

- o Human papilloma virus (HPV2 or HPV4) – Given in three doses and recommended for females up to age 26 who were not vaccinated as children. The second dose should be administered 2 months after the first dose, and the third dose should be administered 6 months after the first dose.

  - ▪ HPV4 – This vaccine is given to males up to age 26.

- o Herpes zoster vaccine – Recommended for all adults over age 60 years.

Purpose

- Expected Pharmacological Action

  - o Immunizations produce antibodies that provide active immunity. Immunizations may take months to have an effect, but provide long-lasting protection against infectious diseases.

- Therapeutic Uses

  - o Eradication of infectious diseases (polio, smallpox)

  - o Prevention of childhood and adult infectious diseases and their complications (measles, diphtheria, mumps, rubella, tetanus, H. influenza)

Complications/Contraindications/Precautions

- An anaphylactic reaction to a vaccine is a contraindication for further doses of that vaccine.

- An anaphylactic reaction to a vaccine is a contraindication to use of other vaccines containing the same substance.

- Moderate or severe illnesses with or without fever are contraindications for use of a vaccine. With acute febrile illness, vaccination is deferred until symptoms resolve. The common cold and other minor illnesses are not contraindications.

  - o Contraindications to vaccinations require the primary care provider to analyze data and weigh the risks that come with or without vaccinating.

  - o Individuals who are immunocompromised are defined by the CDC as those who have hematologic or solid tumors, who have congenital immunodeficiency, or are receiving long-term immunosuppressive therapy, including corticosteroids.

IMMUNIZATIONS	SIDE EFFECTS	CONTRAINDICATIONS
Td or DTaP	• Local reaction at injection site	• Severe febrile illness • A history of prior anaphylactic reaction to the DTaP vaccination • An occurrence of encephalopathy 7 days after the administration of the DTaP immunization • An occurrence of seizures within 3 days of the vaccination • A history of uncontrollable crying and inconsolability by parents after receiving prior vaccination; may last more than 3 hr and occurs within 48 hr of the vaccination
MMR	• Local reactions such as rash; fever; and swollen glands in cheeks, neck, and under the jaw • Possibility of joint pain lasting for days to weeks. • Risk for anaphylaxis and thrombocytopenia	• Pregnancy • Allergy to gelatin and neomycin (Mycifradin) • Clients who are immunocompromised (with HIV infection or from medication administration) • Recent transfusion with blood products

Varicella vaccine	• Varicella-like rash that may be local or generalized, such as vesicles on the body	• Pregnancy
		  ○ Women should not get pregnant for up to 4 weeks after receiving the vaccine.
		  ○ Women who are pregnant should avoid close proximity to children who are recently vaccinated.
		• Cancers of blood and lymphatic system
		• Allergy to gelatin and neomycin
		• Clients who are immunocompromised (with HIV infection or from medication administration)

Pneumococcal vaccine (PCV)	• Mild local reactions, fever, and no serious adverse effects	• Pregnancy

IMMUNIZATIONS	SIDE EFFECTS	CONTRAINDICATIONS

Hepatitis A
Hepatitis B
	• Local reaction at injection site	• Hep A
		  o Pregnancy may be a contraindication
		• Hep B
		  o A prior history of anaphylactic reaction
		  o An allergy to baker's yeast

Seasonal influenza vaccine (one dose annually)	• Inactivated – Mild local reaction and fever • Live attenuated – Headache, cough, and fever • Rare – Risk for Guillain-Barré syndrome, manifested by ascending paralysis beginning with weakness of lower extremities and progressing to difficulty breathing or respiratory arrest	• Live attenuated influenza vaccine administered as a nasal spray is contraindicated for adults who are older than 50, are immunocompromised, or have a chronic disease. • History of Guillain-Barré syndrome
Meningococcal Conjugate vaccine (MCV4)	• Mild local reaction and rare risk of allergic response	• History of Guillain-Barré syndrome
Human papilloma virus (HPV2 or HPV4) vaccine	• Mild local reaction and fever • Fainting has occurred shortly after receiving vaccination • Rare – Risk for Guillain-Barré syndrome	• Pregnancy
Herpes zoster		• Clients who are immunocompromised (with HIV infection or from medication administration)

Medication/Food Interactions

- None significant

Nursing Administration

- For adults

  o Give subcutaneous vaccinations in outer aspect of the upper arm or anterolateral thigh.

  o Give intramuscular vaccinations into the deltoid muscle for adults.

- For clients of all ages

  - Have emergency medications and equipment on standby in case clients experience an allergic response such as anaphylaxis (rare).

  - Follow storage and reconstitution directions. If reconstituted, use within 30 min.

  - Provide written vaccine information sheets and review the content with clients.

  - Instruct clients to observe for complications and to notify the provider if side effects occur.

  - Document administration of vaccines including date, route, site, type, manufacturer, lot number, and expiration of vaccine. Also document the client's name, address, and signature.

Nursing Evaluation of Medication Effectiveness

- Depending on the therapeutic intent of the vaccine, effectiveness may be evidenced by:

  - Improvement of local reaction with absence of pain, fever, and swelling at the site of injection.

  - Development of immunity.

APPLICATION EXERCISES

1. A client is asking about strategies to promote comfort after receiving an immunization. Which of the following strategies should the nurse reinforce? (Select all that apply.)

    _____ Massage the site.

    _____ Apply an antimicrobial ointment.

    _____ Apply cool compresses to the site.

    _____ Take acetaminophen or ibuprofen.

    _____ Use the affected extremity.

2. A client has been exposed to Hepatitis B and has not received the vaccine for this disease. A nurse is preparing to give the client an IM injection of immunoglobulin to impart which of the following types of immunity?

    A. Active-natural

    B. Active-artificial

    C. Passive-natural

    D. Passive-artificial

3. Which of the following data should a nurse collect from a client who is preparing to receive a measles, mumps, and rubella (MMR) vaccine?

    A. "Are you pregnant?"

    B. "Are you allergic to aluminum?"

    C. "Are you allergic to baker's yeast?"

    D. "Are you currently taking an antihistamine?"

APPLICATION EXERCISES ANSWER KEY

1. A client is asking about strategies to promote comfort after receiving an immunization. Which of the following strategies should the nurse reinforce? (Select all that apply.)

    _____ Massage the site.

    _____ Apply an antimicrobial ointment.

    __X___ **Apply cool compresses to the site.**

    __X___ **Take acetaminophen or ibuprofen.**

    __X___ **Use the affected extremity.**

    Cool compresses, administration of acetaminophen or ibuprofen, and encouraging gentle use of the extremity are all comfort strategies useful for discomfort in an injection site. Massaging the site is not recommended for an extended period of time after the injection and use of an antimicrobial ointment is not indicated.

    NCLEX® Connection: Reduction of Risk Potential, Potential for Complications of Diagnostic Tests/Treatments/Procedures

2. A client has been exposed to Hepatitis B and has not received the vaccine for this disease. A nurse is preparing to give the client an IM injection of immunoglobulin to impart which of the following types of immunity?

    A. Active-natural

    B. Active-artificial

    C. Passive-natural

    D. Passive-artificial

    Passive-artificial immunity will allow the client to receive some protection against Hepatitis B sooner than the body would be able to respond. This type of protection is temporary, so a Hepatitis B immunization should be administered when the client is not receiving immunoglobulins.

    NCLEX® Connection: Reduction of Risk Potential, Potential for Alterations in Body Systems

3. Which of the following data should a nurse collect from a client who is preparing to receive a measles, mumps, and rubella (MMR) vaccine?

    A. "Are you pregnant?"

    B. "Are you allergic to aluminum?"

    C. "Are you allergic to baker's yeast?"

    D. "Are you currently taking an antihistamine?"

    Prior to administering a rubella vaccination, the nurse should ask the client if she is pregnant. If so, the client should wait until after the pregnancy to be vaccinated.

    NCLEX® Connection: Reduction of Risk Potential, Potential for Alterations in Body Systems

UNIT 13	NURSING CARE OF CLIENTS WITH IMMUNE SYSTEM AND INFECTIOUS DISORDERS
Chapter 83	Bacterial, Viral, Fungal, and Parasitic Infections

 Overview

- Pathogens are the microorganisms or microbes that cause infections.

    o Bacteria (*Staphylococcus aureus*, *Escherichia coli*, *Mycobacterium tuberculosis*)

    o Viruses – Organisms that use the host's genetic machinery to reproduce (HIV, hepatitis, herpes zoster, herpes simplex)

    o Fungi – Molds and yeasts (*Candida albicans*, aspergillus)

    o Prions – Protein particles (new variant Creutzfeldt-Jakob disease)

    o Parasites – Protozoa (malaria, toxoplasmosis) and helminths (worms [flatworms, roundworms], flukes [Schistosoma])

- Virulence is the ability of a pathogen to invade and injure the host.

- Herpes zoster is a common viral infection that erupts years after the initial exposure to the varicella virus (chickenpox). The virus is dormant and resides in a sensory cranial or spinal nerve.

Infection Process

- The infection process (chain of infection) includes:

    View Media Supplement: Chain of Infection (Image)

    o Causative agent (bacteria, virus, fungus, prion, parasite)

    o Reservoir (human, animal, water, soil, insects)

    o Portal of exit from (means for leaving) the host

      ▪ Respiratory tract (droplet, airborne)

        □ *Myobacterium tuberculosis* and *Streptococcus pneumoniae*

      ▪ Gastrointestinal tract

        □ Shigella, *Salmonella enteritidis*, *Salmonella typhi*, hepatitis A

- Genitourinary tract
  - *Escherichia coli*, hepatitis A, herpes simplex virus (type 1), HIV
- Skin/mucous membranes
  - Herpes simplex virus and varicella
- Blood/body fluids
  - HIV and hepatitis B and C
- Mode of transmission
  - Contact
    - Direct physical contact – Person to person
    - Indirect contact with an inanimate object – Object to person
    - Fecal-oral transmission – Handling food after using a restroom and failing to wash hands
  - Droplet
    - Sneezing, coughing, and talking
  - Airborne
    - Sneezing and coughing
  - Vector borne
    - Animals or insects as intermediaries (ticks transmit Lyme disease; mosquitoes transmit West Nile and malaria)
- Portal of entry to the host
  - May be the same as the portal of exit
- Susceptible host
  - Compromised defense mechanisms (immunocompromised, breaks in skin) leave the host more susceptible to infections.

Immune Defenses

- Nonspecific innate-native immunity is that which allows the body to restrict entry or immediately respond to a foreign organism (antigen) through the activation of phagocytic cells, complement, and inflammation.

  - Nonspecific innate-native immunity provides temporary immunity but does not have memory of past exposures.

  - Intact skin is the body's first line of defense against microbial invasion.

  - The skin, mucous membranes, secretions, enzymes, phagocytic cells, and protective proteins work in concert to prevent infections.

- o Inflammatory response
  - Phagocytic cells (neutrophils, eosinophils, macrophages), the complement system, and interferons are involved.
  - An inflammatory response localizes the area of microbial invasion and limits its spread.
- Specific adaptive immunity is that which allows the body to make antibodies in response to a foreign organism (antigen).
  - o Requires time to react to antigens
  - o Provides permanent immunity due to memory of past exposures
  - o Involves B and T lymphocytes
  - o Produces specific antibodies against specific antigens (immunoglobulins [IgA, IgD, IgE, IgG, IgM]).

Data Collection

- Risk Factors
  - o Environmental factors
    - Excessive alcohol consumption
    - Smoking
    - Malnutrition
  - o Medication therapy (immunosuppressive agents)
    - Glucocorticosteroids
    - Antineoplastics
  - o Chronic diseases
    - Diabetes mellitus
    - Adrenal insufficiency
    - Renal failure
    - Hepatic failure
    - Chronic lung disease
  - Ⓖ o Older adults are at increased risk for infections due to:
    - Slowed response to antibiotic therapy
    - Slowed immune response
    - Loss of subcutaneous tissue and thinning of the skin
    - Decreased vascularity and slowed wound healing
    - Decreased cough and gag reflexes

- Chronic illnesses (diabetes mellitus, COPD, neurological or musculoskeletal impairments)

- Decreased gastric acid production

- Decreased mobility

- Bowel/bladder incontinence

- Dementia

- Greater incidence of invasive devices (urinary catheters, feeding tubes, tracheostomies, intravenous lines)

- Subjective Data

  o Chills

  o Sore throat

  o Fatigue and malaise

  o Change in level of consciousness, nuchal rigidity, photophobia, headache

  o Nausea, vomiting, anorexia, abdominal cramping, and diarrhea

- Objective Data

  o Physical assessment findings

    - Fever

    - Enlarged lymph nodes

    - Dyspnea, cough, purulent sputum, and crackles in lung fields

    - Dysuria, urinary frequency, hematuria, and pyuria

    - Rash, skin lesions, purulent wound drainage, and erythema

    - Odynophagia, dysphagia, hyperemia, and enlarged tonsils

  o Laboratory tests

    - WBC count with differential

    - Culture and sensitivity

    - Erythrocyte sedimentation rate – The rate at which RBCs settle out of plasma

      □ A normal value for adults is 15 to 20 mm/hr.

      □ An increase indicates an active inflammatory process or infection.

    - Immunoglobulin electrophoresis

      □ Determines the presence and quantity of specific immunoglobulins (IgG, IgA, IgM)

      □ Used to detect hypersensitivity disorders, autoimmune disorders, chronic viral infections, immunodeficiency, multiple myeloma, and intrauterine infections

- Antibody screening test
  - Detects the presence of antibodies against specific causative agents (bacteria, fungi, viruses, parasites)
  - A positive antibody test indicates that clients have been exposed to and developed antibodies to a specific pathogen, but it does not provide information about whether or not clients are currently infected (HIV antibodies).
- Auto-antibody screening test
  - Detects the presence of antibodies against a person's own DNA (self-cells)
  - The presence of antibodies against self-cells is associated with autoimmune conditions (systemic lupus erythematosus, rheumatoid arthritis).
- Antigen test
  - Detects the presence of a specific pathogen (HIV)
  - Used to identify certain infections or disorders
- Stool for ova and parasites
  - Detects presence of hookworm ova in stool

○ Diagnostic procedures

- Gallium scan
  - A nuclear scan that uses a radioactive substance to identify hot spots of WBCs within the client's body
  - Radioactive gallium citrate is injected intravenously and accumulates in areas where inflammation is present.
- X-rays, CT scan, magnetic resonance imaging, and biopsies are used to determine the presence of infection, abscesses, and lesions.

Collaborative Care

- Nursing Care

  ○ Monitor

  - Presence of risk factors for infection
  - Recent travel or exposure to an infectious disease
  - Behaviors that may put clients at increased risk
  - Signs and symptoms of fever (increased heart and respiratory rate, thirst, anorexia)
  - Presence of chills, which occur when temperature is rising, and diaphoresis, which occurs when temperature is decreasing
  - Presence of hyperpyrexia (greater than 105.8), which can cause brain and organ damage

- ■ Perform frequent hand hygiene to prevent transmission of infection to other clients.

- ■ Maintain a clean environment.

- ■ Use personal protective equipment/barriers (gloves, masks, gowns, goggles).

- ■ Implement protective precautions as needed and per agency policy.

  - □ Standard (implemented for all clients)

  - □ Airborne (rubeola, varicella, tuberculosis)

  - □ Droplet (Haemophilus influenzae type B, pertussis, plague, *Streptococcal pneumoniae*).

  - □ Contact (*Clostridium difficile*, herpes simplex virus, impetigo)

- o Provide diversional activities if needed.

- o Encourage increased fluid intake.

- o Monitor clients receiving intravenous fluid replacement.

- • Medications

  - o Antipyretics

    - ■ Antipyretics (acetaminophen and aspirin) are used for fever and discomfort as prescribed.

    - ■ Nursing considerations

      - □ Monitor fever to determine effectiveness of medication.

      - □ Graph the client's temperature fluctuations on the medical record for trending.

  - o Antimicrobial therapy

    - ■ Antimicrobial therapy kills or inhibits the growth of microorganisms (bacteria, fungi, viruses, protozoans). Antimicrobial medications either kill pathogens or prevent their growth. Anthelmintics are given for worm infestations. There are currently no treatments for prions.

    - ■ Nursing considerations

      - □ Administer antimicrobial therapy as prescribed.

      - □ Monitor for medication effectiveness (reduced fever, increased level of comfort, decreasing WBC count).

      - □ Maintain a medication schedule to assure consistent therapeutic blood levels of the antibiotic.

      - □ Monitor clients for secondary infections and/or allergic reactions.

- Care After Discharge
  - Client education
    - Teach clients regarding:
      - Any infection control measures needed at home
      - Self-administration of medication therapy
      - Complications that need to be reported immediately
- Client Outcomes
  - The client's fever will be reduced with the administration of an antipyretic.
  - The client's infectious process will resolve in relation to antimicrobial therapy.

Complications

- Multidrug-resistant infection
  - Methicillin-resistant *Staphylococcus aureus* is a strain of *Staphylococcus aureus* that is resistant to all antibiotics, except vancomycin. Vancomycin-resistant *Staphylococcus aureus* is a strain of *Staphylococcus aureus* that is resistant to vancomycin, but so far is sensitive to other antibiotics specific to the client's strain.
  - Nursing actions
    - Obtain specimens for culture and sensitivity prior to initiation of antimicrobial therapy.
    - Monitor antimicrobial levels and ensure that therapeutic levels are maintained.
  - Client education
    - Instruct clients to complete the full course of antimicrobial therapy.
    - Encourage clients to avoid overuse of antimicrobials.
    - Instruct clients regarding food and medication interactions.
- Sepsis
  - A systemic inflammatory response syndrome resulting from the body's response to a serious infection, usually bacterial (peritonitis, meningitis, pneumonia, wound infections, urinary tract infections)
  - Risk factors for sepsis include very young age, very old age, weakened immune system, and severe injuries (trauma). Sepsis can lead to widespread inflammation, blood clotting, organ failure, and shock.
  - Blood cultures definitively diagnose sepsis. Systemic antimicrobials are prescribed accordingly. Vasopressors and anticoagulants may be prescribed for shock and blood clotting symptoms. Mechanical ventilation, dialysis, and other interventions may be needed for treatment of specific organ failure.

Herpes Zoster (Shingles)

- Herpes zoster is a viral infection. The varicella-zoster virus initially produces chickenpox, after which the virus lies dormant in the dorsal root ganglia of the sensory cranial and spinal nerves. It is then reactivated as shingles later in life.

    o Shingles is usually preceded by a prodromal period of several days, during which pain, tingling, or burning may occur along the involved dermatome.

    o Shingles can be very painful and debilitating.

Data Collection

- Risk Factors

    o Stress

    o Compromise to the immune system

    o Fatigue

    o Poor nutritional status

    o Older adult clients are more susceptible to herpes zoster infection. The immune function of older adults may also be compromised, so they should be monitored carefully for local or systemic signs of infection.

- Subjective Data

    o Paresthesia

    o Pain that is unilateral and extends horizontally along a dermatome

- Objective Data

    o Physical assessment findings

        ▪ Vesicular, unilateral rash (the rash and lesions occur on the skin area innervated by the infected nerve)

        ▪ Rash that is erythematous, vesicular, pustular, or crusting (depending on the stage)

        ▪ Rash that usually resolves in 14 to 21 days

        ▪ Low-grade fever

    o Laboratory tests

        ▪ Cultures provide a definitive diagnosis (but the virus grows so slowly that cultures are often of minimal diagnostic use).

        ▪ Occasionally, an immunofluorescence assay can be done.

UNIT 13	NURSING CARE OF CLIENTS WITH IMMUNE SYSTEM AND INFECTIOUS DISORDERS
Chapter 84	General Principles of Cancer

Overview

- Cancer is a neoplastic disease process that involves abnormal cell growth and differentiation.

- The exact cause of cancer is unknown, but viruses, physical and chemical agents, hormones, genetics, and diet are thought to be factors that trigger abnormal cell growth.

- Cancer cells may invade surrounding tissues and/or spread to other areas of the body through lymph and blood vessels (This process is known as metastasis of the cell.).

- Cancers may arise from almost any tissue in the body.

  o Carcinomas arise from epithelial tissue.

  o Adenocarcinomas arise from glandular organs.

  o Sarcomas arise from mesenchymal tissue (a group of cells that make up connective tissue and lymphatic tissue, blood, and blood vessels).

  o Leukemias are malignancies of the blood-forming cells.

  o Lymphomas arise from the lymph tissue.

  o Multiple myeloma arises from plasma cells and affects the bone.

- Screening and early diagnosis are the most important aspects of health education and care.

Data Collection

- Risk Factors

  o Age

    ■ The highest incidence of cancer occurs in older adults. Older adult women most commonly develop colorectal, breast, lung, pancreatic, and ovarian cancers.

    ■ Older adult men most commonly develop lung, colorectal, prostate, pancreatic, and gastric cancers.

- Race

    - Caucasian women over the age of 40 are more likely to develop breast cancer than are African-American, American-Indian, and Hispanic women. However, the death rate for each of these groups is higher than for Caucasian women and may be related to lack of early screening and treatment.

    - Caucasian men are at an increased risk for testicular cancer, whereas African-American men are at an increased risk for prostate cancer.

- Genetic predisposition

- Exposure to chemicals, viruses, tobacco, and alcohol

- Exposure to certain viruses and bacteria

    - Liver cancer can develop after many years of infection with hepatitis B or hepatitis C.

    - Infection with human T-cell leukemia virus increases the risk of lymphoma and leukemia (indigenous to certain areas of the world, such as Africa and Melanesia).

    - Infection with Epstein-Barr virus has been linked to an increased risk of lymphoma.

    - Human papilloma virus (HPV) infection is the main cause of cervical cancer.

    - HIV increases the risk of lymphoma and Kaposi's sarcoma.

    - *Helicobacter pylori* may increase the risk of stomach cancer and lymphoma of the stomach lining.

- A diet high in fat and red meat and low in fiber

- Sun, ultraviolet light, or radiation exposure (radon)

- Sexual lifestyles (multiple sexual partners or STDs)

- Poverty, obesity, and chronic GERD

Subjective and Objective Data

- Findings depend on the type and location of cancer.

    - Seven warning signs (called CAUTION) clients should watch for:

        - C – Change in bowel or bladder habits

        - A – A sore that doesn't heal

        - U – Unusual bleeding or discharge

        - T – Thickening or lump in the breast or elsewhere

        - I – Indigestion or difficulty swallowing

        - O – Obvious change in warts or moles

        - N – Nagging cough or hoarseness

- ○ Weight loss

- ○ Fatigue/weakness

- ○ Pain (may not occur until late in the disease process)

- ○ Nausea/anorexia

Diagnostic Procedures

- Genetic tests (BRCA1, BRCA2) – Mutations in these genes can predispose a woman to a high risk of breast cancer.

- Tissue biopsy – The definitive diagnosis of abnormal cancer cells

- CBC and differential – Screenings for leukemias

- Chest x-ray, CT scan, magnetic resonance imaging, PET scan, and single photon emission computed tomography scans are used to visualize tumors, metastasis, or progression of cancer.

- Tumor marker assays (carcinoembryonic antigen, cancer antigen 125, prostate-specific antigen, human chronic gonadotropin, alpha fetoprotein) – These are blood tests that screen for cancers of the colon, pancreas, liver, prostate, uterus, and ovaries. Elevated values are suggestive of cancer.

Staging

- The tumor-node-metastasis (TNM) system is used to stage cancer.

  - ○ Tumor (T)

    - ■ TX – Unable to evaluate the primary tumor

    - ■ T0 – No evidence of primary tumor

    - ■ Tis – Tumor in situ

    - ■ T1, T2, T3, and T4 – Size and extent of tumor

  - ○ Node (N)

    - ■ NX – Unable to evaluate regional lymph nodes

    - ■ N0 – No evidence of regional node involvement

    - ■ N1, N2, and N3 – Number of nodes that are involved and/or extent of spread

  - ○ Metastasis (M)

    - ■ MX – Unable to evaluate distant metastasis

    - ■ M0 – No evidence of distant metastasis

    - ■ M1 – Presence of distant metastasis

Complications and Nursing Implications

- Oncologic Emergencies

    o Syndrome of inappropriate antidiuretic hormone (SIADH)

        ▪ SIADH occurs when excessive levels of antidiuretic hormones are produced. Because antidiuretic hormones help the kidneys and body to conserve the correct amount of water, SIADH causes the body to retain water. This results in a dilution of electrolytes (such as sodium) in the blood. Most common in lung and brain cancers. Fluid overload may occur quickly and result in death.

        ▪ Nursing Actions

            □ Monitor clients for hyponatremia and low serum osmolality.

            □ Monitor clients receiving furosemide (Lasix), 0.9% sodium chloride, and/or hypertonic saline IV as prescribed for severe hyponatremia.

            □ Obtain baseline vital signs and neurological status. Perform neuro checks every 4 hr or as needed.

            □ Monitor ECG.

    o Hypercalcemia

        ▪ A common complication of leukemia; breast, lung, head, and neck cancers; lymphomas; multiple myelomas; and bony metastases of any cancer

        ▪ Symptoms include anorexia, nausea, vomiting, shortened QT interval, kidney stones, bone pain, and changes in mental status.

        ▪ Nursing Actions

            □ Monitor clients receiving furosemide (Lasix), 0.9% sodium chloride, pamidronate, and phosphates IV as prescribed.

    o Superior vena cava syndrome

        ▪ Results from obstruction (metastases from breast or lung cancers) of venous return and engorgement of the vessels from the head and upper body. Symptoms include periorbital and facial edema, erythema of the upper body, dyspnea, and epistaxis.

        ▪ Nursing Actions

            □ Position clients in a high-Fowler's position initially to facilitate lung expansion. High-dose radiation therapy may be used for emergency temporary relief.

    o Disseminated intravascular coagulation

        ▪ A coagulation complication secondary to leukemia or adenocarcinomas

        ▪ Nursing Actions

            □ Observe clients for bleeding and apply pressure as needed.

            □ Monitor clients who receive plasma transfusions. Heparin may also be used to slow the cascade of events that makes the body overuse its blood clotting factors.

Ⓐ **APPLICATION EXERCISES**

Scenario: A nurse is obtaining a health history from a client who is at the clinic for an annual physical examination. The client is asking questions about signs and symptoms of cancer.

1. The nurse is reinforcing teaching by instructing the client in the seven warning signs that the client should watch for. Identify these seven warning signs.

2. After collecting data about the nutritional habits of the client, the nurse should reinforce limiting or eliminating which of the following foods in order to prevent certain cancers? (Select all that apply.)

    _____ Fish

    _____ Fruits

    _____ Low-fiber foods

    _____ Red meats

    _____ Vegetables

3. Fill in the blank.

    Carcinomas arise from _____.

    Adenocarcinomas arise from _____.

    Leukemias arise from _____.

    Lymphomas arise from _____.

    Multiple myeloma arises from _____.

APPLICATION EXERCISES ANSWER KEY

1. The nurse is reinforcing teaching by instructing the client in the seven warning signs that the client should watch for. Identify these seven warning signs.

   A useful acronym to remember is CAUTION, which includes change in bowel or bladder habits, a sore that doesn't heal, unusual bleeding or discharge, thickening or lump in the breast or elsewhere, indigestion or difficulty swallowing, obvious change in warts or moles, and nagging cough or hoarseness.

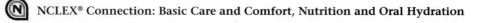 **NCLEX® Connection: Health Promotion and Maintenance, Health Promotion/Disease Prevention**

2. After collecting data about the nutritional habits of the client, the nurse should reinforce limiting or eliminating which of the following foods in order to prevent certain cancers? (Select all that apply.)

   _____ Fish

   _____ Fruits

   __X__ **Low-fiber foods**

   __X__ **Red meats**

   _____ Vegetables

   Low-fiber foods and red meat should be limited or eliminated from the diet because of the increased risk of cancer. A diet with fish, fresh fruits, and vegetables, provides some degree of protection against certain types of cancers.

   NCLEX® Connection: Basic Care and Comfort, Nutrition and Oral Hydration

3. Fill in the blank.

   Carcinomas arise from **epithelial tissue**.

   Adenocarcinomas arise from **glandular organs**.

   Leukemias arise from **blood-forming cells**.

   Lymphomas arise from the **lymph tissue**.

   Multiple myeloma arises from **plasma cells**.

   NCLEX® Connection: Physiological Adaptations, Basic Pathophysiology

UNIT 13	NURSING CARE OF CLIENTS WITH IMMUNE SYSTEM AND INFECTIOUS DISORDERS
Chapter 85	Cancer Treatment Options

Overview

- Cancer treatment options focus on removing or destroying cancer cells and preventing the continued abnormal cell growth and differentiation.

- Cancer treatment options that nurses should be knowledgeable about:

    o Chemotherapy

    o Radiation therapy

    o Hormonal therapy

    o Immunotherapy

- Many cancers are curable when diagnosed early.

Chemotherapy

- Chemotherapy involves the administration of systemic or local cytoxic medications that damage a cell's DNA or destroy rapidly dividing cells.

    o Many of the adverse effects of chemotherapeutic agents are related to the unintentional harm done to normal rapidly proliferating cells, such as those found in the gastrointestinal tract, hair follicles, and bone marrow.

    o Chemotherapy may be administered in an in-patient health care setting, provider's office, clinic, or home.

    o Depending on the agent, it can be given by the oral, parental, intracavitary, or intrathecal route. Implanted ports may be used for long-term therapy. Special training/certification is necessary for the administration of some agents.

- Indications

    o Chemotherapy may be used to cure a disease, control its progression, or to provide palliative treatment.

    o Chemotherapy is most commonly used for treatment of cancer, but it may also be used for other disorders such as autoimmune diseases.

- Client Outcomes

  ○ The client will identify strategies to minimize side effects.

  ○ The client's diagnostic tests will reveal elimination or slowing of disease progression.

  ○ The client will experience relief from cancer symptoms.

- Preprocedure

  ○ Since administration of chemotherapeutic medications is limited to certified individuals, management of adverse effects is the primary focus of health care personnel.

- Complications

  ○ Immunosuppression

    ▪ Immunosuppression due to bone marrow suppression by cytotoxic medications is the most significant adverse effect of chemotherapy.

    ▪ Nursing Actions

      □ Monitor the client's temperature and WBC count.

      □ Immediately report a fever greater than 37.8° C (100° F) to the provider.

      □ Obtain blood cultures prior to initiating antimicrobial therapy.

      □ Initiate neutropenic precautions for clients who have WBC below 1,000/mm³.

        ▸ Place clients in a private room.

        ▸ Minimize time out of room. Have clients wear a mask when leaving the room for a diagnostic procedure or therapy.

        ▸ Protect clients from possible sources of infection (plants, fresh flowers, change water in equipment daily).

        ▸ Have clients, staff, and visitors perform frequent hand hygiene. Restrict visitors who are ill.

        ▸ Avoid invasive procedures that could cause a break in tissue unless necessary (rectal temperatures, injections).

        ▸ Keep designated equipment in the client's room (blood pressure machine, thermometer).

        ▸ Administer colony-stimulating factor filgrastim (Neupogen, Neulasta) as prescribed to stimulate WBC production.

    ▪ Client Education

      □ Encourage clients to avoid crowds while undergoing chemotherapy.

      □ Client instructions

        ▸ Instruct clients to avoid eating fresh fruits and vegetables that could contain bacteria.

- ‣ Recommend for clients to avoid yard work, gardening, or changing a pet's litter box.

- ‣ Instruct clients to avoid fluids that have been sitting at room temperature for greater than 1 hr.

- ‣ Suggest clients wash toothbrush daily in dishwasher or rinse in bleach solution.

- ‣ Have clients report fever greater than 37.8° C (100° F) or other symptoms of bacterial or viral infections immediately to the provider.

- ○ Nausea and vomiting/anorexia

  - ■ Many of the medications used for chemotherapy are emetogenic (induce vomiting) or cause anorexia as well as an altered taste in the mouth.

  - ■ Serotonin blockers, such as ondansetron (Zofran), have been found to be effective and are often given along with corticosteroids, phenothiazines, and antihistamines.

  - ■ Nursing Actions

    - □ Give clients antiemetic medications at times that are appropriate for a chemotherapeutic agent (prior to treatment, during treatment, after treatment).

    - □ Administer antiemetic medications for several days after each treatment.

    - □ Suggest use of visual imagery and relaxation techniques as adjuncts to antiemetics.

    - □ Perform calorie counts to determine intake. Provide liquid supplements as needed. Add protein powders to food or tube feedings.

    - □ Administer megestrol (Megace) to increase the client's appetite if prescribed.

    - □ Perform mouth care prior to serving meals to enhance the client's appetite. Monitor the client for development of mucositis. If noted, request additional treatment immediately to minimize effects.

  - ■ Client Education

    - □ Instruct clients about the administration of antiemetics and to schedule them prior to meals.

    - □ Encourage clients to eat several small meals a day if better tolerated.

    - □ Suggest clients select foods that are served cold and do not require cooking, which can emit odors that stimulate nausea.

    - □ Encourage clients to consume high-protein, high-calorie, nutrient-dense foods and to avoid low- or empty-calorie foods.

    - □ Encourage the use of plastic eating utensils, sucking on hard candy, and avoiding red meats if clients experience a metallic taste in the mouth.

    - □ Suggest use of visual imagery and relaxation techniques as adjuncts to antiemetics.

- ○ Alopecia
  - Alopecia is a side effect of certain chemotherapeutic medications related to their interference with the life cycle of rapidly proliferating cells.
  - Nursing Actions
    - □ Discuss with clients the impact of alopecia on self-image. Discuss options such as hats, turbans, and wigs to deal with hair loss.
    - □ Provide information from the American Cancer Society or a community support group regarding products for clients experiencing alopecia.
    - □ Reinforce with clients that alopecia is temporary and hair should return when chemotherapy is discontinued.
  - Client Education
    - □ Instruct clients to avoid the use of damaging hair-care measures, such as electric rollers, hair dye, and permanent waves. Use of a soft hair brush or wide-tooth comb for grooming is preferred.
    - □ Suggest that clients cut their hair short before treatment to decrease weight on the hair follicle.
    - □ After hair loss, instruct clients to protect the scalp from sun and that they can use a diaper rash ointment/cream for itching.
- ○ Mucositis
  - Mucositis (also referred to as stomatitis) is inflammation of tissues in the mouth, such as the gums, tongue, roof and floor of the mouth, and inside the lips and cheeks.
  - Nursing Actions
    - □ Examine the client's mouth several times a day and inquire about the presence of oral lesions.
    - □ Document the location and size of lesions that are present.
    - □ Avoid using glycerin-based mouthwashes or mouth swabs.
    - □ Administer a topical anesthetic prior to meals.
    - □ Discourage selection of salty, acidic, or spicy foods from the menu.
    - □ Offer mouth care before and after each meal.
  - Client Education
    - □ Encourage clients to rinse the mouth with a solution of half 0.9% sodium chloride and half peroxide at least twice a day, and to brush teeth using a soft-bristled toothbrush.
    - □ Encourage clients to eat soft foods and supplements that are high in calories such as mashed potatoes, scrambled eggs, and cooked cereal. Other appropriate food sources are cold foods such as milk shakes, ice cream, frozen yogurt, bananas, and breakfast mixes.

○ Anemia and thrombocytopenia

- Anemia (decreased number of circulating RBCs) and thrombocytopenia (decreased number of circulating platelets) occur secondary to bone marrow suppression.

- Nursing Actions for Anemia

  □ Monitor clients for fatigue, pallor, dizziness, and shortness of breath.

  □ Help clients manage anemia-related fatigue by scheduling activities with rest periods in between and using energy-saving measures (sitting during showers and ADLs).

  □ Administer erythropoietic medications such as erythropoietin alfa (Epogen) and antianemic medications such as ferrous sulfate (Feosol) as prescribed.

  □ Monitor the client's Hgb to determine response to medications. Be prepared to assist with administering blood if prescribed.

- Nursing Actions for Thrombocytopenia

  □ Monitor the client for petechiae, ecchymosis, bleeding of the gums, nosebleeds, occult or frank blood in stools, urine, and/or vomitus.

  □ Institute bleeding precautions (avoid IVs and injections, apply pressure for approximately 10 min after blood draws, handle client gently and avoid trauma).

  □ Administer thrombopoietic medications such as oprelvekin (Interleukin 11, Neumega), which may decrease the need for platelet transfusions and lessen the risk of bleeding. Monitor platelet count, and be prepared to administer platelets if the count falls below $30,000/mm^3$.

- Client Education

  □ Instruct clients to:

    ▸ Use an electric razor instead of a razor blade when shaving.

    ▸ Use a soft-bristled toothbrush.

    ▸ Blow nose only when necessary.

    ▸ Wear shoes when ambulating.

    ▸ Avoid the use of NSAIDs.

Radiation Therapy

- Radiation therapy involves the use of ionizing radiation to target tissues and destroy cells.

  ○ Side effects include skin changes, hair loss, and debilitating fatigue.

  ○ Radiation therapy can be administered internally with an implant (brachytherapy) or externally with a radiation beam.

- o Radiation therapy is used to cure some cancers, augment the treatment of other cancers, and hopefully increase a client's survival rate and time.

- o Radiation therapy can also be given preoperatively to decrease the size of a tumor or to treat metastatic tumors in clients who are in the terminal stage of their disease.

- Client Outcomes

  - o The client will identify strategies to minimize side effects.

  - o The client's diagnostic tests will reveal elimination or slowing of the disease process.

  - o The client will experience relief from cancer symptoms.

- Internal Radiation Therapy

  - o Brachytherapy is the term used to describe internal radiation that is placed close to the target tissue. This is done via placement in a body orifice (vagina) or body cavity (abdomen) or delivered via IV such as with radionuclide iodine, which is absorbed by the thyroid.

  - o Nursing Actions

    - Ongoing Care

      - □ Place clients in a private room.

      - □ Place appropriate signage on doors warning of the radiation source.

      - □ Wear a dosimeter film badge that records the amount of radiation exposure.

      - □ Limit visitors to 30-min visits and have them maintain a distance of 6 ft.

      - □ Restrict visitors who are pregnant or under the age of 16. Health care personnel who are pregnant should not care for these clients.

      - □ Keep a lead container in the client's room if the delivery method could allow spontaneous loss of radioactive material. Have tongs available to use for placing radioactive material into a lead container.

  - o Client Education

    - Inform clients of the need to remain in a position necessary to prevent dislodgement of the radiation implant.

    - Instruct clients to call the nurse for assistance with elimination.

    - Instruct clients to maintain precautions at home if discharged during therapy.

- External Radiation Therapy

  - o External radiation or teletherapy is delivered over the course of several weeks and aimed at the body from an external source.

  - o Nursing Actions

    - Preparation of clients

      - □ The client's skin over the targeted area is marked with "tattoos" that guide the positioning of the external radiation source.

- Ongoing Care
  - Recommend that clients eat a diet that does not contain red meat. Radiation can cause dysgeusia (distorted sense of taste), making foods such as red meat unpalatable.
  - Help clients manage fatigue by scheduling activities with rest periods in between and using energy-saving measures (sitting during showers and ADLs).
  - Treat symptoms related to the area of the body being irradiated.
    - Mouth – Mucositis, xerostomia
    - Neck – Difficulty swallowing
    - Abdomen – Gastroenteritis
- Client Education
  - Inform clients that fatigue is a common side effect of radiation therapy.
  - Recommend clients gently wash the skin over the irradiated area with mild soap and water. Dry the area thoroughly using patting motions.
  - Instruct clients not to remove radiation "tattoos" that are used to guide therapy.
  - Instruct clients not to apply powders, ointments, lotions, or perfumes to the irradiated skin.
  - Recommend clients wear soft clothing over the irradiated skin and avoid tight or constricting clothes.
  - Recommend clients not expose the irradiated skin to sun or a heat source.

Hormonal Therapy

- Hormone therapy is effective against tumors that are supported or suppressed by hormones.

- Indications
  - Hormone agonists, such as gonadotropin-releasing hormone agonists (GnRH) like leuprolide (Eligard, Lupron), are effective against tumors that require a particular hormone for support.
    - The use of androgenic hormones in a client who has estrogen-dependent cancer can suppress growth of this type of cancer.
    - Conversely, the use of estrogenic hormones for a testosterone-dependent cancer can suppress growth of this type of cancer.
  - Hormone antagonists are also effective against tumors that require a particular hormone for support.
    - The use of an anti-estrogen hormone in a client with estrogen-dependent cancer can suppress growth of this type of cancer.
    - The same is true for anti-testosterone hormones.

- Client Outcomes

  o The client will identify strategies to minimize side effects.

  o The client's diagnostic tests will reveal elimination or slowing of the disease process.

  o The client will experience relief from cancer symptoms.

- Nursing Actions

  o GnRH

    ▪ Ongoing Care

      ▫ Monitor the client's cardiac status, along with blood pressure and the occurrence of pulmonary edema.

    ▪ Client Education

      ▫ Inform male clients about the impact on sexual functioning (decreased libido, erectile dysfunction) and feminizing effects of hormone therapy (gynecomastia, hot flashes, bone loss).

      ▫ Instruct clients to increase intake of calcium and vitamin D.

  o Androgen antagonists – flutamide (Eulexin)

    ▪ Ongoing Care

      ▫ Monitor the client's liver enzymes and CBC.

    ▪ Client Education

      ▫ Warn clients about the feminizing effects of hormone therapy (gynecomastia, erectile dysfunction).

      ▫ Advise clients to notify the provider of sore throat or bruising.

  o Estrogen antagonists – tamoxifen (Nolvadex), anastrozole (Arimidex), trastuzumab (Herceptin)

    ▪ Ongoing Care

      ▫ Monitor the client's CBC, clotting times, lipid profiles, calcium and cholesterol serum levels, and liver function for medication-related changes.

      ▫ Neurologic and cardiovascular functioning should also be monitored for changes.

    ▪ Client Education

      ▫ Inform clients of side effects, which include nausea, vomiting, hot flashes, weight gain, vaginal bleeding, and increased risk of thrombosis.

      ▫ Reinforce the need for yearly gynecologic exams and the need to take calcium and vitamin D supplements.

Immunotherapy

- Immunotherapy, or biologic response modifiers (BMRs), alter a client's biological response to cancerous tumor cells.

  o Interleukins and interferons are the two primary cytokines (immune response modulators) used in immunotherapy.

    ▪ Interleukins help coordinate the inflammatory and immune responses of the body, in particular, the lymphocytes.

    ▪ Interferons, when stimulated, can exert an antitumor effect by activating a variety of responses.

  o Cytokines are the primary BMRs currently used, and they work to enhance the immune system. They help the client's immune system recognize cancer cells and use the body's natural defenses to destroy them.

- Client Outcomes

  o The client will identify strategies to minimize side effects.

  o The client's diagnostic tests will reveal elimination or slowing of the disease process.

  o The client will experience relief from cancer symptoms.

- Nursing Actions

  o Interleukins

    ▪ Ongoing Care

      □ Monitor clients for influenza-like symptoms and edema.

  o Interferons

    ▪ Ongoing Care

      □ Monitor clients for peripheral neuropathy that may affect vision, hearing, balance, and gait.

      □ Take precautions for orthostatic hypotension.

    ▪ Client Education

      □ Instruct clients to immediately report influenza-like symptoms or changes consistent with peripheral neuropathy.

      □ Warn clients that skin rashes are common and use of a perfume-free moisturizer may be helpful.

      □ Instruct clients to avoid the sun and swimming if skin symptoms arise.

APPLICATION EXERCISES

1. A nurse is caring for a client who is undergoing a course of chemotherapy. She is reporting severe nausea and vomiting and has lost 9 lb since her last course of chemotherapy. Which of the following statements is appropriate for the nurse to make? (Select all that apply.)

    _____ "Your nausea will lessen with each course of chemotherapy."

    _____ "Hot food is better tolerated because of the pleasant aroma it produces."

    _____ "Try eating several small meals throughout the day."

    _____ "Eat as much red meat as tolerated to get rid of the metallic taste."

    _____ "Take your antiemetic immediately after you eat."

2. A nurse is caring for a client who is undergoing brachytherapy. Which of the following precautions should be followed? (Select all that apply.)

    _____ The client should have a private room.

    _____ Health care personnel should wear a dosimeter film badge.

    _____ Visitors should stay 4 feet away from the client.

    _____ Visitors can stay as long as they like.

    _____ Children and pregnant women should not visit the client.

    _____ Lead container should be kept in the room.

    _____ Tongs should be kept in the room.

3. A nurse is caring for a client who had a mastectomy for breast cancer. The client has been prescribed tamoxifen (Nolvadex). Which of the following should indicate to the nurse that the client needs further teaching?

    A. "I may experience hot flashes."

    B. "I may experience nausea and vomiting."

    C. "I may lose weight."

    D. "I may have vaginal bleeding."

4. A nurse is caring for a client who is receiving immunotherapy in the outpatient clinic. Which of the following should the nurse recommend for inclusion in the plan of care? (Select all that apply.)

    _____ Get 20 min of direct sunlight a day.

    _____ Monitor for changes in vision.

    _____ Report flu-like symptoms to provider.

    _____ Report changes in hearing.

    _____ Monitor for unsteady gait or balance.

APPLICATION EXERCISES ANSWER KEY

1. A nurse is caring for a client who is undergoing a course of chemotherapy. She is reporting severe nausea and vomiting and has lost 9 lb since her last course of chemotherapy. Which of the following statements is appropriate for the nurse to make? (Select all that apply.)

    _____ "Your nausea will lessen with each course of chemotherapy."

    _____ "Hot food is better tolerated because of the pleasant aroma it produces."

    __X__ **"Try eating several small meals throughout the day."**

    _____ "Eat as much red meat as tolerated to get rid of the metallic taste."

    _____ "Take your antiemetic immediately after you eat."

    Several small meals a day are usually better tolerated than larger meals for a client who has nausea. Nausea usually occurs to the same extent with each course of chemotherapy. Cold foods are tolerated better than warm foods because odors from warm foods can stimulate nausea. Red meat is not tolerated well in clients undergoing chemotherapy as the taste of meat is frequently altered and unpalatable. Antiemetics are prescribed to take before eating.

    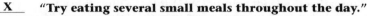 **NCLEX® Connection: Basic Care and Comfort, Nutrition and Oral Hydration**

2. A nurse is caring for a client who is undergoing brachytherapy. Which of the following precautions should be followed? (Select all that apply.)

    __X__ **The client should have a private room.**

    __X__ **Health care personnel should wear a dosimeter film badge.**

    _____ Visitors should stay 4 feet away from the client.

    _____ Visitors can stay as long as they like.

    __X__ **Children and pregnant women should not visit the client.**

    __X__ **Lead container should be kept in the room.**

    __X__ **Tongs should be kept in the room.**

    Brachytherapy is internal radiation administered close to the target tissue. A private room, dosimeter film badge, restricted visitation by children and pregnant women, and keeping a lead container and tongs in the room in case of accidental loss of radioactive material are appropriate precautions. Visitors should stand 6 feet away from the client and limit the time visiting to 30 min.

    NCLEX® Connection: Reduction of Risk Potential, Potential for Complications of Diagnostic Tests/Treatments/Procedures

3. A nurse is caring for a client who had a mastectomy for breast cancer. The client has been prescribed tamoxifen (Nolvadex). Which of the following should indicate to the nurse that the client needs further teaching?

    A. "I may experience hot flashes."

    B. "I may experience nausea and vomiting."

    C. "I may lose weight."

    D. "I may have vaginal bleeding."

    A side effect of Tamoxifen is weight gain not weight loss. Other side effects of this medication can include hot flashes, nausea and vomiting, and vaginal bleeding.

 NCLEX® Connection: Pharmacological Therapies, Adverse Effects/Contraindications/Side Effects/Interactions

4. A nurse is caring for a client who is receiving immunotherapy in the outpatient clinic. Which of the following should the nurse recommend for inclusion in the plan of care? (Select all that apply.)

    _____ Get 20 min of direct sunlight a day.

    __X__ **Monitor for changes in vision.**

    __X__ **Report flu-like symptoms to provider.**

    __X__ **Report changes in hearing.**

    __X__ **Monitor for unsteady gait or balance.**

    Monitoring for changes in vision and hearing, reporting flu-like symptoms, and monitoring for unsteady gait or balance may be an indication of orthostatic hypotension and should be included in the plan of care. Clients receiving immunotherapy should avoid the sun and swimming if skin rashes arise.

 NCLEX® Connection: Reduction of Risk Potential, Potential for Complications of Diagnostic Tests/Treatments/Procedures

UNIT 13	NURSING CARE OF CLIENTS WITH IMMUNE SYSTEM AND INFECTIOUS DISORDERS
Chapter 86	Pain Management for Clients with Cancer

Overview

- The management of cancer pain is necessary to optimize the quality of life of clients who have cancer.

- Clients who have cancer may experience pain from the abnormal tissue growth and/or from cancer treatment (surgery, radiation, chemotherapy).

Identifying Cancer Pain

- Use the client's verbal expression of pain as the most reliable indicator of pain.

- Use standard pain measurement tools to further investigate pain.

- Monitor for:

  - Nonverbal indicators of acute pain

    - Agitation and grimacing

    - Elevated heart rate, respiratory rate, and/or blood pressure

    - Diaphoresis and pupil dilation

    - Splinting of a certain area

  - Nonverbal indicators of chronic pain

    - Depression

    - Lethargy

    - Anger

    - Weakness

Management of Cancer Pain

- Palliative cancer pain management is intended to provide comfort and reduce pain rather than to cure the cancer.

- The goal of palliative pain management is to reduce pain to improve quality of life while maintaining dignity and mental clarity.

- Methods of pain management

  o Removal or reduction in size of cancer

    ▪ Surgery, chemotherapy, and radiation therapy may reduce pain by removing cancer and pressure of tumor on tissues or organs.

      □ Surgical removal of tumor – Removal of cancer may include part of the body and result in change in organ function. Clients may be fearful about survival and anxious about the loss of a body part.

      □ Radiation – Radiation may cause localized hair loss, skin changes, and severe fatigue.

      □ Chemotherapy – Killing of the cells may result in localized complications (stomatitis), or systemic complications (nausea, vomiting, neutropenia).

- Nursing Actions

  o Nursing actions are specific to each surgery or procedure.

  o Client education

    ▪ Include information regarding the specific procedure or treatment.

    ▪ Include families in care and management.

    ▪ Provide information about support groups, such as the American Cancer Society.

    ▪ Radiation – Instruct clients about specific skin care and to avoid sun exposure.

    ▪ Chemotherapy – Include information about avoiding infection and managing other adverse effects.

Medications

- Pharmacological management of pain includes NSAIDS, opioids, antidepressants, anticonvulsants, steroids, and local anesthetics. Some clients who have cancer pain may require regular use of analgesics for pain control.

CLASSIFICATION AND THERAPEUTIC INTENT	MEDICATION	NURSING CONSIDERATION	CLIENT EDUCATION
Nonopioid medications and nonsteroidal anti-inflammatory medications • Given for mild to moderate pain	• Acetaminophen (Tylenol) • Ketorolac (Toradol) • Aspirin (acetylsalicylic acid) • Ibuprofen (Motrin)	• Monitor for signs of gastrointestinal (GI) bleeding, such as bloody stools or emesis that looks like coffee grounds. • Monitor for bruising and bleeding. • Do not give acetaminophen to clients who have liver disease. • Monitor for tinnitus and hearing loss if NSAIDs are prescribed.	• Take with food to prevent GI upset. • Be alert to GI or other bleeding and bruising. • Do not crush or chew enteric-coated products.

CLASSIFICATION AND THERAPEUTIC INTENT	MEDICATION	NURSING CONSIDERATION	CLIENT EDUCATION
Opioids • Given for moderate to severe pain • May be given for breakthrough pain • Fentanyl (Sublimaze) is available for transdermal use.	• Morphine sulfate • Meperidine (Demerol) • Hydromorphone (Dilaudid) • Oxycodone (OxyContin) • Fentanyl (Sublimaze)	• Use with caution in older adult clients. • Monitor for respiratory depression. ○ Have naloxone (Narcan) available to reverse effects.	• Use medication as directed. • Prevent constipation with diet changes and stool softeners if needed. • Be aware that nausea may subside after a few days.
Antidepressants • Given to reduce associated depression, promote sleep, and increase serotonin levels that may improve feelings of well-being • May decrease neuropathic pain	• Amitriptyline (Elavil) • Desipramine (Norpramin) • Imipramine (Tofranil)	• Use with caution in older adult clients. • Do not give to clients who have seizure disorders or a history of cardiac problems. • Use with caution in young adult clients or clients who are at risk for suicide, because antidepressants may increase suicide risk.	• Notify the provider if depression increases or if thoughts of suicide occur. • Be aware that therapeutic effects may take 2 to 3 weeks to become established.
Anticonvulsants • Given to treat neuralgia or neuropathic-type pain	• Gabapentin (Neurontin) • Valproic acid (Depakene) • Pregabalin (Lyrica)	• Monitor electrolytes. • Monitor medications levels. • Monitor for tremors.	• Avoid the use of alcohol. • Do not drive at the start of therapy. • Notify the provider if tremors occur.
Steroids • May reduce pain by reducing swelling	• Prednisolone (Prelone) • Dexamethasone (Decadron)	• Reduce dosage gradually. • Monitor for muscle weakness, joint pain, or fever. • Monitor serum glucose levels.	• Use only as directed. • Do not discontinue suddenly. • Take with food.

CLASSIFICATION AND THERAPEUTIC INTENT	MEDICATION	NURSING CONSIDERATION	CLIENT EDUCATION
Adjunctive agents • Sympatholytic agents – Used to treat neuropathic pain ○ Used in conjunction with bupivacaine in epidural or other local infusions.	• Clonidine (Catapres)	• Monitor for hypotension.	• Change positions slowly, because these medications may cause postural hypotension.
• Skeletal muscle relaxants – May be used along with other pain medications for muscle spasms associated with cancer pain	• Baclofen (Lioresal)	• Monitor for seizure activity.	• Take with food. • Use caution when driving or operating machinery. • These medications may cause drowsiness and dizziness.
Systemic local anesthetics • May be given via an infusion pump directly into the area of pain (intrathecal, intra-articular, intrapleural) to provide pain relief	• Lidocaine (Xylocaine) • Bupivacaine (Marcaine) • Ropivacaine (Naropin)	• Monitor for hypotension. • Monitor for signs of infection at the catheter insertion site. • Evaluate pain status. • Monitor for motor impairment and level of sedation. • May be used in combination with an opioid or another medication, such as clonidine (Catapres).	• Monitor the infusion site for signs of infection, such as redness or swelling. • Monitor for fever. • Notify the provider of increased pain or decreased movement that may indicate a motor block. • Care for and protect the external catheter.
Topical anesthetics • Used to treat oral ulcers that may be caused by radiation or chemotherapy and neuropathic pain, such as in postmastectomy axillary pain	• Lidocaine HCL (Lidoderm patch) • Eutectic mixture of local anesthetic cream	• Monitor for pain relief and local skin reaction.	• Use as directed. • Use only on intact skin.

ADMINISTRATION METHOD	DESCRIPTION
Oral	• First choice for administration • Long-acting formulations are available.
Transdermal – Fentanyl (Sublimaze)	• Easy to administer • Slow onset • Long duration (48 to 72 hr)
Rectal	• Contraindicated for clients with a low WBC or low platelet count
Subcutaneous infusion – Morphine or hydromorphone	• Slow infusion rate (2 to 4 mL/hr) • Requires nursing support • Risk of infiltration • Rapid onset
Intravenous	• Requires nursing support • Risk of infiltration • Rapid onset
Epidural or intrathecal	• Risk of infection, pruritus, and urinary retention • Requires nursing care to monitor, especially with increase in dosage

Anesthetic Interventions

- Regional nerve blocks

    - An anesthetic agent, such as bupivacaine, and/or a corticosteroid, is injected directly into a nerve root to provide pain relief.

        - Used for an isolated area of pain

            - For example, an intercostal nerve block may used to treat chest or abdominal wall pain

        - The procedure may take from 15 min to 1 hr, depending upon the area receiving the block.

- Epidural or intrathecal catheters

    - A local anesthetic or analgesic is injected into the epidural space (the space outside the dura mater of the spinal cord) or intrathecal space (the subarachnoid area within the spinal cord sheath that contains cerebrospinal fluid).

        - An external catheter is surgically placed under the skin with an external port for long-term use.

            - Used for chronic pain management

            - May be attached to a continuous infusion or injected as needed

            - Used for upper abdominal pain, thoracic pain, and pain located below the umbilicus

o   Nursing Actions

- Monitor during insertion/injection and for at least 1 hr following insertion/injection (follow established guidelines) for hypotension, anaphylaxis, seizures, and dura puncture.

- Monitor clients receiving IV fluids.

- Monitor for respiratory depression and sedation.

- Monitor the insertion site for hematoma and signs of an infection.

- Check the level of sensory block.

- Evaluate leg strength prior to ambulating.

- Monitor for signs of systemic infusion (metallic taste, ringing in ears, perioral numbness, seizures).

    o   Client Education

- Advise clients to monitor the injection site for swelling, redness, or drainage.

- Advise clients to protect the area of numbness from injury and to notify the provider of increased pain or signs of systemic infusion (metallic taste, ringing in ears, perioral numbness, seizures).

- Advise clients to notify the provider of signs of infection, (fever, swelling, redness or swelling at injection site, increase in pain or severe headache, sudden weakness to lower extremities, decrease in bowel or bladder control).

- Notify the provider of signs of systemic infusion (metallic taste, ringing in ears, perioral numbness, seizures).

- Inform clients that long-term reactions may include sexual dysfunction or amenorrhea.

Other Invasive Techniques

- Neurolytic ablation

  - Involves interrupting the nerve pathway or destroying the nerve roots that are causing pain; usually involves a CT-guided probe and injection of chemicals, such as phenol or ethanol

    - For example, celiac plexus nerve ablation may be effective for pancreatic, stomach, abdominal, small bowel, and proximal colon pain.

    - The procedure is considered irreversible. However, nerve ablation may provide relief for several months until nerve fibers regenerate.

    - Nerve ablation may cause loss of sensory, motor, and autonomic function.

    - Use only when noninvasive methods are ineffective.

- Radiofrequency ablation

  - Electrical currency creates heat on a probe that is guided to the tumor or nerves and is used to destroy cancer cells or ablate nerve endings. This is often used for lung and bone tumors.

- Cryoanalgesia

  - Uses a needle-like probe to deliver extreme cold to interfere with pain conduction via nerve pathways

  - Nursing Actions

    - Monitor vital signs, especially blood pressure, during and for at least 1 hr following the procedure (follow established guidelines).

    - Monitor for signs of bleeding, such as tachycardia and hypotension.

    - Monitor for skin irritation.

    - Monitor for other effects such as diarrhea, loss of bladder or bowel control, or extremity weakness.

    - Assess pain relief.

  - Client Education

    - Instruct clients to apply ice if needed for pain at the insertion site.

    - Continue to use pain medications as directed if needed.

    - Notify the health care provider of an increase in pain or weakness of extremities.

Alternative Approaches

- Alternative approaches to pain management may be used in addition to pain medications or other techniques. Many of these provide some pain reduction with minimal side effects.

  - Transcutaneous electrical nerve stimulation

    - Low-voltage electrical impulses are transmitted through electrodes that are attached to the skin near or over the area of pain. This is usually used in conjunction with analgesics.

    - Nursing Actions

      - Use with conductive gel.

      - Monitor electrode sites for burns or rash.

      - Offer other pain medications if indicated.

      - Do not use on clients who have pacemakers or infusion pumps.

    - Client Education

      - Advise clients to inspect the skin under the electrodes to monitor for burns or irritation.

      - Advise clients not to use if pregnant.

      - Advice clients not to use near the head or over the heart.

o   Relaxation techniques and imagery

- Useful during a procedure or a period of increased pain.

- Relaxation techniques include deep breathing, progressive relaxation, and meditation.

- Positive imagery involves visualizing a peaceful image and may be used with the aid of audiotapes.

- Relaxation and imagery may help reduce anxiety, stress, and related pain, and they may help clients to feel more in control of the pain.

o   Distraction

- Music, television, exercise, and family and friends may be effective distractions from pain and stress. Other distractions may include repetitive actions or movements or a visual focal point. A change of scenery may offer a distraction from pain.

o   Application of heat or cold, pressure, massage, or vibration

- Heat increases blood flow, relaxes muscles, and reduces joint stiffness. Cold decreases inflammation and causes local analgesia.

    □   Do not use heat or cold directly on skin that is damaged by radiation.

- Massage and vibration may cause relaxation, distraction, and increased surface circulation.

o   Acupuncture

- Acupuncture is a technique that involves the use of small needles inserted into the skin at different depths to stimulate and alter nerve pathways.

o   Hypnosis

- Hypnosis involves using an altered state of awareness to redirect a person's perception of pain. It may be helpful to induce positive imagery, reduce anxiety, and improve coping.

o   Peer group support

- A support group helps provide emotional support for clients and their families. Other benefits to meeting with a support group include the presence of a social network, availability of information, and help in strengthening coping skills.

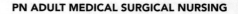

Ⓐ **APPLICATION EXERCISES**

1. A nurse should know that which of the following is the most reliable indicator of pain?

   A. Blood pressure
   B. Facial expression
   C. Pulse
   D. Verbal description of pain

2. A client who has breakthrough cancer pain has been prescribed oxycodone (OxyContin). Which of the following side effects of oxycodone should the nurse monitor for and be prepared to intervene when present? (Select all that apply.)

   _____ Orthostatic hypotension
   _____ Constipation
   _____ Joint pain
   _____ Pruritis
   _____ Respiratory depression

3. A nurse is caring for a client who is to undergo neurolytic ablation. The nurse should recognize that this treatment is used only when other measures have failed due to the risk of

   A. increased pain.
   B. myelosuppression.
   C. thrombocytopenia.
   D. irreversible nerve damage.

4. Match the alternative approach to cancer pain in the left column to its description in the right column.

   _____ Distraction   A. Stimulation of nerve pathways by small needles
   _____ Relaxation   B. Listening to music
   _____ Acupuncture   C. Meditation

APPLICATION EXERCISES ANSWER KEY

1. A nurse should know that which of the following is the most reliable indicator of pain?

   A. Blood pressure

   B. Facial expression

   C. Pulse

   D. Verbal description of pain

   A client's verbal description of pain is the most reliable indicator of pain. Nonverbal and physiological indicators, however, should also be included in the pain assessment.

    NCLEX® Connection: Physiological Adaptation, Alterations in Body Systems

2. A client who has breakthrough cancer pain has been prescribed oxycodone (OxyContin). Which of the following side effects of oxycodone should the nurse monitor for and be prepared to intervene when present? (Select all that apply.)

X	**Orthostatic hypotension**
X	**Constipation**
_____	Joint pain
X	**Pruritis**
X	**Respiratory depression**

   Side effects of oxycodone can include orthostatic hypotension, constipation, respiratory depression, and pruritis. Have naloxone available to reverse the respiratory depression. Adjust diet or use stool softeners if needed for constipation. Pruritis can be treated with an antihistamine or discontinued if an allergic reaction is suspected. Joint pain is not a usual finding with oxycodone.

    NCLEX® Connection: Pharmacological Therapies, Pharmacological Pain Management

3. A nurse is caring for a client who is to undergo neurolytic ablation. The nurse should recognize that this treatment is used only when other measures have failed due to the risk of

   A. increased pain.

   B. myelosuppression.

   C. thrombocytopenia.

   D. irreversible nerve damage.

   Neurolytic ablation causes permanent nerve destruction. It is usually used only after other pain relief methods have been unsuccessful.

    NCLEX® Connection: Reduction of Risk Potential, Potential for Complications of Diagnostic Tests/Treatments/Procedures

. Match the alternative approach to cancer pain in the left column to its description in the right column.

__B__	Distraction	A. Stimulation of nerve pathways by small needles
__C__	Relaxation	B. Listening to music
__A__	Acupuncture	C. Meditation

Alternative approaches to pain management can be used such as hypnosis, biofeedback, acupuncture, acupressure, support groups, massage therapy, and transcutaneous electrical nerve stimulation. Many of these provide some pain reduction with minimal side effects. Alcohol and tobacco are not considered alternative therapies for pain and have side effects that can interfere with certain therapies.

Ⓝ **NCLEX® Connection: Basic Care and Comfort, Nonpharmacological Comfort Interventions**

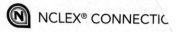

UNIT 14: NURSING CARE OF THE PERIOPERATIVE CLIENT

- Preoperative Nursing Care
- Postoperative Nursing Care

NCLEX® CONNECTIONS

When reviewing the chapters in this section, keep in mind the relevant sections of the NCLEX® outline, in particular:

CLIENT NEEDS: PHARMACOLOGICAL THERAPIES	CLIENT NEEDS: REDUCTION OF RISK POTENTIAL	CLIENT NEEDS: PHYSIOLOGICAL ADAPTATION

...t topics/tasks include:
 	
...se Effects/
...dications/Side
...teractions
 	
...potential and
...mpatibilities
...dications.
 	
...n
 	
...sion-
	Relevant topics/tasks include:
	
	• Changes/Abnormalities in Vital Signs
	  ○ Check and monitor client vital signs.
	• Diagnostic Tests
	  ○ Perform an electrocardiogram.
	• Potential for Complications from Surgical Procedures and Health
	  ○ Identify client response to diagnostic tests/treatments/procedures.
		Relevant topics/tasks include:
		
		• Alterations in Body Systems
		  ○ Provide care for client drainage device.
		• Fluid and Electrolyte Imbalances
		  ○ Monitor client response to interventions to correct fluid and/or electrolyte imbalance.
		• Unexpected Response to Therapies
		  ○ Identify and treat a client intravenous (IV) line infiltration.

993

UNIT 14	NURSING CARE OF THE PERIOPERATIVE CLIENT
Chapter 87	Preoperative Nursing Care

Overview

- Preoperative care takes place from the time clients are scheduled for surgery until care is transferred to the operating suite. Informed consent is obtained by the provider, and at that time all risks and benefits are explained to clients or their surrogate.

- Preoperative care includes thorough data collection of the client's physical, emotional, and psychosocial status prior to surgery.

- Surgical procedures are performed on an inpatient, same-day, or outpatient-admission basis.

Indications

- Surgery may be performed for a restorative, curative, palliative, or cosmetic purpose.

Client Outcomes

- The client will demonstrate appropriate technique to perform postoperative exercises.

- The client will give informed consent.

Data Collection

- Risk Factors for Surgery

  o Infection (risk of sepsis)

  o Anemia (oxygenation, healing impact)

  o Hypovolemia from dehydration or blood loss (circulatory compromise)

  o Electrolyte imbalance through inadequate diet or disease process (dysrhythmias)

  o Age (older adults are at greater risk for adverse reactions to medications, injury due to sensory limitations, development of impaired skin integrity, anesthesia may pose special risks related to cognitive changes and prolonged recovery)

  o Pregnancy (fetal risk with anesthesia)

  o Respiratory disease (COPD, pneumonia, asthma)

  o Cardiovascular disease (cerebrovascular accident, heart failure, myocardial infarction, hypertension, dysrhythmias)

- o Diabetes mellitus (decreased intestinal motility, altered blood glucose levels, delayed healing)

- o Liver disease (altered medication metabolism)

- o Renal disease (altered elimination)

- o Endocrine disorders (hypo/hyperthyroidism, Addison's disease, Cushing's syndrome)

- o Immune system disorders (allergies, immunocompromise)

- o Coagulation defect (increased risk of bleeding)

- o Malnutrition (delayed healing)

- o Obesity (impact on anesthesia, elimination, and wound healing)

- o Use of some medications (antihypertensives, anticoagulants)

- o Substance use (tobacco, alcohol)

- o Family history (malignant hyperthermia)

- o Allergies (latex, anesthetic agents)

- Subjective and Objective Data

  - o Detailed history (including medical problems, allergies, medication use, substance abuse, psychosocial problems, and cultural considerations)

  - o Anxiety level regarding the procedure

  - o Older adult clients may be fearful due to financial concerns and lack of social support.

  - o Laboratory results

  - o Head-to-toe assessment

  - o Vital signs

Diagnostic Procedures

- Urinalysis – Ruling out of infection

- Blood type and cross match – Transfusion readiness

- CBC – Infection/immune status

- Hgb and Hct – Fluid status, anemia

- Pregnancy test – Fetal risk of anesthesia

- Clotting studies (PT, INR, aPTT, platelet count)

- Electrolyte levels – Electrolyte imbalances

- Serum creatinine – Renal status

- ABGs – Oxygenation status

- Chest x-ray – Heart and lung status

- 12-lead ECG – Baseline heart rhythm, dysrhythmias

Nursing Actions

- Verify that the informed consent is accurately completed, signed, and witnessed.

- Once surgery as treatment has been discussed with the client or surrogate, it is the responsibility of the provider to obtain consent after discussing procedure risks and benefits. The nurse is not to obtain the consent for the provider in any circumstance.

- Nurses can clarify any information that remains unclear after the provider's explanation of the procedure. The nurse may not, however, provide any new or additional information not previously given by the provider.

- A legal guardian may need to sign surgical consent forms for older adult clients.

- Ensure consent is signed prior to preoperative medications.

RESPONSIBILITIES FOR INFORMED CONSENT		
THE PROVIDER	THE CLIENT	THE NURSE
Obtains informed consent To obtain informed consent, the provider must give the client: • A complete description of the treatment/procedure. • A description of the professionals who will be performing and participating in the treatment. • A description of the potential harm, pain, and/or discomfort that may occur. • Options for other treatments. • The right to refuse treatment.	Gives informed consent To give informed consent, the client must: • Give it voluntarily (there must be no coercion involved). • Be competent and of legal age or be an emancipated minor. When the client is unable to provide consent, another authorized person must give consent. • Receive enough information to make a decision based on an understanding of what is expected.	Witnesses informed consent To witness informed consent, the nurse must: • Ensure the provider gave the client necessary information, the client understood the information and is competent to give informed consent. • Have the client sign the informed consent document. • Notify the provider if the client has additional questions or appears to not understand. (The provider is responsible for providing clarification.) o The nurse documents client questions and reinforcement of teaching and notifies the provider. • Record use of an interpreter in client's medical record.

- Reinforce preoperative teaching

  o Postoperative pain control techniques

  o Coughing and deep breathing exercises

  o Range-of-motion exercises and early ambulation for prevention of thrombi and respiratory complications

  o Presence of invasive devices (drains, tubes, IV catheters)

  o Postoperative diet to follow

  o Use of the incentive spirometer

 View Media Supplement: Incentive Spirometer Education (Video)

  o Preoperative instructions (avoid cigarette smoking for 24 hr preoperatively, medications to be withheld, bowel preparation)

    ▪ Advise clients who are taking acetylsalicylic acid (Aspirin) should to stop taking it for 1 week before an elective surgery to decrease the risk of bleeding.

  o Care and restrictions relative to surgical procedure performed

  o Administer enemas and/or laxatives for clients undergoing bowel surgery.

  o Regularly check the client's scheduled medication prescriptions. Some medications (antihypertensives, anticoagulants) may be withheld until after the procedure.

  o Ensure that the client remains NPO for at least 6 to 8 hr before surgery with general anesthesia and 3 to 4 hr with local anesthesia to avoid aspiration. Note on the chart the last time any food or fluid is taken.

  o Perform skin preparation, which may include cleansing with antimicrobial soap and clipping hair in areas that will be involved in the surgery.

  o Ensure that jewelry, dentures, prosthetics, makeup, nail polish, and glasses are removed. These items can either be given to the family or inventoried and secured per agency policy.

  o Monitor IV access.

  o Administer preoperative medications (prophylactic antimicrobials, antiemetics, sedatives) as prescribed.

    ▪ Have the client void prior to administration.

    ▪ Monitor the client's response to the medications.

    ▪ Raise side rails following administration to prevent injury.

    ▪ Ensure that the preoperative checklist is complete.

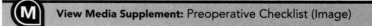 **View Media Supplement:** Preoperative Checklist (Image)

  o Transfer clients to the preanesthesia care unit.

Complications

- Complications during the postoperative period may be related to the medications given preoperatively.

MEDICATION CLASS	POSSIBLE COMPLICATIONS
Sedatives (benzodiazepines, barbiturates)	Respiratory depression, drowsiness, dizziness
Opioids	Respiratory depression, drowsiness, dizziness, constipation
IV infusions (0.9% NaCl, lactated Ringer's)	Heart failure, hypernatremia
Gastrointestinal medications (antiemetics, antacids, H_2 receptor blockers)	Alkalosis, cardiac abnormalities (certain H_2 receptor blockers), drowsiness

- For clients encountering severe anxiety and panic, reassurance will be necessary and sedation medications may be given.

- Be alert for any allergic reactions the client has to medications.

Ⓐ APPLICATION EXERCISES

1. A 68-year-old client is undergoing an endoscopy, which will require moderate sedation. Which of the following findings in the client's history indicates the need for further data collection?

   A. History of gout

   B. Allergic to bee stings

   C. History of GI bleed

   D. Chronic obstructive pulmonary disease

2. An adult woman on a cardiac unit is experiencing episodes of paroxysmal supraventricular tachycardia (PSVT). After performing all other possible interventions, the provider decides to perform cardioversion and to use midazolam (Versed) to relax the client for the procedure. A nurse checks the chart to verify that all the necessary steps have been completed prior to administering the midazolam. Which of the following findings should the nurse expect to see in the chart? (Select all that apply.)

   _____ Signed informed consent

   _____ Allergy history

   _____ Baseline vital signs and cardiac rhythm

   _____ Medications administered

   _____ Documentation of the last time the client ate or drank

   _____ Type and cross match

3. Which of the following preoperative client findings should be reported to the client's provider? (Select all that apply.)

   _____ Serum potassium 3.9 mEq/L

   _____ Serum sodium 145 mEq/L

   _____ Serum creatinine 2.8 mg/dL

   _____ Prothrombin time of 23 seconds

   _____ Blood glucose 235 mg/dL

   _____ WBC 17,850/mm^3

4. The surgeon is behind schedule and asks the licensed practical nurse (LPN) to complete the consent form. Which of the following statements by the LPN is correct?

   A. "I can have surgery personnel discuss the procedure with the client."

   B. "I can have the RN discuss the surgical complications you foresee."

   C. "I can witness the client's signature on the form."

   D. "I can discuss the surgical complications you foresee."

(A) APPLICATION EXERCISES ANSWER KEY

1. A 68-year-old client is undergoing an endoscopy, which will require moderate sedation. Which of the following findings in the client's history indicates the need for further data collection?

    A. History of gout

    B. Allergic to bee stings

    C. History of GI bleed

    D. Chronic obstructive pulmonary disease

    Chronic obstructive pulmonary disease poses a risk for possible airway compromise indicating a need to collect more data. Being allergic to bee stings, having a history of gout, and GI bleed does not indicate a need for further evaluation.

    (N) NCLEX® Connection: Pharmacological Therapies, Adverse Effects/Contraindications/Side Effects/Interactions

2. An adult woman on a cardiac unit is experiencing episodes of paroxysmal supraventricular tachycardia (PSVT). After performing all other possible interventions, the provider decides to perform cardioversion and to use midazolam (Versed) to relax the client for the procedure. A nurse checks the chart to verify that all the necessary steps have been completed prior to administering the midazolam. Which of the following findings should the nurse expect to see in the chart? (Select all that apply.)

    | X | **Signed informed consent** |
    | X | **Allergy history** |
    | X | **Baseline vital signs and cardiac rhythm** |
    | X | **Medications administered** |
    | X | **Documentation of the last time the client ate or drank** |
    | | Type and cross match |

    A signed informed consent, allergy history, baseline vital signs and cardiac rhythm, medications administered, and documentation of last time the client ate or drank, are all necessary prior to administering midazolam for conscious sedation. Because blood loss is unexpected a type and cross match is not necessary.

    (N) NCLEX® Connection: Reduction of Risk Potential, Potential for Complications from Surgical Procedures and Health Alterations

3. Which of the following preoperative client findings should be reported to the client's provider? (Select all that apply.)

_____	Serum potassium 3.9 mEq/L
_____	Serum sodium 145 mEq/L
__X__	**Serum creatinine 2.8 mg/dL**
__X__	**Prothrombin time of 23 seconds**
__X__	**Blood glucose 235 mg/dL**
__X__	**WBC 17,850/mm³**

Potassium and sodium levels are within expected ranges. Creatinine level is elevated, which indicates possible renal dysfunction. Prothrombin time is prolonged, which poses concern for increased risk of bleeding due to delayed coagulation. Glucose level is high and intervention is needed. WBC is elevated and possibly indicative of an ongoing infection that needs treated prior to surgery.

 NCLEX® Connection: Reduction of Risk Potential, Potential for Complications of Diagnostic Tests/Treatments/Procedures

4. The surgeon is behind schedule and asks the licensed practical nurse (LPN) to complete the consent form. Which of the following statements by the LPN is correct?

A. "I can have surgery personnel discuss the procedure with the client."

B. "I can have the RN discuss the surgical complications you foresee."

C. "I can witness the client's signature on the form."

D. "I can discuss the surgical complications you foresee."

The LPN can witness the client's signature on the consent form after the surgeon has discussed the procedure and any possible surgical complications. Surgery personnel or nurses cannot review the procedure with the client as part of obtaining informed consent.

 NCLEX® Connection: Reduction of Risk Potential, Potential for Complications from Surgical Procedures and Health Alterations

UNIT 14	NURSING CARE OF THE PERIOPERATIVE CLIENT
Chapter 88	Postoperative Nursing Care

Overview

- Immediate postoperative care is usually provided in the PACU, where skilled nurses can closely monitor a client's recovery from anesthesia. In some instances, clients are transferred from the operating suite directly to the intensive care unit. Maintaining airway patency and ventilation and monitoring circulatory status are the main priorities for care.

- When clients are stable and able to breathe on their own, they are either discharged to a postsurgical unit or to home if it was a same-day surgical procedure. Priorities of care on the postsurgical unit are the same as for the PACU.

- Clients discharged home must also demonstrate that they can take fluids orally and safely ambulate to the bathroom and wheelchair with assistance. All clients who have had same-day surgery should be accompanied by a significant other, family member, or other caregiver who can receive the discharge instructions and accompany them home.

Indications

- Postoperative care is provided to all clients undergoing surgical procedures and may be offered in a PACU, same-day surgical suite, or on the postsurgical unit.

Client Outcomes

- The client's vital signs will return to baseline levels.

- The client will perform postoperative exercises on a regular basis.

- The client will be free from injury.

Data Collection

- Risk Factors for Postoperative Complications

  - Immobility (respiratory compromise, thrombophlebitis, pressure ulcer)

  - Anemia (blood loss, oxygenation, and healing factors)

  - Hypovolemia (tissue perfusion)

  - Respiratory disease (respiratory compromise)

  - Immune disorder (risk for infection, delayed healing)

- o Diabetes mellitus (gastroparesis, delayed wound healing)
- o Coagulation defect (increased risk of bleeding)
- o Malnutrition (delayed healing)
- o Obesity (wound healing, dehiscence, evisceration)
- Ⓖ o Age-related respiratory, cardiovascular, and renal changes place older adult clients at a greater risk for complications.
- Subjective and Objective Data
  - o Findings indicating clients are ready for transfer from the PACU
    - Stable vital signs
    - No evidence of bleeding
    - Return of reflexes (gag, cough, swallow)
    - Wound drainage that is minimal to moderate
    - Urine output of at least 30 mL/hr
    - Reports of pain (location, quality, quantity, timing)
    - Reports of gastrointestinal discomfort (nausea, vomiting)
  - o Physical assessment findings
    - Airway/breathing – respiratory rate and rhythm, effort, oxygen saturation, lung sounds
    - Circulation – blood pressure, heart rate, peripheral pulses, IV solutions
    - Neuro/musculoskeletal system – level of consciousness, sensation, movement
    - Gastrointestinal system – bowel sounds, emesis, presence of NG tube
    - Genitourinary system – presence of indwelling urinary catheter, amount and quality of output
    - Integumentary system – surgical incisions, drains, drainage
- Diagnostic Procedures
  - o CBC (infection/immune status)
  - o Hgb and Hct (fluid status, anemia)
  - o Electrolyte levels (electrolyte balance)
  - o Serum creatinine (renal status)
  - o ABGs (oxygenation status)
- Laboratory tests (glucose) based on procedure and other health problems

- Nursing Actions
  - Airway/Breathing/Circulation
    - Monitor vital signs per agency policy. Compare to ranges obtained in PACU and baseline.
      - □ Assist clients with coughing and deep breathing every 1 to 2 hr, and provide a pillow or folded blanket so that clients can splint an abdominal incision as necessary.
      - □ Assist clients with the use of an incentive spirometer every 1 to 2 hr.
    - Promote circulation and monitor for thromboembolism (especially following abdominal and pelvic surgeries).
      - □ Apply pneumatic compression stockings and/or elastic stockings.
      - □ Reposition clients every 2 hr and ambulate early and regularly.
      - □ Encourage clients to perform leg exercises every 1 to 2 hr.
      - □ Administer low-level anticoagulants as prescribed.
      - □ Monitor the client's extremities for calf pain, warmth, erythema, and edema.
    - Positioning
      - □ Do not place pillows under knees or elevate the knee gatch on the bed (decreases venous return).
      - □ Maintain clients in midline position to facilitate breathing.
    - Fluid, electrolyte, and acid base balance
      - □ Maintain a patent IV catheter.
      - □ Monitor clients who are receiving isotonic IV solutions (lactated Ringer's solution, 5% dextrose in lactated Ringer's solution).
      - □ Encourage ice chips and fluids as prescribed/tolerated.
      - □ Monitor ABGs and report abnormal findings to the provider.
    - Comfort
      - □ Check the client's pain level frequently, using a standardized pain scale.
      - □ Encourage clients to ask for pain medication before experiencing severe pain.
      - □ Observe clients for signs of pain, such as an increased pulse, respirations, or blood pressure; restlessness; and wincing or moaning during movement.
      - □ Be sure to consider cultural differences when assessing a client's pain.
      - □ Monitor clients for side effects of opioids, such as nausea (encourage the client to change positions slowly), urinary retention, and constipation.

- ☐ Provide analgesia around the clock for the first 24 hr.
- ☐ Provide analgesia 30 min before ambulation or other painful procedures.
  - ▸ Monitor clients who are receiving patient-controlled analgesia.
  - ▸ Provide frequent oral hygiene.
- ■ Renal function (output should equal intake)
  - ☐ Monitor and report urinary outputs of less than 30 mL/hr.
  - ☐ Palpate the client's bladder following voiding to check for bladder distention.
  - ☐ Consider using a bladder scan to identify suspected urinary retention.
- ■ Bowel function
  - ☐ Maintain clients on NPO until return of the gag reflex (risk of aspiration) and peristalsis (risk of paralytic ileus).
  - ☐ Irrigate NG suction tubes with saline as needed to maintain patency.
  - ☐ Monitor the client's bowel sounds in all four quadrants as well as the ability to pass flatus.
  - ☐ Advance the client's diet as prescribed and tolerated (clear liquids to regular).
- ■ Wound care
  - ☐ Monitor the incision site (expected findings include pink wound edges, slight swelling under sutures/staples, slight crusting of drainage). Report any signs of infection, including redness, excessive tenderness, and purulent drainage.
  - ☐ Monitor the client's wound drains (with each vital sign assessment). Empty as often as needed to maintain compression. Report changes in type of drainage as well as sudden increases in drainage (possible hemorrhage).

View Media Supplement:
- ● Penrose Drain (Image)   ● Jackson-Pratt Drain (Image)
- ● Hemovac Drain (Image)

- ☐ Monitor drainage from incisions/drain sites (should progress from sanguineous to serosanguineous to serous).
- ☐ Assist the surgeon with the first dressing change. Perform subsequent dressing changes as prescribed.
- ☐ Use an abdominal binder for clients who are obese or debilitated.
- ☐ Encourage splinting with position changes.

    ☐   Administer prophylactic antibiotics as prescribed.

    ☐   Remove sutures or staples in 6 to 8 days as prescribed.

- Promote wound healing.
  - ☐ Encourage clients to consume a diet that is high in calories, protein, and vitamin C to promote increased wound healing.
  - ☐ Assist clients who have diabetes mellitus to maintain glycemic control.

- Older adult client considerations
  - ☐ Monitor clients closely for appropriate response and possible adverse effects due to age related changes to the cardiovascular and respiratory systems. Responses to medications and anesthetics may delay an older adult client's return to baseline level of orientation postoperatively.
  - ☐ Provide extra blankets for warmth.
  - ☐ Provide meticulous skin care due to greater risk for dry, itchy skin that becomes fragile and easily abraded. Use paper tape for wound dressings. Take special precautions when repositioning clients.
  - ☐ Ensure adequate nutrition for wound healing.

- Care After Discharge
- Client Education
  - ☐ Provide information regarding medication management (purpose, administration guidelines, adverse effects).
  - ☐ Explain activity restrictions (driving, stairs, limits on weight lifting, sexual activity).
  - ☐ Give dietary guidelines, if applicable.
  - ☐ Reinforce wound care instruction, use of durable medical equipment at home including canes, walkers, drains, and catheters.
  - ☐ Provide emergency contact information and findings to report to the provider (elevated temperature, increased pain, swelling, bleeding, nausea and/or vomiting).

Complications

- Airway obstruction

  - o Nursing Actions
    - Monitor clients for choking, noisy, irregular respirations, decreased oxygen saturation values, and cyanosis and intervene accordingly.
    - Keep emergency equipment at the bedside in the PACU.

- Hypoxia

  ○ Hypoxia is evidenced by a decrease in oxygen saturation.

  ○ Nursing Actions

    ▪ Monitor the client's oxygenation status and administer oxygen as prescribed.

    ▪ Encourage clients to cough and deep breathe.

    ▪ Position clients to facilitate respiratory expansion.

- Paralytic ileus

  ○ A paralytic ileus can occur due to the absence of gastrointestinal peristaltic activity.

  ○ Nursing Actions

    ▪ Monitor bowel sounds, encourage ambulation, advance the diet as tolerated, and administer prokinetic agents, such as metoclopramide (Reglan), as prescribed.

- Wound dehiscence or evisceration

  ○ Nursing Actions

    ▪ Monitor risk factors (obesity, coughing, moving without splinting, diabetes mellitus).

    ▪ If wound dehiscence or evisceration occurs, call for help, stay with the client, cover the wound with a sterile towel or dressing that is moistened with sterile saline, do not attempt to reinsert organs, position the client supine with hips and knees bent, monitor the client for shock, and notify the provider immediately.

 View Media Supplement: Wound Evisceration (Video)

Ⓐ APPLICATION EXERCISES

1. A client who had a hysterectomy resumed a regular diet earlier in the day. Now the client is reporting nausea and has vomited once. Which of the following actions should the nurse take first?

   A. Monitor for bowel sounds.

   B. Administer an antiemetic.

   C. Check the client's pain level.

   D. Place the client on NPO status.

2. A nurse is caring for a client who had abdominal surgery 7 days ago. The nurse observes serosanguineous drainage from the incision site. Which of the following are the appropriate nursing actions at this time? (Select all that apply.)

   _____ Report the finding to the charge nurse.

   _____ Reinforce coughing, but avoid forceful coughing.

   _____ Splint the incision upon movement.

   _____ Encourage use of Valsalva maneuver.

   _____ Place the client in high-Fowler's position.

3. A nurse is caring for a client who is postoperative gastric resection. Which of the following actions should the nurse take? (Select all that apply.)

   _____ Reposition the client every 4 hr

   _____ Apply pneumatic compression stockings bilaterally

   _____ Place pillows under the client's knees when in the supine position

   _____ Administer pain medication 30 min prior to ambulation

   _____ Encourage the client to perform leg exercises every 1 to 2 hr

(A) APPLICATION EXERCISES ANSWER KEY

1. A client who had a hysterectomy resumed a regular diet earlier in the day. Now the client is reporting nausea and has vomited once. Which of the following actions should the nurse take first?

   A. Monitor for bowel sounds.

   B. Administer an antiemetic.

   C. Check the client's pain level.

   D. Place the client on NPO status.

   Using the nursing process, the first action the nurse should take is to collect data by listening for bowel sounds. Administering an antiemetic, checking the client's pain level, and placing the client on NPO status are all important but not the first action the nurse should take.

   (N) NCLEX® Connection: Reduction of Risk Potential, Potential for Complications of Diagnostic Tests/Treatments/Procedures

2. A nurse is caring for a client who had abdominal surgery 7 days ago. The nurse observes serosanguineous drainage from the incision site. Which of the following are the appropriate nursing actions at this time? (Select all that apply.)

X	**Report the finding to the charge nurse.**
X	**Reinforce coughing, but avoid forceful coughing.**
X	**Splint the incision upon movement.**
_____	Encourage use of Valsalva maneuver.
_____	Place the client in high-Fowler's position.

   The serosanguineous drainage is an unexpected finding 7 days after surgery and needs to be reported to the charge nurse. Reinforcing coughing but not forceful coughing and splinting the incision when moving are appropriate actions. The client should avoid the Valsalva maneuver as it puts extra strain on the incision. The client should be placed in the supine position with hips and knees bent.

   (N) NCLEX® Connection: Reduction of Risk Potential, Potential for Complications from Surgical Procedures and Health Alterations

3. A nurse is caring for a client who is postoperative gastric resection. Which of the following actions should the nurse take? (Select all that apply.)

_____	Reposition the client every 4 hr
__X__	**Apply pneumatic compression stockings bilaterally**
_____	Place pillows under the client's knees when in the supine position
__X__	**Administer pain medication 30 min prior to ambulation**
__X__	**Encourage the client to perform leg exercises every 1 to 2 hr**

Apply pneumatic compression stockings bilaterally and encourage the client to perform leg exercises every 1 to 2 hr to promote venous return. Administer pain medication 30 min prior to ambulation to facilitate movement for the client. Assist the client to reposition every 1 to 2 hr. Placing pillows under the client's knees will impede venous return.

Ⓝ NCLEX® Connection: Reduction of Risk Potential, Potential for Complications from Surgical Procedures and Health Alterations

References

Berman, A., Snyder, S. J. (2012). *Kozier and Erb's fundamentals of nursing: Concepts, process, and practice* (9th ed.). Upper Saddle River, NJ: Pearson.

Burke, K., & Mohn-Brown, L. (2011). *Medical-surgical nursing care.* Upper Saddle River, NJ: Prentice-Hall.

Centers for Disease Control and Prevention - http://www.cdc.gov

Curren, A. (2008). *Math for meds: Dosages and solutions* (10th ed.). Cliften Park, NY: Delmar.

Dudek, S. G. (2010). *Nutrition essentials for nursing practice* (6th ed.). Philadelphia, PA: Lippincott Williams & Wilkins.

Ebersole, P., Hess, P., Touhy, T. A., Schmidt Logan, A., & Jett, K. (2008) *Toward healthy aging: Human needs and nursing response* (7th ed.). St. Louis, MO: Mosby.

Eliopoulos, C. (2009). *Gerontological nursing.* (7th ed.). Philadelphia, PA: Lippincott Williams & Wilkins.

Grodner, M., Long, S., & Walkingshaw, B. C. (2007). *Foundations and clinical applications of nutrition: A nursing approach* (4th ed.). St. Louis, MO: Mosby.

Ignatavicius, D. D., & Workman, M. L. (2010). *Medical-surgical nursing* (6th ed.). St. Louis, MO: Saunders.

Lehne, R. A. (2010). *Pharmacology for nursing care* (7th ed.). St. Louis, MO: Saunders.

Lilley, L. L., Collins, S., Harrington, S., & Snyder, J. S. (2011). *Pharmacology and the nursing process* (6th ed.). St. Louis, MO: Mosby.

Potter, P. A., & Perry, A. G. (2009). *Fundamentals of nursing* (7th ed.). St. Louis, MO: Mosby.

Roach, S. S., & Ford, S. M. (2008). *Introductory clinical pharmacology.* Philadelphia, PA: Lippincott Williams & Wilkins.

Smeltzer, S. C., Bare, B. G., Hinkle, J. L., & Cheever, K. H. (2010). *Brunner and Suddarth's textbook of medical-surgical nursing* (12th ed.). Philadelphia, PA: Lippincott Williams & Wilkins.

Wilson, B. A., Shannon, M. T., & Shields, K. M. (2011). *Pearson nurse's drug guide 2011.* Upper Saddle River, NJ: Pearson.

United States National Library of Medicine, National Institutes of Health - http://www.nlm.nih.gov

Varcarolis, E. M., Halter, M.J. (2010). *Foundations of psychiatric mental health nursing: A clinical approach* (6th ed.). St. Louis, MO: Saunders.